Emerging Topics in Statistics and Biostatistics

More information about this series at http://www.springer.com/series/16213

Yichuan Zhao • (Din) Ding-Geng Chen
Editors

Modern Statistical Methods for Health Research

Springer

Editors
Yichuan Zhao
Department of Mathematics & Statistics
Georgia State University
Atlanta, GA, USA

(Din) Ding-Geng Chen
School of Mathematics,
Statistics and Computer Science
University of KwaZulu-Natal
South Africa

ISSN 2524-7735 ISSN 2524-7743 (electronic)
Emerging Topics in Statistics and Biostatistics
ISBN 978-3-030-72436-8 ISBN 978-3-030-72437-5 (eBook)
https://doi.org/10.1007/978-3-030-72437-5

This Springer imprint is published by the registered company Springer Nature Switzerland AG
The registered company address is: Gewerbestrasse 11, 6330 Cham, Switzerland

Preface

This book is primarily to discuss the emerging topics in statistical methods for health research in the big data era. The goal of the book was to bring distinguished researchers and applied researchers to present modern statistical procedures, useful methods, and their novel applications in health sciences. We invited leading experts in the frontiers of biomedicine, and health sciences to prepare book chapters, and we received many excellent papers in this topic. Twenty-one high-quality papers were included in this wonderful book. Each book chapter has been peer reviewed by two referees and revised many times before the final acceptance. Therefore, this volume reflects new advances in statistical methods for health research, applications in biostatistics, and interdisciplinary areas. This timely book has high potential to have a great impact in health sciences as authoritative sources and serve as reference. It will identify new directions of health research using modern statistical methods. This book will appeal to readers including statisticians, biostatisticians, data scientists, health-related researchers, and graduate students.

The twenty-one chapters are organized into five parts. Part I includes five chapters, which present health data analysis and applications to EHR data. Part II consists of five chapters on clinical trials, FDR, and applications in health science. Part III is composed of five chapters that present big data analytics and its applications. Part IV outlines survival analysis and functional data analysis. Part V consists of three chapters on statistical modeling in genomic studies. All the chapters are organized as self-contained units. Moreover, the references of each chapter are included at the end of the chapter. In order to make readers to use innovative statistics approaches in practice, computer programs and datasets are included in the book. Readers can also make a request to the chapter authors about their program codes for the facilitation of these new statistical procedures.

Part I: Health Data Analysis and Applications to EHR Data (Chaps. 1–5)

The chapter "The Effective Sample Size of EHR-Derived Cohorts Under Biased Sampling" derives formulas for the mean squared error of an EHR-derived sample as a function of the strength of association between a health outcome of interest, the sampling process, and an underlying unobserved covariate. The authors also give a formula for the effective sample size of an EHR-derived cohort defined as the sample size of a simple random sample with equivalent mean squared error to an EHR-derived sample arising from a biased sampling mechanism. In this chapter, Hubbard, Lou, and Himes demonstrate how the effective sample size can be used to compute confidence intervals that account for the biased sampling scheme.

In the chapter "Non-Gaussian Models for Object Motion Analysis with Time-Lapse Fluorescence Microscopy Images," the authors extend the particle filtering approach by developing non-Gaussian models and the corresponding tracking management strategy. With a gradient-based segmentation algorithm, objects in image sequences are extracted and modeled by states. The authors use the evolution of these states to recover object motion trajectories and quantitatively characterize object motion behaviors.

In the chapter "Alternative Capture-Recapture Point and Interval Estimators Based on Two Surveillance Streams," the authors develop two new multinomial distribution-based estimators that are valid and propose an approach geared toward improved confidence intervals in this setting that utilizes refinements to the posterior distribution of the proposed mean bias-adjusted estimand within a Bayesian credible interval strategy.

In the chapter "A Uniform Shrinkage Prior in Spatiotemporal Poisson Models for Count Data," the authors propose a uniform shrinkage prior (USP) for the variance components of the spatiotemporal random effects. In this chapter, the authors prove that the proposed USP is proper, and the resulting posterior is proper under the proposed USP, an independent flat prior for each fixed effect and a uniform prior for a spatial parameter.

In the chapter "A Review of Multiply Robust Estimation with Missing Data," Chen and Haziza review some existing approaches for multiply robust estimation with missing data and compare them through a simulation study and a real application by using data from the 2015–2016 National Health and Nutrition Examination Survey.

Part II: Clinical Trials, FDR, and Applications in Health Science (Chaps. 6–10)

The chapter "Approaches to Combining Phase II Proof-of-Concept and Dose-Finding Trials" illustrates and explores various practical adaptive design strategies that seamlessly combine the two objectives in one single study. Such adaptive strategies are compared against more traditional approaches of two separate studies or a combined nonadaptive fixed design, with a numerical example in designing a hypothetical phase II clinical program.

In the chapter "Designs of Early Phase Cancer Trials with Drug Combinations," Jimenez, Diniz, Rogatko, and Tighiouart present several innovative phase I and phase I–II designs for early phase cancer clinical trial with drug combinations focusing on continuous dose levels of both agents. The chapter presents the model where a fraction of dose limiting toxicity can be attributed to one or both agents. The authors also study the inclusion of a binary baseline covariate to describe subgroups with different frailty level and discuss binary and time to event endpoints to identify dose combinations along the MTD curve with maximum probability of efficacy in the second stage.

In the chapter "Controlling the False Discovery Rate of Grouped Hypotheses," MacDonalda, Wilson, Liang, and Qin review and compare several competing methods which attempt to approximate the optimal ranking of significance when hypotheses come from known groups and exchangeability is violated. In the simulation and a real data application, the chapter demonstrates the power and false discovery rate (FDR) control properties of these different procedures.

In the chapter "Classic Linear Mediation Analysis of Complex Survey Data Using Balanced Repeated Replication," Mai and Zhang discuss the balanced repeated replication, which is a common variance estimation method for national/international complex surveys. In this chapter, the authors also develop the SAS macro implementing the proposed method that adjusts for complex sampling designs in linear mediation analysis and illustrates the applications.

In the chapter "A Review of Bayesian Optimal Experimental Design on Different Models," Jiang and Zhao provide a general overview on the Bayesian experimental design of various statistical models in the recent years. The Bayesian optimal designs incorporate the prior information and uncertainties of the models by using various utility functions. The fast computational algorithms will bring wider applications of Bayesian experimental design to more complicated models.

Part III: Big Data Analytics and Its Applications (Chaps. 11–15)

In the chapter "A Selective Review on Statistical Techniques for Big Data," Yao and Wang summarize some of new approaches to give an overview of the current development of the big data analysis. This chapter focuses on the case that the number of observations is much larger than the dimension of the unknown parameters. Moreover, the authors discuss methods using subsamples and processing the whole data piece-by-piece.

The chapter "A Selective Overview of Recent Advances in Spectral Clustering and Their Applications" introduces the basics of spectral clustering, the similarity matrix, and conventional methods to identify the total number of clusters. In this chapter, Xu, Srinivasan, and Xue study and investigate extensions of spectral clustering and explore open questions, which may lead to innovative advancements.

In the chapter "A Review on Modern Computational Optimal Transport Methods with Applications in Biomedical Research," Zhang, Zhong, and Ma present some cutting-edge computational optimal transport methods with a focus on the regularization-based methods and the projection-based methods. To meet the big data challenges, the chapter discusses their real-world applications in biomedical research.

The chapter "Variable Selection Approaches in High-Dimensional Space" presents a review of the penalized likelihood approaches, with emphasis on the statistical properties and implementations for different outcomes with high-dimensional covariates. In this chapter, Luo, Yang, and Halabi also introduce independent screening procedures in ultra-high-dimensional variable selection and apply these selection methods to a high-dimensional setting in patients with a time-to-event outcome and high-dimensional inference.

The chapter "Estimation Methods for Item Factor Analysis: An Overview" presents the item factor analysis (IFA) modeling technique and commonly used IFA models. Then Chen and Zhang discuss estimation methods for IFA models and their computation, with a focus on the situation where the sample size, the number of items, and the number of factors are all large. Existing statistical software for IFA is discussed in detail.

Part IV: Survival Analysis and Functional Data Analysis (Chaps. 16–18)

In the chapter "Functional Data Modeling and Hypothesis Testing for Longitudinal Alzheimer Genome-Wide Association Studies," Li, Xu, and Liu propose the use of functional data modeling and inference methods to analyze longitudinal GWAS data, where aging disease-related phenotypes are repeatedly measured over time. The proposed method can be used to analyze both Gaussian-type and non-Gaussian response. In this chapter, the authors compare the effectiveness of two widely used nonparametric tests and show the advantages of the GQLR test over the functional F-test when analyzing sparse functional data from longitudinal GWAS.

In the chapter "Mixed-Effects Negative Binomial Regression with Interval Censoring: a Simulation Study and Application to Aridity and All-Cause Mortality Among Black South Africans Over 1997–2013," the authors contrasted the performance of mixed-effects interval-censored negative binomial regression against three alternative approaches to illustrate how the extent of censoring, between-cluster variation, sample size, and true strength of association can affect model estimates.

The authors assessed the bias in parameter estimates and standard errors, confidence interval coverage, statistical power, and type I error rates.

The chapter "Online Updating of Nonparametric Survival Estimator and Nonparametric Survival Test" proposes an online updating nonparametric estimation method for the cumulative hazard function and proposes an online testing procedure for equality of cumulative hazard functions under a two-group setting via the empirical likelihood. In this chapter, Xue, Schifano, and Hu illustrate the approach with a large lymphoma cancer dataset.

Part V: Statistical Modeling in Genomic Studies (Chaps. 19–21)

The chapter "Graphical Modeling of Multiple Biological Pathways in Genomic Studies" extends the pathway-based approach by combining multiple biological pathways into genomic studies. The topology structures of biological pathways are modeled by a Markov Random Field, which is a graphical model to present the dependence structure in the dataset. In this chapter, the authors construct a Bayesian framework to incorporate the knowledge from topological structures of biological pathways with the evidence from biological experiments. The inference of gene status can be made based on the marginal posterior probability obtained from Bayesian analysis.

In the chapter "A Nested Clustering Method to Detect and Cluster Transgenerational DNA Methylation Sites via Beta Regressions," Wang, Zhang, and Han employ the beta regression to infer the transmission status and, for CpG sites with DNAm transmitted, to cluster transmission patterns at a population level. The transmission status and patterns are inferred under a Bayesian framework. Simulations with different scenarios are used to demonstrate and evaluate the applicability of the proposed method. This chapter also demonstrates the approach using a triad (mother, father, and offspring) dataset with DNA methylation assessed at 4063 CpG sites.

The chapter "Detecting Changepoint in Gene Expressions over Time: An Application to Childhood Obesity" develops a procedure to detect changepoint in gene expression based on a nonparametric method. The proposed procedure performs well for non-normal error distribution and does not require the assumption of normal distribution. In this chapter, Mathur and Sun conduct intensive simulation studies to compare the performance of the proposed procedure with the existing procedure, and the simulation study indicates that the proposed procedure outperforms its competitor.

We sincerely thank the many people who have given us the strong support for the publication of this book with Springer on time. Our deep acknowledgments go to all the chapter authors (in the "List of Contributors") for submitting the excellent works to this book. We deeply appreciate the expertise reviews of many reviewers (in the "List of Chapter Reviewers"). Their comments and suggestions have improved the quality and presentation of the book substantially. Last but not least, we are so grateful to Laura Aileen Briskman (Editor, Statistics, Springer Nature) from Springer and Kirthika Selvaraju (Project Coordinator of Books, Springer Nature) for their full support and useful guidance during the long publication process. We look forward to receiving comments on typos and errors of the book from readers. If readers have any suggestions about improvements of the book, please contact the two editors: Dr. Yichuan Zhao and Dr. Ding-Geng Chen by email.

Atlanta, GA, USA — Yichuan Zhao
Chapel Hill, NC, USA — (Din) Ding-Geng Chen

Contents

About the Editors

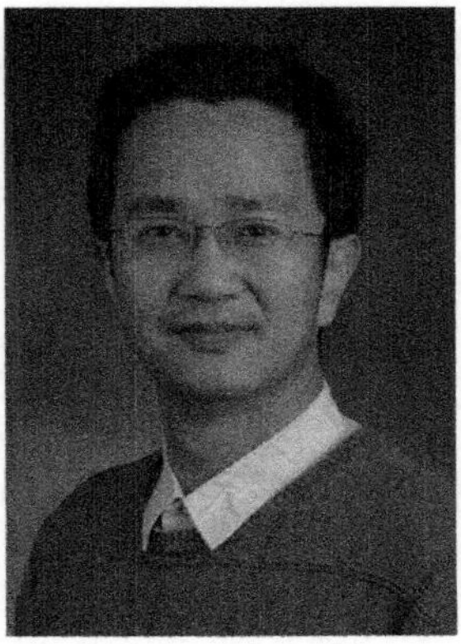

Yichuan Zhao is a Professor of Statistics at Georgia State University in Atlanta. He has a joint appointment as associate member of the Neuroscience Institute, and he is also an affiliated faculty member of the School of Public Health at Georgia State University. His current research interest focuses on survival analysis, empirical likelihood methods, nonparametric statistics, analysis of ROC curves, bioinformatics, Monte Carlo methods, and statistical modeling of fuzzy systems. He has published 100 research articles in statistics and biostatistics, has co-edited four books on statistics, biostatistics, and data science, and has been invited to deliver more than 200 research talks nationally and internationally. Dr. Zhao has organized the Workshop Series on Biostatistics and Bioinformatics since its initiation in 2012. He also organized the 25th ICSA Applied Statistics Symposium in Atlanta as a chair of the organizing committee to great success. He is currently serving as associate editor, or on the editorial board, for several statistical journals. Dr. Zhao is a Fellow of the American Statistical Association, an elected member of the International Statistical Institute, and serves on the Board of Directors, ICSA.

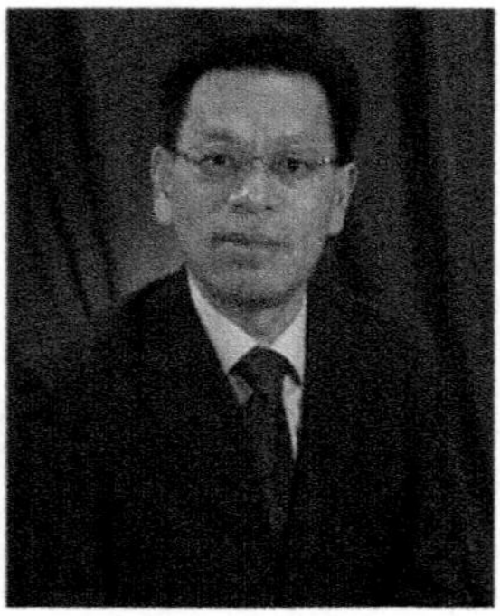

Professor (Din) Ding-Geng Chen is a fellow of the American Statistical Association. He is an honorary professor at the School of Mathematics, Statistics and Computer Science, University of KwaZulu-Natal, South Africa, and an extraordinary professor at the Department of Statistics, University of Pretoria, South Africa. Professor Chen has written more than 200 refereed publications and coauthored/coedited 33 books on clinical trial methodology, meta-analysis, causal inference, and public health statistics. This work is partially supported by the National Research Foundation of South Africa (Grant Number 127727) and the South African National Research Foundation (NRF) and South African Medical Research Council (SAMRC) (South African DST-NRF-SAMRC SARChI Research Chair in Biostatistics, Grant Number 114613).

List of Contributors

Azar M. Abadi Department of Environmental, Agricultural, and Occupational Health, University of Nebraska Medical Center, Omaha, NE, USA

Jesse E. Bell Department of Environmental, Agricultural, and Occupational Health, University of Nebraska Medical Center, Omaha, NE, USA

Rocky G. Bilotta National Oceanic and Atmospheric Administration's National Centers for Environmental Information and ISciences, L.L.C., Asheville, NC, USA

Yujing Cao Department of Mathematical Sciences, University of Texas at Dallas, Dallas, TX, USA

Jiandong Chen Department of Biostatistics and Bioinformatics, The Rollins School of Public Health of Emory University, Atlanta, GA, USA

Min Chen Department of Mathematical Sciences, University of Texas at Dallas, Dallas, TX, USA
Department of Population and Data Sciences, UT Southwestern Medical Center, Richardson, TX, USA

Sixia Chen University of Oklahoma Health Sciences Center, Oklahoma City, OK, USA

Yunxiao Chen Department of Statistics, London School of Economics and Political Science, London, UK

Ying Kuen Cheung Department of Biostatistics, Mailman School of Public Health, Columbia University, New York, NY, USA

Qiqi Deng Boehringer Ingelheim Pharmaceuticals, Inc., Ridgefield, CT, USAWestchester, NY, USA

Marcio Augusto Diniz Samuel Oschin Comprehensive Cancer Institute, Los Angeles, CA, USA

Matthew O. Gribble Department of Environmental Health, Rollins School of Public Health, Emory University, Atlanta, GA, USA
Department of Epidemiology, Rollins School of Public Health, Emory University, Atlanta, GA, USA

Susan Halabi Department of Biostatistics and Bioinformatics, Duke University Medical Center, Durham, NC, USA

Shengtong Han School of Public Health, University of Wisconsin-Milwaukee, Milwaukee, WI, USA

Mathew E. Hauer Department of Sociology, College of Social Sciences and Public Policy, Florida State University, Tallahassee, FL, USA

David Haziza Department of Mathematics and Statistics, Université de Montréal, Montréal, QC, Canada

Blanca E. Himes Department of Biostatistics, Epidemiology and Informatics, University of Pennsylvania, Philadelphia, PA, USA

Rebecca Hubbard Department of Biostatistics, Epidemiology and Informatics, University of Pennsylvania, Philadelphia, PA, USA

Guanyu Hu Department of Statistics, University of Missouri-Columbia, Columbia, MO, USA

Lily Ingsrisawang Faculty of Science, Department of Statistics, Kasetsart University, Bangkok, Thailand

Mohamed Jalloh Ministry of Health and Education, Freetown, Sierra Leone, Leawood, KS, USA,

Amara Jambai Ministry of Health and Education, Freetown, Sierra Leone, Ministry of Health and Sanitation, Freetown, Sierra Leone

Hongyan Jiang Department of Mathematics and Physics, Huaiyin Institute of Technology, Huaian, Jiangsu Province, China

Jose L. Jiménez Novartis Pharma A.G., Basel, Switzerland

Reinhard Kaiser Division of Global Health Protection, Center for Global Health, Centers for Disease Control and Prevention, Freetown, Sierra Leone

Robert Kauffman Department of Pediatrics, Division of Infectious Diseases, Emory University, Atlanta, GA, USA

Jun Kong Department of Mathematics and Statistics, Georgia State University, Atlanta, GA, USA
Department of Computer Science, Georgia State University, Atlanta, GA, USA
Department of Computer Science, Emory University, Atlanta, GA, USA
Department of Biomedical Informatics, Emory University, Atlanta, GA, USA

Christian M. Landon Department of Environmental Health, Rollins School of Public Health, Emory University, Atlanta, GA, USA

Krisada Lekdee Faculty of Science and Technology, Department of Mathematics and Statistics, Rajamangala University of Technology Phra Nakhon, Bangkok, Thailand

Kun Liang Department of Statistics and Actuarial Science, University of Waterloo, Waterloo, ON, Canada

Yehua Li Department of Statistics, University of California, Riverside, CA, USA

Yisheng Li Department of Biostatistics, University of Texas MD Anderson Cancer Center, Houston, TX, USA

Catherine Chunling Liu Department of Applied Mathematics, Hong Kong Polytechnic University, Hong Kong, China

Yutao Liu Department of Biostatistics, Mailman School of Public Health, Columbia University, New York, NY, USA

Carolyn Lou Department of Biostatistics, Epidemiology and Informatics, University of Pennsylvania, Philadelphia, PA, USA

Bin Luo Department of Biostatistics and Bioinformatics, Duke University Medical Center, Durham, NC, USA

Robert H. Lyles Department of Biostatistics and Bioinformatics, The Rollins School of Public Health of Emory University, Atlanta, GA, USA

Peter W. MacDonald Department of Statistics and Actuarial Science, University of Waterloo, Waterloo, ON, Canada

Ping Ma Department of Statistics, University of Georgia, Athens, GA, USA

Yujiao Mai Department of Biostatistics, St. Jude Children's Research Hospital, Memphis, TN, USA

Adam Marcus Department of Hematology and Medical Oncology, Emory University, Atlanta, GA, USA

Sunil Mathur Department of Mathematics and Statistics, Texas A&M University, Corpus Christi, TX, USA

Yingli Qin Department of Statistics and Actuarial Science, University of Waterloo, Waterloo, ON, Canada

Andre Rogatko Samuel Oschin Comprehensive Cancer Institute, Los Angeles, CA, USA

Elizabeth D. Schifano Department of Statistics, University of Connecticut, Storrs, CT, USA

Noah C. Scovronick Department of Environmental Health, Rollins School of Public Health, Emory University, Atlanta, GA, USA

Arun Srinivasan Department of Statistics, Pennsylvania State University, University Park, PA, USA

Jing Sun Department of Biostatistics and Epidemiology, Augusta University, Augusta, GA, USA

Allan W. Taylor Center for Global Health, Centers for Disease Control and Prevention, Atlanta, GA, USA

Mourad Tighiouart Samuel Oschin Comprehensive Cancer Institute, Los Angeles, CA, USA

Naitee Ting Boehringer Ingelheim Pharmaceuticals, Inc., Ridgefield, CT, USA

Fusheng Wang Department of Computer Science, Stony Brook University, Stony Brook, NY, USA

HaiYing Wang Department of Statistics, University of Connecticut, Storrs, CT, USA

Jiajing Wang Department of Mathematical Sciences, University of Memphis, Memphis, TN, USA

Xinlei Wang Department of Statistical Science, Southern Methodist University, Richardson, TX, USA

Amanda L. Wilkinson Center for Global Health, Centers for Disease Control and Prevention, Atlanta, GA, USA

John M. Williamson Center for Global Health, Centers for Disease Control and Prevention, Atlanta, GA, USAAtlanta, GA, USA

Nathan Wilson Department of Statistics and Actuarial Science, University of Waterloo, Waterloo, ON, Canada

Jens Wrammert Department of Pediatrics, Division of Infectious Diseases, Emory University, Atlanta, GA, USA

Ian Xu Department of Applied Mathematics, Hong Kong Polytechnic University, Hong Kong, China

Yang Xu School of Mathematical Sciences, Nankai University, Tianjin, China

Lingzhou Xue Department of Statistics, Pennsylvania State University, University Park, PA, USA

Yishu Xue Department of Statistics, University of Connecticut, Storrs, CT, USA

Chao Yang Department of Biostatistics, University of Texas MD Anderson Cancer Center, Houston, TX, USA

Qian Yang Department of Biostatistics and Bioinformatics, Duke University Medical Center, Durham, NC, USA

Yaqiong Yao Department of Statistics, University of Connecticut, Storrs, CT, USA

Sung Bo Yoon Department of Hematology and Medical Oncology, Emory University, Atlanta, GA, USA

Hanyi Yu Department of Computer Science, Emory University, Atlanta, GA, USA

Hongmei Zhang Division of Epidemiology, Biostatistics, and Environmental Health, School of Public Health, University of Memphis, Memphis, TN, USA

Hui Zhang Feinberg School of Medicine, Northwestern University, Chicago, IL, USA

Jingyi Zhang Center for Statistical Science, Tsinghua University, Beijing, China

Siliang Zhang Department of Statistics, London School of Economics and Political Science, Holborn, London, UK

Yu Zhang Department of Mathematical Sciences, University of Texas at Dallas, Dallas, TX, USA

Yichuan Zhao Department of Mathematics and Statistics, Georgia State University, Atlanta, GA, USA

Wenxuan Zhong Department of Statistics, University of Georgia, Athens, GA, USA

List of Chapter Reviewers

Ash Abebe Department of Mathematics and Statistics, Auburn University, Auburn, AL, USA

Sounak Chakraborty Department of Statistics, University of Missouri, Columbia, MO, USA

Bin Cheng Department of Biostatistics, Mailman School of Public Health, Columbia University, New York, NY, USA

Yichen Cheng Institute for Insight, Georgia State University, Atlanta, GA, USA

Min Chen Department of Mathematical Sciences, University of Texas at Dallas, Richardson, TX, USA

Nelson Chen Division of Epidemiology and Biostatistics, School of Public Health, University of Illinois at Chicago, Chicago, IL, USA

Sixia Chen University of Oklahoma Health Sciences Center, Oklahoma City, OK, USA

Moo Chung Department of Biostatistics and Medical Informatics, University of Wisconsin, Madison, WI, USA

Peisong Han Department of Biostatistics, School of Public Health, University of Michigan, Ann Arbor, MI, USA

Hongyan Jiang Department of Mathematics and Physics, Huaiyin Institute of Technology, Huaian, Jiangsu Province, China

Yuan Ji Department of Public Health Sciences, The University of Chicago, Chicago, IL, USA

Hyeon-Ah Kang Department of Educational Psychology, University of Texas at Austin, Austin, TX, USA

Yuan Ke Department of Statistics, University of Georgia, Athens, GA, USA

Lihua Lei Department of Statistics, Stanford University, Stanford, CA, USA

Zhixiang Lin Department of Statistics, The Chinese University of Hong Kong, Hong Kong, China

Yang Liu Centers for Disease Control and Prevention, Atlanta, GA, USA

Zhonghua Liu Department of Statistics and Actuarial Science, University of Hong Kong, Hong Kong, China

Xiaoou Li School of Statistics, University of Minnesota, Minneapolis, MN, USA

Yehua Li Department of Statistics, University of California, Riverside, CA, USA

Yisheng Li Department of Biostatistics, University of Texas MD Anderson Cancer Center, Houston, TX, USA

Ping Ma Department of Statistics, University of Georgia, Athens, GA, USA

Shiqian Ma Department of Mathematics, University of California, Davis, CA, USA

Roland Matsouaka Department of Biostatistics and Bioinformatics, Duke Clinical Research Institute, Durham, NC, USA

Wei Pan Division of Biostatistics, School of Public Health, University of Minnesota, Minneapolis, MN, USA

Seyoung Park Department of Statistics, Sungkyunkwan University, Seoul, Korea

Ye Shen Department of Epidemiology and Biostatistics, University of Georgia, Athens, GA, USA

Justin Strait Department of Statistics, University of Georgia, Athens, GA, USA

Xiaoxiao Sun Department of Epidemiology and Biostatistics, University of Arizona, Tucson, AZ, USA

HaiYing Wang Department of Statistics, University of Connecticut, Storrs, CT, USA

Asaf Weinstein School of Computer Science and Engineering, Hebrew University of Jerusalem, Jerusalem, Israel

Jing Wu Computer Science and Statistics Department, University of Rhode Island, Kingston, RI, USA

Rui Xie Department of Statistics and Data Science, University of Central Florida, Orlando, FL, USA

Dong Xu Department of Electrical Engineering and Computer Science, University of Missouri, Columbia, MO, USA

Lingzhou Xue Department of Statistics, Pennsylvania State University, University Park, PA, USA

Shu Yang Statistics Department, North Carolina State University, Raleigh, NC, USA

Keying Ye Department of Management Science and Statistics, The University of Texas at San Antonio, San Antonio, TX, USA

Ying Yuan Department of Biostatistics, University of Texas MD Anderson Cancer Center, Houston, TX, USA

Jihnhee Yu Department of Biostatistics, University at Buffalo, Buffalo, NY, USA

Jin-Ting Zhang Department of Statistics and Applied Probability, National University of Singapore, Singapore, Singapore

Xu Zhang Division of Clinical and Translational Sciences, Department of Internal Medicine, Medical School, University of Texas Health Science Center at Houston, Houston, TX, USA

Yichuan Zhao Department of Mathematics and Statistics, Georgia State University, Atlanta, GA, USA

Xiaodong Zhou School of Statistics and Information, Shanghai University of International Business and Economics, Shanghai, China

Part I
Health Data Analysis and Applications to EHR Data

The Effective Sample Size of EHR-Derived Cohorts Under Biased Sampling

Rebecca A. Hubbard, Carolyn Lou, and Blanca E. Himes

1 Introduction

The widespread adoption and use of Electronic Health Records (EHRs) following the Health Information and Technology for Economic and Clinical Health (HITECH) Act of 2009 [1] has increased the amount of medical and administrative information available in computable form, thereby spurring many efforts to use this data to improve health in ways beyond their original purpose [7, 12]. Over the past decade, research conducted using EHR-derived data has proliferated because it offers convenient and low-cost access to longitudinal information for large numbers of patients. Secondary uses of EHR data include understanding demographic and comorbidity relationships [9, 16, 20, 23] and creating biobanks for genomics studies [4, 14, 19]. Many large, multi-site efforts have also been developed to facilitate rapid conduct of observational health studies in populations of unprecedented sizes. For instance, the FDA's Sentinel System conducts post-marketing safety surveillance of medical products by leveraging EHR and administrative claims data for over 100 million individuals and 300 million person-years [3]. Other large databases containing data from hundreds of millions of individuals that are based on EHRs and/or claims data include PCORnet [6], the Healthcare Systems Research Collaboratory [17], and the Observational Medical Outcomes Partnership [21].

Although EHR-derived data has the benefit of capturing a large amount of information corresponding to real-life, diverse patient populations, it is subject to

R. A. Hubbard (✉) · C. Lou · B. E. Himes
Department of Biostatistics, Epidemiology and Informatics, University of Pennsylvania, Philadelphia, PA, USA
e-mail: rhubb@upenn.edu; louc@upenn.edu; bhimes@pennmedicine.upenn.edu

Y. Zhao, (Din) D.-G. Chen (eds.), *Modern Statistical Methods for Health Research*, Emerging Topics in Statistics and Biostatistics,
https://doi.org/10.1007/978-3-030-72437-5_1

many limitations. EHRs provide indirect measures of a patient's true health status, as the process of entering data into EHRs is complex, subject to inaccuracies, and prone to missingness [10, 11]. Because EHRs prioritize clinical care, administration, and billing, their data often do not align with the needs of researchers. Additional limitations of EHR data include the absence of information on key confounders (e.g., behavioral, social, economic, and environmental factors) [23, 24], lack of standardization of outcome and exposure measures, informative observation patterns that arise because EHRs are only generated when a patient interacts with the healthcare system [8, 18], and underrepresentation or, in the case of claims databases, lack of representation of patients without health insurance. Importantly, none of these challenges is ameliorated by increasing the total size of the study sample. In fact, these problems are likely exacerbated by increasing sample size, as the enormous size of the available data leads to highly precise but biased estimates when performing association analyses and, consequently, erroneous inference. Recent studies of this issue have found dramatically inflated type I error rates due to the pernicious combination of bias and high precision in EHR-derived parameter estimates [5, 22].

As the size of EHR datasets available for research increases, concerns about their improper use in epidemiologic studies will increase in parallel. A salient source of bias in EHR-based analyses is the biased sampling scheme that gives rise to the available data. EHRs are generated when a patient chooses to interact with the healthcare system as the result of a specific health concern. Consequently, the presence of an observation will be related to a patient's health status, health literacy, healthcare-seeking tendencies, health insurance or lack thereof, and socio-economic status. On the side of healthcare providers, clinical procedures and laboratory tests are ordered for specific reasons, diagnostic codes and notes may be inaccurate, and health insurance and socio-economic status of patients may bias care choices. This constellation of characteristics and behaviors of patients and providers will also be associated with various health outcomes, resulting in biased samples of patients selected for the study of these outcomes. For modest-sized samples, bias attributable to biased sampling is typically small compared to random error. As a result, mean-squared error is typically dominated by variance rather than bias. However, as the sample size increases, mean-squared error becomes dominated by bias. Use of EHR-based datasets that include tens or hundreds of millions of people's information heightens the need to account for the role of non-random sampling to obtain valid EHR-derived results.

The objective of this chapter is to illustrate the implications of non-random sample selection for mean-squared error of estimates derived from analysis of EHR data. Using recent results from the statistical literature, we provide simple formulas for the effective sample size of a large, but biased, sample. Through simulation, we illustrate the magnitude of bias and mean-squared error as a function of the strength of the biased sampling mechanism, and we demonstrate how confidence intervals acknowledging this bias can be constructed using the effective sample size.

2 Methods

2.1 Notation and Definitions

We consider a setting in which we wish to make inference about some characteristics of a population using either a designed observational study or a convenience sample extracted from a large database of EHRs. We note that the convenience sample could also correspond to an administrative and/or medical claims database, but we refer to it as an EHR database for simplicity. We assume that the designed observational study under consideration takes the form of a simple random sample from the population of interest. We assume that the population we are interested in studying is large but finite with total size N. Let $Y_i = (Y_1, \ldots, Y_N)$ denote a binary health outcome of interest. Let $I_i = 1$ if Y_i is captured in our simple random sample and 0 otherwise, and let $R_i = 1$ if Y_i is captured in the EHR database to be used for research and 0 otherwise. The sample size is denoted as $n_s = \sum_{i=1}^{N} I_i$ for our simple random sample and $n_a = \sum_{i=1}^{N} R_i$ for our EHR sample. Additionally, we let $f_s = n_s/N$ denote the fraction of the total population captured in our simple random sample and $f_a = n_a/N$ denote the sampling fraction of our EHR database.

We assume that because the EHR data were not collected for research purposes, patients were sampled for inclusion in the EHR database through a biased mechanism. Specifically, we assume there exist some underlying characteristics of the population X_i that are associated with both Y_i and R_i. For ease of interpretation of model parameters, we assume that the relationships between X_i and Y_i and X_i and R_i follow logistic functions. Specifically,

$$P(Y_i = 1|X_i) = \exp(\eta + X_i\alpha)/(1 + \exp(\eta + X_i\alpha)) \quad \text{and}$$
$$P(R_i = 1|X_i) = \exp(\mu + X_i\beta)/(1 + \exp(\mu + X_i\beta)).$$

Alternative parameterizations for these relationships could be used. For instance, Meng considers a similar setting using a probit model for the sampling process [15]. Here, we select logistic models solely for the convenience that under this parameterization, the dependence of Y_i and R_i on X_i can be expressed in terms of odds ratios, the magnitude and interpretation of which are generally more familiar to biomedical researchers. In these models, $\exp(\beta)$ represents the odds ratio for the association between X_i and inclusion in the EHR database, and $\exp(\alpha)$ represents the odds ratio for the strength of association between X_i and the health outcome of interest.

In the context of EHR databases, there are many patient characteristics that could play the role of X_i. For instance, household income has a significant impact on the types of healthcare that patients receive and as a result, their presence in these databases. Income is also strongly associated with employment and health insurance status. Consequently, affluent patients tend to be healthier than their poorer peers. If these variables are available in the EHR database, estimates of α could be corrected for selection bias through a standard approach such as inverse probability weighting. In the formulation that follows, we assume that X_i is unobserved and introduce this hypothesized underlying patient characteristic as a device to induce dependence between the outcome and the sampling probabilities. In practice, EHR databases are missing many such characteristics that could be associated with both healthcare utilization and health outcomes including educational attainment and health literacy.

2.2 Bias and Mean-Squared Error of the Simple Random Sample and the EHR-Based Sample

In the setting of biased sampling, how much weight should we place on results from an EHR-based sample of size n_a? One way to answer this question is to consider the size of a simple random sample that would have equivalent mean-squared error (MSE) to a large, but biased, sample from an EHR database. Meng [15] illustrated how MSE can be used to find the effective sample size, defined here as the sample size of a simple random sample with MSE equivalent to an EHR-based sample subject to selection bias, in the setting of outcome-dependent sampling using a probit regression model to link Y_i and sampling probability, $P(R_i = 1|Y_i)$. The formulation presented in the previous section provides an alternative means to connect sampling and the health outcome via the device of an unobserved patient characteristic. Let

$$\bar{Y}_a = \frac{1}{n_a}\sum_{i=1}^{N} Y_i R_i \quad \text{and} \quad \bar{Y}_s = \frac{1}{n_s}\sum_{i=1}^{N} Y_i I_i .$$

Following the arguments of Meng et al., the bias in our EHR database estimate is approximated by

$$\text{Bias}(\bar{Y}_a) = \frac{\sum_{i=1}^{N} P(R_i = 1|X_i)(Y_i - P(Y_i = 1|X_i))}{\sum_{i=1}^{N} P(R_i = 1|X_i)}.$$

If N and f_a are large, then this bias is approximately equivalent to

$$\text{Bias}(\bar{Y}_a) \approx \frac{Cov(Y, P(R = 1|X))}{E(P(R = 1|X))}.$$

To obtain a simple expression for the MSE and effective sample size, we use a first-order Taylor series expansion to linearize $P(R = 1|X)$. Expanding around $P(R = 1|X = 0)$ gives $P(R = 1|X) = P(R = 1|X = 0) + \beta P(R = 1|X = 0)(1 - P(R = 1|X = 0))X$. Thus,

$$\text{Bias}(\bar{Y}_a) \approx \frac{\beta Cov(Y, X)}{(1 - P(R = 1|X = 0))^{-1} + E(X)\beta}. \quad (1)$$

For large values of n_a, MSE($\bar{Y}_a$) is dominated by bias, thus MSE($\bar{Y}_a$) $\approx$ Bias^2($\bar{Y}_a$).

If we postulate a hypothetical standardized covariate with mean = 0 and variance = 1, we can further simplify this expression. By employing a linearization of $P(Y = 1|X)$ using a Taylor series expanded around $P(Y = 1|X = 0)$, we can write the covariance of a standardized covariate, X, and Y as $\alpha P(Y = 1|X = 0)(1 - P(Y = 1|X = 0))$. Thus, for this standardized covariate,

$$\text{Bias}(\bar{Y}_a) \approx \alpha\beta P(Y = 1|X = 0)P(Y = 0|X = 0)P(R = 0|X = 0). \quad (2)$$

Therefore, the bias in our estimate based on an EHR database is directly proportional to the log odds ratio relating sampling to the unobserved covariate, the log odds ratio relating the health outcome to the unobserved covariate, and the probability of being excluded from the sample. As the sampling probability, $P(R = 1|X = 0)$, moves toward 1, bias goes to 0. Using this simple formula, we can envision the magnitude of bias in a given setting by considering a range of plausible values for α and β. We note that this approximate bias formula relies on the Taylor series expansion around $X = 0$ and therefore will only be appropriate for a covariate that can reasonably be assumed to lie near 0.

2.3 *Effective Sample Size of the EHR-Derived Cohort*

By equating the MSE of the simple random sample and the EHR-based sample, we can find the effective sample size of a large EHR-based cohort subject to biased sampling. Since a simple random sample is unbiased, its MSE is equivalent to variance, such that MSE($\bar{Y}_s$) $= \sigma^2/n_s$. Equating the MSE of a simple random sample, which is comprised only of variance, and the MSE of the EHR-based sample, which is dominated by bias, we see that

$$\begin{aligned} n_{eff} &\approx \left(\frac{\sigma^2}{\text{Bias}^2(\bar{Y}_a)}\right) \\ &\approx \left(\frac{\sigma}{\alpha\beta P(Y = 1|X = 0)P(Y = 0|X = 0)P(R = 0|X = 0)}\right)^2, \end{aligned} \quad (3)$$

where n_{eff} is defined as the sample size of an EHR-based cohort subject to biased sampling with equivalent MSE to a simple random sample. The stronger the biased sampling mechanism, due to either α or β, the smaller the EHR-based cohort relative to the total population, and the closer the outcome prevalence is to 0.5, the smaller the effective sample size will be. Note that this formula assumes that MSE of the EHR-based sample is dominated by bias and that the contribution of variance is negligible. If $\alpha = 0$ or $\beta = 0$, there will be no association between the health outcome and the sampling and hence no bias. In that case, Eq. (3) would be inappropriate to use because the denominator is based solely on bias and ignores the contribution of variance to MSE.

Using this conception of effective sample size can help to provide a sense of how "big" an EHR-based cohort truly is. Additionally, we can use the effective sample size to compute more accurate confidence intervals for EHR-derived effect estimates. The very large sample size of EHR databases allows us to estimate quantities of interest with nearly negligible precision. However, naive standard errors and confidence intervals based on the apparent sample size fail to account for the bias associated with using a non-random convenience sample. We can instead compute confidence intervals using the sample size formula provided in Eq. (3), which would acknowledge the bias–variance trade-off associated with using a large, but biased, sample.

In cases where only EHR data are available, it will not be possible to estimate the quantities involved in the effective sample size calculation. Rather, we propose that a sensitivity analysis could be conducted to investigate the magnitude of sample size reduction associated with plausible values for α, β, and $P(R = 0|X = 0)$. In the spirit of other quantitative bias analyses and tipping point analyses, this approach could be used to identify the magnitude of association between sampling and outcome and an unobserved characteristic that would result in a change to inference due to standard error inflation.

Alternatively, in some cases, external data in the form of population-based survey results will be available to augment the results of our EHR-based analyses. For instance, the Behavioral Risk Factors Surveillance System (BRFSS) health survey is a national population-based survey that includes many patient characteristics that may be related to capture in EHR data including education and income. Such an external data source could be used to explicitly estimate $P(X)$. Information on the proportion of a defined geographic region treated within the health system providing EHR data could be used to estimate $P(R)$. In combination with estimates of $P(X|R)$ derived from EHR data, Bayes rule could be used to obtain estimates of $P(R = 0|X)$.

2.4 Simulation Study Design

We conducted simulation studies to illustrate the effective sample size of a large EHR-based cohort subject to biased sampling relative to a simple random sample with equivalent mean-squared error. We first estimated the bias, mean-squared error, and effective sample size of EHR-based samples under varying strengths of association between sampling and covariate (β) and between the outcome and covariate (α). We assumed that the total population from which the sample was drawn included 1,000,000 individuals and that the EHR-based sample was of size 100,000. We simulated a single covariate, X, from a standard normal distribution and fixed the prevalence of the outcome, Y, for individuals with $X = 0$ at 0.5. We varied the odds ratio for sampling ($\exp(\beta)$) and the outcome ($\exp(\alpha)$) from 1.1 to 1.25. Each combination of α and β was repeated 1000 times. For these simulations, we present both the effective sample sizes calculated using the empirical bias and using the approximation to bias given in Eq. (2).

In a second set of simulations, we fixed $\exp(\alpha)$ at 1.2 and varied $\exp(\beta)$ from 1.05 to 1.45. For each simulation, we computed the mean of Y for an EHR-based sample of size 100,000 and a simple random sample of size 1000. We computed 95% confidence intervals (CIs) for each estimate. For the EHR-based sample, we computed both naive confidence intervals using the apparent sample size of 100,000 and effective confidence intervals based on the estimated effective sample size given the magnitude of the biased sampling mechanism.

3 Results

For an EHR-based cohort of size 100,000 selected via a biased sampling mechanism, root mean-squared error (RMSE) is dominated by bias across the range of strengths of association between an unobserved covariate and sampling ($\exp(\alpha)$) and unobserved covariate and outcome ($\exp(\beta)$) investigated (Table 1). The effective sample size is far smaller than the nominal sample size. The approximation to effective sample size provided in Eqs. (3) was reasonably similar to the effective sample size based on empirical bias, although it underestimated the effective sample size slightly for most of the scenarios investigated. For a sample of size 100,000 drawn from a total population of 1,000,000, the effective sample size was less than 60,000 for $\exp(\alpha) = \exp(\beta) = 1.1$. As the magnitude of $\exp(\alpha)$ and $\exp(\beta)$ increases, the effective sample size of the EHR-based cohort decreased to about 2000 for $\exp(\alpha) = \exp(\beta) = 1.25$. Figure 1 presents the percent effective sample size, defined as 100 times the ratio of the effective sample size to the nominal sample size across the range of strengths of association between sampling and outcome investigated. When the value of either $\exp(\alpha)$ or $\exp(\beta)$ was greater than 1.25, the percent effective sample size was less than 5%.

Figure 2 demonstrates the magnitude of bias and resultant inferential error in estimates of the mean of Y for an EHR-based cohort subject to biased sampling. Holding $\exp(\alpha)$ fixed at 1.2, as $\exp(\beta)$ increases, bias in the estimated mean increased. However, due to the large size of the EHR-based cohort, confidence intervals around this point estimate (solid) were narrow and excluded the true value when $\exp(\beta) > 1.05$. In contrast, a simple random sample of size 1000 returned an unbiased estimate but with much broader confidence intervals (dashed). A better sense of the informational content of the EHR sample-based estimate can be obtained by computing confidence intervals using the effective sample size that acknowledges the biased sampling mechanism (dashed and dotted). While the point estimate based on this approach remains biased, the broader confidence interval is more likely to cover the true value of the parameter. This also highlights the

Table 1 Bias, root mean-squared error (RMSE), effective sample size (n_{eff}) based on empirical bias, and effective sample size based on the approximation given in Eq. (3) (n_{eff}^A) for an EHR-based cohort of size 100,000 sampled under a biased mechanism from a total population of size 1,000,000 with strength of odds ratio between covariate and sampling of size exp(α) and between covariate and outcome of size exp(β)

exp(α)	exp(β)	n_{eff}	n_{eff}^A	Bias	RMSE
1.10	1.10	59,221	59,844	0.0021	0.0026
1.15	1.10	28,356	27,830	0.0030	0.0034
1.20	1.10	16,523	16,354	0.0039	0.0042
1.25	1.10	11,234	10,918	0.0047	0.0050
1.10	1.15	27,596	27,830	0.0030	0.0034
1.15	1.15	12,864	12,943	0.0044	0.0047
1.20	1.15	7826	7605	0.0057	0.0059
1.25	1.15	5177	5077	0.0069	0.0071
1.10	1.20	17,233	16,354	0.0038	0.0041
1.15	1.20	7636	7605	0.0057	0.0059
1.20	1.20	4621	4469	0.0074	0.0075
1.25	1.20	3047	2984	0.0091	0.0092
1.10	1.25	10,996	10,918	0.0048	0.0050
1.15	1.25	5232	5077	0.0069	0.0071
1.20	1.25	3088	2984	0.0090	0.0091
1.25	1.25	2054	1992	0.0110	0.0111

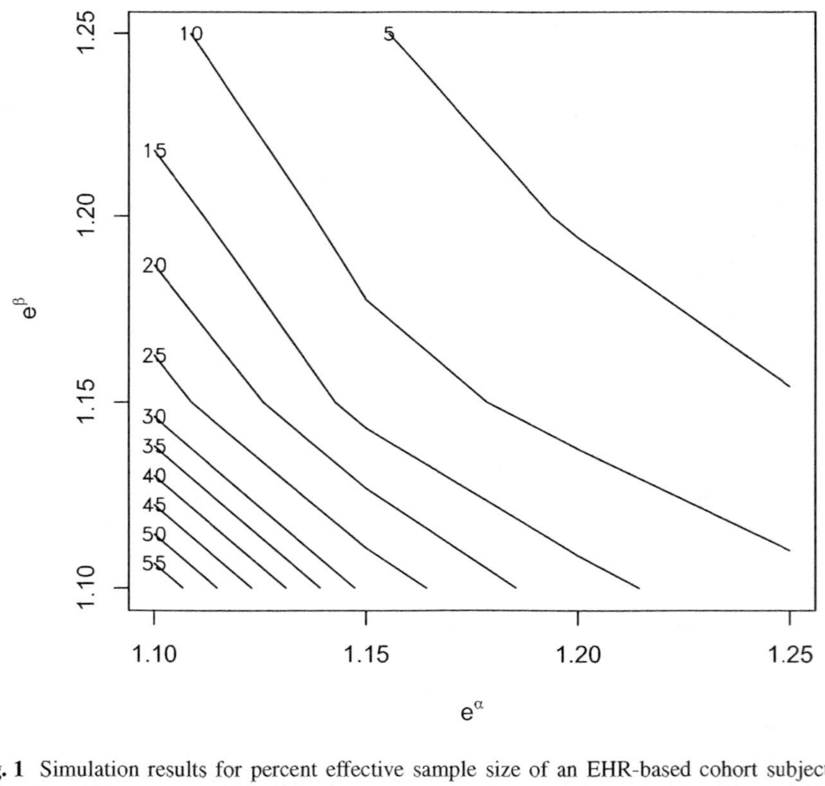

Fig. 1 Simulation results for percent effective sample size of an EHR-based cohort subject to biased sampling with strength of odds ratio between sampling and covariate X of exp(α) and between outcome and X of exp(β)

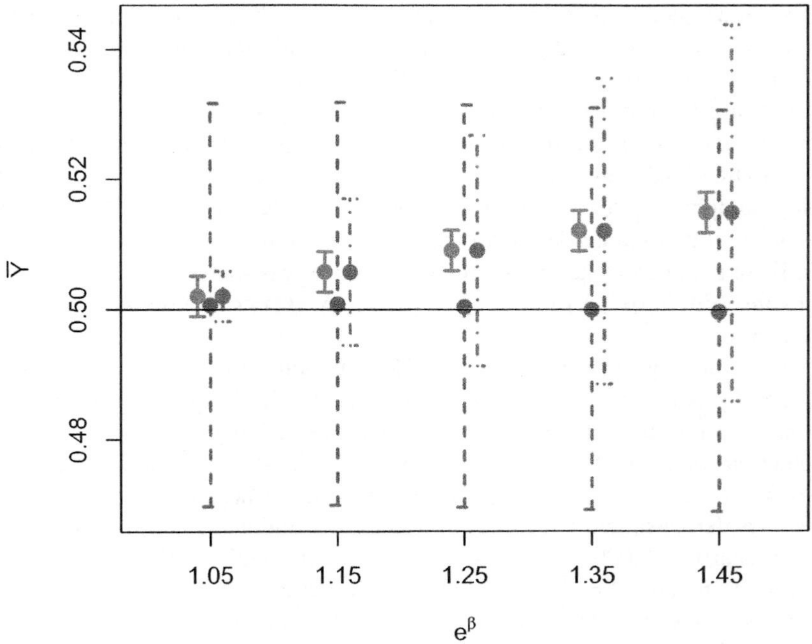

Fig. 2 Point estimates and 95% confidence intervals for an EHR-based sample of size 100,000 (solid), a simple random sample of size 1000 (dashed), and an EHR-based sample of size 100,000 with confidence intervals based on the effective sample size (dashed and dotted). The odds ratio for strength of association between the sampling mechanism and the covariate, X, was 1.2 and between Y and X was varied across a range of values from 1.05 to 1.45 ($\exp(\beta)$)

diminishing value of using an EHR-based cohort relative to a simple random sample as the magnitude of the biased sampling mechanism increases. For $\exp(\beta) = 1.45$, the width of the confidence interval for the simple random sample of size 1000 and the EHR-based sample using the effective sample size were approximately equal.

4 Discussion

While EHR and administrative claims data are readily available, there are several limitations to their use for making inference in observational association studies due to their complex and biased nature. This chapter has focused on one specific challenge arising from the biased sampling mechanism that gives rise to EHR data. Specifically, EHRs are generated by a complex process involving a patient interacting with the healthcare system, health providers making decisions about care, and data being recorded according to requirements of providers, administrators, and billing specialists. The probability of a patient interaction with a health system leading to a specific EHR entry is related to many characteristics of the patient, characteristics of the providers, and the patient's health status, which leads to biased sampling. Because of the large size of EHR and administrative claims datasets, the variance of estimates derived from them may be very small, but the mean-squared error arising due to bias can be large, easily resulting in larger mean-squared error for an EHR-based sample subject to biased sampling than a far smaller simple random sample. Careful consideration should be devoted to the value of using EHR and administrative claims datasets as convenience samples to make inferences about underlying populations, as substantial effort to address sources of bias is required, versus investing resources in conducting primary data collection using traditional approaches.

The availability of information in EHRs and administrative claims datasets is governed by patients' decisions to interact with the healthcare system [8, 10], as well as decisions made by providers and complex data entry processes [11]. Patient decisions are driven by factors that include their health status and healthcare-seeking behavior. At the level of health providers, bias in the presence of information in EHRs was demonstrated effectively in a study by Agniel and colleagues [2]: using data on nearly 670,000 patients from two large hospitals in Boston over 1 year between 2005 and 2006, they showed that the presence of a laboratory test order, regardless of any information about the test result, was significantly associated with survival in 233 of 272 laboratory tests evaluated. Thus, associations between health outcomes and patient characteristics and the timing of ascertainment of outcomes violate the assumption of non-informative observation made by many standard statistical methods. Recent work has investigated a variety of approaches to address informative observation in EHRs and administrative claims data, including models of the observation and outcome process linked by shared random effects [13].

Our work highlights the need for careful consideration of study design and sampling issues when interpreting results of EHR-based studies that make inferences about underlying populations. The nominal sample size of EHR and administrative claims databases may be very large. However, the risk of bias due to a variety of issues including non-random sampling substantially diminishes the strength of inference that can be drawn using these sources. Consideration of the effective sample size of an EHR-derived cohort based on hypothesized strengths of association with an unobserved covariate influencing inclusion in the cohort provides a reality check on the weight that should be placed on these results.

References

1. Adler-Milstein, J., DesRoches, C.M., Furukawa, M.F., Worzala, C., Charles, D., Kralovec, P., Stalley, S., Jha, A.K.: More than half of US hospitals have at least a basic EHR, but stage 2 criteria remain challenging for most. Health Aff. (Millwood) **33**(9), 1664–1671 (2014). https://doi.org/10.1377/hlthaff.2014.0453
2. Agniel, D., Kohane, I.S., Weber, G.M.: Biases in electronic health record data due to processes within the healthcare system: retrospective observational study. BMJ **361**, k1479 (2018). https://doi.org/10.1136/bmj.k1479

3. Ball, R., Robb, M., Anderson, S.A., Pan, G.D.: The FDA's sentinel initiative—a comprehensive approach to medical product surveillance. Clin. Pharmacol. Ther. **99**(3), 265–268 (2016). https://doi.org/10.1002/cpt.320
4. Canela-Xandri, O., Rawlik, K., Tenesa, A.: An atlas of genetic associations in UK Biobank. Nat. Genet. **50**(11), 1593–1599 (2018). https://doi.org/10.1038/s41588-018-0248-z
5. Chen, Y., Wang, J., Chubak, J., Hubbard, R.A.: Inflation of type I error rates due to differential misclassification in EHR-derived outcomes: empirical illustration using breast cancer recurrence. Pharmacoepidemiol. Drug Saf. **28**(2), 264–268 (2019)
6. Fleurence, R.L., Curtis, L.H., Califf, R.M., Platt, R., Selby, J.V., Brown, J.S.: Launching PCORnet, a national patient-centered clinical research network. J. Am. Med. Inform. Assoc. **21**(4), 578–582 (2014)
7. Friedman, C.P., Wong, A.K., Blumenthal, D.: Achieving a nationwide learning health system. Sci. Transl. Med. **2**(57), 5729 (2010). https://doi.org/10.1126/scitranslmed.3001456
8. Goldstein, B.A., Bhavsar, N.A., Phelan, M., Pencina, M.J.: Controlling for informed presence bias due to the number of health encounters in an electronic health record. Am. J. Epidemiol. **184**(11), 847–855 (2016)
9. Greenblatt, R.E., Zhao, E.J., Henrickson, S.E., Apter, A.J., Hubbard, R.A., Himes, B.E.: Factors associated with exacerbations among adults with asthma according to electronic health record data. Asthma Res. Pract. **5**, 1 (2019). https://doi.org/10.1186/s40733-019-0048-y
10. Haneuse, S., Daniels, M.: A General framework for considering selection bias in EHR-based studies: what data are observed and why? EGEMS (Wash DC) **4**(1), 1203 (2016). https://doi.org/10.13063/2327-9214.1203
11. Hripcsak, G., Albers, D.J.: Next-generation phenotyping of electronic health records. J. Am. Med. Inf. Assoc. **20**(1), 117–121 (2013). https://doi.org/10.1136/amiajnl-2012-001145
12. Jensen, P.B., Jensen, L.J., Brunak, S.: Mining electronic health records: towards better research applications and clinical care. Nat. Rev. Genet. **13**(6), 395–405 (2012). https://doi.org/10.1038/nrg3208
13. McCulloch, C.E., Neuhaus, J.M., Olin, R.L.: Biased and unbiased estimation in longitudinal studies with informative visit processes. Biometrics **72**(4), 1315–1324 (2016)
14. McGregor, T.L., Van Driest, S.L., Brothers, K.B., Bowton, E.A., Muglia, L.J., Roden, D.M.: Inclusion of pediatric samples in an opt-out biorepository linking DNA to de-identified medical records: pediatric BioVU. Clin. Pharmacol. Ther. **93**(2), 204–11 (2013). https://doi.org/10.1038/clpt.2012.230
15. Meng, X.L.: A trio of inference problems that could win you a Nobel Prize in statistics (if you help fund it). In: Lin, X., Genest, C., Banks, D., Molenberghs, G., Scott, D., Wang. J.L. (eds.), Past, Present, and Future of Statistical Science, pp. 537–562. Chapman and Hall/CRC (2014). https://doi.org/10.1201/b16720-50
16. Pike, M.M., Decker, P.A., Larson, N.B., St Sauver, J.L., Takahashi, P.Y., Roger, V.L., Rocca, W.A., Miller, V.M., Olson, J.E., Pathak, J., Bielinski, S.J.: Improvement in cardiovascular risk prediction with electronic health records. J. Cardiovasc. Transl. Res. **9**(3), 214–22 (2016). https://doi.org/10.1007/s12265-016-9687-z
17. Richesson, R.L., Green, B.B., Laws, R., Puro, J., Kahn, M.G., Bauck, A., Smerek, M., Van Eaton, E.G., Zozus, M., Ed Hammond, W., et al.: Pragmatic (trial) informatics: a perspective from the NIH Health Care Systems Research Collaboratory. J. Am. Med. Inform. Assoc. **24**(5), 996–1001 (2017)
18. Rusanov, A., Weiskopf, N.G., Wang, S., Weng, C.H.: Hidden in plain sight: bias towards sick patients when sampling patients with sufficient electronic health record data for research. BMC Med. Inform. Decis. Mak. **14**, 51 (2014). https://doi.org/10.1186/1472-6947-14-51
19. Scott, S.A., Owusu Obeng, A., Botton, M.R., Yang, Y., Scott, E.R., Ellis, S.B., Wallsten, R., Kaszemacher, T., Zhou, X., Chen, R., Nicoletti, P., Naik, H., Kenny, E.E., Vega, A., Waite, E., Diaz, G.A., Dudley, J., Halperin, J.L., Edelmann, L., Kasarskis, A., Hulot, J.S., Peter, I., Bottinger, E.P., Hirschhorn, K., Sklar, P., Cho, J.H., Desnick, R.J., Schadt, E.E.: Institutional profile: translational pharmacogenomics at the Icahn School of Medicine at Mount Sinai. Pharmacogenomics **18**(15), 1381–1386 (2017). https://doi.org/10.2217/pgs-2017-0137

20. Siebert, S., Lyall, D.M., Mackay, D.F., Porter, D., McInnes, I.B., Sattar, N., Pell, J.P.: Characteristics of rheumatoid arthritis and its association with major comorbid conditions: cross-sectional study of 502 649 UK Biobank participants. RMD Open **2**(1), e000,267 (2016). https://doi.org/10.1136/rmdopen-2016-000267
21. Stang, P.E., Ryan, P.B., Racoosin, J.A., Overhage, J.M., Hartzema, A.G., Reich, C., Welebob, E., Scarnecchia, T., Woodcock, J.: Advancing the science for active surveillance: rationale and design for the observational medical outcomes partnership. Ann. Intern. Med. **153**(9), 600–606 (2010)
22. Veronesi, G., Grassi, G., Savelli, G., Quatto, P., Zambon, A.: Big data, observational research and P-value: a recipe for false-positive findings? A study of simulated and real prospective cohorts. Int. J. Epidemiol. **49**(3), 876–884 (2019). https://doi.org/10.1093/ije/dyz206
23. Xie, S., Greenblatt, R., Levy, M.Z., Himes, B.E.: Enhancing electronic health record data with geospatial information. AMIA Jt. Summits Transl. Sci. Proc. **2017**, 123–132 (2017). https://www.ncbi.nlm.nih.gov/pubmed/28815121
24. Xie, S., Himes, B.E.: Approaches to link geospatially varying social, economic, and environmental factors with electronic health record data to better understand asthma exacerbations. AMIA Annu. Symp. Proc. **2018**, 1561–1570 (2018). https://www.ncbi.nlm.nih.gov/pubmed/30815202

Non-Gaussian Models for Object Motion Analysis with Time-Lapse Fluorescence Microscopy Images

Hanyi Yu, Sung Bo Yoon, Robert Kauffman, Jens Wrammert, Adam Marcus, and Jun Kong

1 Introduction

The analysis of fluorescence microscopy images has emerged as an effective avenue for a large spectrum of biological and cancer studies. Thanks to modern fluorescence microscopy technologies, a high throughput time-lapse imaging data can be routinely generated to characterize diverse biomedical objects of interest, including cells, vesicles, proteins, and bacteria among others. As numbers of these objects in most biomedical research are large and varying over time, it is infeasible to manually analyze their motion patterns with sufficient accuracy and efficiency. Therefore, development of efficient, accurate, robust, and automated object tracking methods is of great importance to facilitate biomedical investigations.

H. Yu
Department of Computer Science, Emory University, Atlanta, GA, USA
e-mail: hanyi.yu@emory.edu

S. B. Yoon · A. Marcus
Department of Hematology and Medical Oncology, Emory University, Atlanta, GA, USA
e-mail: sung.bo.yoon@emory.edu; adam.marcus@emory.edu

R. Kauffman · J. Wrammert
Department of Pediatrics, Division of Infectious Diseases, Emory University, Atlanta, GA, USA
e-mail: robert.kauffman@emory.edu; jwramme@emory.edu

J. Kong (✉)
Department of Mathematics and Statistics, Georgia State University, Atlanta, GA, USA

Department of Computer Science, Georgia State University, Atlanta, GA, USA

Department of Computer Science, Emory University, Atlanta, GA, USA

Department of Biomedical Informatics, Emory University, Atlanta, GA, USA
e-mail: jkong@gsu.edu

Y. Zhao, (Din) D.-G. Chen (eds.), *Modern Statistical Methods for Health Research*, Emerging Topics in Statistics and Biostatistics,
https://doi.org/10.1007/978-3-030-72437-5_2

Traditional approaches used for tracking low-speed small objects usually consist of two stages. In the first stage, objects in each image frame of an image sequence are detected individually. For example, multi-level threshold methods are efficient when the objects are sparsely distributed and have sharp contrast to the background pixels [13]. Although watershed based methods are useful to deal with clumped objects, they often suffer from the over-segmentation problem [12]. Methods based on the gradient flow are good solutions when image gradient vectors within objects generally point to their centers [9, 11]. In the second stage, detected objects are modeled and linked to recover motion trajectories by various strategies, such as nearest neighbor [2], meanshift [3], and dynamic programming [18]. Additionally, Multiple Hypothesis Tracking (MHT) approaches are widely used to build a graph where vertices representing objects in all image frames are linked by edges for paired objects with possible associations. A set of non-conflicting paths can be identified by either the greedy search [20] or a cost function minimization [19]. However, a common defect shared by tracking methods above is that they only utilize the static object information with such dynamic information as the motion speed omitted. As a result, high speed objects are often either mismatched or ignored by such tracking approaches. Moreover, these approaches do not perform well when objects of interest are overlapped with each other in time-lapse fluorescence image sequences.

More recent investigations [6, 7, 22] have shown that particle filtering (PF) algorithm can produce robust tracking results when objects move at a high motion speed. In these studies, objects captured in images are modeled as blurred spots with their intensity distributions approximated by Gaussian functions. However, due to the complex object shape and limited microscopic image resolution, such object intensities may not always follow the Gaussian distribution. In Fig. 1, we illustrate cases when object intensity can and cannot be modeled as a Gaussian distribution. Although some studies [4, 17, 28] overcome such deficiency by leveraging parametric active contours for more precise object state descriptions, they are vulnerable to large shape variations, especially in the 3D space. Additionally, the larger number of parameters necessary for such models inevitably requires an exponentially increasing number of particles (or random guess) to cover the state space, resulting in a worse computational performance.

As deep neural networks have recently become the state of the art in computer vision research field, more and more efforts have been made to combine object tracking approaches with deep learning algorithms. One strategy is to improve object detection robustness in low signal to noise ratio images by leveraging Convolutional Neural Network (CNN) [8, 10, 15, 27], while others use deep learning algorithms to increase the object tracking accuracy in the linking stage. For example, performance of a particle filtering framework has been improved by CNN enhanced particles before the updating stage [14]. Additionally, unsupervised Denoising AutoEncoder (DAE) [24] has been demonstrated as an effective way for MHT approach improvement to avoid tuning a large number of user-defined parameters [23]. However, all these improvements based on deep learning algorithms require large-scale training samples for optimization of weights in the network

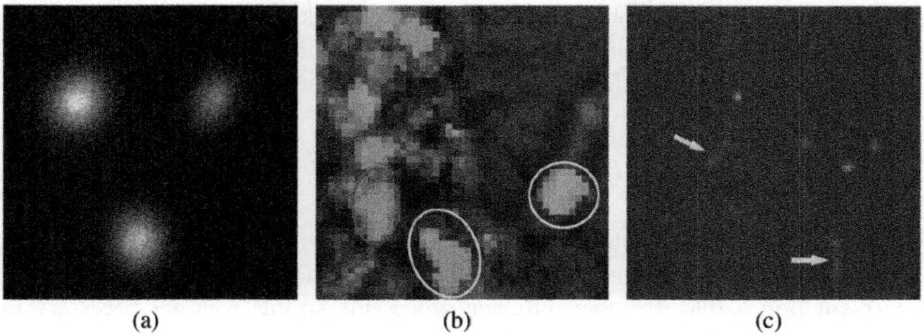

Fig. 1 Illustration of fluorescent images with (a) object intensity following the Gaussian model, (b) objects with sharp edges (yellow) and shifted center (red), and (c) deformed objects due to motion blur

architecture. Meanwhile, the generalizability of a trained network is usually too limited to be applied to different types of image data.

To address these problems, we propose to generalize the traditional particle filtering approaches in this work. Specifically, two different models are presented to improve the tracking performance in non-Gaussian conditions. In addition, we propose a new tracking management strategy to accelerate the model updating. With this new mapping step after updating the particle states, the tracking accuracy can be improved. The performance of our approach is demonstrated with both artificial image sequences and real time-lapse fluorescent image datasets that capture 2D bacteria and 3D lung cancer cells in motion.

2 Method

The proposed tracking approach is based on the particle filtering algorithm. In this section, we first briefly recapitulate the particle filtering tracking framework and introduce the object segmentation method that we use to distinguish objects from background. Next, we present our realization of observation models and dynamics models that are customized for biomedical fluorescent imaging applications. Finally, we explain how we extend the method to accommodate multiple objects. As same methods for 2D images can be directly derived from those for 3D images, we limit our method description to the 3D case.

2.1 Particle Tracking Framework

Particle filtering algorithm is derived from the Bayesian estimation that infers knowledge about the hidden object state $\mathbf{x}_t$ with a sequence of noisy observations

$\mathbf{z}_{1:t} = \{\mathbf{z}_1, \ldots, \mathbf{z}_t\}$. For object tracking, $\mathbf{z}_t$ represents a 2D/3D image, while $\mathbf{x}_t$ is a vector that describes such object properties as location, velocity, and shape. A recursive formula to estimate the evolution of the hidden state is given as follows [5]:

$$p(\mathbf{x}_t|\mathbf{z}_{1:t}) \propto p(\mathbf{z}_t|\mathbf{x}_t) \int p(\mathbf{x}_t|\mathbf{x}_{t-1}) p(\mathbf{x}_{t-1}|\mathbf{z}_{1:t-1}) d\mathbf{x}_{t-1} \tag{1}$$

where $p(\mathbf{x}_t|\mathbf{z}_{1:t})$ is the posterior density function, $p(\mathbf{x}_t|\mathbf{x}_{t-1})$ is the state transition model, and $p(\mathbf{z}_t|\mathbf{x}_t)$ is the likelihood distribution. The merit of the recursion representation is that it enables efficient processing so that it is not necessary to compute with previous data again after a new observation is generated. With the probability density function $p(\mathbf{x}_t|\mathbf{z}_{1:t})$, an estimation of the state can be easily computed by such statistical method as expectation and minimum mean squared error (MMSE) estimate.

One problem with such an approach is that the optimal solution of Eq. 1 is only solvable in some rare cases, such as Gaussian or grid-based modeling [1]. For practical applications, particle filtering algorithm is frequently used by a feasible approximation where the desired posterior density function is estimated with N random samples and associated weights $\{\mathbf{x}_t^{(n)}, w_t^{(n)}\}_{n=1}^{N}$:

$$p(\mathbf{x}_t|\mathbf{z}_{1:t}) \approx \sum_{n=1}^{N} w_t^{(n)} \delta(\mathbf{x}_t - \mathbf{x}_t^{(n)}) \tag{2}$$

These weights are updated and normalized recursively by sequential importance sampling:

$$w_t^n \propto \frac{p(\mathbf{z}_t|\mathbf{x}_t^{(n)}) p(\mathbf{x}_t^{(n)}|\mathbf{x}_{t-1}^{(n)})}{q(\mathbf{x}_t^{(n)}|\mathbf{x}_{t-1}^{(n)}, \mathbf{z}_t)} w_{t-1}^{(n)} \tag{3}$$

where the importance function $q(\mathbf{x}_t|\mathbf{x}_{t-1}, \mathbf{z}_t)$ describes the possibility of the distribution of the new state $\mathbf{x}_t$ in the state space. Therefore, the generation of particle $\mathbf{x}_t^{(n)}$ follows the importance function.

2.2 Object Segmentation

Segmentation is an essential step in our tracking analysis, as both initialization and update of hidden states $\mathbf{x}_t$ require that object voxels are accurately labeled. Either a manually selected or data driven threshold [16] can be used for simple segmentation. Unfortunately, objects in fluorescence microscopy images are often so clumped that it is too challenging to separate them with a single threshold. Therefore, we apply an automated object segmentation method that uses voxel gradient guided information [9].

The segmentation method is based on the assumption that the fluorescent intensity captured by each object of interest declines from its center to its periphery gradually. Thus, the gradient vector $\mathbf{f} = \nabla I = (f_x, f_y, f_z)$ within an object points to the object center. With this property, we can segment an image volume by assigning the same object label to all voxels pointing to the same object center. However, due to varying image noise, directions of gradient vectors are deteriorated, leading to over-segmentation. In order to obtain biologically meaningful results, we regulate the gradient field by gradient vector flow (GVF) [25], a non-irrotational external force field that does not need any prior knowledge about image edges. The GVF field $\mathbf{g} = (u, v, w)$ of a 3D fluorescence image volume $I(x, y, z)$ can be computed by solving the following Euler–Lagrange equations:

$$\begin{aligned}
\mu\nabla^2 u - (u - I_x)(I_x^2 + I_y^2 + I_z^2) &= 0 \\
\mu\nabla^2 v - (v - I_y)(I_x^2 + I_y^2 + I_z^2) &= 0 \\
\mu\nabla^2 w - (w - I_z)(I_x^2 + I_y^2 + I_z^2) &= 0
\end{aligned} \tag{4}$$

where μ is a weight coefficient and ∇^2 is the Laplacian operator. As GVF can be used directly without training and is resistant to image noise, we use GVF algorithm in this work.

After computing the GVF field $\mathbf{g}$, we group voxels into sub-volumes with distinct object labels by finding paths in the GVF field. Given a voxel $\mathbf{r}^{(i)} = (x^{(i)}, y^{(i)}, z^{(i)})^T$, it is linked to the next voxel $\mathbf{r}^{(i+1)}$ by

$$\mathbf{r}^{(i+1)} = \mathbf{r}^{(i)} + S(\mathbf{g}(\mathbf{r}^{(i)}), \xi) + S(\mathbf{g}(\mathbf{r}^{(i)}), -\xi) - (1, 1, 1)^T \tag{5}$$

where $S(\mathbf{g})$ is a vector of step functions

$$S(\mathbf{g}, \xi) = \begin{pmatrix} \varepsilon(u + \xi) \\ \varepsilon(v + \xi) \\ \varepsilon(w + \xi) \end{pmatrix}, \varepsilon(a) = \begin{cases} 1, & a \geq 0 \\ 0, & a < 0 \end{cases}$$

Equation 5 suggests that the next voxel to be linked, i.e. $\mathbf{r}^{(i+1)}$, is found by moving along all directions by the signs of the individual GVF components at $\mathbf{r}^{(i)}$, i.e. $\mathbf{g}(\mathbf{r}^{(i)}) = (u(\mathbf{r}^{(i)}), v(\mathbf{r}^{(i)}), w(\mathbf{r}^{(i)}))$. When the absolute value of a certain GVF field component is greater than or equal to ξ, the voxel is moved in that component direction. If a voxel cannot move in any direction further, such a linking process is terminated. Thus, the parameter ξ controls the scope of the linking process. This linking process is repeated until all voxels are connected to some center voxels. Further, we assign the same but unique label to all voxels connected with the same center voxel and consider the space by all voxels sharing the same label a distinct sub-volume. By this approach, background voxels would be linked to some center voxel for each sub-volume. To remove such background voxels, we use Otsu algorithm [16] and compute a global threshold and a local threshold for each sub-volume. Voxels with intensity either lower than the global threshold or the corresponding local threshold would be labeled as zero, i.e. the label for background.

2.3 *Observation and Dynamics Models*

To apply the particle filtering algorithm to time-lapse fluorescence microscopy images, we consider our observations as time series of gray-scale image volumes of size $A \times B \times C$. Thus, observation $\mathbf{z}_t = \{z_t(i, j, k) \mid i \in [1, A], j \in [1, B], k \in [1, C]\}$ is interpreted as the voxel intensity at location (i, j, k) and time t, while the state vector $\mathbf{x}_t$ characterizes a vector of status properties of an object of interest at time t. As shown in Eq. 3, particle filtering algorithm requires the computation of the likelihood function $p(\mathbf{z}_t|\mathbf{x}_t^{(n)})$ that assesses the appropriateness of observation $\mathbf{z}_t$ for the particle $\mathbf{x}_t^{(n)}$, and the transition prior $p(\mathbf{x}_t|\mathbf{x}_{t-1})$ that describes the state evolution used for particle generation. A common state space vector for fluorescence microscopy image is $\mathbf{x}_t = (\mathbf{r}_t, \mathbf{v}_t, \mathbf{s}_t, I_t)$, where $\mathbf{r}_t = (x_t, y_t, z_t)$, $\mathbf{v}_t = (\dot{x}_t, \dot{y}_t, \dot{z}_t)$, $\mathbf{s}_t = (\sigma_{max,t}, \sigma_{min,t}, \sigma_{z,t}, \theta_t)$, and I_t denote the spatial position, velocity, shape, and object intensity, respectively [21, 22]. This model assumes that the observation intensity distribution can be well characterized by a Gaussian function with parameters given by the state $\mathbf{x}_t$:

$$h_t(i, j, k; \mathbf{x}_t) = I_t \exp(-\frac{1}{2}\mathbf{m}^T \mathbf{R}^T \Sigma^{-1} \mathbf{R}\mathbf{m}) + b_t \quad (6)$$

where b_t denotes the estimated background intensity; $\Sigma = \text{diag}(\sigma_{max,t}^2, \sigma_{min,t}^2, \sigma_{z,t}^2)$ is the covariance matrix; $\mathbf{R} = \mathbf{R}(\theta_t)$ is the rotation matrix on the x-y plane, and $\mathbf{m}^T = (i - x_t, j - y_t, k - z_t)$. The likelihood function can be defined in multiple ways, such as Sum of Absolute Difference (SAD) [21], Normalized Cross Correlation (NCC) [2], or other intensity-based similarity metrics.

However, due to diverse factors in the imaging acquisition process, objects of interest in fluorescence microscopy images do not always fit the Gaussian model. To address this issue, we propose two models that are designed for non-Gaussian cases.

Ellipsoid Model

Illustrated in Fig. 1b, the transition between object foreground and background could be abrupt and bright voxels could deviate from the object center in fluorescence microscopy image data of real biomedical research. For such cases, we propose an ellipsoid model to characterize such 3D object voxel intensity distribution. By this model, we first extract object volumes from gray-scale image $\mathbf{z}_t$ with our segmentation method described in Sect. 2.2. The resulting object volumes are denoted as $G(\mathbf{z}_t)$. Next, each object volume $g_t \in G(\mathbf{z}_t)$ is fitted by an ellipsoid $\mathcal{E}_t$ in a way such that the overlap between volume g_t and the ellipsoid is maximized. Since most objects are noticed to have a small range along the z direction in a large number of biomedical applications, the elevation angle is ignored. Thus, the ellipsoid $\mathcal{E}_t$ has two axes $\sigma_{max,t}, \sigma_{min,t}$ parallel to the x-y plane, and the third axis $\sigma_{z,t}$ perpendicular to the x-y plane. With the ellipsoid $\mathcal{E}_t$, we define the state vector $\mathbf{x}_t = (\mathbf{r}_t, \mathbf{v}_t, \mathbf{s}_t)$ where $\mathbf{r}_t = (x_t, y_t, z_t)$, $\mathbf{v}_t = (\dot{x}_t, \dot{y}_t, \dot{z}_t)$, and $\mathbf{s}_t$ represent the ellipsoid centroid, velocity, and the shape vector, respectively. For shape characterization, $\mathbf{s}_t$ includes the half principal axis length $\sigma_{max,t}, \sigma_{min,t}, \sigma_{z,t}$ and the rotation angle θ_t around the z-axis.

The likelihood function computes the degree of overlap between the state vector specified volume and the segmented object volume. We describe such overlapping effect by the ratio of the intersection to the union of such two volumes. With the ellipsoid model, the likelihood function is defined as

$$p(\mathbf{z}_t|\mathbf{x}_t^{(n)}) = \max_{g_t \in G(z_t)} \frac{\left|g_t \cap E\left(\mathbf{x}_t^{(n)}\right)\right|}{\left|g_t \cup E\left(\mathbf{x}_t^{(n)}\right)\right|} \tag{7}$$

where $E(\mathbf{x}_t^{(n)}) = \{e(i, j, k; \mathbf{x}_t^{(n)})\}$ represents a 3D volume with an ellipsoid mask specified by the state vector $\mathbf{x}_t^{(n)}$ and $|\cdot|$ represents the cardinality of the voxel coordinate set. Additionally, the voxel value $e(i, j, k; \mathbf{x}_t^{(n)})$ can be either 0 or 1 determined by the formula modified from Eq. 6:

$$e(i, j, k; \mathbf{x}_t^{(n)}) = \epsilon(\mathbf{m}^T \mathbf{R}^T \Sigma^{-1} \mathbf{R}\mathbf{m} - 1), \tag{8}$$

where $\epsilon(\cdot)$ is the unit step function.

Meanwhile, we assume that changes in object motion and shape are independent. Thus, we can factorize the transition prior as

$$p(\mathbf{x}_t|\mathbf{x}_{t-1}) = p(\mathbf{y}_t|\mathbf{y}_{t-1})p(\mathbf{s}_t|\mathbf{s}_{t-1}), \tag{9}$$

where the motion vector $\mathbf{y}_t = (x_t, \dot{x}_t, y_t, \dot{y}_t, z_t, \dot{z}_t)$.

Further, the transition prior for the motion vector is given by

$$p(\mathbf{y}_t|\mathbf{y}_{t-1}) = \mathcal{N}(\mathbf{P}\,\mathbf{y}_{t-1}, \mathbf{q}_1) \tag{10}$$

where $\mathcal{N}(\mu, \Sigma)$ is the normal distribution with mean μ and covariance matrix Σ. The process transition matrix $\mathbf{P}$ is defined as follows:

$$\mathbf{P} = \begin{pmatrix} \mathbf{P}' & 0 & 0 \\ 0 & \mathbf{P}' & 0 \\ 0 & 0 & \mathbf{P}' \end{pmatrix}, \quad \mathbf{P}' = \begin{pmatrix} 1 & 1 \\ 0 & 1 \end{pmatrix}.$$

Similarly, the transition prior for the shape vector is given by the following normal distribution:

$$p(\mathbf{s}_t|\mathbf{s}_{t-1}) = \mathcal{N}(\mathbf{s}_{t-1}, \mathbf{q}_2) \tag{11}$$

In Eqs. 10 and 11, $\mathbf{q}_1$ and $\mathbf{q}_2$ represent the noise level vectors for motion and shape, respectively. Note both parameters can be tuned during experiments.

Voxel-Based Model

Although the ellipsoid model can be used to characterize objects with non-Gaussian intensity distribution, it assumes objects are approximately ellipsoidal by shape. As presented in Fig. 1c, objects from images of real biomedical studies can be deformed in shape due to motion blur. To improve the performance of particle filtering algorithm for such cases, we propose a voxel-based (VB) model that accommodates such shape aberrations. Instead of using a shape vector for shape representation, VB model records voxel coordinates of objects. The resulting state vector is defined as $\mathbf{x}_t = (\mathbf{r}_t, \mathbf{v}_t, C_t) = (\mathbf{y}_t, C_t)$ where C_t denotes the object voxel coordinate set. Therefore, $E(\mathbf{x}_t^{(n)})$ in Eq. 7 is replaced by C_t and the likelihood function in this model is given as

$$p(\mathbf{z}_t|\mathbf{x}_t^{(n)}) = \max_{g_t \in G(z_t)} \frac{\left|g_t \cap C_t^{(n)}\right|}{\left|g_t \cup C_t^{(n)}\right|}. \tag{12}$$

Note that we only consider the change of motion vector $\mathbf{y}_t$ and spatial shift of the coordinate set C_t for the transition prior computation. Thus, we can update the spatial coordinate set by the following equation:

$$C_t = C_{t-1} + \mathbf{r}_t - \mathbf{r}_{t-1} \tag{13}$$

Therefore, unlike the factorization in Eq. 9 for the ellipsoid model, the transition prior in this case is simplified as

$$p(\mathbf{x}_t|\mathbf{x}_{t-1}) = p(C_t|C_{t-1}) = p(\mathbf{y}_t|\mathbf{y}_{t-1}) \tag{14}$$

The VB model can effectively describe objects in arbitrary shapes at the cost of more memory expense. It is an appropriate model to use when (1) image sequences contain a large number of objects not in ellipsoidal shapes and (2) computing

Algorithm 1 Proposed multiple object tracking management framework

Input: time lapse image volumes $\{\mathbf{z}_t\},\ t \in [1, T]$
Output: object state sets $\{\mathbf{x}_{t,k} |\ k \in [1, M_t],\ t \in [1, T]\}$
Initialize state set $\{\mathbf{x}_{1,k}\}$ with $\mathbf{z}_1$
for $t = 2 : T$ **do**
  Extract states $\{\mathbf{x}_{t,k}\}$ from $\mathbf{z}_t$ and set their labels to 0
  for $j = 1 : M_{t-1}$ **do**
    Generate particles $\{\mathbf{x}_{t,j}^{(n)}\}$ according to the state $\mathbf{x}_{t-1,j}$
    Compute weight $\pi_{t,j}^{n}$ for each particle $\mathbf{x}_{t,j}^{(n)}$
    Normalize weights such that $\sum_{n=1}^{N} \pi_{t,j}^{n} = 1$
    Compute the estimated state $\mathbf{x}'_{t,j}$
  end for
  Map labels of estimated states $\{\mathbf{x}'_{t,j}\}$ to detected states $\{\mathbf{x}_{t,k}\}$
end for

resources are sufficient. By contrast, the ellipsoid model is more economic in memory usage and is appropriate to use when objects of interest are in ellipsoidal shapes.

As the proposed VB model does not take into account shape information in the updating process, we next present a new tracking management strategy that we have developed to play the role of the shape information update absent in the VB model.

2.4 *Multiple Object Tracking Management*

We have developed a new and automatic tracking management strategy for multiple object tracking problems. This strategy includes four steps: initialization, prediction, updating, and mapping. The complete workflow is illustrated in a diagram in Fig. 2. Note that all steps but initialization can be executed recurrently, thus leading to a reduced computational complexity. An algorithmic description of our approach is presented in Algorithm 1. In addition, we provide details of each step as follows:

(1) **Initialization**: In this step, we initialize global parameters: particle number N, noise levels $\mathbf{q}_1$ and $\mathbf{q}_2$. A larger N in general results in a higher tracking precision, but at a higher computational time cost. Additionally, a higher noise level helps track drastic changes in object states but decreases the resistance to interference when objects are densely distributed. In this step, the time-lapse image data $\mathbf{z}_t$ is segmented as a temporal volume set $\{G(\mathbf{z}_t)\}$ by the gradient-based algorithm presented in Sect. 2.2. We denote the number of volumes in $G(\mathbf{z}_t)$ as $|G(\mathbf{z}_t)| = M_t$. Therefore, states $\mathbf{x}_{1,1}, \mathbf{x}_{1,2}, \ldots, \mathbf{x}_{1,M_1}$ are extracted from the first image volume when $t = 1$. In addition to the basic information of an object, i.e. location, speed, intensity among others, a state vector $\mathbf{x}_{t,k}$ contains

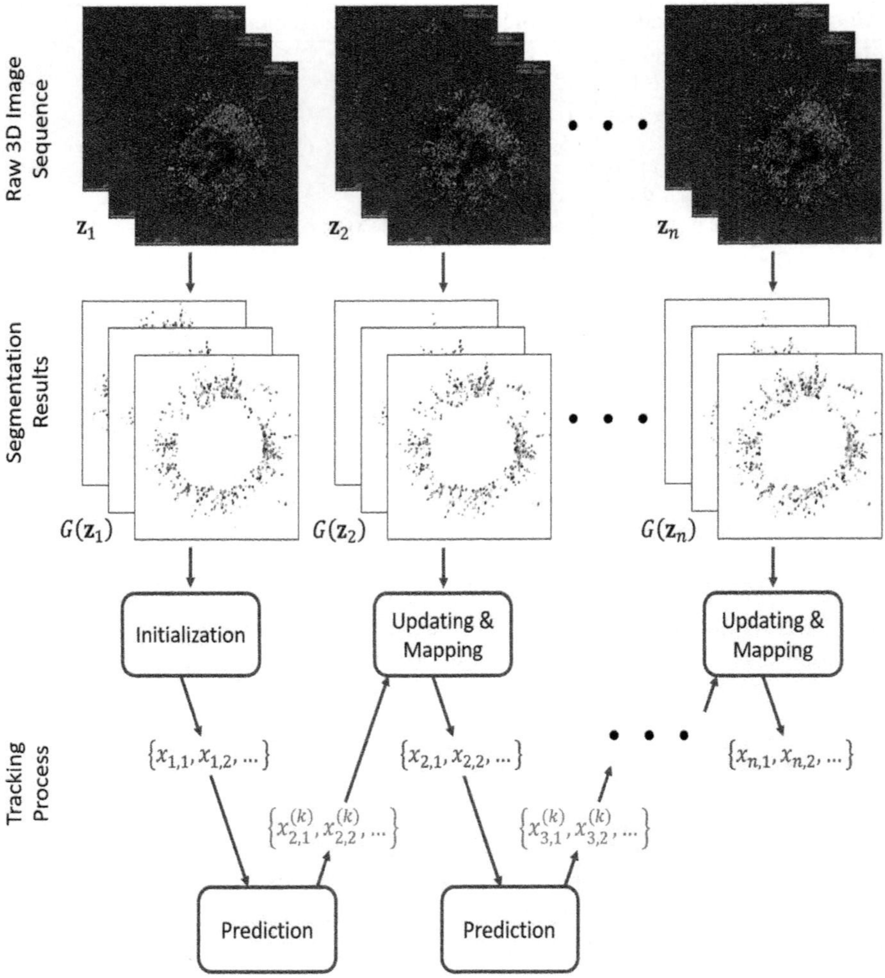

Fig. 2 Overall schema for multiple object tracking management method. Raw 3D images (first row) are first processed to assign each object of interest a unique label (second row). Labels are further modified by the tracking process (remaining rows) such that each object of interest retains the same unique label in temporal imaging data. For the tracking process, the estimated states are represented in red, while produced particles are in blue

an object label. This is designed to facilitate the identification of the same object traversing image volumes at different time points.

(2) **Prediction**: In the prediction step, particles $\{\mathbf{x}_{t,k}^{(n)} \mid n \in [1, N],\ k \in [1, M_{t-1}]\}$ are generated according to Eqs. 9, 10, and 11 when the ellipsoid model is used. When the VB model is adopted, Eqs. 10, 13, and 14 are used for particle generation instead. As each state has N particles, the total number of particles in each iteration is $N \times M_{t-1}$.

(3) **Updating**: The likelihood of each particle is updated by Eqs. 7 and 12 when the ellipsoid model and the VB model are used respectively. We use the likelihood as particle weight $\pi^n_{t,k}$ and normalize such weights with $\sum_{n=1}^{N} \pi^n_{t,k} = 1$. The estimated state $\mathbf{x}'_{t,j}$ inherits its label from the state $\mathbf{x}_{t-1,j}$. The remaining components in $\mathbf{x}'_{t,j}$ are computed by

$$\mathbf{x}'_{t,k} = \sum_{n=1}^{N} \pi^n_{t,k} \mathbf{x}^{(n)}_{t,k}$$

(4) **Mapping**: Finally, the relationship between estimated state $\mathbf{x}'_{t,k}$ and all detected states $\{\mathbf{x}_{t,j}\}$ can be characterized by the likelihood function. For each estimated state $\mathbf{x}'_{t,k}$, we assign its label to the detected state with the highest likelihood. Note when the highest likelihood is less than a specified threshold D, such labeling process does not occur. Objects without any matched estimated state are treated as disappearing objects, while the ones without any matched detected state are treated as newly emerged objects receiving new labels. In the traditional particle filtering framework, two cells C_t^1 and C_t^2 may be linked to the same cell C_{t+1}^1 in the next frame when the object density is high. As a result, the second cell C_{t+1}^2 in the next frame that should have been linked from the cell C_t^2 could be considered as a new cell, leading to a decreased tracking accuracy. By our method, such erroneous cases are avoided because of our proposed mapping step. Thus, it is an important step to improve tracking accuracy.

3 Experiments and Results

To assess our proposed tracking method performance, we apply our workflow to multiple time-lapse fluorescence microscopy image datasets, including one artificial dataset with known ground truth, as well as real biological image datasets from two time-lapse microscopy studies on bacteria motility and 3D lung cancer spheroid analysis.

3.1 Validation with Artificial Data

Our proposed tracking approach is first tested and validated with a synthetic 2D image dataset with each image of 1000×1000 pixels in size. This dataset is generated by artificially initializing object states, updating states with the Gaussian model, and producing individual temporal image frames with evolving object states and noise background. In the dataset, 10 objects are produced initially with speed subject to a uniform distribution between 8 and 11 pixels per frame. Each object can split into two child objects with probability 0.02 in each frame. Parameters of the approach with the ellipsoid model are set with the following values: $N = 200$ for each object, $\mathbf{q}_1 = (10, 1, 10, 1)$, and $\mathbf{q}_2 = (0.5, 0.5, 0.2)$. As objects in our synthetic images are sparse and move relatively slow, almost all objects in all frames are correctly tracked in reference to their ground truth, with the overall tracking accuracy 99.7%. Additionally, the root mean square error (RMSE), a frequently used metric computed with the ground truth and estimated object positions, is 1.91 ± 0.32 pixels for those correctly tracked objects. Figure 3 demonstrates typical tracking results where object motion trajectories are illustrated. When objects are split, trajectories of parents and children are represented by forked chains in the same color. With Fig. 3, we notice that both objects with crossing trajectories and divisions are correctly tracked. For example, object 1 and 2 are partially overlapped in frame 3 and 4. However, our method manages to track them after their collision. Additionally, object 3 is proliferated into two child objects, i.e. object 4 and 5, in frame 17. The resulting two child objects are correctly linked to the parent object 3 as suggested by the same trajectory color. All results above suggest the effectiveness and robustness of our approach in simple cases where objects are sparse and present a good contrast to the background.

3.2 Bacteria Motility Analysis

We further test our method with a real time-lapse 2D fluorescence image dataset of the bacterial pathogen *Vibrio cholerae* after treatment with bacteria-specific motility inhibiting monoclonal antibodies. In this experiment design, the inhibition of bacteria average speed is considered as the metric of bacteria vitality. This is inversely proportional to the potential protective efficacy of cholera vaccines that aim, in part, to induce antibodies able to inhibit bacterial motility. With a high speed confocal microscope, motility of bacteria is observed at 100 ms intervals for 5 s, with 5 min post treatment on six types of antibodies in various dose concentrations. The resulting dataset consists of 23 image sequences. Each includes 50 temporal image frames of 512×512 pixels in image resolution. Figure 4a presents an image frame from a typical image sequence that captures both active bacteria with high speeds and in deformed shapes, as well as slow-moving bacteria with vitality significantly reduced by vaccine. We have applied the proposed tracking method to bacteria image sequences. We present in Fig. 4b the bacteria segmentation result of Fig. 4a. In Fig. 4c, bacteria tracking results are illustrated. Specifically, the motion trajectories of bacteria are plotted in colors. For each bacterium, its trajectory is visualized from the frame of its occurrence to the current example frame shown in Fig. 4a. Additionally, we present the dynamic tracking results frame by frame in Fig. 5 where the tracking result of each bacterium over eight temporal frames is illustrated. In particular, we demonstrate the motion trajectory of one specific bacterium in an inset.

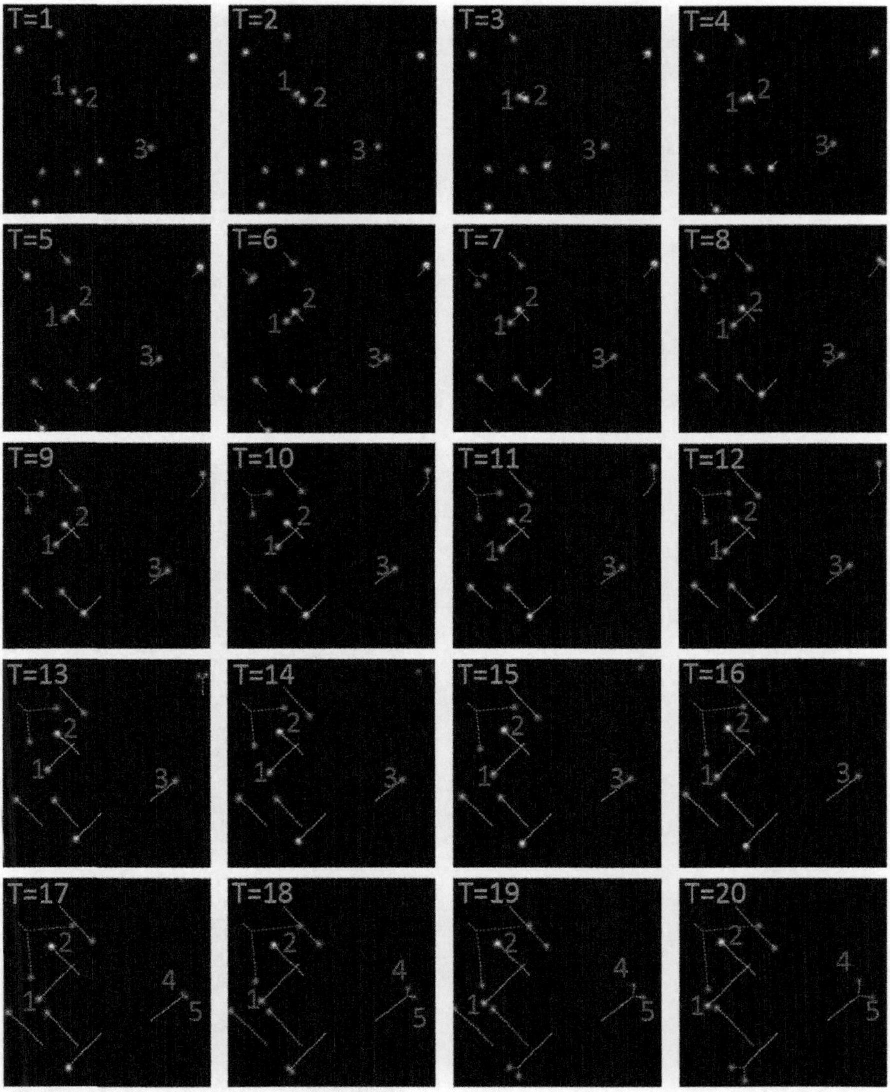

Fig. 3 Experimental results of artificial data with left to right and top to bottom time order. Trajectories are color coded and overlaid on original images. Note that object 1 and 2 are overlapped in frame 3 and 4. Additionally, object 3 is split into two child objects, i.e. object 4 and 5, in frame 17. In both cases, our method can track objects correctly

We quantitatively assess our tracking method by comparing manually annotated and machine produced bacteria trajectories. Two metrics, i.e. precision and recall, are used to evaluate the tracking performance:

Fig. 4 (**a**) A typical raw image frame from a dataset for bacteria motility study; (**b**) Segmented bacteria from (**a**); (**c**) Tracking result demonstrated with all bacteria trajectories overlaid on the image

(a)

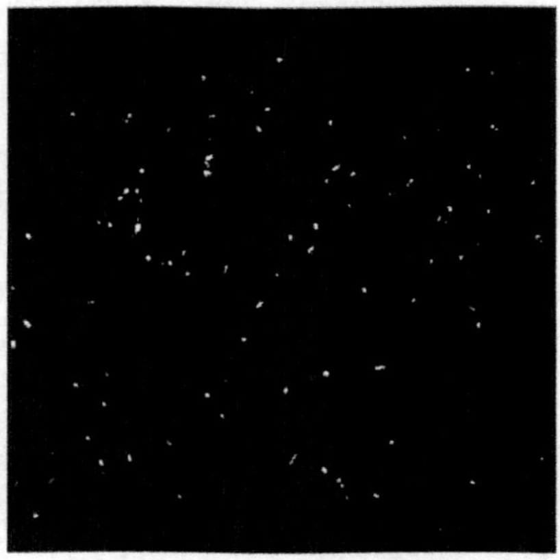

(b)

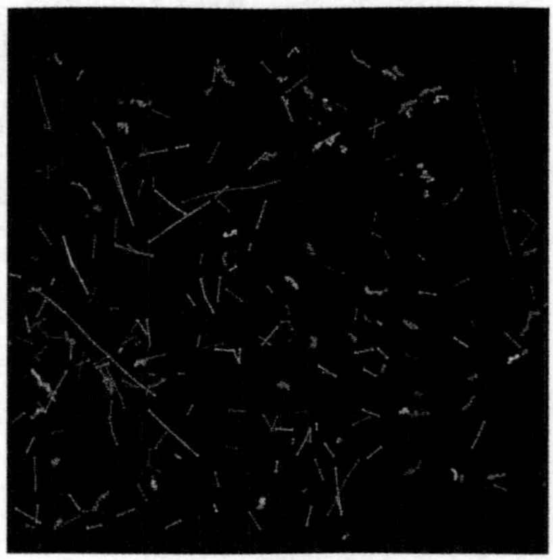

(c)

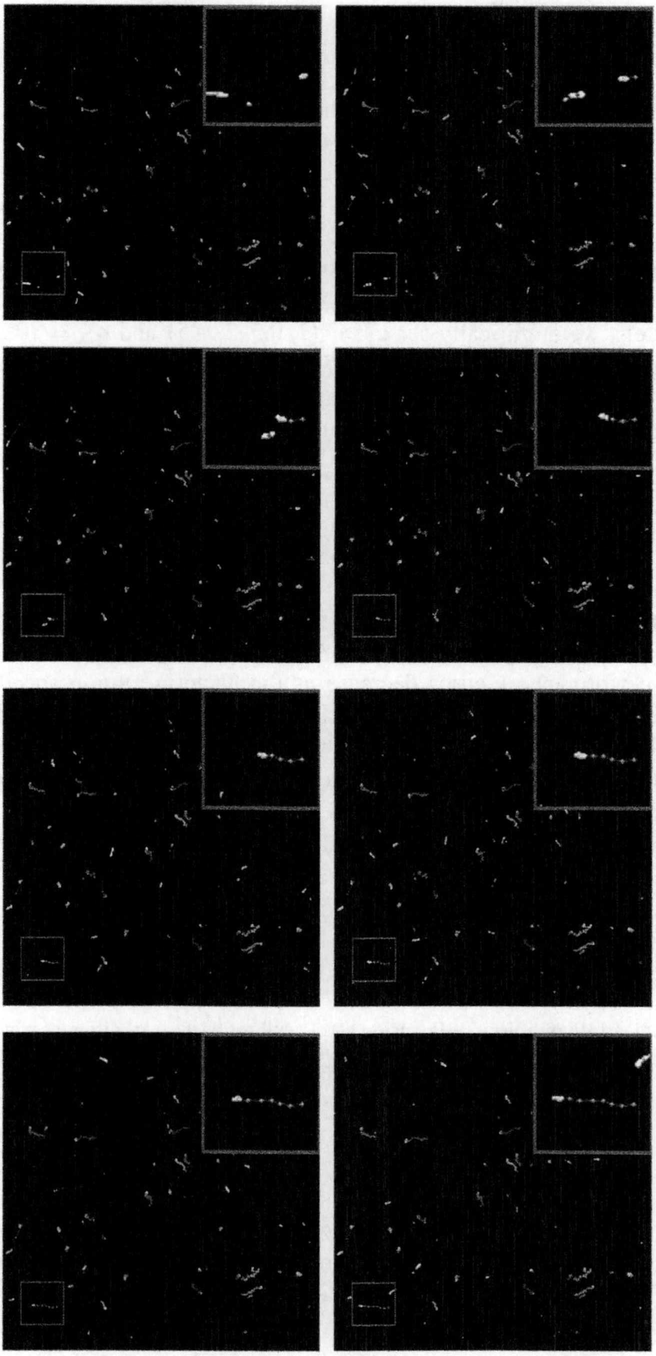

Fig. 5 Illustration of the tracking result dynamics of a 2D bacteria motility dataset. With the image inset, one typical bacterium from a local region is enlarged for its trajectory demonstration in detail

$$\text{Precision} = \frac{L_1}{L_2}, \qquad \text{Recall} = \frac{L_1}{L_3}$$

where L_1, L_2, and L_3 represent the number of frames with correct tracking results, total number of frames tracked by our method, and the number of frames with human annotations for each object, respectively.

To assess our method performance, we apply the classical particle filtering method [6], the particle filtering method improved by data-dependent importance sampling [22], and our method with two proposed models to bacteria image sequences. The particle numbers for all methods are set to $N = 200$ per object. In our models, we empirically set $\mathbf{q}_1 = (2, 0.5, 2, 0.5)$ and $\mathbf{q}_2 = (0.2, 0.2, 0.2)$. Our validation set includes 50 low and 50 high speed bacteria randomly selected from image sequences at each time point. The cutoff value between low and high speed populations is three pixels per frame. We compute the trajectory Precision and Recall for bacteria populations with low and high speed and present tracking results from different methods in Table 1. For the low speed bacteria population, all methods present good performance with minor difference. However, our method, especially with the VB model, is superior to other two state-of-the-art methods for tracking the high speed population.

We further present tracking Precision and Recall of 460 randomly selected individual bacteria using our VB model. As shown in Fig. 6a and b, it is noticeable that these performance metrics decrease as the bacteria motion speed increases. Meanwhile, we investigate the trajectory length distribution for high and low speed bacteria with the speed cutoff value of three pixels per frame. We notice in Fig. 6c that most high speed bacteria are captured in less than 10 image frames, with an average of 6.6 frames. These analyses explain why the trajectory Precision and Recall of most high speed bacteria tend to be substantially deteriorated even if there is only one erroneously tracked image frame. Additionally, the comparisons between low and high speed bacteria populations by Precision and Recall are presented in Figs. 7 and 8, respectively. It is noticed that Precision and Recall of

Table 1 Comparison of trajectory Precision and Recall for bacteria of different motion speeds

		Precision		Recall	
Population	Method	Mean	Std	Mean	Std
High speed	Classical [6]	0.6338	0.1415	0.7393	0.1699
	Improved [22]	0.7327	0.1577	0.7410	0.1738
	Ellipsoid model	0.7768	0.1904	0.7586	0.2173
	VB model	0.8032	0.1679	0.7970	0.1698
Low speed	Classical [6]	0.9450	0.1177	0.9647	0.0626
	Improved [22]	0.9544	0.0784	0.9670	0.0596
	Ellipsoid model	0.9591	0.1076	0.9615	0.0961
	VB model	0.9594	0.0575	0.9562	0.0964

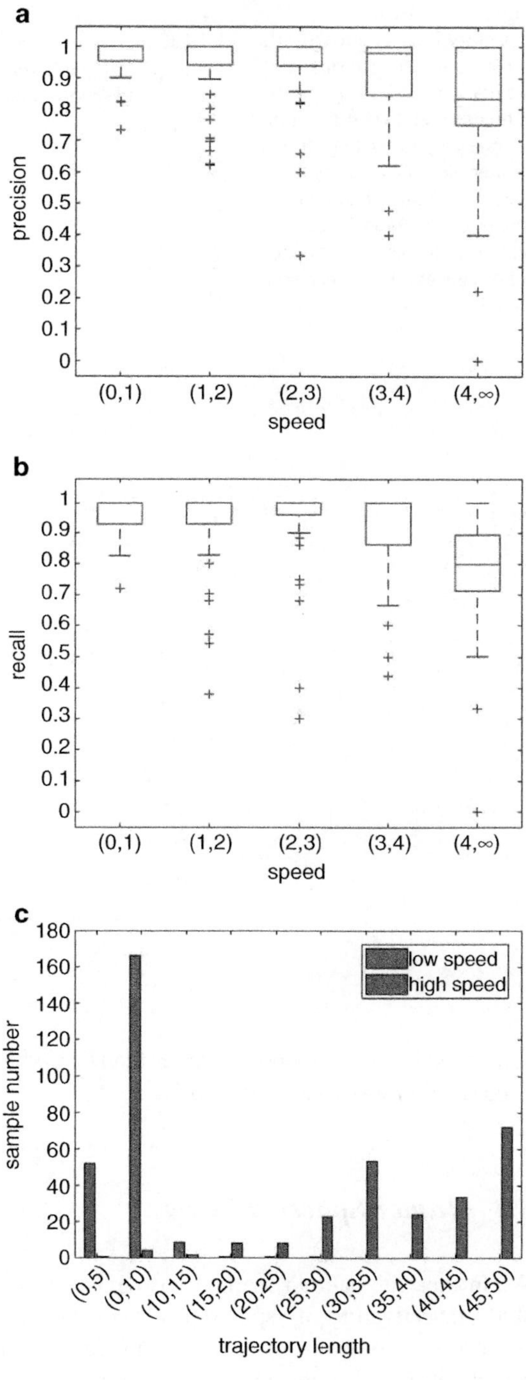

Fig. 6 (**a**) Tracking Precision grouped by bacteria motion speed; (**b**) Tracking Recall grouped by bacteria motion speed; (**c**) Distribution of bacteria trajectory length for low and high speed bacteria populations with speed threshold of 3 pixels per frame

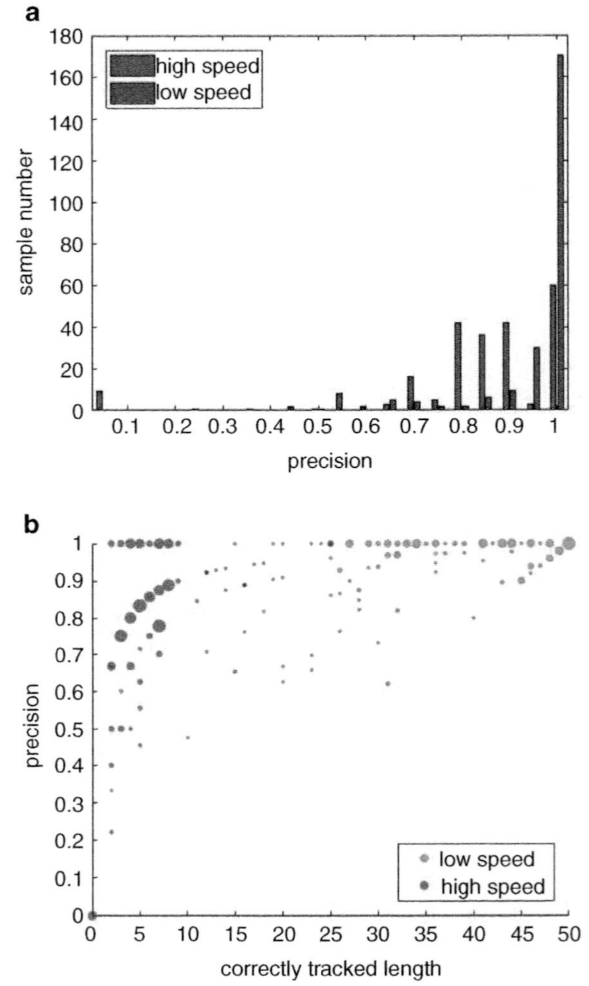

Fig. 7 Comparison of trajectory Precision for low and high speed bacteria populations in the 2D validation set. (**a**) Distribution of trajectory Precision; (**b**) Scatter plot of trajectory Precision. Note the unit of trajectory length is frame number, and size of each dot represents number of bacteria samples

low speed bacteria are mostly larger than 0.9, while these two metrics of high speed bacteria are mostly larger than 0.66.

3.3 Tumor Spheroid Study

We further validate our method with 3D time-lapse imaging data from an in vitro study investigating 3D spheroid invasion in the 4T1 mouse carcinoma cell line. In vitro spheroids are formed by centrifuging 3000 4T1 murine cancer cells in a round bottom, ultra-low attachment 96-well plate (Corning). After 72 h, compacted spheroids are collected and embedded in 3.0 mg/ml rat tail collagen type-I (Corning)

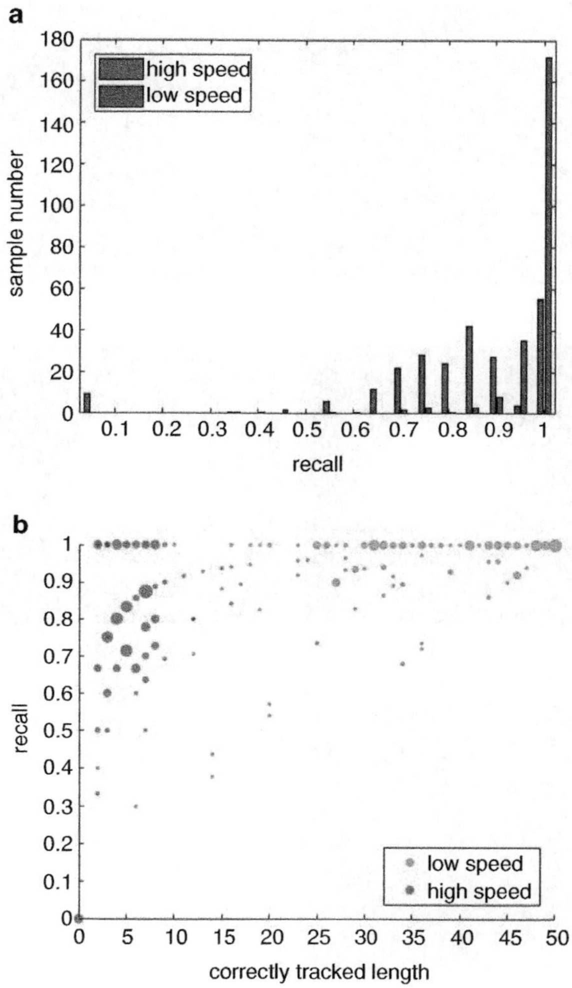

Fig. 8 Comparison of trajectory Recall for low and high speed bacteria populations in the 2D validation set. (**a**) Distribution of trajectory Recall; (**b**) Scatter plot of trajectory Recall. Note the unit of trajectory length is frame number, and size of each dot represents number of bacteria samples

in a μ-Slide 8 well chamber slide (Ibidi). Images are taken every 10 min for 16 h post-embedding using a Leica SP8 confocal microscope at 10× magnification. Time-lapse data show that these cancer cells invade with different behaviors, i.e. either collectively (in chain-like cellular protrusions) or individually. Cancer cells moving in collective chains are termed "in-chain" cells, while the invading cells not in chains are termed "single" cells. Through our analysis, we want to quantitatively characterize distinct moving patterns for each cancer cell population.

The dataset for analysis in this study consists of four longitudinal 3D image sequences acquired at 93 time points. Each image volume at one time point includes $24 \sim 32$ image planes of 512×512 pixels in resolution. Figure 9a presents an x-y slice of a typical RGB-model fluorescent image volume at a time point. For computation convenience, we prefer to transform each RGB 3-channel image to a

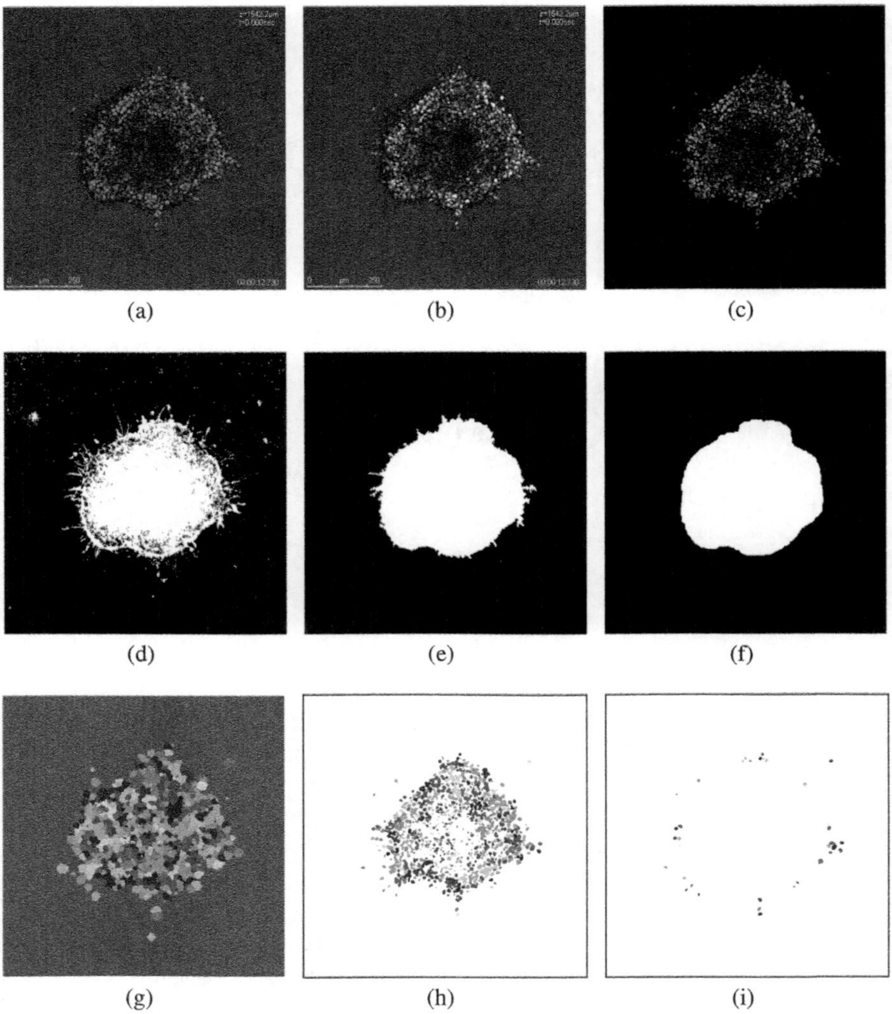

Fig. 9 2D x-y cross section views of preprocessing and segmentation results for a 3D tumor spheroid dataset. (**a**) Original image; (**b**) Gray-scale green channel; (**c**) Improved gray-scale image by mapping in the RGB color space; (**d**) Binary image after thresholding; (**e**) Binary mask with holes filled and outliers removed; (**f**) Final mask after mask contour regulation; (**g**) Rough segmentation result; (**h**) Refined segmentation result with a global and a local Otsu threshold applied to each block; (**i**) Final segmentation result with removed mask-specified spheroid

gray-scale image. As cells in this study are captured by fluorescent signals from the green channel, we extract the green channel from the original images and use it as the derived gray-scale image. Shown in Fig. 9b, the background surrounding the central spheroid is noisy and has similar intensity values to that of cancer cells, resulting in poor algorithm performance. To address this problem, we identify a feasible mapping formula to effectively distinguish cells from background: $I_{gray} = -0.5r + g - 0.5b$, where r, g, and b represent the red, green, and blue channel, respectively. The enhanced image is demonstrated in Fig. 9c.

In this study, we are only interested in tracking and characterizing cells invading outward from the central spheroid core. Thus, we implement a mask to remove cells of non-interest within the spheroid core before the tracking process, which substantially increases the computation efficiency. For automatic mask identification, we convert the resulting gray-scale image to a binary image by thresholding (Fig. 9d), fill holes in the mask by morphological algorithms, remove outliers (Fig. 9e), and smooth the resulting mask contour (Fig. 9f). We present the rough cell segmentation result of Fig. 9c in Fig. 9g where each color coded block contains a cell of interest and its surrounding background. Figure 9h presents the refined segmentation result after a global and a local Otsu threshold are applied to each block. With the spheroid mask illustrated in Fig. 9f, we remove the volume of the spheroid core from further tracking analysis. The final segmentation result is illustrated in Fig. 9i. As this dataset captures cancer cells in 3D, we present a 3D view of a typical 3D image volume before and after our segmentation analysis in Fig. 10a and b, respectively. After segmentation, all cells of interest are uniquely labeled at each time point. Next, we apply the proposed tracking method with the ellipsoid model to the time-lapse 3D labeled imaging volumes with the following empirical parameter setup: $N = 500$ per object, $\mathbf{q}_1 = (5, 1, 5, 1, 1, 1)$, and $\mathbf{q}_2 = (2, 2, 0.5, 0.2)$. Figure 11 demonstrates 3D views of the tracking result of a longitudinal image dataset where all cell trajectories are recovered. We share our tracking codes on GitHub [26] and provide a video in the supplement presenting the growing dynamics of these trajectories.

To assess the tracking performance, we generate the validation set with 50 cells of interest from each population by the same strategy described in Sect. 3.2. After reviewing trajectories of "in-chain" cells and "single" cells shown in Fig. 11, we notice that the former population moves radially outward from the spheroid center to peripheral areas at a moderate speed, while the latter group moves either at a near to zero speed or at a relatively high speed with frequently varying directions, leading to zig-zag trajectories. Typical examples of "single" cells, typically with z-axis value $z > 20$, can be clearly observed from the y-z view in Fig. 11b. Additionally, we visualize in Fig. 12 cells of interest with color codes representing motion speed. From this figure, it is salient that spatial invasion patterns of "in-chain" and "single" cells are different. Insets of each 3D plot enlarge sub-volumes that capture representative cell chains color coded in purple for moderate speed. These sub-volumes also capture representative "single" cells in cyan and yellow, suggesting low and high motion speed, respectively. For better illustration of motion dynamics, we provide a video in the supplement to show the different cell motion patterns.

We further quantitatively evaluate the tracking quality with the metrics defined in Sect. 3.2. As the vast majority of cells in this study are in the ellipsoidal shape, the VB model does not prevail over the ellipsoid model. Considering the memory cost, we apply the ellipsoid model to the validation set and compare with two state-of-the-

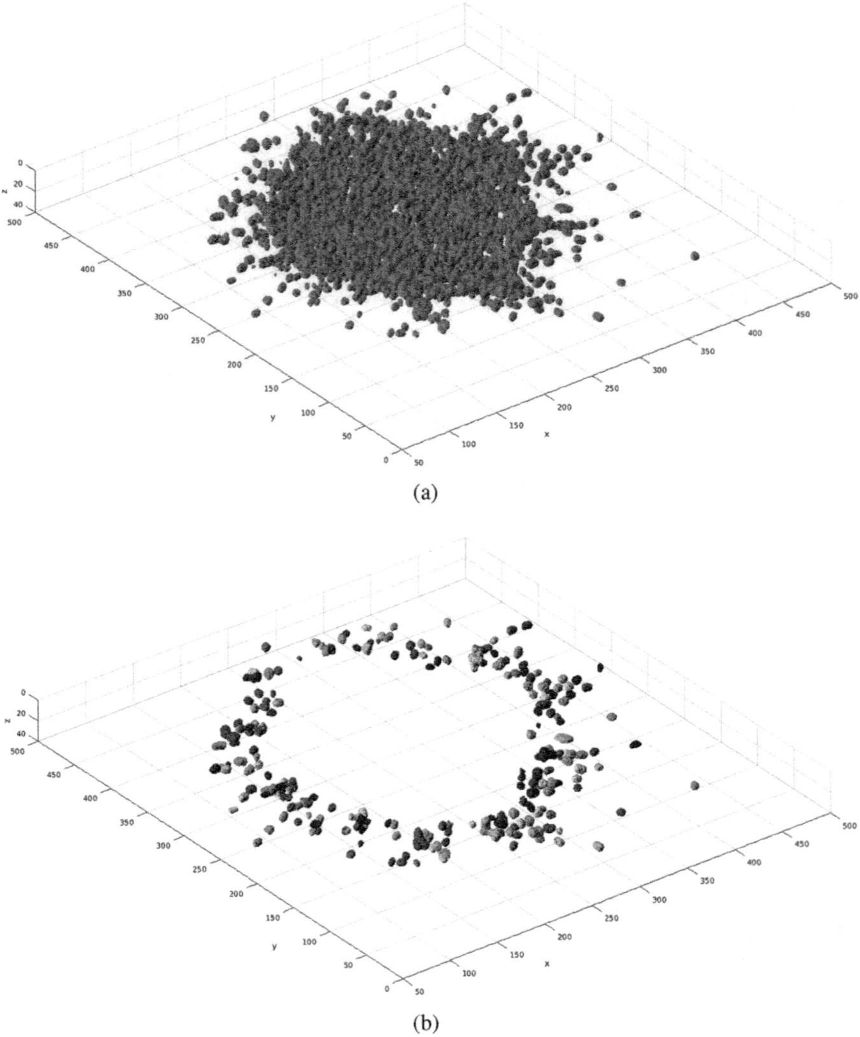

Fig. 10 (**a**) 3D view of the preprocessed tumor spheroid image volume; (**b**) 3D segmentation result of the 3D image volume

art algorithms [6, 22]. The evaluation results are presented in Table 2. Note that our approach presents the best trajectory Precision. A higher tracking Precision results from fewer incorrect segments in trajectories. Therefore, this experimental result suggests the efficacy of our new mapping step for cell state mismatch reduction when certain cells disappear from a field of view. Overall, our experimental results suggest the promising potential of our framework for automated cell invasion tracking and quantitative motion pattern characterization for cancer research.

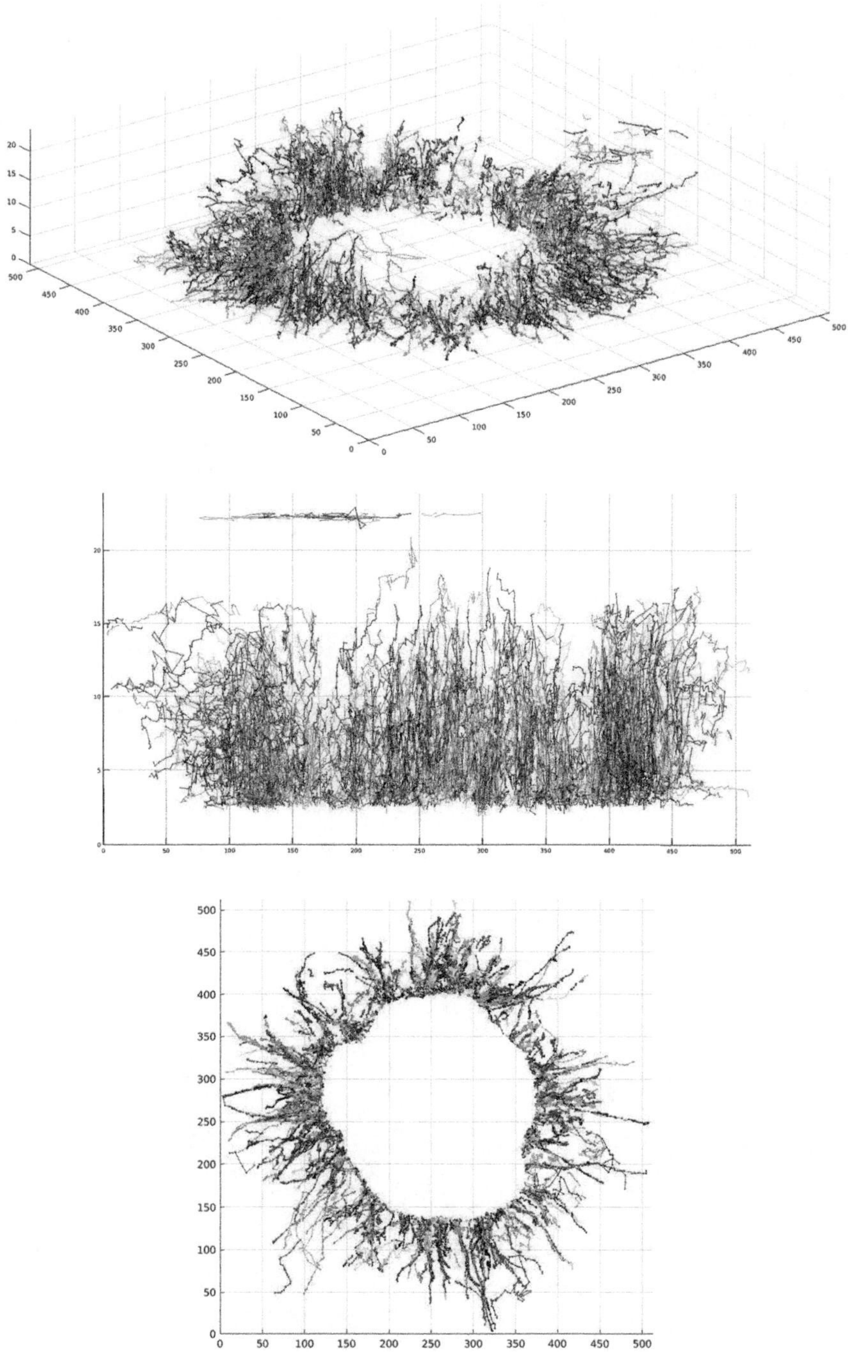

Fig. 11 Cancer cell tracking results of a 3D tumor spheroid dataset presented in three different views. (Top) 3D view; (Middle) y-z view; (Bottom) x-y view

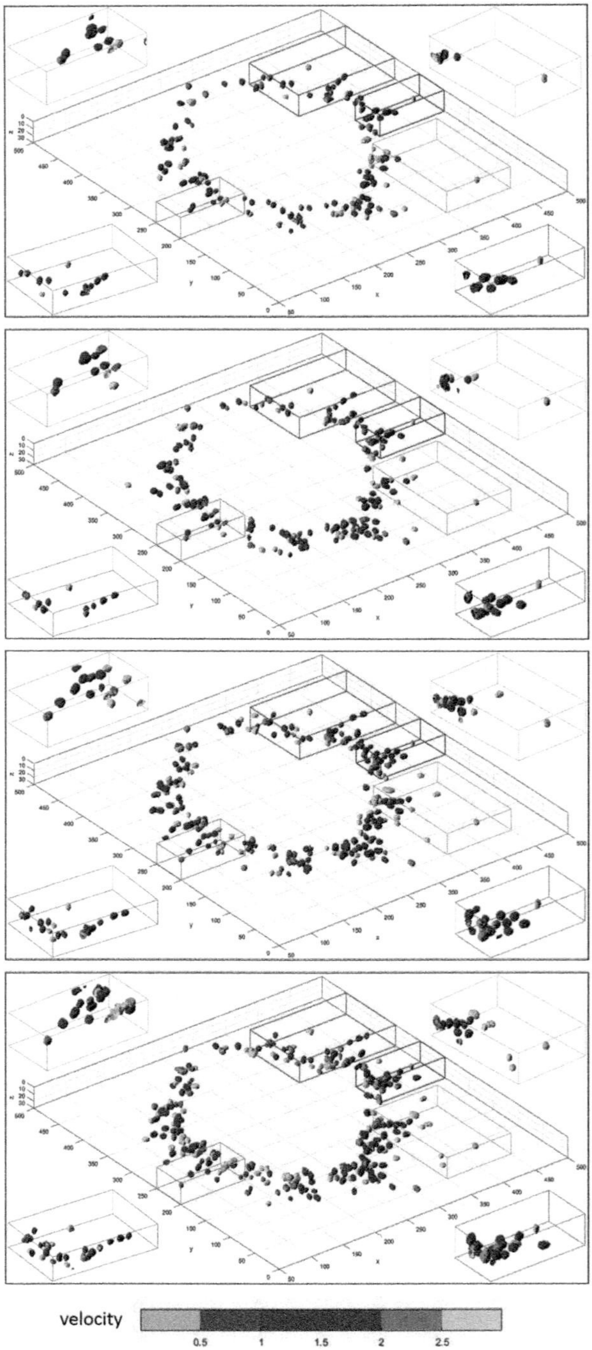

Fig. 12 3D view of tracking results with 3D cancer cells color coded by motion speed. The frame interval for visualization is five for enhanced motion effect. The figure insets present enlarged details sub-volumes capturing representative "in-chain" and "single" cells

Table 2 Comparison of trajectory Precision and Recall for cancer cells of different populations

		Precision		Recall	
Population	Method	Mean	Std	Mean	Std
Single	Classical [6]	0.9014	0.1114	0.8973	0.1011
	Improved [22]	0.9190	0.0909	0.9135	0.0923
	Ellipsoid model	0.9342	0.0794	0.9097	0.0969
In-chain	Classical [6]	0.9364	0.0596	0.9519	0.0347
	Improved [22]	0.9388	0.0573	0.9592	0.0402
	Ellipsoid model	0.9578	0.0451	0.9584	0.0314

4 Conclusions

In this work, we present a complete, automatic, and promising object tracking and motion pattern analysis approach for time-lapse fluorescence microscopy image data. We present two specific non-Gaussian state models to extend the applicability of the particle filtering tracking algorithm to biomedical research. Our proposed tracking management strategy combines the advantages of prior two-step tracking methods and fundamental particle filtering approaches. Notably, our tracking strategy can avoid object state mismatch commonly seen in particle filtering when certain objects disappear from the scope of view. We test our method with both synthetic and real biomedical datasets. The experimental results are promising, suggesting the potential of the application of our approach to diverse biological and cancer research.

Acknowledgments This research is supported in part by grants from National Institute of Health 7K25CA181503, 1U01CA242936, 5R01EY028450, 5R01CA214928, and 1R01CA236369, the Winship cancer Institute of Emory University pilot award under award number P30CA138292, and It's The Journey & GA CORE breast cancer award.

References

1. Arulampalam, M.S., Maskell, S., Gordon, N., Clapp, T.: A tutorial on particle filters for online nonlinear/non-Gaussian Bayesian tracking. IEEE Trans. Signal Process. **50**(2), 174–188 (2002)
2. Cheezum, M.K., Walker, W.F., Guilford, W.H.: Quantitative comparison of algorithms for tracking single fluorescent particles. Biophys. J. **81**(4), 2378–2388 (2001)
3. Debeir, O., Van Ham, P., Kiss, R., Decaestecker, C.: Tracking of migrating cells under phase-contrast video microscopy with combined mean-shift processes. IEEE Trans. Med. Imaging **24**(6), 697–711 (2005)
4. Delgado-Gonzalo, R., Chenouard, N., Unser, M.: A new hybrid Bayesian-variational particle filter with application to mitotic cell tracking. In: 2011 IEEE International Symposium on Biomedical Imaging: From Nano to Macro, pp. 1917–1920. IEEE, Piscataway (2011)
5. Doucet, A., Godsill, S., Andrieu, C.: On sequential Monte Carlo sampling methods for Bayesian filtering. Stat. Comput. **10**(3), 197–208 (2000)

6. Genovesio, A., Liedl, T., Emiliani, V., Parak, W.J., Coppey-Moisan, M., Olivo-Marin, J.C.: Multiple particle tracking in 3-d+ t microscopy: method and application to the tracking of endocytosed quantum dots. IEEE Trans. Image Process. **15**(5), 1062–1070 (2006)
7. Godinez, W., Rohr, K.: Tracking multiple particles in fluorescence time-lapse microscopy images via probabilistic data association. IEEE Trans. Med. Imaging **34**(2), 415–432 (2015)
8. Gudla, P.R., Nakayama, K., Pegoraro, G., Misteli, T.: Spotlearn: Convolutional neural network for detection of fluorescence in situ hybridization (fish) signals in high-throughput imaging approaches. In: Cold Spring Harbor Symposia on Quantitative Biology, vol. 82, pp. 57–70. Cold Spring Harbor Laboratory Press, New York (2017)
9. Kong, J., Wang, F., Teodoro, G., Liang, Y., Zhu, Y., Tucker-Burden, C., Brat, D.J.: Automated cell segmentation with 3d fluorescence microscopy images. In: 2015 IEEE 12th International Symposium on Biomedical Imaging (ISBI), pp. 1212–1215. IEEE, Piscataway (2015)
10. Krizhevsky, A., Sutskever, I., Hinton, G.E.: ImageNet classification with deep convolutional neural networks. In: Advances in Neural Information Processing Systems, pp. 1097–1105 (2012)
11. Li, G., Liu, T., Tarokh, A., Nie, J., Guo, L., Mara, A., Holley, S., Wong, S.T.: 3d cell nuclei segmentation based on gradient flow tracking. BMC Cell Biol. **8**(1), 40 (2007)
12. Lin, G., Adiga, U., Olson, K., Guzowski, J.F., Barnes, C.A., Roysam, B.: A hybrid 3d watershed algorithm incorporating gradient cues and object models for automatic segmentation of nuclei in confocal image stacks. Cytometry A **56**(1), 23–36 (2003)
13. Luo, D., Barker, J., McGrath, J., Daly, C.: Iterative multilevel thresholding and splitting for three-dimensional segmentation of live cell nuclei using laser scanning confocal microscopy. J. Comput.-Assist. Microsc. **10**(4), 151–162 (1998)
14. Mozhdehi, R.J., Medeiros, H.: Deep convolutional particle filter for visual tracking. In: 2017 IEEE International Conference on Image Processing (ICIP), pp. 3650–3654. IEEE, Piscataway (2017)
15. Newby, J.M., Schaefer, A.M., Lee, P.T., Forest, M.G., Lai, S.K.: Convolutional neural networks automate detection for tracking of submicron-scale particles in 2d and 3d. Proc. Natl. Acad. Sci. **115**(36), 9026–9031 (2018)
16. Otsu, N.: A threshold selection method from gray-level histograms. IEEE Trans. Syst. Man Cybern. **9**(1), 62–66 (1979)
17. Rathi, Y., Vaswani, N., Tannenbaum, A., Yezzi, A.: Tracking deforming objects using particle filtering for geometric active contours. IEEE Trans. Pattern Anal. Mach. Intell. **29**(8), 1470 (2007)
18. Sage, D., Neumann, F.R., Hediger, F., Gasser, S.M., Unser, M.: Automatic tracking of individual fluorescence particles: application to the study of chromosome dynamics. IEEE Trans. Image Process. **14**(9), 1372–1383 (2005)
19. Sbalzarini, I.F., Koumoutsakos, P.: Feature point tracking and trajectory analysis for video imaging in cell biology. J. Struct. Biol. **151**(2), 182–195 (2005)
20. Shafique, K., Shah, M.: A noniterative greedy algorithm for multiframe point correspondence. IEEE Trans. Pattern Anal. Mach. Intell. **27**(1), 51–65 (2005)
21. Smal, I., Niessen, W., Meijering, E.: Advanced particle filtering for multiple object tracking in dynamic fluorescence microscopy images. In: 2007 4th IEEE International Symposium on Biomedical Imaging: From Nano to Macro, pp. 1048–1051. IEEE, Piscataway (2007)
22. Smal, I., Meijering, E., Draegestein, K., Galjart, N., Grigoriev, I., Akhmanova, A., Van Royen, M., Houtsmuller, A.B., Niessen, W.: Multiple object tracking in molecular bioimaging by Rao-Blackwellized marginal particle filtering. Med. Image Anal. **12**(6), 764–777 (2008)
23. Smal, I., Yao, Y., Galjart, N., Meijering, E.: Facilitating data association in particle tracking using autoencoding and score matching. In: 2019 IEEE 16th International Symposium on Biomedical Imaging (ISBI 2019), pp. 1523–1526. IEEE, Piscataway (2019)
24. Vincent, P., Larochelle, H., Bengio, Y., Manzagol, P.A.: Extracting and composing robust features with denoising autoencoders. In: Proceedings of the 25th International Conference on Machine Learning, pp. 1096–1103. ACM, New York (2008)

25. Xu, C., Prince, J.L.: Snakes, shapes, and gradient vector flow. IEEE Trans. Image Process. **7**(3), 359 (1998)
26. Yu, H.: Object tracking. https://github.com/hyu88/object_tracking_3d.git
27. Zhang, Y., Cheng, Z., Jin, Y., Si, K., Jin, X.: Detection and recognition of micro-nano fluorescent particle array based on AlexNet. In: IOP Conference Series: Materials Science and Engineering, vol. 504, p. 012035. IOP Publishing, Bristol (2019)
28. Zimmer, C., Labruyere, E., Meas-Yedid, V., Guillén, N., Olivo-Marin, J.C.: Segmentation and tracking of migrating cells in videomicroscopy with parametric active contours: A tool for cell-based drug testing. IEEE Trans. Med. Imaging **21**(10), 1212–1221 (2002)

Alternative Capture-Recapture Point and Interval Estimators Based on Two Surveillance Streams

Robert H. Lyles, Amanda L. Wilkinson, John M. Williamson, Jiandong Chen, Allan W. Taylor, Amara Jambai, Mohamed Jalloh, and Reinhard Kaiser

1 Introduction

Capture-recapture methods are commonly applied for estimating the size of animal populations, as well as in social science or epidemiological contexts for quantifying unique or vulnerable human populations [1–3]. The classic capture-recapture paradigm originated in tag and release experiments, e.g., in the effort to estimate the number of fish in a lake or animals of a given species in a geographic region [4–6]. A seminal text by Seber [7] records a broad synopsis of theoretical results that underlie the classical analytic approaches, primarily stemming from hypergeometric or multinomial models for data obtained in specific capture-recapture sampling scenarios. Fundamentally, the problem is one of missing count data arising from the application of $T \geq 2$ capture efforts (or, in epidemiology, surveillance streams),

---

Disclaimer: The findings and conclusions in this report are those of the author(s) and do not necessarily represent the official position of the Centers for Disease Control and Prevention.

R. H. Lyles (✉) · J. Chen
Department of Biostatistics and Bioinformatics, The Rollins School of Public Health of Emory University, Atlanta, GA, USA
e-mail: rlyles@sph.emory.edu

A. L. Wilkinson · J. M. Williamson · A. W. Taylor · M. Jalloh
Center for Global Health, Centers for Disease Control and Prevention, Atlanta, GA, USA

A. Jambai
Ministry of Health and Education, Freetown, Sierra Leone

R. Kaiser
Division for Global Health Protection, Center for Global Health, Centers for Disease Control and Prevention, Freetown, Sierra Leone

Y. Zhao, (Din) D.-G. Chen (eds.), *Modern Statistical Methods for Health Research*, Emerging Topics in Statistics and Biostatistics,
https://doi.org/10.1007/978-3-030-72437-5_3

involving 2^T possible capture profiles. The number of units in the final profile category (captured in none of the T efforts) is unobserved. The goal is to use the capture profile data, together with assumptions and perhaps augmented by covariate information on the observed units, to infer an estimate of the total population size.

Research to extend standard capture-recapture methodology remains vibrant, due in part to the practical need to enumerate populations, the allure of doing so non-exhaustively, and the vexing but intriguing nature of the associated statistical challenges. In the latter regard, a taxonomy of conceivable capture-recapture models labeled M_{tbh} (e.g., [8, 9]) has arisen and spawned a vast literature. In this notation, the t subscript refers to the notion that the model should acknowledge that the T different capture efforts may have varying overall success in terms of the population proportion identified. Models in the class including the b subscript make an attempt to account for the possibility that behavioral characteristics of individual units may affect their likelihood of recapture, while those with the h subscript incorporate the notion that individual units could be heterogeneous with respect to their capture probability profiles.

Our current work derives motivation from a collaborative effort conducted by members of the Child Health and Mortality Surveillance (CHAMPS) study team, in which the goal was to quantify under-5 deaths that occurred during the years 2015–2016 in Bombali Shebora chiefdom, Sierra Leone, based on multiple surveillance streams [10]. In such settings designed to assess human mortality or morbidity, the behavioral ("b") component of the general capture-recapture paradigm can often be ignored. This is logically the case as long as surveillance efforts operate in such a way that individuals or their associates are contacted directly through no more than one stream without referrals or other connections, as was the case in the motivating study and as we will assume throughout. However, surveillance will typically induce the "t" component, as separate streams are unlikely to sample equivalent proportions of the population. While one should in general also consider the "h" component (and thus the M_{th} class of models), there are conditions under which the M_t class of models can be defended. We refer to these as the "LP conditions" when $T = 2$, as when they hold it is justifiable to utilize the Lincoln-Petersen estimator [4, 5, 11] to estimate population size (N). The LP estimator is the most classic and best known estimator in the two-stream case, perhaps rivaled only by a bias-corrected alternative proposed by Chapman [12].

In the current article, our focus is on the "two-catch" (or two surveillance stream) setting, which is common in epidemiologic and demographic settings. We begin with a section designed to clarify the LP conditions and explain why in our view they remain the central and pivotal ones in the two-catch scenario despite justifying only one specific subset of the broad conceivable class of M_{tbh} models. This involves a focus on the parameter identifiability issue that generates the fundamental challenge associated with capture-recapture methods and because of which a valid estimate of N can never be justified solely by statistical means. It allows a consideration of how best to incorporate covariates and some risks and misconceptions associated with the popular use of estimation methods designed to incorporate model heterogeneity

[13–15]. Finally, it provides the motivation for our subsequent efforts to propose two new alternatives to the LP and Chapman estimators, along with a new approach to interval estimation for use under the LP conditions. Those developments follow a brief review of the classical LP and related estimators, which are then included along with the new proposals in comparative simulation studies and an analysis of the motivating Sierra Leone surveillance data. A SAS macro-program to facilitate most of the relevant calculations is available on the website for the volume or from the authors by request.

2 Methods

2.1 The LP Conditions and Their Central Role

Table 1A reflects a completely general individual-level model for the $T = 2$ case, where the capture-recapture experience of each unit is obtained by a single draw from a multinomial distribution specific to that unit. Specifically, (Y_{i11}, Y_{i10}, Y_{i01}, Y_{i00}) ~ *Multinomial* $(1, p_{i11}, p_{i10}, p_{i01}, p_{i00})$, where the ($0 =$ no, $1 =$ yes) subscripts j and k in p_{ijk}, respectively, indicate capture or not by means of the first and second surveillance streams. Applying that process to each unit in a population of size N yields the cell counts (N_{11}, N_{10}, N_{01}, N_{00}). Consider now any admissible joint distribution $f(\mathbf{p}) = f(p_{i11}, p_{i10}, p_{i01}, p_{i00})$, and imagine repeating this same capture-recapture data generation mechanism for arbitrarily many populations of size N that share the same $f(\mathbf{p})$. This yields the population-level model (N_{11}, N_{10}, N_{01}, N_{00}) ~ *Multinomial*(N, p_{11}, p_{10}, p_{01}, p_{00}) (see Table 1B). In other words, regardless of the distribution of individual-level capture event probabilities, the multinomial can be motivated as a natural model for the population-level cell counts. This explains our focus on multinomial capture-recapture models, which is consistent with preferences expressed by others (e.g., [16, 17]) in epidemiological surveillance scenarios. For a similar discussion of the extrapolation from individual- to population-level capture probabilities without explicitly invoking the multinomial, see Chao, Pan, and Chiang [18].

The challenge in the capture-recapture setting, of course, is that the cell count N_{00} is not observed. In fact, it must be understood that N_{00} (and therefore N) cannot be estimated without assumptions that are completely unverifiable based

Table 1 Multinomial random variables and probabilities underlying the two-catch capture-recapture scenario at the individual and population levels

A. Individual-level			B. Population-level		
	Found in second capture			Found in second capture	
Found in first capture	Yes	No	Found in first capture	Yes	No
Yes	$Y_{i11}(p_{i11})$	$Y_{i10}(p_{i10})$	Yes	$N_{11}(p_{11})$	$N_{10}(p_{10})$
No	$Y_{i01}(p_{i01})$	$Y_{i00}(p_{i00})$	No	$N_{01}(p_{01})$	$N_{00}(p_{00})$

on the observed data alone. To make this fully clear, consider the three observed cell counts under the population multinomial model (N_{11}, N_{10}, N_{01}; Table 1B). Define $p_1 = p_{11} + p_{10}$, $p_2 = p_{11} + p_{01}$, $p_{2|1} = \frac{p_{11}}{p_1}$, and $p_{2|\bar{1}} = \frac{p_{01}}{1-p_1}$ as the marginal probabilities of identification by the first and second surveillance streams and the conditional probabilities of identification by the second stream given identified and not identified by the first, respectively. Under the population-level multinomial model, the three types of observed units make the following likelihood contributions, where $p_c = p_1 + p_{2|\bar{1}}(1 - p_1)$ is the overall probability of being identified:

$$Units\ identified\ twice: \quad p_c^{-1} p_{2|1} p_1$$

$$Units\ identified\ in\ the\ first\ but\ not\ the\ second\ capture\ effort: \quad p_c^{-1}\left(1 - p_{2|1}\right) p_1$$

$$Units\ identified\ in\ the\ second\ but\ not\ the\ first\ capture\ effort: \quad p_c^{-1} p_{2|\bar{1}}(1 - p_1)$$

Note now that while $p_{2|1}$ is estimable, the observed data alone contain no information about the parameters p_1, p_2, $p_{2|\bar{1}}$ and therefore about p_c and N. The only way to make N estimable is thus to make at least one unverifiable assumption. In surveillance, this requires expertise that is epidemiological or demographic in nature rather than statistical. That is, it calls for incorporating a grassroots-level understanding of the operating features characterizing one or more of the surveillance efforts (e.g., geographic and temporal coverage); we return to this notion later. Suppose for the moment that the epidemiologist specifies a best guess of the parameter $\psi = p_{2|\bar{1}}$, and assume this guess is correct. It is then readily verified that the maximum likelihood estimator (MLE) for N under the population-level multinomial model is given by

$$\hat{N} = N_{11} + N_{10} + N_{01}/\psi \tag{1}$$

Alternatively, suppose a correct guess of the ratio $\phi = p_{2|1}/p_{2|\bar{1}}$ is supplied. In that case, the MLE is found to be

$$\hat{N} = N_{11} + N_{10} + \phi\left[\frac{N_{01}\left(N_{11} + N_{10}\right)}{N_{11}}\right] \tag{2}$$

The complete lack of information for estimating N based solely on the observed data is now clear in light of the following fact: *the maximized log-likelihood value is identical for any admissible value of ψ or ϕ that one chooses to specify*. As a result, any value of N greater than or equal to the number of distinct units identified by the two streams is as consistent with the observed data as any other.

The parameter ϕ is clearly a measure (akin to a relative risk) of the population-level dependency between the first and second capture events. Some authors (e.g., [19]) focus on ϕ. Others (e.g., [20]) prefer to focus on the population-level odds ratio (OR), i.e., $p_{11}p_{00}(p_{10}p_{01})^{-1}$. Chao et al. [18] introduce a similar measure that they call the coefficient of covariation (CCV), where CCV $= p_{11}(p_1p_2)^{-1} - 1$. Here we favor ϕ, as in our view that ratio is most easily conceptualized by an epidemiologist or demographer for characterizing population-level dependency. Note that the condition $\phi = 1$ holds if and only if OR $= 1$ and CCV $= 0$. Note also that taking $\phi = 1$ in (Eq. 2) yields the LP estimator (reviewed in Sect. 2.5), as does replacing ψ by the MLE of $p_{2|1}$ in (Eq. 1).

The literature reflects a surprising level of variation surrounding the perceived assumptions required to validate the LP estimator in practice. For example, practitioners are sometimes led to believe that if it is reasonable to assume any variation in subject-specific capture probabilities across subjects (i) and/or unreasonable to assume that capture events are independent for all i, then the LP conditions are violated. Seber [7] provided a somewhat more flexible set of guidelines for capture-recapture in the animal abundance context; these include the assumption that all units in the population have the same probability of being "caught" in the second sample and that "tagging" does not affect subsequent catchability so that unit-specific capture events are independent. Chao et al. [18] recognized that the necessary conditions can be further relaxed. They acknowledge that Seber's first condition of a random second sample is in itself sufficient for validity of the LP estimator while noting the potential importance of temporality, that is, a random first sample may not be sufficient in the presence of local dependence whereby individual units captured the first time may be more or less likely to be captured the second time. We note here that in epidemiological contexts, two surveillance efforts often overlap temporally. However, when one of the two surveillance mechanisms occurs without the knowledge of specific units or their associates (e.g., by an agnostic examination of health records), this temporality distinction should not matter and the LP estimator can be defended if either stream constitutes a random sample.

In light of the aforementioned connection between the individual- and population-level multinomial models (Table 1), we offer a crystallization of the criteria under which the LP estimator is valid. Specifically, this is the case *whenever* $\phi = 1$ *at the population level, regardless of the distribution* $f(\mathbf{p})$ *of individual-level capture probabilities*. Note, for example, that this does occur in the absence of local dependence if either sample is taken randomly from the population. However, defining ϕ_i as the capture relative risk specific to unit i based on his or her individual capture profile ($\mathbf{p_i}$), it could also occur if the population contains a mixture of "trap happy" ($\phi_i > 1$) and "trap averse" ($\phi_i < 1$) individuals.

Such a mixture of "happy" and "averse" units is conceivable in ecological studies of animal abundance based on behavioral characteristics of animals, while we have argued that the behavioral component should be negligible in surveillance when either stream is implemented agnostically with respect to the other. Nevertheless, surveillance creates a clear pathway for such a mixture to happen as a result of heterogeneity of the two sampling efforts and their levels of success across subgroups of the population (e.g., [20, 21]). Consider, for example, two surveillance streams designed to identify deaths or cases of a disease over a fixed period of time (e.g., 1 year). Suppose the first stream operates most effectively due to available staffing and resources over the first 6 months, while the second operates inefficiently early on but effectively during the latter half of the year. This would induce a tendency toward an overall negative association ($\phi < 1$) between the two streams. A tendency toward ($\phi < 1$) might also occur if the two streams happen to focus on different geographic subsets of the region of interest (e.g., if one operates primarily in urban and the other in rural areas). On the other hand, if both streams tend to be more effective in identifying cases in urban (as opposed to rural or remote) geographic areas of the population catchment area, this would introduce a tendency toward positive association ($\phi > 1$). Without knowledge or control of design and implementation aspects of one or both streams, there is of course never any guarantee that such tendencies would cancel. The point, however, is that the LP estimator may be as defensible as any other when such competing forces are likely at play.

2.2 Some Cautionary Notes on Alternatives to the LP Estimator

When surveying the extensive literature on capture-recapture, one finds a great deal of skepticism about the LP conditions and a general tendency for statisticians to advocate methods allowing for heterogeneity of capture profiles. In this regard, two of the most prominent alternative estimators are found in Chao [14] and Zelterman [15]. While we examine Zelterman's estimator $\left(\hat{N}_{\text{Zelt}}\right)$ empirically in Sects. 3 and 4, we restrict primary attention to Chao's given the close connection between the two proposals in the two-capture case [22]. In particular, Chao [14] developed an estimator for the T-catch case that was demonstrated to yield a lower bound for N under certain mathematical conditions. A close look at these conditions reveals that the estimator was proposed for the case of "large" T (i.e., it was never originally intended for the two-catch case) and "small" capture probabilities ($\mathbf{p}_i$). It was derived under the assumption that capture probabilities vary arbitrarily across units (lending a nonparametric feel to the method) but remain the same for a given unit at every capture occasion (which is restrictive and, as previously noted, unrealistic in typical surveillance scenarios). Nevertheless, subsequent literature has promulgated the notion that the Chao estimator provides a reasonable lower bound for N and/or serves as a particularly robust point estimator in two-catch surveillance settings (e.g., [23, 24]). For insight into why this may be problematic and misleading to the epidemiologist seeking an estimator to use, one needs only to consider implications about the population parameter ϕ.

In the notation of Table 1B, Chao's estimator is given by

$$\hat{N}_{\text{Chao}} = N_c + \frac{(N_{10} + N_{01})^2}{2N_{11}} \tag{3}$$

where N_c is the total number of units identified at least once by the two surveillance streams; for a standard error, see Chao [14]. With simple algebra, one can verify that using $\hat{N}_{\text{Chao}}$ is equivalent to inserting the following estimate for ϕ into Eq. (2):

$$\hat{\phi}_{\text{Chao}} = \frac{2N_{01}N_{11} + (N_{10} + N_{01})^2}{2N_{01}\left(N_{11} + N_{10}\right)} \tag{4}$$

It is readily shown that $\hat{\phi}_{\text{Chao}}$ is always larger than 1, which also means that Chao's estimate for N always exceeds the LP estimate. On the surface, these points may be unsurprising given the motivation for Chao's approach. However, two cautionary notes quickly emerge: (a) the notion that $\hat{N}_{\text{Chao}}$ provides a lower bound in the two-capture case is patently false and (as we will see) can be highly misleading and (b) the notion that $\hat{N}_{\text{Chao}}$ is "robust" is also misleading. With regard to (b), note from Eqs. (2) and (4) that $\hat{N}_{\text{Chao}}$ (as any estimator must) projects a specific assumption about ϕ that is in no way supported by the observed data alone. This assumption is also impossible to target by design or to justify by defensible means, particularly given the aforementioned issues with the mathematical assumptions in the two-catch case. Specifically, use of the estimator is equivalent to assuming that ϕ equals the expression on the right side of (Eq. 4), with N_{ij} replaced by p_{ij} $(i,j = 0,1)$. Note that such concerns are not limited to $\hat{N}_{\text{Chao}}$ but apply to Zelterman's [15] proposal, to loglinear model-based estimators (next section), and in fact to any estimator that infers an estimate for ϕ based on mathematical constructs without expert opinion to consider and vet that estimate.

Attempts to promote the Chao [14] estimator for epidemiological surveillance are no doubt influenced by the notion that two streams may often operate in a way that corresponds to "trap happiness" ($\phi > 1$) at the population level. Clearly, though, if one assumes this to be the case, then it is the LP estimator (not $\hat{N}_{\text{Chao}}$) that provides a natural lower bound for N [25]. We acknowledge evidence suggestive of the $\phi > 1$ condition in the literature, e.g., Brittain and Böhning [24] offer examples in which a modified version of $\hat{N}_{\text{Chao}}$ approximated the truth more closely than the LP estimate upon conditioning on units identified by a third stream. However, as noted in the previous section, forces operating in the opposite direction (toward $\phi < 1$) are quite conceivable in surveillance. Correspondingly, in Sect. 3, we apply the Brittain and Böhning assessment to the CHAMPS motivating example and obtain the opposite conclusion. We also note that, despite such anecdotal evidence, there is no guarantee the LP estimator will be inferior to $\hat{N}_{\text{Chao}}$ even if one is fully committed to the notion that $\phi > 1$. Instead, what is guaranteed is that the LP estimator will always be superior whenever $\phi \leq 1$. Again, this point relates to the specific unverifiable assumption embodied in (Eq. 4) and will be illustrated in the context of the CHAMPS example.

2.3 Loglinear Models and a Perspective on the Use of Covariates

One common approach to capture-recapture analysis that incorporates covariate data and is widely available to practitioners through software is the loglinear model [13, 26, 27]. Agresti [28] provides useful insight about the connections between loglinear and other approaches that have been used in capture-recapture settings, such as the Rasch model [29] and latent class modeling (e.g., [30]). For an introduction, assume initially that there are no useful covariates available so that the data for analysis consist solely of the three observed cell counts (N_{11}, N_{10}, N_{01}) in Table 1B. Letting the random variable $N_{\mathbf{x}}$ denote the number of units with capture pattern $\mathbf{x} = (x_1, x_2)$ where $x_t \in (0,1)$ indicates capture status in stream t, the standard loglinear model for the two-catch case ($T = 2$) is

$$\ln\left[E(N_{\mathbf{x}})\right] = \alpha + \beta_1 x_1 + \beta_2 x_2 + \beta_3 x_1 x_2 \quad (5)$$

The counts $N_{\mathbf{x}}$ are typically treated as independent Poisson variates conditional on $\mathbf{x}$. With N_{00} unobserved, the four parameters in (Eq. 5) clearly cannot all be identified. Standard practice is to impose one or more restrictions on the model parameters that make N_{00} estimable as $\hat{N}_{00} = \exp\left(\hat{\alpha}\right)$, with $\hat{\alpha}$ typically taken to be the MLE based on a submodel of (Eq. 5).

A common strategy in loglinear capture-recapture modeling is to drop the highest-order interaction term and undertake a comparative fit of possible remaining models (e.g., [31–33]), by means of Akaike's information criterion (AIC; [34]) or similar measures. However, we agree with others [35] who point out pitfalls associated with both of these practices. As a simple illustration, it is instructive to consider the implications of each of the possible models that can be fit based on Eq. (5), particularly with respect to what untestable assumption each one projects with respect to the population parameter ϕ.

Table 2 displays the closed-form fitted (by ML) cell counts for each candidate loglinear model in the two-catch case without covariates, together with the corresponding MLEs for ϕ and N based on the motivating example data introduced in Sect. 2.5. The exercise is conceptually instructive about what loglinear modeling actually does and does not accomplish in the capture-recapture setting. First, note that even with the inclusion of those that incorporate the X_1X_2 interaction, there are only seven possible models. Models 5–7 are saturated, in that they fit the three observed cell counts (N_{11}, N_{10}, N_{01}) perfectly. A quandary with the common practice of selecting a model based on AIC is thus immediately apparent, since those models yield vastly different estimates of N. The problem goes deeper, however: loglinear models applied to capture-recapture data can mislead practitioners into a false notion that AIC can be trusted to decide which estimate of N is most defensible, as well as a false sense of security that a large or exhaustive set of contingencies

Table 2 Possible loglinear models for two-catch capture-recapture without covariates

		Fitted cell counts[a]						
Model [b]	Predictors	$\hat{N}_{11}$	$\hat{N}_{10}$	$\hat{N}_{01}$	$\hat{N}_{00}$	$\hat{\phi}_{ML}$	$\hat{N}_{ML}$ [c]	AIC[c]
1	None	$n_c/3$	$n_c/3$	$n_c/3$	$n_c/3$	1	1180	−8294
2	X_1	$n_{1\bullet}/2$	$n_{1\bullet}/2$	n_{01}	n_{01}	1	1520	−8836
3	X_2	$n_{\bullet 1}/2$	n_{10}	$n_{\bullet 1}/2$	n_{10}	1	1087	−8339
4	X_1X_2	n_{11}	$\frac{n_{10}+n_{01}}{2}$	$\frac{n_{10}+n_{01}}{2}$	$\frac{n_{10}+n_{01}}{2}$	$\frac{4n_{11}}{2n_{11}+n_{10}+n_{01}}$	1304	−8703
5	X_1, X_2	n_{11}	n_{10}	n_{01}	$\frac{n_{10}n_{01}}{n_{11}}$	1	3557	−8936
6	X_1, X_1X_2	n_{11}	n_{10}	n_{01}	n_{01}	$\frac{2n_{11}}{n_{1\bullet}}$	1520	−8936
7	X_2, X_1X_2	n_{11}	n_{10}	n_{01}	n_{10}	$\frac{n_{11}(n_{10}+n_{01})}{n_{01}n_{1\bullet}}$	1087	−8936

[a]ML estimators; $n_c = n_{11} + n_{10} + n_{01} =$ # unique units captured, $n_{1\bullet} = n_{11} + n_{10}$, $n_{\bullet 1} = n_{11} + n_{01}$; $\hat{N}_{00} = e^{\hat{\alpha}} =$ ML projection for # units uncaptured based on Poisson loglinear model
[b]All models include the intercept (α)
[c]MLE for N and AIC values based on motivating example data in Table 3A

has been considered. With regard to the latter, note that the seven possible models project only four unique assumptions about ϕ. Yet we have seen (Eq. (2) and related discussion) that, in fact, the observed data are equally consistent with a continuum of possible values for ϕ. Note, for example, that models 1–3 correspond to assuming the LP conditions ($\phi = 1$) in addition to one or more statistically assessable constraints on the population-level proportions (p_{11}, p_{10}, p_{01}), while model 5 does so under no constraints and hence yields $\hat{N}_{LP}$ as the MLE for N. Some implications about the proper role of AIC in capture-recapture modeling should be clear. While it can justify such assessable constraints, it actually has nothing trustworthy to say about what the projected value for N_{00} (and thus N) should be. Practitioners need to understand that the "winning" model in an AIC competition could quite conceivably be the worst of the lot in terms of the most crucial fitted value $\left(\hat{N}_{00}\right)$ and in fact that none of the candidates may provide a reasonable estimate for N.

In response to the preceding illustration, one might argue that loglinear models can be far more general than (Eq. 5) because they can incorporate covariates measured on the observed units. While this is true, it does little to ease our concerns. Suppose, for example, that two binary covariates are measured on each observed unit. In that case, the full array of loglinear models essentially just produces the analogous subset of possible scenarios within each of the four strata formed by those covariates (along with an opportunity for further assessable constraints involving estimable parameters across strata). The pitfalls, particularly in terms of the lack of fundamentally useful information in AIC as a metric for projecting N_{00} overall or within any stratum, remain.

2.4 A Rationale for Renewed Statistical Interest Under the LP Conditions

The above discussion brings us to some realizations that color and motivate our work in subsequent sections. Clearly, there is no truly robust estimator for N in the two-catch case, as a valid estimator would have to infer the correct population-level value for ϕ (see Eq. (2)). Because there is no information about that correct value of ϕ in the observed data, no statistical model can ferret it out on its own. As such, we believe the defensible use of capture-recapture methods in surveillance should hinge on the epidemiologist's expert opinion about the implementation and geographic coverage properties of the two streams and the corresponding implications about ϕ. A best estimate for N would arguably be obtained by inserting his or her best guess for ϕ into Eq. (2).

Nevertheless, there is one specific value ($\phi = 1$) that can be targeted by design, e.g., by implementing the second stream as a random sample of the population [18] or either stream as random if the two data collection efforts are conducted agnostically. It is also the only specific value for which the epidemiologist might be able to argue theoretically, either as an overall measure of dependence between the two streams or as a stratum-specific one. In particular, we subscribe to the notion [11] that the most promising use of covariates is to apply expert opinion (if possible at the design stage) such that a cogent argument can be made for assuming $\phi = 1$ within specified strata. Given sufficient information to allocate each identified unit to his/her unique stratum, the overall estimate for N then becomes the sum of stratum-specific estimates made under the LP conditions. In the absence of any grounds for such expert opinion and with nothing but the observed data to go by, we agree with others (e.g., [19]) that uncertainty in the non-identifiable parameter ϕ should by rights be a key component in capture-recapture (see Discussion). An important implication is that, except when the LP conditions are defensible, there is no estimator for which a standard statistical measure of variability or corresponding confidence interval legitimately accounts for uncertainty (see [36] for relevant discussion in the loglinear model context).

Given our expressed view that they remain central in two-stream capture-recapture, we focus the remainder of this article on estimation and inference under the LP conditions. Specifically, despite the long history of statistical work in this setting, we believe the potential remains for further refinements to both point and interval estimation.

2.5 Review of Classical Point Estimators in the Two-Capture Case

Table 3A shows motivating data on recorded counts of under-5 deaths (excluding stillbirths) during the 23-month period from January 2015 through November 2016

Table 3 Motivating data on under-5 mortality and generic notation for two-capture cell counts

A. Motivating data				B. Notation for two-capture case			
	Identified by phone alert				Found in second capture		
Identified by health facility	Yes	No	Total	Found in first capture	Yes	No	Total
Yes	48	202	250	Yes	n_{11}	n_{10}	$n_{1\bullet}$
No	635	?	?	No	n_{01}	$N_{00} = ?$	?
Total	683	?	$N = ?$	Total	$n_{\bullet 1}$	?	$N = ?$

in Sierra Leone's Bombali Shebora chiefdom, based on two surveillance streams: (1) health facility records from Bombali Shebora and (2) toll-free phone alert notifications of deaths based on a system implemented during the Ebola epidemic of 2014–2015 [10]. When referring generically to the observed data, we replace (N_{11}, N_{10}, N_{01}) by (n_{11}, n_{10}, n_{01}) as shown in Table 3B; however, we continue to denote the number unidentified in either capture as N_{00} in that it remains a random variable conditional on the observed sample. The goal is to estimate the population total $N = n_{11} + n_{10} + n_{01} + N_{00}$. Under the LP conditions clarified in Sect. 2.1, it is well known (e.g., [7]) that one derives the same MLE for N under a hypergeometric or a multinomial model for the population-level data; this simple closed-form estimator is the Lincoln-Petersen estimator [4, 5]:

$$\hat{N}_{\text{LP}} = \frac{n_{1\bullet} \times n_{\bullet 1}}{n_{11}} \tag{6}$$

where $n_{1\bullet} = n_{11} + n_{10}$ and $n_{\bullet 1} = n_{11} + n_{01}$. The same corresponding multivariate delta method variance also applies under either model [7]:

$$\hat{\text{Var}}\left(\hat{N}_{\text{LP}}\right) = \frac{n_{1\bullet} \times n_{\bullet 1} \times n_{10} \times n_{01}}{n_{11}{}^3} \tag{7}$$

One well-recognized issue with (Eq. 6) is its bias in small to moderate sample sizes and/or under conditions in which identification by both streams is relatively rare; in fact, the MLE is undefined when $n_{11} = 0$ and has infinite mean and variance whenever Pr($N_{11} = 0$) is non-null. Efforts to reduce the bias include an adjustment due to Darroch [16] and an expedient approach analogous to that of Gart [37] in contingency table analysis whereby one adds 0.5 to each observed cell in Table 3B prior to calculating (Eq. 1) and subtracts 1.5 from the result ([38]; we refer to this estimator as $\hat{N}_{\text{EB}}$ in Tables 4 and 5). Darroch's bias-adjusted estimator, derived under a generalized hypergeometric model, applies under the analogue to the LP conditions in the $T \geq 2$ capture event setting. In the two-catch case, it is written as:

Table 4 Point and interval estimates of number of under-5 deaths (N) based on data in Table 3A

Estimator [a]	Point estimate (std. error)	
$\hat{N}_{\mathrm{LP}}$	3557 (445)	
$\hat{N}_{\mathrm{EB}}$	3538	
$\hat{N}_{\mathrm{Chap}}$	3503 (428)	
$\hat{N}_{\mathrm{BC}}$	3502	
$\hat{N}_{\mathrm{BC2}}$	3503	
$\hat{N}_{\mathrm{BC3}}$	3504	
$\hat{N}_{\mathrm{Med}}$	3550	
$\hat{N}_{\mathrm{Chao}}$	8183 (1171)	
$\hat{N}_{\mathrm{Zelt}}$	8167	
CI method	Interval estimate	Width
Wald-type centered on $1/\hat{N}_{\mathrm{LP}}$ [b]	(2857, 4713)	1856
Wald-type centered on $1/\hat{N}_{\mathrm{Chap}}$ [b]	(2842, 4563)	1721
Proposed Wald-type (Eq. 14)	(2822, 4618)	1796
Transformed logit (Eq. 15)	(2802, 4557)	1756
Unadjusted credible interval[c]	(2825, 4611)	1786
Proposed (Eq. 20)[c]	(2794, 4546)	1752

[a]Estimators reviewed and/or introduced in Sects. 2.5–2.8
[b]CI for N based on inverted limits of CI for $1/N$
[c]Based on 100,000 posterior draws

$$\hat{N}_{\mathrm{Darr}} = \hat{N}_{\mathrm{LP}} - \frac{\left[\hat{N}_{\mathrm{LP}}^{-1} - \sum_{j=1}^{2}\left(\hat{N}_{\mathrm{LP}} - n_j\right)^{-1}\right]^2 + \left[\hat{N}_{\mathrm{LP}}^{-2} - \sum_{j=1}^{2}\left(\hat{N}_{\mathrm{LP}} - n_j\right)^{-2}\right]}{2\left[\left(\hat{N}_{\mathrm{LP}} - n_c\right)^{-1} + \hat{N}_{\mathrm{LP}}^{-1} - \sum_{j=1}^{2}\left(\hat{N}_{\mathrm{LP}} - n_j\right)^{-1}\right]^2} \tag{8}$$

where $n_c = n_{11} + n_{10} + n_{01}$, $n_1 = n_{1\bullet}$ and $n_2 = n_{\bullet 1}$ [7, 16].

While Darroch's result is of historical significance, the best known and most widely used bias-reduced estimator is that of Chapman [12]; this estimator and its accompanying delta method-based variance are as follows:

$$\hat{N}_{\mathrm{Chap}} = \frac{(n_{1\bullet}+1)\times(n_{\bullet 1}+1)}{n_{11}+1} - 1, \quad \widehat{\mathrm{Var}}\left(\hat{N}_{\mathrm{Chap}}\right) = \frac{(n_{1\bullet}+1)\times(n_{\bullet 1}+1)\times n_{10}\times n_{01}}{(n_{11}+1)^2\times(n_{11}+2)} \tag{9}$$

The Chapman estimator is unbiased when $n_{1\bullet} + n_{\bullet 1} \geq N$ [39]; it can exhibit negative bias otherwise, but in many cases this bias remains negligible. In general, we recommend avoiding use of the variance estimator in (Eq. 9) when constructing confidence intervals (see Sect. 4).

Table 5 Simulations evaluating point estimates of N with cell probabilities mimicking conditions of motivating example data in Table 3A[a,b]

True N	Estimator	Mean [median] (SD)	True N	Estimator	Mean [median] (SD)
3500	$\hat{N}_{\mathrm{LP}}$	3559 [3508] (469)	500	$\hat{N}_{\mathrm{LP}}$	587 [507] (343)
	$\hat{N}_{\mathrm{EB}}$	3539 [3488] (461)		$\hat{N}_{\mathrm{EB}}$	549 [488] (284)
	$\hat{N}_{\mathrm{Chap}}$	**3501** [3453] (451)		$\hat{N}_{\mathrm{Chap}}$	**500** [456] 198
	$\hat{N}_{\mathrm{BC}}$	**3500** [3451] (450)		$\hat{N}_{\mathrm{BC}}$	**471** [446] (158)
	$\hat{N}_{\mathrm{BC2}}$	**3501** [3453] (451)		$\hat{N}_{\mathrm{BC2}}$	**502** [457] (205)
	$\hat{N}_{\mathrm{BC3}}$	**3502** [3454] (451)		$\hat{N}_{\mathrm{BC3}}$	**520** [464] (243)
	$\hat{N}_{\mathrm{Med}}$	3552 [**3501**] (466)		$\hat{N}_{\mathrm{Med}}$	569 [**499**] (281)
	$\hat{N}_{\mathrm{Chao}}$	8219 [8078] (1233)		$\hat{N}_{\mathrm{Chao}}$	1399 [1177] (927)
	$\hat{N}_{\mathrm{Zelt}}$	8204 [8064] (1235)		$\hat{N}_{\mathrm{Zelt}}$	1396 [1174] (927)
1000	$\hat{N}_{\mathrm{LP}}$	1067 [1007] (308)	250	$\hat{N}_{\mathrm{LP}}$	343 [257] (262)
	$\hat{N}_{\mathrm{EB}}$	1041 [988] (283)		$\hat{N}_{\mathrm{EB}}$	307 [239] (251)
	$\hat{N}_{\mathrm{Chap}}$	**1000** [954] (255)		$\hat{N}_{\mathrm{Chap}}$	**244** [211] 128
	$\hat{N}_{\mathrm{BC}}$	**993** [950] (246)		$\hat{N}_{\mathrm{BC}}$	**191** [177] (119)
	$\hat{N}_{\mathrm{BC2}}$	**1000** [954] (256)		$\hat{N}_{\mathrm{BC2}}$	**249** [212] (134)
	$\hat{N}_{\mathrm{BC3}}$	**1006** [958] (264)		$\hat{N}_{\mathrm{BC3}}$	**274** [223] (160)
	$\hat{N}_{\mathrm{Med}}$	1057 [**999**] (297)		$\hat{N}_{\mathrm{Med}}$	305 [**249**] (173)
	$\hat{N}_{\mathrm{Chao}}$	2491 [2329] (820)		$\hat{N}_{\mathrm{Chao}}$	848 [602] (729)
	$\hat{N}_{\mathrm{Zelt}}$	2487 [2325] (821)		$\hat{N}_{\mathrm{Zelt}}$	846 [601] (726)

[a]Multinomial cell probabilities (Table 2A) for data generation were $p_{11} = 0.0135, p_{10} = 0.0568, p_{01} = 0.1785, p_{00} = 0.7512$
[b]Bold type highlights performance criteria targeted by bias-adjusted estimators

2.6 A Class of Estimators Including $\hat{N}_{\mathrm{LP}}$ and $\hat{N}_{\mathrm{Chap}}$ as Special Cases

A viable estimator for N under the LP conditions (whereby $\psi = p_{2|\bar{1}} = p_{2|1}$) can be obtained by replacing ψ in Eq. (1) by any valid estimator for $p_{2|1}$. Naturally, $\hat{N}_{\mathrm{LP}}$ is obtained by inserting the MLE $\hat{\psi} = \hat{p}_{2|1} = n_{11}/n_{1\bullet}$, but as noted it is undefined in the event that $n_{11} = 0$. Other estimators reviewed above (e.g., $\hat{N}_{\mathrm{Darr}}$ and $\hat{N}_{\mathrm{Chao}}$) share this same limitation. Bolfarine et al. [40] considered Bayesian alternatives to circumvent this problem. Along similar lines, one can consider classes of estimators for ψ defined as the posterior mean (or median or mode) based on a set of Beta(φ_1, φ_2) priors for the parameter $\psi = p_{2|1}$, yielding conjugate Beta$(\varphi_1 + n_{11}, \varphi_2 + n_{10})$ posterior distributions with mean $(\varphi_1 + n_{11})/(\varphi_1 + \varphi_2 + n_{1\bullet})$.

Taking the posterior mean as the estimator for ψ, one finds algebraically that $\hat{N}_{\mathrm{LP}}$ and $\hat{N}_{\mathrm{Chap}}$ correspond to the use of Beta$(0, 0)$ and Beta$(1, 0)$ priors, respectively, where the former is known as the prior of "complete uncertainty" [41]. Thus, we see that a class of estimators for N under the LP conditions can be obtained by inserting into (Eq. 1) the posterior means for $\psi = p_{2|1}$ based on Beta$(\eta, 0)$ priors, where

η is a tuning parameter over the (0,1) range. The resulting estimates for N would lie between $\hat{N}_{\text{LP}}$ and $\hat{N}_{\text{Chap}}$ whenever $n_{11} \neq 0$ while yielding finite values when $n_{11} = 0$ for all positive choices of η. We note, however, that while the resulting class of estimators may be of interest to explore, it is difficult to target an optimal value of η in this framework except with bias in expectation as a focal performance criterion.

2.7 A New Estimator Targeting Median Bias as a Criterion

Typically, capture-recapture estimators designed to reduce bias (e.g., $\hat{N}_{\text{Darr}}$ in (Eq. 8) and $\hat{N}_{\text{Chap}}$ in (Eq. 9)) focus on the traditional criterion of bias in terms of expectation. While such adjustments typically reduce variability as well, a seldom considered drawback is that they often introduce a strong tendency toward negative *median bias* (i.e., more often than not, the estimate will fall below the true value of N). As this could be undesirable in epidemiological surveillance, we propose a new capture-recapture estimator specifically targeting reduced median bias under the LP conditions (where $\psi = p_{2|\bar{1}} = p_{2|1}$). To do so, we insert an essentially median unbiased estimator for $\psi = p_{2|1}$ into Eq. (1). When both n_{11} and n_{10} exceed 0, this estimator is given by

$$\tilde{\psi}_{\text{Med}} = \frac{\tilde{p}^U + \tilde{p}^L}{2}$$

where $\tilde{p}^U$ and $\tilde{p}^L$ are the 50th percentiles of the Beta($n_{11} + 1, n_{10}$) and Beta($n_{11}, n_{10} + 1$) distributions, respectively (see [42, 43] for details). In the event that $n_{11} > 0$ and $n_{10} = 0$, we follow Carter et al. [42] and set $\tilde{\psi}_{\text{Med}} = \left(0.5^{n_{1\bullet}^{-1}} + 1\right)/2$. On the other hand, in the event that $n_{11} = 0$, we default to Chapman's estimator as a means of reducing overall variability with no likely effect on median bias. The new proposed estimator targeting median unbiasedness thus becomes

$$\hat{N}_{\text{Med}} = \begin{pmatrix} N_{11} + N_{10} + N_{01}/\tilde{\psi}_{\text{Med}}, & \text{if} \quad n_{11} > 0 \\ \hat{N}_{\text{Chap}}, & \text{if} \quad n_{11} = 0 \end{pmatrix} \tag{10}$$

2.8 New Alternatives to the Chapman Estimator Aimed at Reduced Mean Bias

As noted in Sect. 2.5, Darroch [16] derived the bias correction leading to Eq. (8) in a hypergeometric framework. Here, we leverage the population-level multinomial model for the unobservable four-cell complete data to obtain a first-order bias adjustment to the MLE $\left(\hat{N}_{\text{LP}}\right)$ in (Eq. 6). We consider the random variables corresponding to the four cell counts in Table 1B upon conditioning on the true population size (N) and work with the induced multinomial for the three observable cell counts (N_{11}, N_{10}, N_{01}) conditional on the number (N_c) identified in both captures.

To be specific, the multinomial capture-recapture model (e.g., [17]) assumes that $(N_{11}, N_{10}, N_{01}, N_{00}|N = n) \sim$ *Multinomial* $(n, p_{11}, p_{10}, p_{01}, p_{00})$ and consequently that $(N_{11}, N_{10}, N_{01}|N_c = n_c) \sim$ *Multinomial* $(n_c, p_{11}{*}, p_{10}{*}, p_{01}{*})$, where $N_c = N_{11} + N_{10} + N_{01}$, $n_c = n_{11} + n_{10} + n_{01}$, $p_{ij}{*} = p_{ij}/p_c$, and $p_c = p_{11} + p_{10} + p_{01}$ is the probability of identification in at least one of the two captures. Defining the vector $\mathbf{p}^* = \left(p_{11}^*, p_{10}^*, p_{01}^*\right)'$, note that the inverse of p_c can be written in terms of the three conditional probabilities ($p_{ij}{*}$) as follows:

$$f\left(\mathbf{p}^*\right) = p_c^{-1} = \frac{\left(p_{11}^* + p_{10}^*\right) \times \left(p_{11}^* + p_{01}^*\right)}{p_{11}^*}$$

Further, the MLE in (Eq. 6) can be rewritten as

$$\hat{N}_{\text{LP}} = n_c \times f\left(\hat{\mathbf{p}}^*\right) = n_c \times \hat{p}_{c,\text{ML}}^{-1} = n_c \times \frac{\left(\hat{p}_{11}^* + \hat{p}_{10}^*\right) \times \left(\hat{p}_{11}^* + \hat{p}_{01}^*\right)}{\hat{p}_{11}^*}$$

where $\hat{p}_{ij}^* = n_{ij}/n_c$. To derive a bias-corrected (BC) estimator for N as $n_c \times \hat{p}_{c,\text{BC}}^{-1}$, we use a Taylor series expansion that has proven useful in odds ratio estimation scenarios in cross-sectional or pair-matched sampling scenarios [44, 45]:

$$\hat{p}_{c,\text{ML}}^{-1} = f\left(\hat{\mathbf{p}}^*\right) = f\left(\mathbf{p}^*\right) + g\left(\mathbf{p}^*\right) + O\left(n^{-2}\right),$$

where $g\left(\mathbf{p}^*\right) = E\left[\frac{1}{2}\left(\hat{\mathbf{p}}^* - \mathbf{p}^*\right)'\mathbf{D}_2\left(\mathbf{p}^*\right)\left(\hat{\mathbf{p}}^* - \mathbf{p}^*\right)\right]$ and $\mathbf{D}_2(\mathbf{p}^*)$ is the Jacobian of f evaluated at $\mathbf{p}^*$. After some considerable algebra and subtraction of the term $\hat{g}\left(\mathbf{p}^*\right)$, we arrive at the following bias-corrected estimator:

$$\hat{N}_{\text{BC}} = \hat{N}_{\text{LP}} - \frac{n_{10} \times n_{01}}{n_{11}{}^2} \tag{11}$$

Though written more compactly in terms of the observable cell counts, Eq. (11) is in fact algebraically identical to $\hat{N}_{\text{Darr}}$ in Eq. (8). However, the re-expression in (Eq. 11) makes clear that the estimator due to Darroch [16] is subject to the same problems that malign the MLE $\left(\hat{N}_{\text{LP}}\right)$ itself, with regard to potential instability for small values of p_{11} and failure to be defined when $n_{11} = 0$. To combat this, we define two additional bias-corrected estimators by adjusting only the denominator of the term subtracted in (Eq. 11) (somewhat in the spirit of Gart [37] and Agresti [46]):

$$\hat{N}_{\text{BC2}} = \hat{N}_{\text{LP}} - \frac{n_{10} \times n_{01}}{\left(n_{11} + 0.5\right)^2} \text{ and } \hat{N}_{\text{BC3}} = \hat{N}_{\text{LP}} - \frac{n_{10} \times n_{01}}{\left(n_{11} + 1\right)^2} \tag{12}$$

As in (Eq. 10), we recommend setting $\hat{N}_{\mathrm{BC2}}$ and $\hat{N}_{\mathrm{BC3}}$ equal to Chapman's estimate ($\hat{N}_{\mathrm{Chap}}$; Eq. (9)) in the special case that $n_{11} = 0$. We use the two proposed bias-reduced estimators in (Eq. 12) in Sect. 2.10 as part of a proposed technique for interval estimation, and we compare them with alternative estimators via simulation in Sect. 4.

2.9 Closed-Form Confidence Interval Estimation in the Two-Capture Case

With a consistent estimator $\hat{N}$ and corresponding valid estimator $\hat{\mathrm{SE}}\left(\hat{N}\right)$ of its standard error in hand, a basic confidence interval (CI) of the form $\hat{N} \pm 1.96\hat{\mathrm{SE}}\left(\hat{N}\right)$ is a logical first candidate. However, most authors reject this approach due to a tendency for asymmetry in the distribution of $\hat{N}$. If such a CI is to be used, it is generally deemed best to employ a normalizing transformation like the log [14] or the inverse [3, 47]. Empirical comparisons (not reported here) tend to favor the inverse, whereby we invert limits obtained via $1/\hat{N} \pm 1.96\hat{\mathrm{SE}}\left(1/\hat{N}\right)$. Since delta method-based standard errors $\hat{\mathrm{SE}}\left(\hat{N}\right)$ are more readily found in the literature, one can use them in conjunction with another delta method approximation to obtain

$$\hat{\mathrm{SE}}\left(1/\hat{N}\right) = \hat{N}^{-2} \times \hat{\mathrm{SE}}\left(\hat{N}\right) \tag{13}$$

A further concern about Wald-type intervals, however, is that $\hat{\mathrm{SE}}\left(\hat{N}\right)$ often tends to be overly optimistic. We have found this particularly problematic in the case of the well-known standard error estimate that accompanies $\hat{N}_{\mathrm{Chap}}$ in Eq. (9). As such, we recommend using the point estimate $\hat{N}_{\mathrm{Chap}}$ in conjunction with the typically larger standard error estimate based on the variance of the LP estimator in Eq. (7) to obtain a Wald-type CI for 1/*N*, i.e.

$$1/\hat{N}_{\mathrm{Chap}} \pm 1.96\hat{\mathrm{SE}}\left(1/\hat{N}_{\mathrm{LP}}\right) \tag{14}$$

Asymptotically this is equivalent to using $\hat{\mathrm{SE}}\left(1/\hat{N}_{\mathrm{Chap}}\right)$ within the same interval, but the use of $\hat{\mathrm{SE}}\left(1/\hat{N}_{\mathrm{LP}}\right)$ confers a beneficial measure of conservatism. When calculating the CI in (Eq. 14), we replace $\hat{N}$ on the right side of (Eq. 13) by $\hat{N}_{\mathrm{LP}}$ in (Eq. 6), where 0.5 is used in the denominator of (Eq. 6) in the event that $n_{11} = 0$. To further avoid numerical problems, we replace any zero cell count (n_{11}, n_{10}, or n_{01}) by 0.5 when calculating $\hat{\mathrm{SE}}\left(1/\hat{N}_{\mathrm{LP}}\right)$ in (Eq. 14). Should the lower limit in (Eq. 14) be ≤ 0, we calculate the upper limit of the corresponding CI for

N without the inverse transformation as $\hat{N}_{\text{Chap}} + 1.96\hat{\text{SE}}\left(\hat{N}_{\text{LP}}\right)$. These conventions are followed in our simulation studies (Sect. 4); results indicate that the use of (Eq. 14) with these caveats tends to improve overall CI coverage and balance relative to more conventional Wald-type CIs for N regardless of whether they employ the inverse transformation.

Sadinle [48] conducted an extensive simulation study of alternative approaches to confidence interval estimation in the two-capture setting. This study included bootstrap and related Monte Carlo-based methods [49], a profile likelihood approach [50], and Wald-type intervals involving delta method-based standard errors with and without first applying an inverse transformation to the population size estimator [3, 47]. Across a variety of conditions with small and large population sizes, it was found that an adaptation of a transformed logit confidence interval [37, 46] offered the most consistently reliable performance in terms of coverage [48, 51], although interval width was not directly considered as a criterion. The transformed logit-based CI is computed as follows:

$$\left[(n_c - 0.5) + h(\mathbf{n})\exp\left(-1.96\hat{\sigma}_{\text{TL}}\right), (n_c - 0.5) + h(\mathbf{n})\exp\left(1.96\hat{\sigma}_{\text{TL}}\right)\right] \quad (15)$$

where $\hat{\sigma}_{\text{TL}} = \sqrt{(n_{11}+0.5)^{-1} + (n_{10}+0.5)^{-1} + (n_{01}+0.5)^{-1} + (n_{11}+0.5)(n_{10}+0.5)^{-1}(n_{01}+0.5)^{-1}}$ and $h(\mathbf{n}) = (n_{10}+0.5)(n_{01}+0.5)(n_{11}+0.5)^{-1}$.

2.10 An Adapted Bayesian Credible Interval Approach

Our objective in this section is to propose a new approach that competes favorably with the transformed logit interval in (Eq. 15), based on adaptations of a Bayesian Dirichlet-multinomial paradigm. It seems natural to explore this framework, given our motivation for the population-level multinomial and the fact that Bayesian credible intervals based on weakly or non-informative priors often exhibit favorable frequentist properties (e.g., [52]).

The proposed technique begins as if the goal were to obtain Bayesian credible intervals (e.g., [53, 54]) for the conditional probabilities $\mathbf{p}^* = \left(p_{11}^*, p_{10}^*, p_{01}^*\right)'$ using a weakly informative Jeffreys prior. This Dirichlet(½, ½, ½) prior yields the following posterior distribution:

$$\mathbf{p}^* \mid \mathbf{n} \sim \text{Dirichlet}\left(n_{11} + \frac{1}{2}, n_{10} + \frac{1}{2}, n_{01} + \frac{1}{2}\right) \quad (16)$$

where $\mathbf{n} = (n_{11}, n_{10}, n_{01})'$ is the vector of observed cell counts in Table 3B. One readily obtains a large sample of D draws from this posterior through appropriate sequences of gamma random variates. From each draw $\tilde{\mathbf{p}}_j^*$ ($j = 1, \ldots, D$), we generate the corresponding posterior probability of identification in at least one of the two captures which is a sum of posterior unconditional probabilities, i.e.,

$\tilde{p}_{cj} = \tilde{p}_{11j} + \tilde{p}_{10j} + \tilde{p}_{01j}$. From this we obtain a draw from the posterior distribution of N given that N_c equals the observed value n_c, i.e.

$$\tilde{N}_{j|n_c} = \text{round}\left(\frac{n_c}{\tilde{p}_{cj}}\right) \tag{17}$$

While it may appear at first glance that the posterior distribution obtained via (Eq. 17) provides an appropriate basis for a Bayesian credible interval, it will be too narrow due to conditioning on the observed value n_c. Thus for the jth draw $\tilde{p}_{cj}$, we generate a new value n_{cj} from the Binomial $(\tilde{N}_{j|n_c}, \tilde{p}_{cj})$ distribution. A draw from the posterior distribution of N is obtained as

$$\tilde{N}_j = \frac{n_{cj}}{\tilde{p}_{cj}} \tag{18}$$

($j = 1, \ldots, D$). At this point, a standard approach to constructing a 95% credible interval is to utilize the 2.5th and 97.5th sample percentiles of the resulting distribution.

While the credible interval based on (Eq. 18) is principled in terms of achieving nominal coverage asymptotically under the same conditions required for other intervals (e.g., Eq. (14)), to do so, its draws essentially reflect a mimicking in spirit of the LP estimator in (Eq. 6). As such, one might expect achievable improvements in terms of interval width. In this direction, we propose first generating posterior draws $\tilde{\mathbf{n}}_j = (\tilde{n}_{11j}, \tilde{n}_{10j}, \tilde{n}_{01j})' = n_{cj}\left(\tilde{p}^*_{11j}, \tilde{p}^*_{10j}, \tilde{p}^*_{01j}\right)'$. These draws are then used in Eqs. (6) and (9) to replace the cell counts (n_{11}, n_{10}, n_{01}) and create posterior versions $\tilde{N}_{\text{LP},j}$ and $\tilde{N}_{\text{Chap},j}$ of the Lincoln-Petersen and Chapman estimates and ultimately of the proposed bias-corrected estimate $\hat{N}_{\text{BC2}}$ in (Eq. 12), i.e.

$$\tilde{N}_{\text{BC2},j} = \begin{pmatrix} \tilde{N}_{\text{LP},j} - \frac{\tilde{n}_{10j} \times \tilde{n}_{01j}}{(\tilde{n}_{11j}+0.5)^2}, & \text{if } \tilde{n}_{11j} \geq 0.5 \\ \tilde{N}_{\text{Chap},j}, & \text{if } \tilde{n}_{11j} < 0.5 \end{pmatrix} \tag{19}$$

While a (2.5%, 97.5%) interval using the posterior sample based on (Eq. 19) should typically be narrower than that based on (Eq. 18) and tend toward nominal coverage under the same conditions, we implement asymptotically negligible adjustments to stabilize its performance in practice. For this purpose, we borrow the notion of the bias-corrected bootstrap percentile interval [55] and apply it to adjust for asymmetry in the posterior distribution of $\tilde{N}_{\text{BC2},j}$ ($j = 1, \ldots, D$). That is, rather than the 2.5th and 97.5th, we take the $100(\alpha_1)$th and $100(\alpha_2)$th percentiles of the posterior, where

$$\alpha_1 = \Phi\left(2\widehat{z}_0 + z_{0.025}\right), \alpha_2 = \Phi\left(2\widehat{z}_0 + z_{0.975}\right), \widehat{z}_0 = \Phi^{-1}\left(\lambda^*\right)$$

and λ^* is the proportion of posterior $\tilde{N}_{BC2}$ draws that fall below the value estimated by $\hat{N}_{BC3}$ in (Eq. 12). As a measure designed to reduce the risk of upper lack of coverage errors without significant impact on interval width, we set α_1 back to 0.025 in the event that $\widehat{z}_0 > 0$. That is, if the interval adjustment dictates a shift to the right, we adjust only the upper bound. We denote the resulting proposed interval as

$$\left(\tilde{N}_{BC2}^{\alpha_1}, \tilde{N}_{BC2}^{\alpha_2}\right) \tag{20}$$

Note that the percentile adjustments used in (Eq. 20) have no effect asymptotically, as $\widehat{z}_0$ converges to 0.5 and α_1 and α_2 to 0.025 and 0.975, respectively. However, extensive simulation studies suggest that the asymmetry adjustment is highly effective for improving coverage properties. While other valid estimators under the LP conditions (e.g., $\hat{N}_{LP}$, $\hat{N}_{Chap}$, or $\hat{N}_{BC2}$) could have been used as the benchmark for calculating $\widehat{z}_0$, we prefer $\hat{N}_{BC3}$ based on empirical studies. In Sect. 4, we compare our proposed adaptation with the more standard Bayesian credible interval based on (Eq. 18) as well as with other methods (including the transformed logit-based interval in (Eq. 15)).

3 Motivating Example Data and Results

Table 4 provides point and interval estimates of the total number of under-5 deaths in the Sierra Leone Bombali Shebora chiefdom during the 23-month period from January 2015 through November 2016, based on the motivating data in Table 3A. The nine population size estimators considered are reviewed or proposed in Sect. 2; reported estimates and standard errors are rounded to the nearest integer. Table 4 also displays the results of several candidate interval estimation methods. These include intervals based on inverse transforming the limits of standard Wald-type CIs for $1/\hat{N}_{LP}$ and $1/\hat{N}_{Chap}$, the altered Wald-type interval in Eq. (14), the modified logit CI of Sadinle [48] in (Eq. 15), an unadjusted credible interval using posterior draws based on (Eq. 18), and the proposed adjusted credible interval in (Eq. 20). We report estimated standard errors to accompany a select few of the point estimates in Table 4, though that associated with $\hat{N}_{LP}$ based on Eq. (6) could defensibly accompany any of the first seven estimates that assume the LP conditions.

The LP estimator is known to exhibit positive bias under the LP conditions, particularly when the probability p_{11} associated with the (1,1) cell (Table 1B) is relatively small. Note that $\hat{N}_{EB}$ appears to slightly mitigate this tendency in Table 4, while $\hat{N}_{Chap}$, $\hat{N}_{BC}$, $\hat{N}_{BC2}$, and $\hat{N}_{BC3}$ all yield approximately 3500 as the estimate based on the data in Table 3A. In terms of interval estimates, the standard CIs based on inverse transforming $\hat{N}_{LP}$ and $\hat{N}_{Chap}$ are noticeably the widest and narrowest, respectively. The transformed logit CI favored by Sadinle [48] yields a similar result to our proposed variant on a credible interval obtained via (Eq. 20). The latter result

(2794, 4546) was obtained based on 100,000 posterior draws, as was the (wider) standard credible interval based on (Eq. 18). The latter is very close to the proposed Wald-type interval in Eq. (14).

Two point estimates that stand out as vastly different from the others in Table 4 are $\hat{N}_{\text{Chao}} = 8183$ and $\hat{N}_{\text{Zelt}} = 8167$; as indicated in Sect. 2.2, this is because those estimators assume a rather extreme level of "trap happiness" at the population level. From Eq. (4), note that the projected value $\hat{\phi}_{\text{Chao}}$ based on the data in Table 3A is 2.40; inserting this value into Eq. (2) yields 8183. That is, $\hat{N}_{\text{Chao}}$ in this case is equivalent to the MLE for N assuming that the population-level ratio $\phi = p_{2|1}/p_{2|\bar{1}}$ is 2.4.

Unfortunately, while it seems unlikely that identification or not through health facility records would induce any local dependence with respect to capture by phone alerts, we cannot confidently claim that either surveillance stream achieved an overall random sampling of under-5 deaths in Bombali Shebora during the specified period. From an epidemiological perspective (see Sect. 2.1), we believe the likely scenario is that opposing forces toward $\phi > 1$ (e.g., a tendency toward more efficient capture both by health facility records and phone alerts in urban as opposed to rural areas) and $\phi < 1$ (e.g., misalignment of subsets of the sampling period over which each stream most efficiently identified cases) were at play. In the effort to vet the notion that ϕ may be close to 1, we took three available approaches: (1) We considered covariates for stratification to see how well a sum of estimates over strata agreed with the overall estimates under LP conditions; (2) we conditioned on capture by a third surveillance stream (vital records from the Makeni Office of Births and Deaths) to estimate the value of ϕ conditional on that event; and (3) we enlisted the expert opinion of an epidemiologist to obtain a comparative estimate of N based on other means.

Although locations of residence and death were not available to us, we did have access to date of death and the gender of each identified case. We deemed gender unnecessary to account for, given little evidence or reason for variation from the rough expectation of 50% males and females in the overall as well as the identified population. However, stratifying into quarterly periods based on date of death revealed temporal variation in the apparent relative efficiency of the two streams. In fact, we found that no health facility record-based deaths were recorded in the first quarter (January to March of 2015) and only seven in the second quarter. We thus combined the first three quarters of 2015 into one stratum and treated the remaining five quarters separately, for a total of six temporal strata. The observed cell counts (n_{11}, n_{10}, n_{01}) for each stratum (in temporal order) were as follows: (18, 70, 377), (11, 41, 65), (2, 22, 51), (5, 13, 72), (8, 37, 51), and (4, 19, 19). Summing the LP estimates across these six strata yields the following overall estimate and standard error:

$$\hat{N}_{\text{LP,sum}} = 3667 \text{ and } \hat{\text{SE}}\left(\hat{N}_{\text{LP,sum}}\right) = 605.6,$$

with the SE obtained as the square root of the summed variances based on (Eq. 7). Summing the Chapman estimates (which adjust for mean bias) naturally yielded a somewhat smaller value, $\hat{N}_{\text{Chap,sum}} = 3308$. For a corresponding approximate confidence interval, we applied the approach in Eqs. (13) and (14) as follows: $1/\hat{N}_{\text{Chap,sum}} \pm 1.96\hat{\text{SE}}\left(1/\hat{N}_{\text{LP,sum}}\right) = (2560, 4672)$. The larger standard error and wider interval compared to those in Table 4 are to be expected, but the summed estimates agree well with their counterparts ($\hat{N}_{\text{LP}} = 3557$ and $\hat{N}_{\text{Chap}} = 3503$, respectively). While this cannot be seen as definitive evidence in favor of the overall or summed stratified estimates under the LP conditions in this case, we note that such agreement is not guaranteed and would in fact serve as a vetting of the overall LP estimate if the assumption that the LP conditions hold within strata is correct (e.g., [20]).

Conditioning on identification by vital records, the cell counts for the complete 2×2 table for capture by health records and phone alerts were as follows: $n_{11} = 8$, $n_{10} = 15$, $n_{01} = 35$, $n_{00} = 45$. Note that this permits a conditional estimate of ϕ as (8/23)/(35/80) = 0.795 < 1. While one cannot legitimately infer specifics about the unconditional ϕ, this supplies the sort of anecdotal evidence considered by Brittain and Böhning [24]. In this case, one comes far closer to the true conditional total ($N = 103$) by applying the LP ($\hat{N}_{\text{LP}} = 124$) as opposed to the Chao estimator ($\hat{N}_{\text{Chao}} = 214$) to what would be the three observable cell counts ($n_{11} = 8$, $n_{10} = 15$, $n_{01} = 35$).

Finally, an alternate approach to approximate N was applied by an epidemiologist (MJ) directly connected with the Sierra Leone surveillance efforts. It was noted that Bombali Shebora chiefdom included rural areas (population 36,413) and Makeni City (125,970), resulting in a total chiefdom population of about 162,000 in 2016 (Statistics Sierra Leone; https://www.statistics.sl). A rough estimate of the population of children <5 years in the chiefdom was given as 24,000 with an approximate U-5 mortality rate in Sierra Leone of 120/1000 live births, yielding a 2016 projection of 2880 deaths. Over the 23-month surveillance period represented by the data, one might then expect about 5500 deaths. From (Eq. 2) and the observed data in Table 3A, this estimate would correspond to a value $\phi = p_{2|1}/p_{2|\bar{1}}$ of approximately 1.59. The external estimate of N thus lies between the original values $\hat{N}_{\text{LP}} = 3557$ and $\hat{N}_{\text{Chao}} = 8183$ (Table 4) and closer to the former. However, this estimate is subject to its own uncertainties (e.g., the accuracy of the Sierra Leone U-5 mortality rate and percentage of U-5 children as extrapolations to Bombali Shebora).

Figure 1 uses the Table 3A data to plot the MLE for N in Eq. (2) against the unknown true value of ϕ (see footnotes for details). As a whole, the figure represents a sensitivity analysis through which we emphasize again that the observed three cell counts in themselves are equally consistent with all values of N reflected on the plot (and, technically, with increasing values beyond the cutoff for ϕ employed). Thus, the example illustrates the drawbacks of two-stream capture-recapture when implementation cannot be controlled in such a way as to ensure defense of the LP conditions. We suspect in this case that $\hat{N}_{\text{Chao}}$ is an overestimate, while $\hat{N}_{\text{LP}}$ and

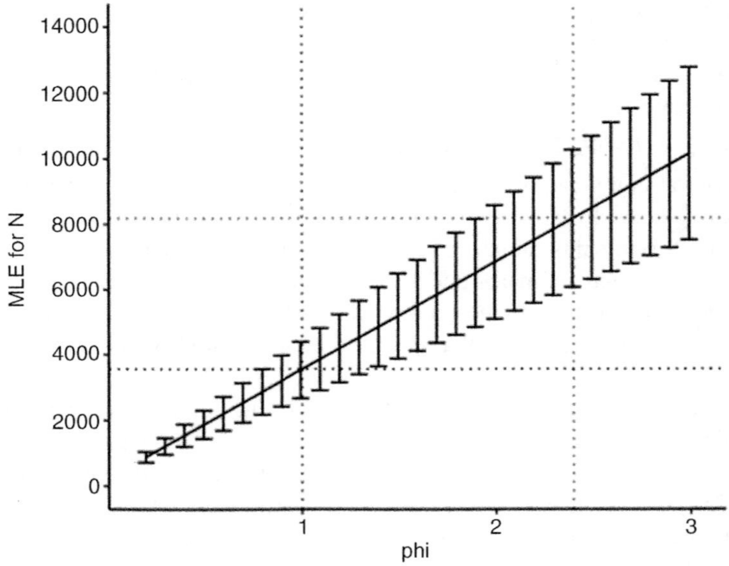

Fig. 1 The MLE for N in Eq. (2) as a function of the assumed value $\phi = p_{2|1}/p_{2|\bar{1}}$, based on observed data in Table 3A. MLEs obtained from Eq. (2); error bars indicate ± 1.96 times estimated standard errors. Dashed lines drawn to indicate estimates of N (3557 and 8183) and ϕ (1 and 2.399) corresponding to the LP and Chao [14] estimates. Error bars reflect ± 1.96 SE, with SE estimated via delta method

$\hat{N}_{\text{LP,sum}}$ may be underestimates due in part to lack of access to a measure of location (urban vs. rural) for each case. If urban cases were more efficiently captured by both streams, this would introduce a tendency toward $\phi > 1$ that could have been further mitigated by stratifying on the location variable.

4 Simulation Studies

In this section, we summarize the results of simulations designed to compare the properties of the alternative point and interval estimates in Table 4 under the LP conditions. When evaluating point estimates of population size, we generated 100,000 datasets under each simulation scenario. We reduced this number to 10,000 simulation runs when evaluating interval estimates, in light of computational time required to obtain the proposed unadjusted and adjusted credible intervals.

Tables 5 and 6 show the results for scenarios reflecting conditions designed to mimic the motivating example data. Specifically, multinomial data were generated with cell probabilities equal to the MLEs based on the data in Table 3A, i.e., $p_{11} = 0.0135, p_{10} = 0.0568, p_{01} = 0.1785, p_{00} = 0.7512$. Note that this corresponds to probabilities of identification at the first and second capture of $p_1 = 0.0703$ and

Table 6 Simulations evaluating interval estimates for N with cell probabilities mimicking conditions of motivating example data in Table 3A[a]

N	CI method	Median (mean) width	Overall coverage (%)	% Missed low (%), high (%)
3500	Wald-type centered on $1/\hat{N}_{LP}$[b]	1853 (1927)	94.6	1.3, 3.7
	Wald-type centered on $1/\hat{N}_{Chap}$[b]	1715 (1774)	93.8	2.9, 3.3
	Proposed Wald-type (Eq. 14)	1791 (1858)	94.8	2.4, 2.8
	Transformed logit (Eq. 15)	**1750 (1812)**	**95.1**	2.8, 2.1
	Unadjusted credible interval[c]	1778 (1845)	94.9	2.4, 2.7
	Proposed (Eq. 20)[c]	**1746 (1809)**	**95.1**	2.9, 2.0
1000	Wald-type centered on $1/\hat{N}_{LP}$[b]	1193 (1616)	93.6	1.6, 4.8
	Wald-type centered on $1/\hat{N}_{Chap}$[b]	863 (955)	90.5	4.2, 5.4
	Proposed Wald-type (Eq. 14)	1041 (1246)	94.5	2.7, 2.8
	Transformed logit (Eq. 15)	**955 (1092)**	**95.5**	3.2, 1.3
	Unadjusted credible interval[c]	1015 (1187)	94.9	2.6, 2.5
	Proposed (Eq. 20)[c]	**931 (1058)**	**94.8**	3.8, 1.4
500	Wald-type centered on $1/\hat{N}_{LP}$[b]	1166 (1902)	92.4	1.7, 5.9
	Wald-type centered on $1/\hat{N}_{Chap}$[b]	531 (577)	85.8	6.2, 8.0
	Proposed Wald-type (Eq. 14)	840 (18,168)	93.9	2.9, 3.2
	Transformed logit (Eq. 15)	**695 (1025)**	**96.2**	3.4, 0.5
	Unadjusted credible interval[c]	783 (6292)	94.6	2.9, 2.5
	Proposed (Eq. 20)[c]	**652 (839)**	**94.4**	4.6, 1.0
250	Wald-type centered on $1/\hat{N}_{LP}$[b]	781 (6215)	90.4	1.5, 8.2
	Wald-type centered on $1/\hat{N}_{Chap}$[b]	245 (260)	76.2	10.5, 13.3
	Proposed Wald-type (Eq. 14)	833 (1297)	93.7	3.1, 3.2
	Transformed logit (Eq. 15)	**519 (1460)**	**96.7**	3.3, 0.0
	Unadjusted credible interval[c]	663 (42,579)	94.6	2.9, 2.5
	Proposed (Eq. 20)[c]	**476 (564)**	**94.2**	5.1, 0.7

[a]Multinomial cell probabilities (Table 2A) for data generation were $p_{11} = 0.0135$, $p_{10} = 0.0568$, $p_{01} = 0.1785$, $p_{00} = 0.7512$; Bold type highlights comparative properties of best performing methods

[b]CI for N based on inverted limits of CI for $1/N$

[c]Based on 10,000 posterior draws for each simulation

$p_2 = 0.1920$, respectively. For calculating the unadjusted credible interval based on (Eq. 18) and the proposed adjusted credible interval in (Eq. 20), 10,000 posterior draws were obtained based on each simulated dataset. Simulations were conducted for a variety of true population sizes (N). When evaluating methods for interval estimation, we applied the convention of setting any calculated lower limit equal to the number captured (n_c) if its value fell below n_c. This should be an angst-free practice in any capture-recapture setting, as all intervals are data driven and the clearest signal in the data is that $N \geq n_c$.

The upper left section of Table 5 summarizes mean estimates and empirical standard deviations (SDs) for $N = 3500$, to most closely mimic the example data. The positive bias of the LP estimator is evident, while all four mean bias-adjusted estimators ($\hat{N}_{\text{Chap}}$, $\hat{N}_{\text{BC}}$, $\hat{N}_{\text{BC2}}$, and $\hat{N}_{\text{BC3}}$) are virtually unbiased. Note, however, that all four of these estimators display negative median bias. In contrast, the proposed estimator $\hat{N}_{\text{Med}}$ in Eq. (10) is essentially median unbiased as designed, with smaller mean and median bias and SD than that of $\hat{N}_{\text{LP}}$. As the true population size decreases in Table 5, note that $\hat{N}_{\text{BC}}$ begins to exhibit negative bias, while (to a lesser extent) $\hat{N}_{\text{BC3}}$ begins to exhibit positive bias, respectively. With $N = 250$, $\hat{N}_{\text{Chap}}$ begins to suffer from negative bias as well. The most consistent maintenance of the targeted properties is offered by $\hat{N}_{\text{BC2}}$ and $\hat{N}_{\text{Med}}$, which remain essentially mean and median unbiased, respectively, under all Table 5 conditions.

Standard Wald-type CIs centered around $\hat{N}_{\text{LP}}$ and $\hat{N}_{\text{Chap}}$ markedly undercovered the true value of N in many scenarios and were often found to miss exclusively on the low side (i.e., had very poor coverage balance; data not shown). As a result, we only summarize Wald-type CIs that incorporate the approximately normalizing inverse transformation (Sect. 2.9). Table 6 compares coverage and width properties of these CIs centered on $1/\hat{N}_{\text{LP}}$ and $1/\hat{N}_{\text{Chap}}$, together with the proposed adjusted Wald-type interval in (Eq. 14), the transformed logit interval (Eq. 15), the unadjusted credible interval, and the proposed adjusted credible interval (Eq. 20).

Note in Table 6 that the Wald-type CI centered on $1/\hat{N}_{\text{Chap}}$ with SE approximation based on Eqs. (9) and (13) yielded sub-nominal coverage in all cases; this problem became acute for smaller values of N. The analogous interval centered on $1/\hat{N}_{\text{LP}}$ exhibited much better coverage but was far wider; it was in turn outperformed by the proposed Wald-type interval in Eq. (14) in all cases. Nevertheless, the best CIs were those based on the transformed logit (Eq. 15) and the newly proposed adjusted credible interval approaches (Eq. 20). Note that while the former was conservative for all values of N, the latter achieved overall coverage in excess of 94% in all cases and was always considerably narrower. While the unadjusted Bayesian credible interval based on (Eq. 18) exhibited excellent coverage, it became inordinately wide for smaller N in some cases due to extremely high upper limits. The importance of the proposed adjustments underlying Eq. (20) in terms of interval width is clearly reflected throughout Table 6.

Tables 7 and 8 extend the mean [median] (SD) comparisons of point estimators ($\hat{N}_{\text{LP}}$, $\hat{N}_{\text{Chap}}$, $\hat{N}_{\text{BC2}}$, and $\hat{N}_{\text{Med}}$) across a broader range of conditions. Table 7 considers large population sizes ($N = 1000$, 2500, 5000, 10,000), with a cross-classification of the capture probabilities (p_1, p_2) over the values (0.025, 0.05, 0.1, 0.2). Table 8 examines moderate to small population sizes ($N = 100$, 200, 350, 500), with a cross-classification of (p_1, p_2) over the values (0.05, 0.1, 0.2, 0.3). The tables are somewhat compacted because reversal of (p_1, p_2) is redundant, e.g., results for $(p_1, p_2) = (0.1, 0.05)$ are the same as those for $(p_1, p_2) = (0.05, 0.1)$ and hence are not shown. Values of p_1 and p_2 larger than 0.3 are omitted, as in such cases $\hat{N}_{\text{Chap}}$ and $\hat{N}_{\text{BC2}}$ were identical and unbiased for all values of N considered.

Tables 7 and 8 reflect the expected positive bias and inflated SD of the LP estimator under all tabulated scenarios. Scanning down the columns, we initially see negative mean bias associated with $\hat{N}_{\text{Chap}}$ and $\hat{N}_{\text{BC2}}$ that quickly diminishes and then disappears as the capture probabilities (p_1, p_2) become larger. When $\hat{N}_{\text{Chap}}$

Table 7 Simulations evaluating point estimates for large population sizes (N) over a range of first and second capture probabilities[a–c]

		True population size			
Capture probabilities	Estimator	10,000	5000	2500	1000
0.025, 0.025	$\hat{N}_{LP}$	12,471 [10,258] (9018)	7490 [5243] (6261)	3573 [3050] (2343)	—
	$\hat{N}_{Chap}$	**9993** [8882] (4774)	**4799** [3989] (2843)	**2001** [1674] (1089)	—
	$\hat{N}_{BC2}$	**10,064** [8890] (4993)	**4941** [4017] (2975)	**2076** [1792] (1091)	—
	$\hat{N}_{Med}$	11,825 [**9999**] (6943)	6297 [**4974**] (3777)	2585 [**2575**] (1129)	—
0.025, 0.05	$\hat{N}_{LP}$	10,895 [10,117] (3737)	6200 [5121] (4393)	3708 [2622] (3062)	1307 [1144] (786)
	$\hat{N}_{Chap}$	**9994** [9412] (2963)	**4994** [4445] (2338)	**2400** [2005] (1402)	**734** [620] (380)
	$\hat{N}_{BC2}$	**9998** [9413] (2974)	**5029** [4449] (2447)	**2470** [2021] (1467)	**759** [671] (377)
	$\hat{N}_{Med}$	10,736 [**9997**] (3557)	5892 [**4998**] (3413)	3134 [**2494**] (1865)	922 [**921**] (375)
0.025, 0.1	$\hat{N}_{LP}$	10,390 [10,056] (2136)	5435 [5057] (1868)	3061 [2552] (2086)	1477 [1056] (1138)
	$\hat{N}_{Chap}$	**10,006** [9714] (1957)	**5005** [4722] (1466)	**2494** [2235] (1127)	**928** [773] (532)
	$\hat{N}_{BC2}$	**10,006** [9414] (1958)	**5007** [4723] (1472)	**2511** [2236] (1177)	**957** [785] (549)
	$\hat{N}_{Med}$	10,330 [**10,003**] (2105)	5362 [**5003**] (1761)	2922 [**2497**] (1635)	1208 [**997**] (661)
0.025, 0.2	$\hat{N}_{LP}$	10,164 [10,020] (1321)	5170 [5021] (994)	2689 [2516] (840)	1271 [1020] (929)
	$\hat{N}_{Chap}$	**10,001** [9866] (1272)	**4999** [4868] (915)	**2499** [2369] (679)	**996** [882] (474)
	$\hat{N}_{BC2}$	**10,001** [9866] (1272)	**4999** [4868] (915)	**2500** [2369] (681)	**1007** [883] (498)
	$\hat{N}_{Med}$	10,143 [**10,001**] (1313)	5147 [**5001**] (981)	2661 [**2496**] (806)	1193 [**999**] (685)
0.05, 0.05	$\hat{N}_{LP}$	10,421 [10,003] (2321)	5437 [5055] (1863)	3081 [2557] (2145)	1493 [1060] (1155)
	$\hat{N}_{Chap}$	**10,022** [9656] (2102)	**4997** [4711] (1472)	**2495** [2228] (1148)	**925** [768] (534)
	$\hat{N}_{BC2}$	**10,023** [9656] (2103)	**4999** [4711] (1478)	**2512** [2230] (1201)	**956** [780] (552)
	$\hat{N}_{Med}$	10,355 [**9945**] (2281)	5359 [**4996**] (1771)	2932 [**2497**] (1676)	1210 [**997**] (662)
0.05, 0.1	$\hat{N}_{LP}$	10,181 [9999] (1416)	5185 [5025] (1046)	2707 [2525] (892)	1294 [1026] (992)
	$\hat{N}_{Chap}$	**10,003** [9831] (1361)	**4999** [4859] (960)	**2499** [2362] (713)	**993** [873] (496)
	$\hat{N}_{BC2}$	**10,003** [9831] (1361)	**4999** [4859] (960)	**2500** [2363] (716)	**1005** [875] (522)
	$\hat{N}_{Med}$	10,154 [**9973**] (1407)	5156 [**5000**] (1031)	2672 [**2499**] (855)	1203 [**999**] (718)

(continued)

Table 7 (continued)

		True population size			
Capture probabilities	Estimator	10,000	5000	2500	1000
0.05, 0.2	$\hat{N}_{LP}$	10,075 [9997] (901)	5078 [5009] (652)	2584 [2510] (492)	1101 [1010] (430)
	$\hat{N}_{Chap}$	**9998** [9922] (885)	**4999** [4934] (628)	**2501** [2437] (453)	**1001** [939] (310)
	$\hat{N}_{BC2}$	**9998** [9922] (885)	**4999** [4934] (628)	**2501** [2437] (453)	**1002** [939] (314)
	$\hat{N}_{Med}$	10,066 [**9987**] (898)	5068 [**4999**] (648)	2573 [**2501**] (485)	1085 [**1000**] (396)
0.1, 0.1	$\hat{N}_{LP}$	10,083 [10,002] (932)	5087 [5000] (687)	2587 [2510] (508)	1010 [1026] (453)
	$\hat{N}_{Chap}$	**10,001** [9922] (915)	**5003** [4921] (661)	**2499** [2430] (467)	**999** [935] (322)
	$\hat{N}_{BC2}$	**10,001** [9922] (915)	**5003** [4921] (661)	**2499** [2430] (467)	**1000** [935] (326)
	$\hat{N}_{Med}$	10,071 [**9990**] (930)	5074 [**4988**] (683)	2573 [**2497**] (501)	1086 [**998**] (411)
0.1, 0.2	$\hat{N}_{LP}$	10,038 [10,000] (611)	5037 [5000] (439)	2539 [2506] (316)	1041 [1005] (221)
	$\hat{N}_{Chap}$	**10,001** [9964] (605)	**5000** [4964] (432)	**2501** [2471] (305)	**1000** [970] (199)
	$\hat{N}_{BC2}$	**10,001** [9964] (605)	**5000** [4964] (432)	**2501** [2471] (305)	**1000** [970] (199)
	$\hat{N}_{Med}$	10,033 [**9995**] (610)	5033 [**4995**] (438)	2534 [**2502**] (315)	1035 [**1001**] (199)
0.2, 0.2	$\hat{N}_{LP}$	10,017 [10,001] (404)	5016 [5000] (287)	2517 [2500] (206)	1017 [1001] (135)
	$\hat{N}_{Chap}$	**10,001** [9985] (402)	**5000** [4984] (285)	**2500** [2484] (202)	**1000** [985] (129)
	$\hat{N}_{BC2}$	**10,001** [9985] (402)	**5000** [4984] (285)	**2500** [2484] (202)	**1000** [985] (129)
	$\hat{N}_{Med}$	10,015 [**9999**] (403)	5014 [**4998**] (287)	2514 [**2498**] (205)	1015 [**999**] (134)

[a]Numbers tabulated are mean [median] (SD) of estimates over 250,000 simulation runs
[b]Empty cells (−) denote cases in which $E(N_{11}) < 1$ and/or more than 50% of runs yielded $n_{11} = 0$
[c]Bold type highlights performance criteria targeted by bias-adjusted estimators

Table 8 Simulations evaluating point estimates for moderate to small population sizes (N) over a range of first and second capture probabilities[a–c]

		True population size			
Capture probabilities	Estimator	500	350	200	100
0.05, 0.05	$\hat{N}_{LP}$	646 [558] (393)	378 [340] (208)	—	—
	$\hat{N}_{Chap}$	**371** [314] (194)	**218** [191] (108)	—	—
	$\hat{N}_{BC2}$	**383** [338] (193)	**224** [203] (106)	—	—
	$\hat{N}_{Med}$	462 [**449**] (195)	260 [**251**] (103)	—	—
0.05, 0.1	$\hat{N}_{LP}$	732 [527] (557)	492 [378] (336)	228 [198] (134)	—
	$\hat{N}_{Chap}$	**465** [389] (263)	**298** [251] (164)	**137** [119] (71)	—
	$\hat{N}_{BC2}$	**479** [395] (271)	**308** [260] (166)	**141** [125] (70)	—
	$\hat{N}_{Med}$	601 [**497**] (327)	379 [**340**] (183)	165 [**156**] (71)	—
0.05, 0.2	$\hat{N}_{LP}$	631 [510] (454)	477 [360] (365)	276 [210] (193)	108 [90] (67)
	$\hat{N}_{Chap}$	**497** [442] (233)	**341** [295] (178)	**180** [152] (97)	**72** [62] (38)
	$\hat{N}_{BC2}$	**503** [443] (245)	**349** [297] (187)	**185** [156] (99)	**73** [65] (38)
	$\hat{N}_{Med}$	594 [**499**] (336)	426 [**349**] (244)	226 [**196**] (114)	85 [**77**] (39)
0.05, 0.3	$\hat{N}_{LP}$	565 [504] (278)	427 [355] (278)	268 [204] (193)	123 [99] (81)
	$\hat{N}_{Chap}$	**499** [463] (173)	**349** [315] (149)	**193** [168] (98)	**85** [74] (44)
	$\hat{N}_{BC2}$	**501** [463] (178)	**352** [316] (156)	**198** [169] (102)	**87** [75] (45)
	$\hat{N}_{Med}$	554 [**499**] (239)	407 [**350**] (213)	239 [**199**] (129)	103 [**91**] (50)
0.1, 0.1	$\hat{N}_{LP}$	640 [510] (476)	488 [361] (386)	282 [210] (198)	111 [96] (67)
	$\hat{N}_{Chap}$	**497** [440] (241)	**342** [293] (185)	**178** [150] (97)	**70** [60] (37)
	$\hat{N}_{BC2}$	**503** [440] (253)	**349** [295] (194)	**183** [155] (99)	**72** [63] (37)
	$\hat{N}_{Med}$	598 [**498**] (349)	430 [**348**] (252)	226 [**197**] (114)	83 [**78**] (38)
0.1, 0.2	$\hat{N}_{LP}$	547 [504] (209)	404 [354] (221)	263 [204] (196)	136 [105] (93)

(continued)

Table 8 (continued)

		True population size			
Capture probabilities	Estimator	500	350	200	100
	$\hat{N}_{Chap}$	**500** [470] (151)	**349** [321] (131)	**197** [174] (98)	**90** [77] (48)
	$\hat{N}_{BC2}$	**500** [470] (153)	**351** [321] (136)	**201** [174] (103)	**93** [79] (49)
	$\hat{N}_{Med}$	540 [**500**] (192)	393 [**349**] (184)	241 [**199**] (137)	112 [**97**] (57)
0.1, 0.3	$\hat{N}_{LP}$	524 [502] (127)	377 [352] (126)	235 [202] (136)	132 [102] (93)
	$\hat{N}_{Chap}$	**500** [482] (109)	**350** [332] (95)	**200** [183] (77)	**97** [85] (48)
	$\hat{N}_{BC2}$	**500** [482] (109)	**350** [332] (96)	**201** [183] (80)	**99** [85] (50)
	$\hat{N}_{Med}$	522 [**500**] (124)	373 [**349**] (118)	239 [**199**] (129)	119 [**100**] (63)
0.2, 0.2	$\hat{N}_{LP}$	518 [501] (104)	369 [351] (95)	223 [201] (101)	128 [101] (89)
	$\hat{N}_{Chap}$	**500** [486] (94)	**350** [337] (80)	**200** [187] (66)	**99** [88] (46)
	$\hat{N}_{BC2}$	**500** [486] (94)	**350** [337] (80)	**200** [187] (67)	**100** [88] (48)
	$\hat{N}_{Med}$	516 [**499**] (102)	366 [**349**] (92)	217 [**199**] (87)	118 [**99**] (64)
0.2, 0.3	$\hat{N}_{LP}$	510 [501] (74)	360 [351] (65)	211 [201] (57)	115 [101] (62)
	$\hat{N}_{Chap}$	**500** [492] (70)	**350** [342] (59)	**200** [192] (47)	**100** [92] (36)
	$\hat{N}_{BC2}$	**500** [492] (70)	**350** [342] (59)	**200** [192] (47)	**100** [92] (37)
	$\hat{N}_{Med}$	509 [**500**] (74)	359 [**350**] (64)	210 [**200**] (55)	112 [**100**] (50)
0.3, 0.3	$\hat{N}_{LP}$	506 [500] (55)	356 [350] (47)	206 [201] (38)	107 [100] (36)
	$\hat{N}_{Chap}$	**500** [495] (53)	**350** [345] (45)	**200** [195] (35)	**100** [95] (26)
	$\hat{N}_{BC2}$	**500** [495] (53)	**350** [345] (45)	**200** [195] (35)	**100** [95] (26)
	$\hat{N}_{Med}$	505 [**500**] (55)	355 [**350**] (47)	206 [**200**] (38)	106 [**99**] (33)

[a]Numbers tabulated are mean [median] (SD) of estimates over 250,000 simulation runs
[b]Empty cells (–) denote cases in which $E(N_{11}) < 1$ and/or more than 50% of runs yielded $n_{11} = 0$
[c]Bold type highlights performance criteria targeted by bias-adjusted estimators

is noticeably biased downward, the new proposed estimator $\hat{N}_{\text{BC2}}$ in (Eq. 12) is somewhat less biased in almost all cases. However (as in Table 5), both $\hat{N}_{\text{Chap}}$ and $\hat{N}_{\text{BC2}}$ demonstrate marked negative median bias in all cases, meaning that they underestimate the true N more than half the time. As designed, this continues to be mitigated quite successfully by the proposed estimator $\hat{N}_{\text{Med}}$. This estimator outperforms $\hat{N}_{\text{LP}}$ in terms of mean bias and SD in all cases, although there are some cases in Table 7 in which $\hat{N}_{\text{LP}}$ displays the least median bias.

Tables 9 and 10 summarize a similar expansion of our simulation studies to evaluate competing interval estimation methods (the proposed adjusted Wald-type interval in (Eq. 14), the transformed logit interval (Eq. 15), and the proposed adjusted credible interval (Eq. 20)) across a wide variety of large (Table 9) and small to moderate (Table 10) population sizes. In Table 9, the proposed credible interval achieves the smallest median width in the vast majority of cases together with coverage close to nominal and always exceeding 94%. Scanning down the column for $N = 1000$ in Table 10, note that the three methods performed very similarly in terms of both width and overall coverage. The only noteworthy exceptions are the cases of the lowest capture probabilities (0.1, 0.1) and (0.2, 0.2), in which the adjusted Wald-type interval (Eq. 14) tends to be widest and the proposed adjusted credible interval narrowest. For a more moderate true population size ($N = 250$) and especially for $N = 50$, a tendency toward sub-nominal coverage for the Wald-type CI persists over the full range of capture probabilities (p_1, p_2), while the transformed logit and adjusted credible interval achieve close to the nominal 95% coverage in nearly all cases. The transformed logit CI is nearly always conservative, although Table 10 reveals a few exceptions in which its coverage strays from nominal and its width becomes excessive. All three intervals have performance issues when $N = 50$ and capture probabilities are smallest (0.1, 0.1), while a somewhat pathological tendency with respect to width of the transformed logit interval occurs in that case and also for $N = 50$ and 250 when capture probabilities are highest (0.9, 0.9).

5 Discussion

In this article focused on the standard closed population single-recapture scenario, we first set out to review and clarify the fundamental challenge in terms of the population parameter ϕ. We expressed our view that surveillance can set up competing forces toward $\phi > 1$ and $\phi < 1$ driven by variations in efficiency of the two streams (e.g., across geographical or temporal strata). We argue for the perspective that the LP conditions (i.e., $\phi = 1$) remain central, as that population-level state of nature is the only one that can specifically be targeted by design or defended epidemiologically. In light of popular estimation techniques [e.g., loglinear models and estimators like that of Chao [14] that make hidden, arbitrary, or at least questionable (in the two-catch case) assumptions about the non-identifiable parameter ϕ], we point out the ease with which the practitioner can be misled. No

Table 9 Simulations evaluating interval estimates for large population sizes (N) over a range of first and second overall capture probabilities[a]

		True population size		
Capture probabilities	CI method[b]	10,000	5000	2500
0.025, 0.05	A	12,56394.8 [2.2, 3.0]	10,62594.4 [1.9, 3.8]	11,38794.4 [1.8, 3.8]
	B	10,86595.2 [3.9, 0.9]	777295.6 [4.3, 0.1]	564595.5 [4.5, 0.0]
	C	10,65794.7 [4.1, 1.3]	734394.1 [4.8, 1.1]	529894.3 [5.5, 0.3]
0.025, 0.1	A	790295.0 [2.3, 2.7]	607094.3 [2.4, 3.3]	508793.9 [2.2, 3.9]
	B	742095.4 [3.3, 1.3]	531595.2 [3.8, 1.0]	382495.7 [4.2, 0.1]
	C	737595.1 [3.4, 1.4]	518894.4 [4.2, 1.4]	359994.1 [4.8, 1.1]
0.025, 0.2	A	505495.5 [2.0, 2.5]	369194.4 [2.7, 2.9]	280794.6 [2.6, 2.8]
	B	493395.6 [2.5, 1.9]	351295.1 [3.3, 1.6]	253495.6 [3.2, 1.2]
	C	491095.5 [2.7, 1.8]	347594.8 [3.6, 1.6]	244494.7 [3.9, 1.4]
0.05, 0.05	A	800594.6 [1.8, 3.6]	613194.8 [2.1, 3.1]	514294.4 [1.8, 3.8]
	B	748695.1 [2.8, 2.1]	533695.2 [3.7, 1.0]	382096.0 [3.9, 0.1]
	C	745894.8 [2.8, 2.4]	523294.7 [3.9, 1.3]	360794.7 [4.4, 1.0]
0.05, 0.1	A	530595.2 [2.2, 2.7]	389894.3 [2.4, 3.3]	295294.1 [2.7, 3.3]
	B	515095.4 [2.8, 1.8]	366894.8 [3.4, 1.8]	260895.2 [3.8, 1.1]
	C	515795.4 [2.9, 1.7]	365394.6 [3.5, 1.9]	255394.6 [4.2, 1.3]
0.05, 0.2	A	505495.5 [2.0, 2.5]	250195.1 [2.2, 2.7]	182294.6 [2.6, 2.8]
	B	493395.6 [2.5, 1.9]	244595.4 [2.6, 2.1]	174195.1 [3.1, 1.8]
	C	491095.5 [2.7, 1.8]	243995.2 [2.9, 1.9]	172494.9 [3.4, 1.7]
0.1, 0.1	A	356795.0 [2.3, 2.7]	256994.4 [2.3, 3.3]	189194.7 [2.5, 2.8]
	B	352195.1 [2.7, 2.2]	250294.6 [2.8, 2.6]	179295.3 [3.1, 1.6]
	C	353695.0 [2.8, 2.1]	250394.6 [2.9, 2.5]	178395.0 [3.4, 1.6]
0.1, 0.2	A	237095.3 [2.1, 2.6]	168994.9 [2.5, 2.6]	120694.7 [2.7, 2.6]
	B	235995.5 [2.2, 2.3]	167294.9 [2.8, 2.3]	118395.0 [3.0, 2.0]
	C	236795.5 [2.2, 2.3]	167595.0 [2.9, 2.2]	118494.9 [3.3, 1.8]

[a]Table entries are median interval width, overall coverage %, [% missed low, % missed high]
[b]A, Adjusted Wald-type CI, Eq. (14); B, transformed logit CI, Eq. (15); C, proposed adjusted credible interval, Eq. (20)

Table 10 Simulations evaluating interval estimates for moderate to small population sizes (N) over a range of first and second overall capture probabilities[a]

		True population size		
Capture probabilities	CI method[b]	1000	250	50
0.1, 0.1	A	1338 (1980) 94.3 [2.2, 3.5]	1036 (1383) 94.6 [2.7, 2.7]	88 (115) 82.2 [17.8, 0.0]
	B	1158 (1475) 96.0 [3.1, 0.9]	622 (2229) 95.9 [4.1, 0.0]	580 (672) 97.2 [2.8, 0.0]
	C	1122 (1355) 94.9 [3.7, 1.4]	567 (617) 94.6 [4.7, 0.8]	69 (74) 80.3 [19.7, 0.0]
0.2, 0.2	A	511 (534) 94.6 [3.0, 2.4]	281 (379) 94.0 [3.5, 2.5]	164 (206) 94.7 [4.4, 0.9]
	B	504 (524) 95.1 [2.9, 2.0]	262 (317) 95.7 [2.9, 1.4]	148 (509) 98.0 [2.0, 0.0]
	C	502 (523) 95.1 [3.3, 1.7]	260 (310) 95.1 [3.8, 1.1]	102 (119) 94.1 [5.8, 0.1]
0.3, 0.3	A	292 (297) 94.4 [3.1, 2.5]	152 (165) 94.7 [3.2, 2.1]	83 (154) 92.2 [5.3, 2.5]
	B	292 (298) 94.7 [2.5, 2.8]	153 (164) 95.4 [2.2, 2.5]	81 (167) 97.5 [1.3, 1.2]
	C	292 (298) 94.7 [3.1, 2.3]	150 (161) 95.3 [3.0, 1.7]	70 (94) 94.4 [4.7, 1.0]
0.4, 0.4	A	186 (188) 95.3 [2.9, 1.9]	94 (98) 94.8 [3.6, 1.6]	45 (66) 93.3 [5.5, 1.2]
	B	187 (189) 95.5 [2.2, 2.4]	97 (100) 95.4 [1.9, 2.7]	51 (64) 96.7 [0.8, 2.5]
	C	187 (189) 95.5 [2.7, 1.9]	95 (98) 95.3 [3.0, 1.7]	44 (55) 94.9 [4.2, 1.0]
0.5, 0.5	A	124 (125) 95.3 [2.9, 1.8]	62 (64) 94.8 [3.7, 1.4]	28 (33) 93.0 [6.1, 0.9]
	B	125 (126) 95.5 [1.9, 2.6]	65 (66) 95.2 [1.8, 3.0]	34 (38) 96.1 [0.5, 3.4]
	C	125 (126) 95.6 [2.4, 2.0]	63 (64) 95.2 [3.0, 1.7]	29 (33) 95.0 [3.9, 1.1]
0.6, 0.6	A	83 (83) 95.0 [3.1, 1.9]	41 (42) 94.8 [3.7, 1.5]	18 (20) 93.4 [6.1, 0.4]
	B	83 (84) 95.2 [2.0, 2.9]	43 (44) 95.1 [1.4, 3.4]	23 (25) 95.4 [0.3, 4.4]
	C	83 (83) 95.3 [2.6, 2.1]	42 (42) 95.0 [3.1, 2.0]	19 (21) 94.9 [4.1, 1.0]

(continued)

Table 10 (continued)

		True population size		
Capture probabilities	CI method[b]	1000	250	50
0.7, 0.7	A	53 (53) 95.2 [3.1, 1.7]	26 (27) 94.8 [4.1, 1.1]	11 (11)93.0 [6.7, 0.3]
	B	54 (54) 95.3 [1.7, 3.0]	28 (29) 95.0 [1.2, 3.8]	16 (17) 94.0 [0.1, 5.9]
	C	53 (54) 95.4 [2.5, 2.1]	27 (27) 95.0 [3.4, 1.7]	12 (12) 94.1 [5.1, 0.9]
0.8, 0.8	A	31 (31) 94.9 [3.4, 1.7]	15 (16) 94.7 [4.4, 1.0]	5 (6) 92.4 [7.6, 0.0]
	B	32 (32) 94.9 [1.5, 3.6]	17 (17) 94.6 [0.8, 4.6]	11 (12) 94.1 [0.0, 5.9]
	C	31 (31) 95.1 [2.8, 2.1]	16 (16) 94.8 [4.0, 1.2]	6 (6) 94.9 [5.1, 0.1]
0.9, 0.9	A	14 (14) 94.9 [4.0, 1.1]	6 (6) 94.7 [5.2, 0.0]]	2 (2) 90.3 [9.7, 0.0]
	B	15 (15) 95.2 [0.8, 4.0]	9 (9) 93.0 [0.1, 7.0]	11 (141) 99.9 [0.0, 0.1]
	C	14 (14) 95.2 [3.3, 1.6]	6 (6) 93.7 [6.3, 0.0]	3 (3) 96.0 [4.0, 0.0]

[a]Table entries are median (mean) interval width, overall coverage %, [% missed low, % missed high]
[b]A, Adjusted Wald-type CI, Eq. (14); B, transformed logit CI, Eq. (15); C, proposed adjusted credible interval, Eq. (20)

statistical information to identify ϕ in fact exists without assumptions best judged by those with a true understanding of the operating characteristics of the two streams, and we suggest at minimum that any reported estimate for N should be accompanied by clear consideration and disclosure of its implications about ϕ. Our view is that the best point estimate for N in the two-stream setting is essentially the one obtained by inserting the epidemiologist's best guess for ϕ into Eq. (2). To validate such a guess, it seems clear that by far the most effective design in two-stream surveillance is to target one stream as an overall or stratified random sample that is implemented in agnostic fashion relative to the other. In that case, the $\phi = 1$ assumption can be made with confidence either overall or within strata, so that both the validity of point estimation and accompanying measures of variance are assured under the LP conditions. Short of such control at the design stage, we believe the proper role of covariates is to use them judiciously to define strata within which a defensible case might be made for the $\phi = 1$ assumption based on expert opinion (e.g., [11]).

While we have emphasized the need for caution in their use, we recognize the historical significance of the Chao [14] and Zelterman [15] estimators. As noted, Chao's estimator was developed under mathematical assumptions (e.g., "large" T and "small" $\mathbf{p}_i$ that vary across units but remain homogeneous for a given unit across captures) that we see as highly unlikely to apply to surveillance but perhaps more defensible in ecological or other settings with many capture events. The unfortunate thing is that the perception of robustness and the misguided notion that $\hat{N}_{\text{Chao}}$ can be defended as a general lower bound for N in the two-capture surveillance setting has made its way into practice due in part to a promulgation of literature determined to promote alternatives to the classical LP and Chapman estimators. As we have seen, if one is convinced that $\phi > 1$ at the population level, then it is $\hat{N}_{\text{LP}}$ (or a bias-adjusted alternative like $\hat{N}_{\text{Chap}}$ or $\hat{N}_{\text{BC2}}$) that serves as a defensible lower bound. $\hat{N}_{\text{Chao}}$ then becomes just one of a continuum of estimates across the feasible range of ϕ that are equally consistent with the data (see Fig. 1 for illustration). On the other hand, if one can defend the LP conditions based on the design and implementation of surveillance streams, then $\hat{N}_{\text{Chao}}$ is always biased upward (potentially to an extreme; see Table 5). If the prevailing belief is that $\phi < 1$, then $\hat{N}_{\text{LP}}$ in fact provides an upper bound and the upward bias of $\hat{N}_{\text{Chao}}$ becomes even more severe. These comments are not to discount empirical evidence (e.g., [24]), in favor of the notion that surveillance studies may often operate in an overall "trap happy" ($\phi > 1$) fashion. Interestingly, those authors promote an estimator derivable as an MLE based on a truncated binomial model that they refer to as "Chao's," in which 4 takes the place of 2 in the denominator on the right side of Eq. (3). Clearly, this would mitigate some positive bias associated with the original $\hat{N}_{\text{Chao}}$ and might have contributed to some of the empirical evidence Brittain and Böhning presented in which "Chao's" was often closer than the LP estimate to a true count after conditioning on capture by a third surveillance stream. Of course, as seen in Sect. 3, our motivating example presented a conditional estimate of ϕ below 1 and therefore the opposite sort of non-conclusive empirical evidence.

With regard to the use of loglinear models, our view is that a similar set of misconceptions have contributed to their widespread use and interpretation. Practitioners are understandably thrilled to apply a modeling approach and a metric like AIC that they perceive as useful both to account for covariates and to sort out the mystery of what the "best" estimate for N should be based on the observed data. Unfortunately, as Table 2 illustrates clearly in the two-capture case, this perception is misguided in crucial ways (see also [35]). With regard to Table 2, note that it is only the fitted values corresponding to the observed cell counts (n_{11}, n_{10}, n_{01}) that AIC is legitimately informative about. The projections made for the last and (by far) most crucial column $\left(\hat{N}_{00}\right)$ by any given model are essentially an arbitrary mathematical construct. We suggest that the effort to identify one of the seven loglinear models as "best" should be almost exclusively in light of examining that model's fundamental assumption about ϕ and determining whether that assumption is defensible based on how the two-capture efforts were designed and implemented. A legitimate role for AIC might then come into play in terms of distinguishing (in terms of parsimony) between a set of models that make the most defensible assumption about ϕ. Nevertheless, as Eq. (2) and Fig. 1 clearly illustrate, the complete set of available loglinear models covers a small subset of the continuum of possible ϕ values. To further emphasize this restrictiveness, note that none of the models summarized in Table 4 in fact corresponds to a projected $\phi > 1$ for our example (and correspondingly, none yields an estimate in excess of $\hat{N}_{\text{LP}}$).

Given our arguments for the enduring central role of the LP conditions, the second component of our work has been to seek possible improvements in both point and interval estimation under those conditions. We have proposed a bias-corrected estimator in $\hat{N}_{\text{BC2}}$ (Eq. 12) that provides to our knowledge the first truly competitive and potentially preferable alternative to the classic estimator of Chapman [12] in terms of mean bias. The estimator $\hat{N}_{\text{BC2}}$ arose from applying first principles (e.g., [44]) to develop a bias correction under the population-level multinomial model, leading initially to an adjustment to the MLE that is equivalent (for $T = 2$) to the general proposal of Darroch [16]. However, the algebraic form of this equivalent multinomial-based estimator suggested a way to mitigate instability in the bias correction factor, by simply adding a constant to the observed value n_{11} in the squared denominator term (Eq. 12). Our empirical study shows the necessity of such mitigation to avoid negative bias in Darroch's estimator and suggests near optimality of the constant 0.5 with respect to the mean bias criterion. We found that $\hat{N}_{\text{BC2}}$ quickly becomes equivalent to the Chapman estimator as N and/or (p_1, p_2) increases. Nevertheless, in situations where the negative bias in $\hat{N}_{\text{Chap}}$ is not negligible (Tables 5, 7, and 8), $\hat{N}_{\text{BC2}}$ tended to be less biased. This appears noteworthy given the stature of $\hat{N}_{\text{Chap}}$ in the pantheon of closed population single-recapture estimators, although we note that the mediation of negative bias exhibited by $\hat{N}_{\text{BC2}}$ was often minor. Thus, there may yet be further room for improvement, perhaps facilitated by the algebraic form of the MLE for N given a known fixed value for the parameter $\psi = p_{2|\bar{1}}$ that we present in Eq. (1). We used that expression to motivate a class of estimators for N that includes $\hat{N}_{\text{LP}}$ and $\hat{N}_{\text{Chap}}$ as bookend special cases (Sect.

2.6) and to propose a novel estimator ($\hat{N}_{\text{Med}}$) that targets median bias as a criterion (Sect. 2.7). Specifically, we point out a seldom discussed potential drawback to mean bias-adjusted estimators in that they naturally tend to induce negative median bias (and thus a potentially high risk of underestimating the true population size). Our simulation studies demonstrate that $\hat{N}_{\text{Med}}$ effectively targets reduced median bias while maintaining smaller mean bias as well as variability relative to $\hat{N}_{\text{LP}}$.

Much like the Chapman point estimator, our review of the literature suggests that the transformed logit CI in Eq. (15) represents an arguably best previously available choice for an interval estimator in the single-recapture setting under LP conditions. This view is in light of extensive coverage comparisons given by Sadinle [48], though we note that those omitted interval width as a criterion. As an alternative closed-form option, we considered an adjusted Wald-type interval in which one centers about the inverse of the Chapman estimate but incorporates the SE that corresponds to the LP estimate as a conservative measure. This adjustment (Eq. 14) empirically outperformed all other Wald-type CIs considered yet remained noticeably inferior to the transformed logit method. We then proposed a new CI approach that generally outperformed the transformed logit interval in terms of the joint criteria of coverage and width, although it requires more computational effort. Our initial goal was to apply the Dirichlet-multinomial model-based Bayesian credible interval approach as directly as possible, but it quickly became apparent that adjustments would be necessary in order to compete with the performance of the transformed logit-based CI. We developed an approach that first mimics the $\hat{N}_{\text{BC2}}$ estimand based on each Dirichlet draw and then borrows the principle of the bias-corrected bootstrap percentile interval [55] in order to adjust for asymmetry in the posterior distribution of that estimand. The adjustments become negligible under the same conditions required for $\hat{N}_{\text{LP}}$ and $\hat{N}_{\text{BC2}}$ to approach the truth, but the effect in terms of improved interval width can be pronounced. The resulting adjusted credible interval (Eq. 20) maintained favorable coverage across a wide range of simulation scenarios (Tables 6, 9, and 10) and nearly always produced narrower intervals than those based on the transformed logit approach. Nevertheless, our study confirms the outstanding overall properties of the latter method, and we would agree with Sadinle [48] in that to our knowledge Eq. (15) offers the best available closed form interval under the LP conditions.

With regard to the motivating example involving U-5 mortality data from Bombali Shebora, we acknowledge that we cannot claim sufficient control of the design and implementation of the two streams to be confident in assuming the LP conditions. Summing over temporal strata, we obtained a similar estimate (3667) to the original LP estimate (3557) based on the overall data in Table 3A. While this adds a small measure of reassurance, our sense is that additional stratification by variables unavailable to us (especially urban vs. rural geographic location of residence) might have mitigated some residual tendency toward $\phi > 1$. This is despite empirical evidence somewhat in the opposite direction based on conditioning on cases identified by a third stream and in light of the somewhat larger estimate (5520) projected based on other sources of Sierra Leone population and mortality rate data (see Sect. 3). The truth is unknown, and of course we cannot definitively claim that any one of the point estimates considered comes closest. The example thus helps to emphasize the need to collect sufficient covariate data to account for strata that might explain variations in the efficiency of the surveillance streams and within which the LP conditions seem reasonable to assume. Ideally, of course, one of the surveillance streams would be purposefully implemented as an overall or stratified random sample in a manner that does not impact identification by the other.

As noted in Sect. 2.4, we believe that unless the LP conditions can defensibly be assumed overall or within strata, one would do best to acknowledge the fundamental (not statistical) uncertainty in ϕ when characterizing the variability of any estimate of N. While Bayesian methods (e.g., [19, 56]) have been explored in this direction, we are currently working to develop more accessible analogues for the purposes of sensitivity and uncertainty analysis that epidemiologists might find easier to visualize and apply. Additional avenues for future work include the application of the insights gained here toward surveillance settings involving $T \geq 3$ streams. In particular, we believe the same sort of focus toward the fundamentally non-identifiable parameters that stand in the way of a defensible estimate of N may uncover a clearer roadmap for analysis as well as the need for similar cautions with respect to common practice. We hope that such further work will help alleviate some of the concerns (e.g., [57]) that may stand as a barrier to more widespread use of capture-recapture methodology in epidemiological surveillance settings.

Acknowledgments We thank Dr. Kevin Clarke for his contributions to the motivating study and helpful input. The CHAMPS study is funded by the Bill and Melinda Gates Foundation (OPP1126780), and partial support was also provided through the Emory Center for AIDS Research (P30AI050409). We thank the following agencies for their support of the motivating project: Ministry of Health and Sanitation, Sierra Leone; eHealth Africa, Sierra Leone; and CDC Country Office, Sierra Leone.

References

1. Böhning, D., van der Heijden, P.G.M., Bunge, J. (eds.): Capture-recapture methods for the social and medical sciences. Taylor and Francis Group LLC, Milton Park (2018)
2. Borchers, D.L., Buckland, S.T., Zucchini, W.: Estimating animal abundance: closed populations. Springer-Verlag, London (2002)
3. Krebs, C.J.: Ecological methodology. Benjamin/Cummings, Menlo Park, CA (1998)
4. Lincoln, F.C.: Calculating waterfowl abundance on the basis of banding returns. U.S. Depart. Agricult. Circul. **118**, 1–4 (1930)
5. Petersen, C.G.J.: The yearly immigration of young plaice into the Limfjord from the German sea. Rep. Danish Biol. Station. **6**, 5–48 (1896)
6. Schnabel, Z.E.: The estimation of the total fish population of a lake. Am. Math. Mon. **45**, 348–352 (1938)
7. Seber, G.A.F.: The estimation of animal abundance and related parameters. The Blackburn Press, Caldwell, NJ (1982)

8. Evans, M.A., Bonett, D.G., McDonald, L.L.: A general theory for modeling capture-recapture data from a closed population. Biometrics. **50**, 396–405 (1994)
9. Otis, D.L., Burnham, K.P., White, G.C., Anderson, D.R.: Statistical inference from capture data on closed animal populations. Wildl. Monogr. **62**, 1–135 (1978)
10. Alpren, C., Jallow, M.F., Kaiser, R., Diop, M., Kargbo, S., Castle, E., Dafae, E., Hersey, S., Redd, J.T., Jambai, A.: The 117 call alert system in Sierra Leone: from rapid Ebola notification to routine death reporting. BMJ Global Health. **2**, e000392 (2017). https://doi.org/10.1136/bmjgh-2017-0003
11. Chandra Sekar, C., Deming, W.E.: On a method of estimating birth and death rates and the extent of registration. J. Am. Stat. Assoc. **44**, 101–115 (1949)
12. Chapman, D.G.: Some properties of the hypergeometric distribution with applications to zoological simple censuses. Univ. Calif. Publ. Statis. **1**, 131–160 (1951)
13. Baillargeon, S., Rivest, L.-P.: Rcapture: loglinear models for capture-recapture in R. J. Stat. Softw. **19**, 1–31 (2007)
14. Chao, A.: Estimating the population size for capture-recapture data with unequal catchability. Biometrics. **43**, 783–791 (1987)
15. Zelterman, D.: Robust estimation in truncated discrete distributions with application to capture-recapture experiments. J. Statis. Plan. Inference. **18**, 225–237 (1988)
16. Darroch, J.N.: The multiple recapture census. I. Estimation of a closed population. Biometrika. **45**, 343–359 (1958)
17. Wittes, J.T.: Applications of a multinomial capture-recapture model to epidemiological data. J. Am. Stat. Assoc. **69**, 93–97 (1974)
18. Chao, A., Pan, H.-Y., Chiang, S.-C.: The Petersen-Lincoln estimator and its extension to estimate the size of a shared population. Biom. J. **6**, 957–970 (2008)
19. Chatterjee, K., Mukherjee, D.: On the estimation of homogenous population size from a complex dual-record system. J. Stat. Comput. Simul. **86**(17), 3562–3581 (2016)
20. Hook, E.B., Regal, R.R.: Effect of variation in probability of ascertainment by sources ("variable catchability") upon "capture-recapture" estimates of prevalence. Am. J. Epidemiol. **137**, 1148–1166 (1993)
21. Chao, A., Tsay, P.K., Lin, S.-H., Shau, W.-Y., Chao, D.-Y.: The applications of capture-recapture models to epidemiological data. Stat. Med. **20**, 3123–3157 (2001)
22. Böhning, D.: Some general comparative points on Chao's and Zelterman's estimators of the population size. Scand. J. Stat. **37**, 221–236 (2010)
23. Béguinot, J.: An algebraic derivation of Chao's estimator of the number of species in a community highlights the condition allowing Chao to deliver centered estimates. Int. Scholar. Res. Notice. **2014**, 847328 (2014). https://doi.org/10.1155/2014/847328
24. Brittain, S., Böhning, D.: Estimators in capture-recapture studies with two sources. Adv. Statis. Anal. **93**, 23–47 (2009)
25. Nour, E.-S.: On the estimation of the total number of vital events with data from duel collection systems. J. Roy. Statis. Soc. Ser. A. **145**, 106–116 (1982)
26. Fienberg, S.E.: The multiple-recapture census for closed populations and incomplete contingency tables. Biometrika. **59**, 591–603 (1972)
27. Rivest, L.-P., Levesque, T.: Improved log-linear model estimators of abundance in capture-recapture experiments. Can. J. Stat. **29**(4), 555–572 (2001)
28. Agresti, A.: Simple capture-recapture models permitting unequal catchability and variable sampling effort. Biometrics. **50**, 494–500 (1994)
29. Rasch, G.: On general laws and the meaning of measurement in psychology. In: Neyman, J. (ed.) Proceedings of the 4th Berkeley symposium on mathematical statistics and probability, vol. 4, pp. 321–333. University of California Press, Berkeley, California (1961)
30. Goodman, L.A.: Exploratory latent structure analysis using both identifiable and unidentifiable models. Biometrika. **61**, 215–231 (1974)
31. Bassili, A., Grant, A.D., El-Mohgazy, E., Galal, A., Glaziou, P., Seita, A., Abubakar, I., Bierrenbach, A.L., Crofts, J.P., van Hest, N.A.: Estimating tuberculosis case detection rate in resource-limited countries: a capture-recapture study in Egypt. Int. J. Tubercul. Lung Dis. **14**, 727–732 (2010)

32. Ma, Z., Mao, C.X., Yang, Y.: Performance of hierarchical log-linear models for a heterogeneous population with three lists. In: Böhning, D., van der Heijden, P.G.M., Bunge, J. (eds.) Capture-recapture methods for the social and medical sciences, pp. 305–313. Taylor and Francis Group LLC, Milton Park (2018)
33. Poorolajal, J., Mohammadi, Y., Farzinara, F.: Using the capture-recapture method to estimate the human immunodeficiency virus-positive population. Epidemiol. Health. **39**, 1–5 (2017)
34. Akaike, H.: A new look at the statistical model identification. IEEE Trans. Autom. Control. **19**, 716–723 (1974)
35. Jones, H.E., Hickman, M., Welton, N.J., De Angelis, D., Harris, R.J., Ades, A.E.: Recapture or precapture? Fallibility of standard capture-recapture methods in the presence of referrels. Am. J. Epidemiol. **11**, 1383–1393 (2014)
36. Regal, R.R., Hook, E.B.: The effects of model selection on confidence intervals for the size of a closed population. Stat. Med. **10**, 717–721 (1991)
37. Gart, J.J.: Alternative analyses of contingency tables. J. Roy. Statis. Soc. Ser. B. **28**, 164–179 (1966)
38. Evans, M.A., Bonett, D.G.: Bias reduction for multiple-recapture estimators of closed population size. Biometrics. **50**, 388–395 (1994)
39. Wittes, J.T.: On the bias and estimated variance of Chapman's two-sample capture-recapture population estimate. Biometrics. **28**, 592–597 (1972)
40. Bolfarine, H., Leite, J.G., Rodrigues, J.: On the estimation of the size of a finite and closed population. Biom. J. **5**, 577–593 (1992)
41. Haldane, J.B.S.: *A note on inverse probability. Math. Proc. Camb. Philos. Soc.**28**, 55–61 (1932)*
42. Carter, R.E., Lin, Y., Lipsitz, S.R., Newcombe, R.G., Hermayer, K.L.: Relative risk estimated from the ratio of two median unbiased estimates. J. Roy. Statis. Soc. Ser. C. **59**, 657–671 (2010)
43. Hirji, K., Tsiatis, A., Mehta, C.: Median unbiased estimation for binary data. Am. Stat. **43**, 7–11 (1989)
44. Jewell, N.P.: Small-sample bias of point estimators of the odds ratio from matched sets. Biometrics. **40**, 421–435 (1984)
45. Lyles, R.H., Guo, Y., Greenland, S.: Reducing bias and mean squared error associated with regression-based odds ratio estimators. J. Statis. Plan. Inference. **142**, 3235–3241 (2012)
46. Agresti, A.: On logit confidence intervals for the odds ratio with small samples. Biometrics. **55**, 597–602 (1999)
47. Jensen, A.L.: Confidence intervals for nearly unbiased estimators in single-mark and single-recapture experiments. Biometrics. **45**, 1233–1237 (1989)
48. Sadinle, M.: Transformed logit confidence intervals for small populations in single capture-recapture estimation. Commun. Statis. Simulat. Comput. **38**, 1909–1924 (2009)
49. Buckland, S.T., Garthwaite, P.H.: Quantifying precision of mark-recapture estimates using the bootstrap and related methods. Biometrics. **47**, 255–268 (1991)
50. Evans, M.A., Kim, H.-M., O'Brien, T.E.: An application of profile-likelihood based confidence interval to capture-recapture estimators. J. Agric. Biol. Environ. Stat. **1**, 131–140 (1996)
51. Wikipedia Contributors. (2018, August 7). Mark and recapture. In *Wikipedia, The Free Encyclopedia*. Retrieved 14:02, August 7, 2018, from https://en.wikipedia.org/w/index.php?title=Mark_and_recapture&oldid=853831908.
52. Carlin, B.P., Louis, T.A.: Bayesian methods for data analysis, 3rd edn. Chapman & Hall/CRC, Boca Raton, FL (2009)
53. Brown, L.D., Cai, T.T., DasGupta, A.: Interval estimation for a binomial proportion. Stat. Sci. **16**, 101–133 (2001)
54. Sangeetha, U., Subbiah, M., Srinivasan, M.R.: Estimation of confidence intervals for multinomial proportions of sparse contingency tables using Bayesian methods. Int. J. Sci. Res. Publ. **3**, 1–7 (2013)

55. Efron, B.: Nonparametric standard errors and confidence intervals. Can. J. Stat. **9**, 139–158 (1981)
56. Lee, S.M., Hwang, W.H., Huang, L.H.: Bayes estimation of population size from capture-recapture models with time variation and behavior response. Stat. Sin. **13**, 477–494 (2003)
57. Tilling, K.: Capture-recapture methods—useful or misleading? Int. J. Epidemiol. **30**, 12–14 (2001)

A Uniform Shrinkage Prior in Spatiotemporal Poisson Models for Count Data

Krisada Lekdee, Chao Yang, Lily Ingsrisawang, and Yisheng Li

1 Introduction

Data collected across both time and space are found in various applications, such as agriculture, climatology, ecology, economy, epidemiology, geography, and geology. These data are usually collected in each area at different points of time. Therefore, the analysis should take into account the spatial correlation across the areas and temporal correlation within each area. In Thailand, the Ministry of Public Health [1] releases a yearly report for all common infectious diseases, such as cholera, dengue fever, hepatitis, leptospirosis, malaria, rabies, and tuberculosis. Disease maps are useful tools to present these data to the reader in an intuitive as well as informative manner [2].

Disease mapping has played a key role in spatial epidemiology. It is useful for several purposes, such as identifying suspected areas at elevated disease risk, assisting in the formulation of hypotheses about disease etiology, and assessing potential needs for follow-up studies on geographic variation, preventive measures,

Krisada Lekdee and Chao Yang co-first author.

K. Lekdee
Faculty of Science and Technology, Department of Mathematics and Statistics, Rajamangala University of Technology Phra Nakhon, Bangkok, Thailand

C. Yang · Y. Li (✉)
Department of Biostatistics, University of Texas MD Anderson Cancer Center, Houston, TX, USA
e-mail: ysli@mdanderson.org

L. Ingsrisawang
Faculty of Science, Department of Statistics, Kasetsart University, Bangkok, Thailand

Y. Zhao, (Din) D.-G. Chen (eds.), *Modern Statistical Methods for Health Research*, Emerging Topics in Statistics and Biostatistics,
https://doi.org/10.1007/978-3-030-72437-5_4

or other forms of health resource allocation [3]. A number of models have been developed for disease mapping. For example, Kleinschmidt [4] used a generalized linear mixed model (GLMM) with spatial and temporal random effects for modeling and mapping malaria risks in Africa. Kazembe et al. [5] applied a bivariate ordinary logistic regression model including a spatial component to predict and map malaria risks in Malawi, using point-referenced prevalence of infection data.

Our focus in this paper is not to develop new models to account for the spatial effects for spatiotemporal data. Rather, our main focus is to develop default priors for the variance components of the spatiotemporal random effects in a common GLMM for count data, namely, one with proper conditional autoregressive (CAR) spatial effects to account for the spatial correlation.

The CAR model has been commonly used in Bayesian disease mapping, in part due to its computational convenience in Gibbs sampling. Clayton and Kaldor [6] proposed empirical Bayesian methods built from Poisson regression with random intercepts defined with spatial correlation. The approach provided a conceptual framework that induces positive spatial correlation across the local disease rates via a CAR model. Besag et al. [7] extended the models of Clayton and Kaldor [6] to a fully Bayesian setting for mapping the disease risks. Sun et al. [8] examined the properties of the CAR models through Bayesian analysis of mortality rates. They considered Bayesian hierarchical linear mixed models where the fixed effects have vague priors, such as flat priors, and the random effects follow a class of CAR models. The resulting joint prior distribution of the regional effects is improper. Pettitt et al. [9] used a CAR formulation that permits the modelling of spatial dependence and dependence between multivariate random variables at irregularly spaced sites. They demonstrated the use of models in analysis of bivariate binary data where the observed data are modeled as the sign of a hidden CAR process. Johnson [10] used the model of Besag et al. [7] for prostate cancer incidence data in New York State. Zhu et al. [11] also used the model of Besag et al. [7] for alcohol availability, drug "hot spots," and violent crime. Zacarias and Andersson [12] used a GLMM with spatial and temporal effects to analyze the spatial and temporal patterns of malaria incidence in Maputo province, Mozambique. The spatial dependence is introduced through the CAR process. Lekdee and Ingsrisawang [13] used GLMMs with spatial CAR effects to estimate the dengue fever risks in Thailand and used the estimated risks for the dengue fever mapping.

In a conventional Bayesian GLMM with proper CAR spatial effects, the most commonly used priors for the variance components of the spatiotemporal random effects are the inverse gamma (IG) or inverse Wishart (IW) priors, due to the computational convenience associated with the use of the Gibbs sampler for posterior inference. However, Daniels [14], Natarajan and Kass [15], and Gelman [16], among others, noted difficulties in using vague IG or IW priors for the variance components or covariance matrix in GLMMs. In particular, in the limit that the two hyperparameters of an IG prior approach zero, the posterior distribution becomes improper [17]. Therefore, a lack of default recommendation on the use of the scale and shape parameters of the IG prior becomes a concern. Similarly, posterior inference may be sensitive to the choice of the scale and shape parameters in the IW priors for the random-effect covariance matrix in the GLMMs [15].

To address the above difficulties with the IG and IW priors, Daniels [14] and Natarajan and Kass [15] proposed uniform shrinkage priors (USPs) for the variance components or covariance matrix in GLMMs where the observations from different clusters (subjects) are assumed independent. The USP is attractive because it is noninformative and proper (thus may yield a proper posterior) and has a default specification (unlike the "vague" IG or IW priors). Both Daniels [14] and Natarajan and Kass [15] have demonstrated desirable performance of the posterior inference resulting from the use of the USPs. However, due to the restriction in their applicable model structure, namely, that the random effects are assumed independent and the associated random-effect design matrix needs to be block-diagonal, wide use of USPs is limited in practice. To address the above limitation in the required model structure, Li et al. [18] extended USPs to semiparametric mixed models for longitudinal data in which the smoothing spline-induced scalar random effects are allowed to have a non-diagonal design matrix. However, to the best of our knowledge, USPs for variance components in spatiotemporal GLMMs have not been developed.

In this paper, we develop default Bayesian inference for a Poisson GLMM with proper CAR spatial effects by developing a USP for the variance components of the spatiotemporal random effects. In particular, the definition of a USP for the variance component of the spatial effects conditional on the covariance matrix of the temporal random effects is made possible by the fact that the scalar spatial effects allow us to use a Cholesky decomposition along with an additional orthogonal transformation to transform a shrinkage matrix to diagonal, thus reducing the model to a similar case of Li et al. [18], where a USP can be defined. Vague priors are also proposed for the fixed-effect and other model parameters as part of the default inference approach, which is also justified with a lack of prior information available on these model parameters in the data example considered in this paper.

In most GLMMs for spatiotemporal data, there is an identifiability issue between the temporal random effects capturing heterogeneity across regions and spatial effects for modeling spatial correlations, as only the sums of these random effects are typically identifiable [19]. The same issue is present in the Poisson GLMM with CAR spatial effects considered in this paper. Our focus, however, is on the development of default priors for the variance components and the resulting inference on the identifiable part of the model parameters, namely, the fixed effects that are used for estimating disease incidence rates that also involve the prediction of the sums of the temporal and spatial random effects.

The proposed method is motivated by disease mapping using a leptospirosis dataset of Thailand [1]. Leptospirosis is one of the major public health problems in Thailand. The outcome data are the numbers of leptospirosis patients in 17 northern Thai provinces across 4 quarters in 2011. The researchers are also interested in learning whether rainfall and temperature are associated with the leptospirosis risks.

The paper is organized as follows. In Sect. 2, we present the proposed Poisson default Bayesian GLMM with CAR spatial effects for spatiotemporal data. Specifically, we develop a USP for the variance components of the spatiotemporal random effects. We apply the proposed model to analyze the leptospirosis data of Thailand to draw the disease maps in Sect. 3. OpenBUGS and R2OpenBUGS are used to implement the posterior inference. We compare the performance of the developed USP with the conventional IG priors for the variance components using the deviance information criterion (DIC) [20, 21]. In Sect. 4, we conduct a simulation study to evaluate the accuracy of the parameter estimates under the proposed USP. The RStan package is used for posterior inference in the simulation study. In Sect. 5, we conclude with a discussion.

2 Derivation of a USP for the Variance Components in GLMM with Proper CAR and Its Properties

2.1 Derivation of the USP

A Poisson GLMM with proper CAR spatial effects is defined as follows. Conditional on the temporal random effects $\boldsymbol{b}_i$ and spatial random effects v_i, y_{it} are assumed independent and follow a Poisson distribution

$$y_{it} \mid \boldsymbol{b}_i, v_i \sim \text{Pois}\left(\mu_{it}\right), \tag{1}$$

where

$$\log\left(\mu_{it}\right) \triangleq \eta_{it} = \mathbf{x}_{it}^T \boldsymbol{\beta} + \mathbf{z}_{it}^T \mathbf{b}_i + v_i, \tag{2}$$

with $E(y_{it}|\boldsymbol{b}_i, v_i) = \mu_{it}$, $\boldsymbol{\beta}$ being a $p \times 1$ vector of fixed-effect coefficients for covariates $\boldsymbol{x}_{it}$, $\boldsymbol{b}_i$ being a $q \times 1$ vector of temporal random-effect coefficients for covariates z_{it}, and y_{it} being marginally correlated counts from area $i = 1, \ldots, m$, at time $t = 1, \ldots, n_i$, respectively. For simplicity, we assume $\boldsymbol{b}_i \overset{\text{iid}}{\sim} N\left(\mathbf{0}, \boldsymbol{D}\right)$. However, the proposed method can be extended to cases where $\boldsymbol{b}_i$ are assumed to have a nonparametric distribution, e.g., with a Dirichlet process prior [22].

Let $\boldsymbol{v} = (v_1, \ldots, v_m)^T$, where the spatial effects v_i are assumed to follow a zero-centered proper CAR model [23, 24]:

$$v_i \mid v_{(-i)} \sim N\left(\rho \sum\nolimits_{j=1}^{m} \frac{w_{ij} v_j}{w_{i+}}, \frac{{\tau_v}^2}{w_{i+}}\right) \tag{3}$$

with $v_{(-i)} = \{v_j : j \neq i\}$. Through Brook's Lemma [25], we have

$$\boldsymbol{v} \sim N\left(\mathbf{0}, {\tau_v}^2 (\boldsymbol{D}_w - \rho \boldsymbol{W})^{-1}\right),$$

where $\boldsymbol{W} = (w_{ij})$ is a neighborhood matrix for areal units, defined as

$$w_{ij} = \begin{cases} 1 \text{ if subregions } i \text{ and j share a common boundary}, i \neq j \\ 0 \text{ otherwise} \end{cases},$$

$\boldsymbol{D}_w =$ diag (w_{i+}) is a diagonal matrix with the (i, i)-th entry equal to $w_{i+} = \sum_j w_{ij}$, ${\tau_v}^2$ is the variance of v_i, and ρ is a spatial parameter with value in (0,1). The model does not include an offset term. However, this can be straightforwardly incorporated, as necessary.

For prior specification, an independent normal distribution with a zero mean and a large variance, such as 10^6, is assigned to each element of the fixed-effect vector $\boldsymbol{\beta}$; a uniform$(0, 1)$ prior is assumed for the spatial parameter ρ. Following the work of Daniels [14], Natarajan and Kass [15], and Li et al. [18], USP for the variance components in a GLMM with proper CAR spatial effects can be developed as follows.

For each area, Eq. (2) can be rewritten as

$$\boldsymbol{\eta}_i = \boldsymbol{X}_i\boldsymbol{\beta} + \boldsymbol{Z}_i\boldsymbol{b}_i + \mathbf{1}v_i, \tag{4}$$

where $\mathbf{1}\,(n_i \times 1) = \left(1, \ldots, 1\right)_{n_i}^T$, $\boldsymbol{X}_i\,(n_i \times p) = \left[\boldsymbol{x}_{i1}{}^T; \ldots; \boldsymbol{x}_{in_i}{}^T\right]$, a vertical concatenation of $\boldsymbol{x}_{i1}{}^T$, …, $\boldsymbol{x}_{in_i}{}^T$, and $\boldsymbol{Z}_i(n_i \times q)$, $\boldsymbol{\eta}_i(n_i \times q)$, and $\boldsymbol{y}_i(n_i \times 1)$ are defined similarly. Across all areas, we have

$$\boldsymbol{\eta} = \boldsymbol{X\beta} + \boldsymbol{Zb} + \boldsymbol{Sv} \tag{5}$$

where

$$\boldsymbol{S}\,(n \times m) = \begin{pmatrix} \mathbf{1}_{n_1} & \mathbf{0}_{n_1} & . & . & . & \mathbf{0}_{n_1} \\ \mathbf{0}_{n_2} & \mathbf{1}_{n_2} & \mathbf{0}_{n_2} & . & . & \mathbf{0}_{n_2} \\ \mathbf{0}_{n_3} & \mathbf{0}_{n_3} & \mathbf{1}_{n_3} & \mathbf{0}_{n_3} & . & \mathbf{0}_{n_3} \\ . & . & . & . & . & . \\ \mathbf{0}_{n_m} & . & . & . & . & \mathbf{1}_{n_m} \end{pmatrix}, \mathbf{1}\,(n_i \times 1) = \left(1, \ldots, 1\right)_{n_i}^T, \mathbf{0}\,(n_i \times 1)$$
$$=(0, \ldots, 0)_{n_i}{}^T, \boldsymbol{X}\,(n \times p) = \left(\boldsymbol{X}_1{}^T, \ldots, \boldsymbol{X}_p{}^T\right)^T, n = \textstyle\sum_{i=1}^m n_i,$$

and $\boldsymbol{Z}(n \times mq)$, $\boldsymbol{v}(m \times 1)$, $\boldsymbol{b}(mq \times 1)$, $\boldsymbol{\eta}(n \times 1)$, and $\boldsymbol{y}(n \times 1)$ are defined similarly.

In a Poisson GLMM with proper CAR spatial effects, a shrinkage matrix for each individual random effect vector $(\boldsymbol{b}_i)$ cannot be readily defined because the observations are correlated across areas due to the spatial CAR effects. Therefore, there is no shrinkage matrix associated with each $\boldsymbol{b}_i$. Because the v_i's are correlated, there is no readily defined shrinkage coefficient associated with each v_i, either. Following the work of Li et al. [18], we define a new joint USP for $(\boldsymbol{D}, {\tau_v}^2, \rho)$ as $\pi(\boldsymbol{D}, {\tau_v}^2, \rho) = \pi(\mathbf{D}, {\tau_v}^2 | \rho)\pi(\rho) = \pi({\tau_v}^2 | \boldsymbol{D}, \rho)\pi(\mathbf{D})\pi(\rho)$, with $\pi(\boldsymbol{D})$ being a marginal USP for $\boldsymbol{D}$ and $\tau_v^2 \mid \boldsymbol{D}, \rho$ being a conditional USP for τ_v^2 given $\boldsymbol{D}$ and ρ. Following Banerjee et al. [26], we assume $\pi(\rho) \sim$ uniform(0, 1).

To develop $\pi(\boldsymbol{D})$, Eq. (4) is simplified by temporarily removing the spatial effects ($\mathbf{1}v_i$) from the model [18, 27]. Then we get

$$\boldsymbol{\eta}_i = \boldsymbol{X}_i\boldsymbol{\beta} + \boldsymbol{Z}_i\boldsymbol{b}_i. \tag{6}$$

Based on the work of Natarajan and Kass [15], an average shrinkage matrix for the posterior mean of $\boldsymbol{b}_i$ conditional on $\boldsymbol{\beta}$ in Eq. (6) can be defined as

$$\left(\boldsymbol{D}^{-1} + \frac{1}{m}\sum\nolimits_{i=1}^{m} \boldsymbol{Z}_i^{\,T}\boldsymbol{E}_i^{\,-1}\boldsymbol{Z}_i\right)^{-1} \frac{1}{m}\sum\nolimits_{i=1}^{m} \boldsymbol{Z}_i^{\,T}\boldsymbol{E}_i^{\,-1}\boldsymbol{Z}_i, \tag{7}$$

where $\mathbf{E}_i$ is the diagonal weight matrix from the generalized linear model (GLM) based off Eq. (4), i.e., $\boldsymbol{\eta}_i = \boldsymbol{X}_i\boldsymbol{\beta}$ [15]. By placing a uniform prior on expression (7), an approximate USP for $\boldsymbol{D}$ results as

$$\pi\left(\boldsymbol{D}\right) \propto \left|\boldsymbol{I} + \left\{\frac{1}{m}\sum\nolimits_{i=1}^{m} \boldsymbol{Z}_i^{\,T}\boldsymbol{E}_i^{\,-1}\boldsymbol{Z}_i\right\}\boldsymbol{D}\right|^{-q-1}.$$

To derive a USP for $\tau_v^2 \mid \boldsymbol{D}, \rho$, we use Eq. (5). To make the elements of $\boldsymbol{v}$ uncorrelated, a Cholesky decomposition is applied. For a covariance matrix $\boldsymbol{A}$, the Cholesky decomposition is defined as

$$\boldsymbol{A} = \boldsymbol{L}\boldsymbol{L}^T = \boldsymbol{U}^T\boldsymbol{U},$$

where $\boldsymbol{L}$ is a lower triangular matrix, while $\boldsymbol{U}$ is an upper triangular matrix. $\boldsymbol{L}$ and $\boldsymbol{U}$ are interpreted as the square root of $\boldsymbol{A}$ and are called the Cholesky factor of $\boldsymbol{A}$. It is much easier to compute the inverse of a triangular matrix, and there exist numerical solutions. Then the inverse of the original matrix is computed simply by multiplying the two inverses as

$$\boldsymbol{A}^{-1} = \left(\boldsymbol{L}\boldsymbol{L}^T\right)^{-1} = \left(\boldsymbol{U}^T\boldsymbol{U}\right)^{-1}$$

$$\boldsymbol{A}^{-1} = \left(\boldsymbol{L}^{-1}\right)^T\left(\boldsymbol{L}^{-1}\right) = \left(\boldsymbol{U}^{-1}\right)\left(\boldsymbol{U}^{-1}\right)^T.$$

Thus, to make the elements of $\boldsymbol{v}$ uncorrelated, we transform $\boldsymbol{v}$ to $\boldsymbol{u}$ by defining

$$\boldsymbol{u} = (\boldsymbol{D}_w - \rho\boldsymbol{W})^{\frac{1}{2}}\boldsymbol{v}.$$

One can easily verify that cov($\mathbf{u}$) $= \tau_v^2\boldsymbol{I}$, which implies that the elements of $\boldsymbol{u}$ are uncorrelated. Equation (5) can thus be rewritten as

$$\boldsymbol{\eta} = \boldsymbol{X\beta} + \boldsymbol{Zb} + \boldsymbol{S}\Big((\boldsymbol{D}_w - \rho \boldsymbol{W})^{-1}\Big)^{\frac{1}{2}}\boldsymbol{u}. \tag{8}$$

Since $\boldsymbol{S}\big((\boldsymbol{D}_w - \rho \boldsymbol{W})^{-1}\big)^{\frac{1}{2}}$ is not diagonal, the posterior mean of each u_i conditional on $(\boldsymbol{\beta}, \boldsymbol{D}, \rho)$ cannot be expressed as a shrinkage estimator toward its prior mean ($\boldsymbol{0}$). In other words, the classical shrinkage matrix associated with $\boldsymbol{u}$ does not exist. Therefore, the methods proposed by Daniels [14] and Natarajan and Kass [15] do not apply in this case.

However, because u_i is a scalar, we can apply the approach of Li et al. [18] to define a conditional USP for $\tau_v{}^2$ given $\boldsymbol{D}$ and ρ, as follows. First, the shrinkage matrix for the posterior mean of $\boldsymbol{u}$ is obtained as

$$\left(\frac{1}{\tau_v{}^2}\boldsymbol{I} + \left(\boldsymbol{S}(\boldsymbol{D}_w - \rho\boldsymbol{W})^{-1/2}\right)^T \boldsymbol{R}^{-1}\boldsymbol{S}(\boldsymbol{D}_w - \rho\boldsymbol{W})^{-1/2}\right)^{-1}\frac{1}{\tau_v{}^2}\boldsymbol{I},$$

where $\boldsymbol{R} = \text{var}(\mathbf{y}|\,\mathbf{u}) = \mathbf{ZDZ}^T + \boldsymbol{E}$, with $\boldsymbol{E} = \text{var}(\mathbf{y})$ based on the GLM $\boldsymbol{\eta} = \boldsymbol{X\beta}$ [15]. Let $\boldsymbol{P}$ be the orthogonal matrix ($\boldsymbol{P}^T = \boldsymbol{P}^{-1}$) that satisfies

$$\left(\boldsymbol{S}(\boldsymbol{D}_w - \rho\boldsymbol{W})^{-1/2}\right)^T \boldsymbol{R}^{-1}\boldsymbol{S}(\boldsymbol{D}_w - \rho\boldsymbol{W})^{-1/2} = \boldsymbol{PAP}^T,$$

where $\boldsymbol{A}$ is a diagonal matrix with diagonal elements $\lambda_i \geq 0,\ i = 1, \ldots, m$. Hence, the shrinkage matrix is

$$\left(\frac{1}{\tau_v{}^2}\boldsymbol{I} + \boldsymbol{PAP}^T\right)^{-1}\frac{1}{\tau_v{}^2}\boldsymbol{I},$$

which is equal to

$$\boldsymbol{P}\left(\frac{1}{\tau_v{}^2}\boldsymbol{I} + \boldsymbol{A}\right)^{-1}\frac{1}{\tau_v{}^2}\boldsymbol{P}^T. \tag{9}$$

Note that the orthogonal matrix $\boldsymbol{P}$ does not depend on $\tau_v{}^2$. Therefore, a uniform prior on expression (9) is equivalent to a uniform prior on expression (10):

$$\left(\frac{1}{\tau_v{}^2}\boldsymbol{I} + \boldsymbol{A}\right)^{-1}\frac{1}{\tau_v{}^2}. \tag{10}$$

Conditional on $(\boldsymbol{D}, \rho)$, a uniform shrinkage prior for $\tau_v{}^2 \mid \boldsymbol{D}, \rho$ can thus be defined by placing a uniform prior on

$$\left(\frac{1}{\tau_v{}^2} + \bar{\lambda}\right)^{-1}\frac{1}{\tau_v{}^2}, \tag{11}$$

with $\bar{\lambda}$ being the average of the diagonal elements of $\boldsymbol{A}$ or the average of the eigenvalues λ_i of

$$\left(\boldsymbol{S}(\boldsymbol{D}_w - \rho\boldsymbol{W})^{-1/2}\right)^T \boldsymbol{R}^{-1}\boldsymbol{S}(\boldsymbol{D}_w - \rho\boldsymbol{W})^{-1/2},$$

i.e., $\bar{\lambda} = \frac{1}{m}\sum_{i=1}^{m}\lambda_i$. The reason is that the diagonalized shrinkage matrix in Eq. (10) corresponds to m shrinkage coefficients $\left(\frac{1}{\tau_v^2} + \lambda_i\right)^{-1}\frac{1}{\tau_v^2}$ along its diagonal with each being a transformation of $\tau_v{}^2$ from $(0, \infty)$ to $(0, 1)$. As a result, a uniform prior on Eq. (11) leads to a USP for $\tau_v{}^2 \mid \boldsymbol{D}, \rho$ as

$$\pi\left(\tau_v{}^2 | \boldsymbol{D}, \rho\right) \propto \frac{1}{\left(1 + \bar{\lambda}\tau_v{}^2\right)^2}.$$

2.2 Motivation of the Derived USP

1. In linear mixed models, the best linear unbiased predictor (BLUP) of the random effects is a shrinkage estimator from the least squares estimator toward the mean of the random effects ($\mathbf{0}$). The shrinkage coefficient for each individual scalar random effect predictor is a ratio between 0 and 1, as determined by the relative magnitude of the random effect variance and residual variance. The same is true for vector random effect predictors where the shrinkage coefficients are replaced by shrinkage matrices, with each shrinkage matrix being a positive-definite matrix with all eigenvalues being in (0,1).
2. Placing a uniform prior on the average shrinkage coefficient (or shrinkage matrix) across all independent and identically distributed (i.i.d.) random effect scalars (or vectors) reflects vague prior information on the anticipated random effect predictors lying between $\mathbf{0}$ and the least squares estimator, thus inducing vague prior distribution on the random effect variance (or covariance matrix). This idea has first been proposed by Strawderman [28] and later used or generalized by Christiansen and Morris [29], Daniels [14], and Natarajan and Kass [15], among others.
3. In Li et al. [18], the design matrix for the i.i.d. scalar random effects resulting from the linear mixed model representation of the cubic spline estimate of a nonparametric function of time, $f(t)$, is not block-diagonal. As a result, there does not exist a natural shrinkage coefficient associated with the BLUP of each individual random effect, making the methods proposed by Daniels [14] and Natarajan and Kass [15] inapplicable. Li et al. [18] thus propose an orthogonal transformation of the shrinkage matrix for the combined random effect vector to a diagonal matrix, made possible by the fact that the random effects are scalars (rather than vectors). Based on the idea that placing a uniform prior on a shrinkage matrix is "equivalent" to placing a uniform prior on its orthogonal

transformation, a USP can then be defined by placing a uniform prior on the average shrinkage coefficient resulting from the diagonalized shrinkage matrix for the combined random effect vector associated with the spline function estimation.

4. In a Poisson GLMM with CAR spatial effects as considered in this paper, the spatial random effects are not i.i.d. Therefore, a transformation using Cholesky decomposition may transform the scalar spatial random effects to be i.i.d., yet with a non-block-diagonal design matrix, reducing the model to a case similar to that in Li et al. [18]. Therefore, using a similar approach based on an orthogonal transformation from Li et al. [18], we are able to develop a conditional USP for the variance of the spatial random effects v_i; we can also develop a USP for the variance or covariance matrix of the temporal random effects $\boldsymbol{b}_i$ using the approach of Natarajan and Kass [15].

As for the motivation of developing a USP, as pointed out by previous authors, such as Daniels [14] and Natarajan and Kass [15], diffuse IG or inverse Wishart priors for the variance components or covariance matrix of the random effects may suffer from the following issues. First, the posteriors may be sensitive to the choice of the hyperparameters in the inverse Wishart prior even in applications with moderate sample sizes. Second, when exceedingly small specifications of the shape and scale for IG priors are used, the convergence of the Markov chains may become problematic due to the "near" impropriety of the resulting posteriors [30].

2.3 *Analytical Properties of the Derived USP*

Next we prove that $\pi(\mathbf{D}, \tau_v{}^2 | \rho)$ is proper and the resulting posterior is also proper under suitable conditions.

Theorem 1 The joint conditional USP, $\pi(\boldsymbol{D}, \tau_v{}^2 | \rho)$, is proper.

Proof By Theorem 2 of Natarajan and Kass [15], $\pi(\boldsymbol{D})$ and $\pi(\tau_v{}^2 | \boldsymbol{D}, \rho)$ are proper; then $\pi(\boldsymbol{D}, \tau_v{}^2 | \rho) = \pi(\tau_v{}^2 | \boldsymbol{D}, \rho)\pi(\boldsymbol{D})$ is proper.

Below we extend the proofs of Natarajan and Kass [15] to show that the posterior distribution is proper under the proposed USP, an independent flat prior for each fixed effect, and a uniform (0,1) prior for the spatial parameter, under suitable conditions.

Theorem 2 In a Poisson GLMM with proper CAR spatial effects as in Eq. (8), the joint posterior distribution resulting from a prior $\pi(\boldsymbol{\beta}, \boldsymbol{D}, \tau_v{}^2, \rho) \propto \pi(\boldsymbol{D}, \tau_v{}^2 | \rho)$ is proper if there exists p full rank vectors $\boldsymbol{x}_k{}^T (k = 1, \ldots, p)$ such that the integral

$$\varepsilon = \iiint \iint \prod_{k=1}^{p} \int_{-\infty}^{\infty} f\left(y_k | r_k, \boldsymbol{b}, \boldsymbol{v}, \rho\right) dr_k f\left(\boldsymbol{b} | \boldsymbol{D}\right) d\boldsymbol{b}$$
$$\pi\left(\mathbf{D}\right) d\boldsymbol{D}\; f\left(\mathbf{v} | \tau_v{}^2, \rho\right) d\boldsymbol{v}\; \pi\left(\tau_v{}^2 | \boldsymbol{D}, \rho\right) d\tau_v{}^2\; \pi\left(\rho\right) d\rho$$

is finite, where $r_k = \boldsymbol{x}_k{}^T\boldsymbol{\beta}$, and *f(.) generically denotes the density function of a random variable or vector.*

Proof The proof rests on bounding the marginal distribution of the data, $m(\boldsymbol{y})$, from above by ε.

$m(\boldsymbol{y}) = \iiint\iint\int\prod_{i=1}^{m}\prod_{t=1}^{n_i} f\left(y_{it}|\boldsymbol{\beta},\boldsymbol{b},\boldsymbol{v},\tau_v{}^2,\rho\right) f(\boldsymbol{b}|\boldsymbol{D})\, d\boldsymbol{b}\, f\left(\boldsymbol{v}|\tau_v{}^2,\rho,\right)$ $d\boldsymbol{v}\pi(\boldsymbol{D})\, d\boldsymbol{D}\pi\left(\tau_v{}^2|\boldsymbol{D},\rho\right) d\tau_v{}^2\pi(\rho)\, d\rho\pi(\beta)d\beta$ is integrable. We first examine

$$L^* \propto \iiint\prod_{i=1}^{m}\prod_{t=1}^{n_i} f(y_{it}|\boldsymbol{\beta},\boldsymbol{b},\boldsymbol{v})\, f(\boldsymbol{b}|\boldsymbol{D})\, d\boldsymbol{b}\, f\left(\boldsymbol{v}|\tau_v{}^2,\rho,\right) d\boldsymbol{v}\, d\boldsymbol{\beta}.$$

Make the transformation $r_k = \boldsymbol{x}_k{}^T\boldsymbol{\beta}$ for any p full-rank design vectors $\boldsymbol{x}_k{}^T$ (which are assumed to exist because rank($\mathbf{X}$) = p). The Jacobian of this transformation is $det(\boldsymbol{X}_*{}^{-1})$, where $\boldsymbol{X}_*(p \times p)$ has rows $\boldsymbol{x}_k{}^T$. Then ignoring the indices k that are not in $\boldsymbol{X}_*$ (because the individual components in the likelihood are bounded, these indices can be ignored), we see that $m(\boldsymbol{y})$ is bounded above by an expression proportional to ε.

Corollary 1 Under the assumptions of Theorem 2, a Poisson distribution with canonical link $log(\mu_k) = \boldsymbol{x}_k{}^T\boldsymbol{\beta} + z_k{}^T\boldsymbol{b} + v$ leads to a proper posterior distribution $\pi(\boldsymbol{\beta},\boldsymbol{D},\tau_v{}^2,\rho|\boldsymbol{y})$.

Proof We can write

$$f(y_k|r_k,\boldsymbol{b},v) \propto \exp\left(y_k\left(r_k + z_k{}^T\boldsymbol{b} + v\right) - \exp\left(r_k + z_k{}^T\boldsymbol{b} + v\right)\right).$$

Then

$$\varepsilon = \iiint\iint\left[\prod_{k=1}^{p}\int_{-\infty}^{\infty}\exp\left(y_k\left(r_k+z_k{}^T\boldsymbol{b}+v\right) - \exp\left(r_k+z_k{}^T\boldsymbol{b}+v\right)\right) dr_k\right]$$
$$\left[f(\boldsymbol{b}|\mathbf{D})\, d\boldsymbol{b}\ \pi(\mathbf{D})\, d\boldsymbol{D}.\right.$$

$$\left.\mathrm{f}\left(\mathbf{v}|\tau_v{}^2,\rho,\right) d\boldsymbol{v}\ \pi\left(\tau_v{}^2|\boldsymbol{D},\rho\right) d\tau_v{}^2\ \pi(\rho)\, d\rho\right].$$

Making the transformation $u_k = exp\left(r_k + z_k{}^T\boldsymbol{b} + v\right)$, we obtain

$$\varepsilon = \iiint\iint\prod_{k=1}^{p}\int_{-\infty}^{\infty} u_k{}^{y_k-1}\exp(-u_k)\, du_k f(\boldsymbol{b}|\boldsymbol{D})\, d\boldsymbol{b}\pi(\boldsymbol{D})$$
$$d\boldsymbol{D} f\left(\boldsymbol{v}|\tau_v{}^2,\rho,\right) d\boldsymbol{v}\pi\left(\tau_v{}^2|\boldsymbol{D},\rho\right) d\tau_v{}^2\pi(\rho)\, d\rho,$$

which is finite, if the y corresponding to the full-rank $\mathbf{x}_k{}^T$ are nonzero.

3 Application to the Leptospirosis Data

Leptospirosis [31] is an infectious disease caused by pathogenic organisms belonging to the genus *Leptospira* that are transmitted directly or indirectly from animals to humans. Virtually all mammalian species can harbor leptospires in their kidneys which act as a source of infection to human beings and other animals. However, cattle, buffaloes, horses, sheep, goats, pigs, dogs, and rodents are common reservoirs of leptospires. In particular, rodents were the first recognized carriers of leptospirosis. Leptospirosis occurs worldwide, but it is most common in tropical and subtropical areas with heavy rainfall. The disease is found mainly wherever humans come into contact with the urine of infected animals or a urine-polluted environment. Leptospirosis is endemic in many countries, and it often has a seasonal distribution, increasing with increased rainfall. However, the disease can occur throughout the year. In Thailand, leptospirosis is one of the major public health problems. According to the Thai Ministry of Public Health, Bureau of Epidemiology [32] report on leptospirosis, available in Thai, between January 2012 and August 2012, a total of 1779 cases and 27 fatalities were found in 70 provinces. The morbidity rate was 2.80 (per 100,000 population). The case fatality rate was 0.04%.

A Poisson GLMM with proper CAR spatial effects using the proposed USP for the variance components of the spatiotemporal random effects is used to analyze the quarterly leptospirosis data in 2011 from 17 northern provinces of Thailand. The dataset contains the mid-year population and the number of leptospirosis patients in each province collected from the Ministry of Public Health [1], as well as related factors, rainfall and average temperature, as collected from the Thai Meteorological Department [33]. The number of repeated measures in each area is the same and there are no missing data. Let y_{it}, $i = 1, \ldots, 17$, $t = 1, \ldots, 4$, denote the number of leptospirosis patients in province i and in quarter (Q)t. Each province contributes four quarterly observations over time. The Poisson GLMM with spatial effects is expressed as $y_{it} \mid b_i, v_i \sim \text{Pois}(\mu_{it})$, with

$$\log(\mu_{it}) = \log(pop_i) + \beta_0 + \beta_1 \text{rain}_{it} + \beta_2 \text{temp}_{it} + b_i + v_i. \tag{12}$$

Here, $\log(\text{pop}_i)$ is an offset where pop_i are the mid-year population in province i; rain_{it} are the amounts of rainfall (in mm) in province i and quarter t; temp_{it} are the average temperatures (in Celsius) in province i and quarter t; b_i are the random intercepts capturing provincial heterogeneity, or equivalently, correlation within provinces; and v_i are spatial effects capturing spatial correlation across provinces [34]. The morbidity rates in which the mid-year population of each province is used for calculation [1, 35] are defined as

$$\text{MR}_{it} = \frac{\mu_{it}}{\text{pop}_i} = \exp(\beta_0 + \beta_1 \text{rain}_{it} + \beta_2 \text{temp}_{it} + b_i + v_i).$$

We assume $N(0, \tau_b{}^2)$ for b_i, a proper CAR model in Eq. (3) for v_i, independent $N(0, 10^6)$ priors for all fixed effects (β_0, β_1, β_2), and a uniform(0, 1) prior for ρ. The proposed USP is used for $\tau_b{}^2$ and $\tau_v{}^2 \mid \tau_b{}^2, \rho$.

To implement posterior inference, we write source code in OpenBUGS and R2OpenBUGS. The OpenBUGS source code is called to be run in R2OpenBUGS. A built-in Gibbs sampler is used for posterior simulation. The potential scale reduction factor [36], or R-hat, is used for assessing the convergence of the Markov chains of the posterior samples.

To evaluate model performance, the proposed model using the USP for the variance components is compared with that using the conventional IG priors, based on the DIC [21]. Similar comparisons between the prior distributions for a model based on DIC have been shown in the GeoBUGS user manual [37]. In the method for comparison, an IG(0.5,0.0005) prior (yielding a mode of 0.0005/(0.5+1)) is assumed for both $\tau_v{}^2$ and $\tau_b{}^2$. The estimated leptospirosis morbidity rates are used to construct the disease maps, which are divided into intervals, ordered from the smallest to the largest. The disease maps for the 17 northern provinces are colored differently according to the posterior means of their morbidity rates, using a simple Paint software.

We perform Gibbs sampling with three Markov chains. Each chain contains a total of 55,000 iterations including a burn-in of 5000 iterations. Every tenth sample is stored in each chain after burn-in (a thinning of 10), resulting in a total of 15,000 samples (5000 samples from each chain) to be used to draw posterior inference. The convergence of the stored Markov chains is diagnosed by the R-hats, as follows: β_0 (R-hat = 1.0163), β_1 (R-hat = 1.0021), β_2 (R-hat = 1.0160), $\tau_b{}^2$ (R-hat = 1.0549), $\tau_v{}^2$ (R-hat = 1.0209), ρ (R-hat = 1.0017). Each R-hat is around 1.0, not greater than 1.1, indicating that the Markov chains for each of the parameters, β_0, β_1, β_2, $\tau_b{}^2$, $\tau_v{}^2$, ρ, have converged [38]. See, also, the trace plots of the stored Markov chains of the posterior samples of all parameters in Fig. 1. The posterior summaries of the fixed-effect parameters and variance components of the random effects from the Poisson GLMM with proper CAR using the proposed USP as well as IG priors are presented in Table 1.

Table 1 (under the USP) suggests that the amount of rainfall and the leptospirosis morbidity rates appear to be positively correlated. In contrast, the temperature and leptospirosis morbidity rates appear to be negatively correlated. If the amount of rainfall increases by 1 mm, the morbidity rate (per 100,000 population) increases by 0.48% (exp(0.0048) – 1.0 = 0.0048); if the temperature increases by 1 °C, the morbidity rate decreases by 1.03% (1 – exp(−0.0104) = 0.0103). However, caution needs to be taken in the interpretation of the effect of temperature as this association does not appear to be significant in the sense that the 95% posterior credible interval of its coefficient contains 0. The spatial parameter ρ is not close to zero ($\hat{\rho} = 0.5343$), suggesting that there is likely a spatial association across provinces. The variance of the spatial effects is quite large ($\tau_v{}^2 = 2.517$), as compared to the variance of the temporal random effects ($\tau_b{}^2 = 0.4281$), suggesting a relatively strong spatial correlation among adjacent provinces. In other words, the

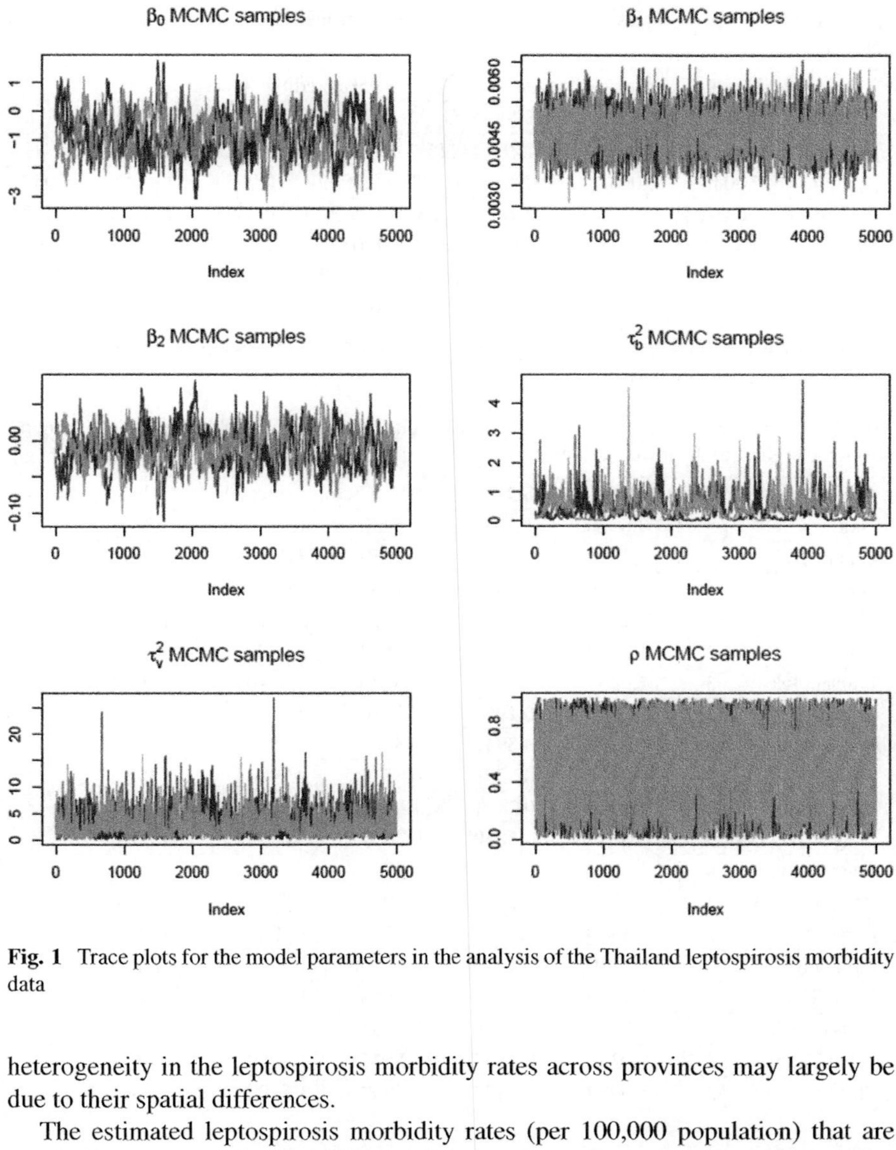

Fig. 1 Trace plots for the model parameters in the analysis of the Thailand leptospirosis morbidity data

heterogeneity in the leptospirosis morbidity rates across provinces may largely be due to their spatial differences.

The estimated leptospirosis morbidity rates (per 100,000 population) that are higher than 1.00 are shown in Table 2. The top ten estimated provincial morbidity rates, ranging from the highest to the lowest, are in Nan (Q3, 9.8060), Chiang Rai (Q3, 3.1010), Nan (Q2, 3.0190), Nan (Q4, 2.2370), Nan (Q1, 2.2330), Phitsanulok (Q3, 2.2240), Lampang (Q3, 1.7890), Uttaradit (Q3, 1.5230), Phrae (Q3, 1.4720), and Phetchabun (Q3, 1.4380), respectively.

Table 1 also presents the parameter estimates under the proposed USP versus the IG priors for the variance components of the spatiotemporal random effects, as well as the DIC for each model. The DIC of 286.2 (USP) and 342.8 (IG) for the two models suggest that the Poisson GLMM with proper CAR spatial effects using the

Table 1 Parameter estimates from Poisson GLMM with proper CAR using the proposed USPs and IG priors

	Mean		SD		95% credible interval			
Parameter	USP	IG	USP	IG	USP		IG	
β_0	−0.8024	−0.9454	0.7592	0.7691	−2.1530	0.6922	−2.4560	0.5549
β_1 (rain)	0.0048	0.0048	0.0005	0.0005	0.0039	0.0057	0.0039	0.0057
β_2 (temp)	−0.0104	−0.0069	0.0260	0.0258	−0.0621	0.0398	−0.0584	0.0437
$\tau_b{}^{2a}$	0.4281	1.1610	0.3940	0.6948	0.0120	1.3990	0.0281	2.8500
$\tau_v{}^{2a}$	2.5170	0.2835	1.9460	1.0680	0.1149	7.4430	0.0002	3.7565
ρ^a	0.5343	0.5000	0.2762	0.2860	0.0323	0.9654	0.0274	0.9709

[a]Note: Due to the model identifiability issue, inference for the variance parameters and spatial correlation may not be reliable

Table 2 Estimated provincial leptospirosis morbidity rates (per 100,000 population) ranging from the highest to the lowest values

Province	Q	Mean	SD	95% Credible interval		R-hat (mean)
Nan	3	9.8060	1.2050	7.5730	12.2700	1.0011
Chiang Rai	3	3.1010	0.4415	2.3030	4.0290	1.0010
Nan	2	3.0190	0.4643	2.1950	4.0080	1.0042
Nan	4	2.2370	0.3461	1.6170	2.9610	1.0020
Nan	1	2.2330	0.3200	1.6540	2.9000	1.0012
Phitsanulok	3	2.2240	0.3366	1.6170	2.9240	1.0014
Lampang	3	1.7890	0.2960	1.2610	2.4130	1.0013
Uttaradit	3	1.5230	0.3949	0.8529	2.3830	1.0011
Phrae	3	1.4720	0.3751	0.8374	2.2990	1.0013
Phetchabun	3	1.4380	0.2421	1.0080	1.9480	1.0010
Phayao	3	1.3740	0.3050	0.8455	2.0340	1.0010
Phitsanulok	4	1.3370	0.2041	0.9730	1.7650	1.0021
Phichit	3	1.1990	0.2987	0.7021	1.8520	1.0010
Lampang	2	1.1300	0.2159	0.7513	1.5940	1.0046
Lampang	4	1.1150	0.1990	0.7666	1.5400	1.0016
Uthai Thani	2	1.1090	0.3147	0.5868	1.8180	1.0020
Phitsanulok	2	1.0720	0.1815	0.7535	1.4590	1.0026
Uthai Thani	3	1.0350	0.2867	0.5547	1.6740	1.0011
Phayao	2	1.0080	0.2402	0.5999	1.5400	1.0021

proposed USP has a better performance. The results also show moderate differences in the parameter estimates for β_0 and β_2.

While our proposed model assumes a Poisson distribution for the disease count conditional on the temporal and spatial random effects, we have also explored additional models that account for potential overdispersion of the spatiotemporal data, namely, the negative binomial (NB), zero-inflated Poisson (ZIP), and zero-inflated negative binomial (ZINB) models [39]. The same IG(0.5,0.0005) prior for both variances $\tau_v{}^2$ and $\tau_b{}^2$ is used in each of these models. In addition, a gamma(0.0001, 0.0001) prior (with a prior mean of 0.0001/0.0001 = 1.0) is used for the real-valued version of the parameter of number of failures in the NB distribution (or Polya distribution) in the NB and ZINB models [39]. The results suggest that the ZIP and ZINB models perform worse than the proposed Poisson model with IG priors, possibly due to the small sample size (17 provinces) that limits the ability of the models to identify the probability of zero inflation, if any. In the meantime, the NB model performs similarly to (slightly better than) the proposed Poisson model with IG priors. All these models perform worse than our proposed Poisson model with USPs. Specifically, the DICs are 339.7 (NB + IG), 364.5 (ZIP + IG), 405.8 (ZINB + IG), 342.8 (Poisson + IG), and 286.2 (Poisson + USP), respectively, the last one being our proposed model.

While there is a slight improvement in the performance of the NB model over the Poisson model when both using IG priors for the random-effect variances, we emphasize that the main contribution of the paper is the introduction of USPs for the variance components of a Poisson GLMM for spatiotemporal data and that the same approach could be extended to the NB or other models that account for potential overdispersion of the data. These extensions, however, are beyond the scope of this paper.

The leptospirosis maps of the northern provinces of Thailand in Q1 to Q4 constructed from the estimated leptospirosis morbidity rates are shown in Fig. 2, which depicts the "hot spots" of the leptospirosis morbidity rates across provinces and in each quarter. It is easily seen that for every quarter the highest morbidity rate is in Nan.

4 Simulation Study

We perform a simulation study to assess the accuracy of the parameter estimates, using the relative bias as a criterion. A total of 100 datasets with 100 areas each are generated according to the spatiotemporal model (Eq. 12), with the true parameter values for β_0, β_1, β_2, τ_b^2, τ_v^2 and ρ being −0.9454, 0.8, −0.21, 1.161, 1.5, and 0.5, respectively, and the 100 offsets being simulated as i.i.d. observations from a lognormal (2.5, 1) distribution. Sampling from the posteriors is implemented using the RStan package with the No-U-Turn sampler (NUTS; [40]). Three Markov chains of 2000 iterations each were simulated with the first 1000 iterations as burn-in and thinned at every tenth for each simulated dataset, resulting in a total of 300 samples used for posterior inference. For each of a few randomly selected datasets, the R-hat is very close to 1.0 for each of the fixed-effect parameters and is slightly larger for the variance parameters (still <1.1), suggesting convergence of the chains for all parameters. The inspection of the trace plots suggests that the chains for these parameters mix well after burn-in. The relative bias for the posterior mean for each of the fixed-effect parameters is presented in Table 3. (For the variance parameters and spatial correlation, our model suffers from weak identifiability issue as mentioned in Sect. 1; thus the corresponding estimates are not reliable and

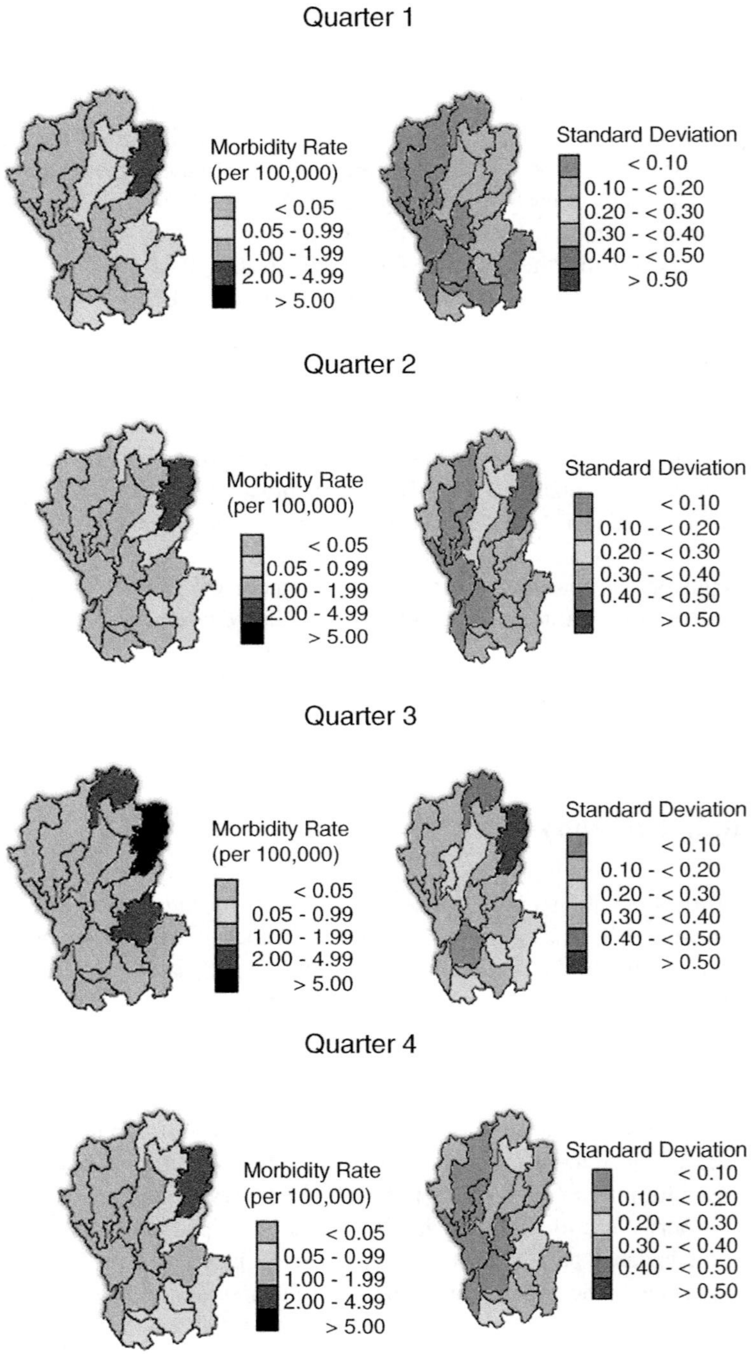

Fig. 2 Estimated leptospirosis morbidity rates and standard deviations in Q1–Q4

Table 3 Simulation results for the fixed-effect parameters

Parameter	RB	MSE	Mean of SD	SD of posterior mean	CIW	CP
β_0	−0.0153	0.0196	0.1746	0.1399	0.6690	0.9700
β_1 (rain)	0.0023	0.0002	0.0158	0.0140	0.0607	0.9800
β_2 (temperature)	−0.0050	0.0003	0.0145	0.0159	0.0561	0.9300

Note: *RB* relative bias, *MSE* mean squared error, *SD* standard deviation, *CIW* mean credible interval width, *CP* coverage probability

omitted.) For each fixed-effect parameter, the relative bias is considered small if it does not exceed 0.05 [41].

We used the NUTS for posterior sampling in the simulation study. Hamiltonian Monte Carlo (HMC) is a gradient-based MCMC method that proposes a new value through simulating trajectories according to the Hamiltonian dynamics to efficiently explore the target distribution [40, 42]. The NUTS implemented in RStan is a variant of the HMC that automatically tunes the two key hyperparameters for HMC algorithm, the step size, and trajectory length [43].

Comparing with a Gibbs sampler or a random walk Metropolis-Hastings sampler, NUTS can effectively produce less-correlated samples from a high-dimensional target distribution with strong correlations [40]. That is why convergence may be achieved even with a moderate number of posterior samples from the Markov chains for each simulated dataset.

5 Discussion

We have proposed a uniform shrinkage prior (USP) for the variance components of the spatiotemporal random effects in a Poisson GLMM with CAR spatial effects. The proposed USP is proper, has a default specification and a noninformative interpretation, and yields a proper posterior under flat priors for the fixed effects and a uniform (0,1) prior for the spatial parameter, under suitable conditions. An application of the proposed method to analyze a leptospirosis dataset that spans 17 northern provinces in Thailand across 4 quarters in 2011 suggests a good performance of the proposed USP based on the DIC, as compared with the IG priors. The analysis suggests a potentially positive and negative relationship between each of rainfall and temperature and the leptospirosis count, respectively, and a considerable spatial correlation across provinces relative to the within-province correlation over time. A simulation study suggests that the posterior estimation of the fixed-effect parameters is accurate.

It is considered an advantage to implement posterior inference for the proposed model using the noncommercial software packages OpenBUGS and R2OpenBUGS. These packages are popular for analyzing complex Bayesian statistical models using MCMC methods, sparing the need for heavy problem-specific programming. However, there are limitations in that these packages do not have a built-in function to calculate the inverse of a matrix when the elements of the matrix are not prespecified. Under a USP for the variance components, inverse operations on the matrices the elements of which are not constants are required in the model specification in OpenBUGS. Therefore, the matrix inversion must be done outside the OpenBUGS and R2OpenBUGS, i.e., in a powerful mathematical software, such as Mathematica or Maple, with the results then being taken back to the OpenBUGS. Another minor issue encountered in the model specification in OpenBUGS is that an overly long algebraic expression may not be allowed. However, in such cases, a long expression may be broken into shorter pieces. Nonetheless, all the above issues can be dealt with when another computer language, such as R, RStan, C, or C++, is used for posterior simulation and inference. That is also why the RStan package is used in posterior inference in our simulation study with a larger number of areas specified than in our data example.

Multiple extensions of the proposed methods are possible. First, the proposed method can be extended to models with additional serial correlations. For example, Eq. (2) can be extended to $\eta_{it} = \boldsymbol{x}_{it}{}^T\boldsymbol{\beta} + z_{(1)it}{}^T\boldsymbol{b}_i + z_{(2)it}{}^T\boldsymbol{u}_i + v_i$ where, in the example of quarterly data, $z_{(2)it}{}^T = (1, 1, 1, 1)$ and $\boldsymbol{u}_i = (u_{i1}, u_{i2}, u_{i3}, u_{i4})^T$. In this model, we may assume $\boldsymbol{b}_i \overset{iid}{\sim} N(\boldsymbol{0}, \boldsymbol{D})$ and $\boldsymbol{u}_i \sim N(\boldsymbol{0}, \boldsymbol{R})$, with $\boldsymbol{R}$ having a temporal autoregressive (AR)(1) correlation structure. A conditional USP for the variance of u_{it}, given the fact that each u_{it} is a scalar, can be defined using a similar approach for deriving a USP for $\tau_v{}^2 \mid \boldsymbol{D}, \rho$ as used in this paper.

Second, while we have assumed a normal distribution for $\boldsymbol{b}_i$ in the paper, future work can relax this assumption and allow for a Dirichlet process prior for the distribution of $\boldsymbol{b}_i$. The analysis process will remain similar except in two aspects. Firstly, posterior sampling of the full conditionals of $\boldsymbol{b}_i$ will follow a similar Pólya urn scheme as in the literature, e.g., in Li et al. [22] and Kleinman and Ibrahim [44]. Secondly, inference for the fixed-effect intercept β_0 needs to address an additional identifiability issue, e.g., by following a center-adjusted inference procedure proposed by Li et al. [22] or alternatively, by using an approximation approach based on truncation of the stick-breaking representation of the Dirichlet process [45], which may be implemented using DPpackage v1.1-7.4 [46].

Third, the USPs may be extended to other models for spatiotemporal count data, such as the negative binomial models, zero-inflated Poisson models, and zero-inflated negative binomial models (e.g., [47]), all of which are potentially useful candidates for modeling overdispersion of the data as compared with the Poisson models. Other extensions of the USP may include for GLMMs for binary or other non-normal outcome data.

References

1. MOPH: Report on leptospirosis (2011). Available Source: http://www.boe.moph.go.th/boedb/surdata/506wk/y55/d43_3155.pdf. Accessed 8 Nov 2012.
2. Lawson, A.B.: Bayesian disease mapping: hierarchical modeling in spatial epidemiology, 2nd edn. Chapman & Hall/CRC Interdisciplinary Statistics, New York (2013)

3. Bailey, T.C.: Spatial statistical methods in health. Cae. Saude Ppublica, Rio de Janeiro. **17**(5), 1083–1098 (2001)
4. Kleinschmidt, I.: Spatial statistical analysis, modelling and mapping of malaria in Africa. Ph.D thesis. Faculty of Philosophy and Natural Sciences, University of Basel (2001).
5. Kazembe, L.N., Kleinschmidt, I., Holtz, T.H., Sharp, B.L.: Spatial analysis and mapping of malaria risk in Malawi using point referenced prevalence of infection data. Int. J. Health Geogr. **5**, 41 (2006)
6. Clayton, D.G., Keldor, J.: Empirical Bayes estimates of age-standardized relative risks for use in disease mapping. Biometrics. **43**, 671–691 (1987)
7. Basag, J., York, J., Mollie, A.: Bayesian image restoration with two applications in spatial statistics. Ann. Inst. Stat. Math. **43**, 1–59 (1991)
8. Sun, D., Sutakawa, R.K., Kim, H., He, Z.: Spatiotemporal interaction with disease mapping. Stat. Med. **19**, 2015–2035 (2000)
9. Pettitt, A., Weir, I., Hart, A.: Conditional autoregressive Gaussian process for irregularly spaced multivariate data with application to modelling large sets of binary data. Stat. Comput. **12**, 353–367 (2002)
10. Johnson, G.D.: Smoothing small area maps of prostate cancer incidence in New York State (USA) using fully Bayesian hierarchical modelling. Int. J. Health Geogr. **3**, 29 (2004)
11. Zhu, L., Gorman, D.M., Horel, S.: Hierarchical Bayesian spatial models for alcohol availability, drug "hot spots" and violent crime. Int. J. Health Geogr. **5**, 54 (2006)
12. Zacarias, O.P., Andersson, M.: Spatial and temporal patterns of malaria incidence in Mozambique. Malar. J. **10**, 189 (2011)
13. Lekdee, K., Ingsrisawang, L.: Generalized linear mixed models with spatial random effects for spatiotemporal data: an application to dengue fever mapping. J. Math. Stat. **9**, 137–143 (2013)
14. Daniels, M.J.: A prior for the variance in hierarchical models. Can. J. Stat. **27**, 569–580 (1999)
15. Natarajan, R., Kass, R.E.: Reference Bayesian methods for generalized linear mixed models. J. Am. Stat. Assoc. **95**, 227–237 (2000)
16. Gelman, A.: Prior distributions for variance parameters in hierarchical models. Bayesian Anal. **1**, 515–533 (2006)
17. Hobert, J., Casella, G.: The effect of improper priors on Gibbs sampling in hierarchical linear mixed models. J. Am. Stat. Assoc. **91**, 1461–1473 (1996)
18. Li, Y., Lin, X., Müller, P.: Bayesian inference in semiparametric mixed models for longitudinal data. Biometrics. **66**(1), 70–78 (2010)
19. Eberly, L.E., Carlin, B.P.: Identifiability and convergence issues for Markov chain Monte Carlo fitting of spatial models. Stat. Med. **19**, 2279–2294 (2000)
20. Spiegelhalter, D., Thomas, A., Best, N., Lunn, D.: WinBUGS Version 1.4 User Manual. MRC Biostatistics Unit. Institute of PublicHealth, London (2004)
21. WinBUGS: The BUGS Project: DIC. MRC Biostatistics Unit, Cambridge (2012). Available Source: http://dvorak.mrc-bsu.cam.ac.uk/bugs/winbugs/dicpage.shtml. Accessed 8 Dec 2012.
22. Li, Y., Müller, P., Lin, X.: Center-adjusted inference for a nonparametric Bayesian random effect distribution. Stat. Sin. **21**(3), 1201–1223 (2011)
23. Basag, J.: Spatial interaction and the statistical analysis of lattice systems (with Discussion). J. R. Stat. Soc. Ser. B. **36**, 192–236 (1974)
24. Cressie, N.A.C.: Statistics for Spatial Data. Wiley, New York (1993)
25. Brook, D.: On the distinction between the conditional probability and the joint probability approaches in the specification of nearest-neighbour systems. Biometrika. **51**, 481–483 (1964)
26. Banerjee, S., Carlin, B.P., Gelfand, A.E.: Hierarchical modeling and analysis for spatial data. Chapman and Hall/CRC Press, FL (2004)
27. Breslow, N.E., Clayton, D.G.: Approximate Inference in Generalized Linear Mixed Models. J. Am. Stat. Assoc. **88**, 9–25 (1993)
28. Strawderman, W.E.: Proper Bayes minimax estimators of the multivariate normal mean. Ann. Math. Stat. **42**, 385–388 (1971)
29. Christiansen, C.L., Morris, C.N.: Hierarchical Poisson regression modeling. J. Am. Stat. Assoc. **92**, 618–632 (1997)

30. Natarajan, R., McCulloch, C.: Gibbs sampling with diffuse proper priors: a valid approach to data-driven inference? J. Comput. Graph. Stat. **7**, 267–277 (1998)
31. WHO: Leptospirosis. (2013). Available Source: http://www.searo.who.int/about/administration_structure/cds/CDS_leptospirosis-Fact_Sheet.pdf?ua=1. Accessed 9 Feb 2013.
32. BOE: Leptospirosis (2012). Available Source: http://www.boe.moph.go.th/boedb/surdata/disease.php?dcontent=old&ds=43. Accessed 18 Jan 2013.
33. TMD: Weather. (2011). Available Source: http://www.tmd.go.th/en/. Accessed 8 Nov 2012.
34. Bernardinelli, L., Clayton, D.G., Pascutto, C., Montomoli, C., Ghislandi, M., Songini, M.: Bayesian analysis of space-time variation in disease risk. Stat. Med. **14**, 2433–2443 (1995)
35. PHE: Quarterly analyses: mandatory MRSA, MSSA and E. coli Bacteraemia and CDI in England (up to July-September 2013). (2013). Available Source: http://www.hpa.org.uk/webc/hpawebfile/hpaweb_c/1284473407318. Accessed 15 Dec 2013.
36. Gelman, A., Rubin, D.B.: Inference from iterative simulation using multiple sequences. Stat. Sci. **7**, 457–472 (1992)
37. Thomas, A., Best, N., Lunn, D., Arnold, R., Spiegelhalter, D.: Geobugs User Manual. (2004). Available Source: http://www.openbugs.net/Manuals/GeoBUGS/Manual.html.
38. SAS: SAS/STAT(R) 9.2 User's Guide. 2nd ed. (2012). Available Source: https://support.sas.com/documentation/cdl/en/statug/63033/HTML/default/viewer.htm#statug_introbayes_sect007.htm. Accessed 9 Feb 2013.
39. Ntzoufras, I.: Bayesian modeling using WINBUGS, vol. 698, pp. 282–295. John Wiley & Sons, New York (2011)., Chapter 8.3
40. Hoffman, M.D., Gelman, A.: The No-U-Turn sampler: adaptively setting path lengths in Hamiltonian Monte Carlo. J. Mach. Learn. Res. **15**(1), 1593–1623 (2014)
41. Moineddin, R., Matheson, F.I., Glazier, R.H.: A simulation study of sample size for multilevel logistic regression models. BMC Med. Res. Methodol. **7**, 34 (2007)
42. Wang, Z., Mohamed, S., Freitas, N.: Adaptive Hamiltonian and Riemann Manifold Monte Carlo. In International Conference on Machine Learning. (2013), pp. 1462–1470.
43. Robert, C.P., Elvira, V., Tawn, N., Wu, C.: Accelerating MCMC algorithms. Wiley Interdiscip. Rev. Comput. Statis. **10**(5), e1435 (2018)
44. Kleinman, K.P., Ibrahim, J.G.: A semi-parametric Bayesian approach to generalized linear mixed models. Stat. Med. **17**(22), 2579–2596 (1998)
45. Yang, M., Dunson, D.B.: Semiparametric Bayes hierarchical models with mean and variance constraints. Computat. Statis. Data Anal. **54**, 2172–2186 (2010)
46. Jara, A., Hanson, T., Quintana, F.A., Müller, P., Rosner, G.L.: DPpackage: Bayesian Semi- and Nonparametric Modeling in R. J. Stat. Softw. **40**, 5 (2011)
47. Neelon, B.: Bayesian Zero-inflated negative binomial regression based on Pólya-gamma mixtures. Bayesian Anal. **14**(3), 829–855 (2019)

A Review of Multiply Robust Estimation with Missing Data

Sixia Chen and David Haziza

1 Introduction

Missing values are virtually certain to occur in clinical trials, epidemiology, economics, and sample surveys. Simply ignoring the missing values in statistical analyses may lead to invalid inferences due to the inherent nonresponse bias. Adjusting for the bias can be achieved through different approaches, including imputation and propensity score weighting. Regardless of the approach used to handle the missing values, the validity of the resulting estimators relies on the validity of an underlying model. Estimators based on propensity score weighting require the specification of a propensity score model, which is a set of assumptions about the mechanism generating the missing values. Estimators based on imputation require the specification of an imputation model, which is a set of assumptions about the distribution of the study variable subject to missingness. To improve the robustness against model misspecification, one can incorporate both models at the estimation stage, which leads to doubly robust (DR) estimation procedures; see [2, 17, 19, 20], among others. DR procedures are attractive because the resulting estimators are consistent if either the propensity score model or the imputation model is correctly specified.

To further improve the robustness of DR estimation procedures, Han and Wang [15] proposed a multiply robust (MR) approach based on the empirical likelihood method. The idea is to combine the information from multiple propensity

S. Chen (✉)
University of Oklahoma Health Sciences Center, Oklahoma City, OK, USA
e-mail: sixia-chen@ouhsc.edu

D. Haziza
Department of Mathematics and Statistics, University of Ottawa, Ottawa, ON, Canada
e-mail: dhaziza@uottawa.ca

Y. Zhao, (Din) D.-G. Chen (eds.), *Modern Statistical Methods for Health Research*, Emerging Topics in Statistics and Biostatistics,
https://doi.org/10.1007/978-3-030-72437-5_5

score models and/or multiple imputation models to construct point estimators. MR estimators are consistent if all but one model are misspecified. While Han and Wang [15] proposed to combine the model information through a calibration procedure, [10] used refitting procedures to achieve the same goal. Chen and Haziza [5] extended the procedure of [15] to handle survey data. Chen and Haziza [6] extended the approach of [10] in the context of zero-inflated distributions in surveys. Chen and Haziza [7] proposed a nonparametric multiply robust multiple imputation procedure, where one can safely use Rubin's point and variance formula [23], which is attractive from a secondary user's perspective.

Some motivations of using multiply robust procedures are listed as follows. In particular, MR procedures may be useful in the presence of a large number of predictors. In this case, it may be difficult to build a model describing the relationship between study variable and predictors that makes all other models out of consideration. Even with the recent techniques of variable selection, different levels of tuning may lead to different models. Building an enlarged model would be an option, but the estimation of model parameters may be problematic if the dimension of predictors is large. In practice, we propose to select a set of reasonable candidate models through different variable selection procedures, each based on different levels of tuning, and to incorporate the selected models simultaneously. MR procedures are also useful when it is required to transform the data prior to imputation. Selecting an appropriate transformation may be difficult unless the sample size is very large. In this case, one may use several imputation models, each based on a different transformation. Finally, we give the example of a binary variable. In practice, the imputation procedures are often based on a logistic regression model. However, if the functional is misspecified, then the resulting estimator may be biased. MR procedures allow the use of multiple models, each based on a different functional. In the context of survey data, it is important to account for the characteristics of the survey design such as stratification, sampling weights, and clustering. With multiple models, it is possible to postulate some models that include the sampling weights and other models that do not include them. One does not have to decide whether or not to use the sampling weights, which is an attractive property.

In this paper, we review three MR procedures for handling missing data: Calibration approach, Projection approach, and Multiple imputation approach. We compare the three methods in a simulation study and a real application. The paper is organized as follows. The setup and some notation are introduced in Sect. 2. Three MR procedures are described in Sect. 3. The results of a limited simulation study, which compares the three approaches in terms of bias and efficiency, are presented in Sect. 4. We present a real application based on 2015–2016 NHANES data in Sect. 5. Section 6 contains some further discussions of MR approaches and future research directions.

2 Basic Setups

Let $(\mathbf{X}_i, Y_i), i = 1, 2, \ldots, n$, be a random sample generated from the following regression model:

$$Y_i = m(\mathbf{X}_i; \boldsymbol{\beta}) + \epsilon_i, \tag{1}$$

where $\mathbf{X}$ is a q dimensional predictor, Y denotes the study variable, and $m(\cdot; \boldsymbol{\beta})$ is an unknown function with unknown parameter $\boldsymbol{\beta}$. The errors ϵ_i are assumed to be independent with $E(\epsilon_i|\mathbf{X}_i) = 0$ and $V(\epsilon_i|\mathbf{X}_i) = \sigma^2 h(\mathbf{X}_i)$, where $h(\cdot)$ is a known function and σ^2 is an unknown parameter. Denote s as the set of sampled units and we assume that the vector $\mathbf{X}_i$ is observed for all $i \in s$ but that the study variable Y may be subject to missingness. Let R_i be a response indicator associated with unit i such that $R_i = 1$ if Y_i is observed and $R_i = 0$, otherwise. We assume that

$$\Pr(R_i = 1|\mathbf{X}_i, Y_i) = \Pr(R_i = 1|\mathbf{X}_i) \triangleq p(\mathbf{X}_i; \boldsymbol{\alpha}), \tag{2}$$

where $p(\mathbf{X}_i; \boldsymbol{\alpha})$ is an unknown function with unknown parameter $\boldsymbol{\alpha}$. Assumption (2) is the customary Missing At Random assumption [22]. Let $s_r = \{i \in s : r_i = 1\}\}$ and $s_m = \{i \in s : r_i = 0\}\}$ denote the set of respondents and nonrespondents to item Y, respectively.

We are interested in estimating the population mean of Y, denoted by $\theta_0 = E(Y)$. The imputed estimator of θ_0 based on the working model $\tilde{m}(\mathbf{X}; \boldsymbol{\beta})$ is defined as

$$\widehat{\theta}_I = \frac{1}{n} \sum_{i \in s} \left\{ R_i Y_i + (1 - R_i)\tilde{m}(\mathbf{X}_i; \widehat{\boldsymbol{\beta}}) \right\}, \tag{3}$$

where $\widehat{\boldsymbol{\beta}}$ can be obtained by solving the following estimating equations:

$$S_m(\boldsymbol{\beta}) = \frac{1}{n} \sum_{i \in s_r} \{Y_i - \tilde{m}(\mathbf{X}_i; \boldsymbol{\beta})\} \frac{1}{h(\mathbf{X}_i)} \frac{\partial \tilde{m}(\mathbf{X}_i; \boldsymbol{\beta})}{\partial \boldsymbol{\beta}} = 0. \tag{4}$$

The validity of (3) depends on the validity of the imputation model. Alternatively, we can use the propensity score weighted estimator

$$\widehat{\theta}_P = \frac{1}{n} \sum_{i \in s} \frac{R_i}{\tilde{p}(\mathbf{X}_i; \widehat{\boldsymbol{\alpha}})} Y_i, \tag{5}$$

where $\tilde{p}(\mathbf{X}; \boldsymbol{\alpha})$ is a working propensity score model and $\widehat{\boldsymbol{\alpha}}$ can be obtained by solving the following estimating equations:

$$S_p(\boldsymbol{\alpha}) = \frac{1}{n} \sum_{i \in s} \frac{R_i - \tilde{p}(\mathbf{X}_i; \boldsymbol{\alpha})}{\tilde{p}(\mathbf{X}_i; \boldsymbol{\alpha}) \{1 - \tilde{p}(\mathbf{X}_i; \boldsymbol{\alpha})\}} \frac{\partial \tilde{p}(\mathbf{X}_i; \boldsymbol{\alpha})}{\partial \boldsymbol{\alpha}} = 0. \tag{6}$$

The validity of the above propensity score weighted estimator depends on the validity of the propensity score model. To improve the robustness against the failure of underlying model assumptions, one can use the following doubly robust estimator of θ_0:

$$\widehat{\theta}_{DR} = \frac{1}{n}\sum_{i\in s}\frac{R_i}{\tilde{p}(\mathbf{X}_i;\boldsymbol{\alpha})}Y_i + \frac{1}{n}\sum_{i\in s}\left\{1 - \frac{R_i}{\tilde{p}(\mathbf{X}_i;\boldsymbol{\alpha})}\right\}\tilde{m}(\mathbf{X}_i;\boldsymbol{\beta}). \tag{7}$$

The estimator (7) is consistent if either the outcome regression model or the propensity score model is correctly specified; see [1, 18, 21, 24–26] and [3], among others.

3 Multiply Robust Estimation Procedure

In this section, we consider three multiply robust procedures: Calibration approach, Projection approach, and Multiple imputation approach.

Let $\mathscr{C}_1 = \left\{m^{(j)}(\mathbf{X}_i;\boldsymbol{\beta}^{(j)}) : j = 1, \ldots, J\right\}$ be a set of J candidate imputation models and $\mathscr{C}_2 = \left\{p^{(k)}(\mathbf{X}_i;\boldsymbol{\alpha}^{(k)}) : k = 1, \ldots, K\right\}$ be a set of K propensity score models. The corresponding estimators $\widehat{\boldsymbol{\beta}}^{(j)}$ and $\widehat{\boldsymbol{\alpha}}^{(k)}$ can be obtained by solving the following estimating equations:

$$S_m^{(j)}(\boldsymbol{\beta}^{(j)}) = \frac{1}{n}\sum_{i\in s_r}\left\{Y_i - m^{(j)}(\mathbf{X}_i;\boldsymbol{\beta}^{(j)})\right\}\frac{1}{h(\mathbf{X}_i)}\frac{\partial m(\mathbf{X}_i;\boldsymbol{\beta}^{(j)})}{\partial\boldsymbol{\beta}^{(j)}} = 0, \tag{8}$$

and

$$S_p^{(k)}(\boldsymbol{\alpha}^{(k)}) = \frac{1}{n}\sum_{i\in s}\frac{R_i - p^{(k)}(\mathbf{X}_i;\boldsymbol{\alpha}^{(k)})}{p^{(k)}(\mathbf{X}_i;\boldsymbol{\alpha}^{(k)})\left\{1 - p(\mathbf{X}_i;\boldsymbol{\alpha}^{(k)})\right\}}\frac{\partial p(\mathbf{X}_i;\boldsymbol{\alpha}^{(k)})}{\partial\boldsymbol{\alpha}^{(k)}} = 0. \tag{9}$$

For each unit $i \in s$, we thus have the following two vectors:

$$\widehat{\mathbf{U}}_{mi} = \left(m^{(1)}(\mathbf{X}_i;\widehat{\boldsymbol{\beta}}^{(1)}), \ldots, m^{(J)}(\mathbf{X}_i;\widehat{\boldsymbol{\beta}}^{(J)})\right),$$

$$\widehat{\mathbf{U}}_{pi} = \left(p^{(1)}(\mathbf{X}_i;\widehat{\boldsymbol{\alpha}}^{(1)}), \ldots, p^{(K)}(\mathbf{X}_i;\widehat{\boldsymbol{\alpha}}^{(K)})\right).$$

In the following sections, we discuss how to combine this information arising from the $J + K$ models.

3.1 Calibration Approach

Han and Wang [15] proposed a multiply robust estimation procedure by using an empirical likelihood approach. Chen and Haziza [5] extended their method to complex survey data with a general calibration function. According to [5], the multiply robust estimator $\widehat{\theta}_{MRC}$ can be obtained as follows. We seek calibrated weights $\mathbf{w} = (w_1, w_2, \ldots, w_{n_r})$ such that

$$D(\mathbf{w}) = \sum_{i \in s_r} G(w_i/(1/n_r)) \tag{10}$$

is minimized subject to the following constraints:

$$\sum_{i \in s_r} w_i = 1, \tag{11}$$

$$\sum_{i \in s_r} w_i m^{(j)}(\mathbf{X}_i; \widehat{\boldsymbol{\beta}}^{(j)}) = \frac{1}{n} \sum_{i \in s} m^{(j)}(\mathbf{X}_i; \widehat{\boldsymbol{\beta}}^{(j)}), \tag{12}$$

and

$$\sum_{i \in s_r} w_i L\left\{1/p^{(k)}(\mathbf{X}_i; \widehat{\boldsymbol{\alpha}}^{(k)})\right\} = \frac{1}{n} \sum_{i \in s} L\left\{1/p^{(k)}(\mathbf{X}_i; \widehat{\boldsymbol{\alpha}}^{(k)})\right\}, \tag{13}$$

for $j = 1, \ldots, J$ and $k = 1, \ldots, K$. The function $G(\cdot)$ in (10) is a strictly convex function, differentiable with respect to w_i with continuous derivative function $g(t)$ with $g(0) = 0$. Furthermore, the function satisfies $G(t) \geq 0$ and $G(1) = 0$; see [9]. Popular distance functions include the generalized chi-square distance $G(t) = (1/2)(t-1)^2$, the generalized pseudo-empirical likelihood distance $G(t) = -\log t + t - 1$, and the generalized exponential tilting distance $G(t) = t \log t - t + 1$; see [27] for further details. The function $L(\cdot)$ in (13) is the inverse function of $F(t)$, which is a calibration function defined in (14) below. The resulting weights w_i are given by

$$w_i = n_r^{-1} F(\widehat{\boldsymbol{\lambda}}_r^{\top} \mathbf{h}_i), \tag{14}$$

where $F(t)$ is defined as the inverse function of $g(t)$ and $\widehat{\boldsymbol{\lambda}}_r$ is the solution of constraints (11)–(13). A multiply robust estimator of θ_0 is given by

$$\widehat{\theta}_{MRC} = \sum_{i \in s_r} w_i Y_i. \tag{15}$$

Chen and Haziza [5] showed that $\widehat{\theta}_{MRC}$ is consistent if at least one of the models in $\mathscr{C}_1$ or $\mathscr{C}_2$ is correctly specified and established its asymptotic properties. In finite population sampling, Chen and Haziza [5] proposed a generalized jackknife variance estimator that works well for negligible sampling fractions. Recently, Chen et al. [8] proposed a multiply robust pseudo-population bootstrap procedure that can be used for large sampling fractions.

3.2 Projection Approach

Duan and Yin [10] and Chen and Haziza [6] considered a projection approach for constructing a multiply robust estimator. Instead of using a calibration approach, one can summarize the working models information by regressing Y_i on $\widehat{\mathbf{U}}_{mi}$ and R_i on $\widehat{\mathbf{U}}_{pi}$ to obtain the regression coefficients

$$\widehat{\boldsymbol{\eta}}_m = \left(\sum_{i=1}^{n} R_i \widehat{\mathbf{U}}_{mi} \widehat{\mathbf{U}}_{mi}^{\top}\right)^{-1} \left(\sum_{i=1}^{n} R_i \widehat{\mathbf{U}}_{mi} Y_i\right) \tag{16}$$

and

$$\widehat{\boldsymbol{\eta}}_p = \left(\sum_{i=1}^{n} \widehat{\mathbf{U}}_{pi} \widehat{\mathbf{U}}_{pi}^{\top}\right)^{-1} \left(\sum_{i=1}^{n} \widehat{\mathbf{U}}_{pi} R_i\right). \tag{17}$$

Define the standardized predictions of $m_i = m(\mathbf{X}_i; \boldsymbol{\beta})$ and $p_i = p(\mathbf{X}_i; \boldsymbol{\alpha})$ as

$$\widehat{m}_i = \widehat{\mathbf{U}}_{mi} \times \frac{\widehat{\boldsymbol{\eta}}_m^2}{\widehat{\boldsymbol{\eta}}_m^{\top} \widehat{\boldsymbol{\eta}}_m}, \quad \widehat{p}_i = \widehat{\mathbf{U}}_{pi} \times \frac{\widehat{\boldsymbol{\eta}}_p^2}{\widehat{\boldsymbol{\eta}}_p^{\top} \widehat{\boldsymbol{\eta}}_p}, \tag{18}$$

where $\mathbf{a}^2$ denotes the column vector $\left(a_1^2, \ldots, a_q^2\right)$ for a given vector $a = (a_1, \ldots, a_q)^{\top}$. It can be shown that $\widehat{m}_i$ converges to m_i if one of the imputation models is correctly specified and $\widehat{p}_i$ converges to p_i is one of the propensity score models is correctly specified, see [10]. A multiply robust estimator based on the projection approach is given by

$$\widehat{\theta}_{MRP} = \frac{1}{n} \sum_{i=1}^{n} \frac{R_i}{\widehat{p}_i} Y_i + \frac{1}{n} \sum_{i=1}^{n} \left(1 - \frac{R_i}{\widehat{p}_i}\right) \widehat{m}_i. \tag{19}$$

Duan and Yin [10] showed that $\widehat{\theta}_{MRP}$ is consistent if at least one of the models in $\mathscr{C}_1$ and $\mathscr{C}_2$ is correctly specified and derived its asymptotic expansion for variance estimation purposes. Alternatively, one can use the generalized jackknife variance estimation procedure described in [5]. Chen and Haziza [6] extended the idea to handle zero-inflated distributions in finite population sampling.

In the presence of near-zero estimated $\widehat{p}_i$, the estimator (19) may be highly unstable. In this case, one can use a calibration procedure (similar to that described in Sect. 3.1) using the compressed scores $\widehat{p}_i$ and $\widehat{m}_i$. More specifically, we seek calibrated weights $\mathbf{w} = (w_1, w_2, \ldots, w_{n_r})$ such that (10) is minimized subject to

$$\sum_{i \in s_r} w_i = 1,$$

$$\sum_{i \in s_r} w_i \widehat{m}_i = \frac{1}{n} \sum_{i \in s} \widehat{m}_i,$$

and

$$\sum_{i \in s_r} w_i L\{1/\widehat{p}_i)\} = \frac{1}{n} \sum_{i \in s} L\{1/\widehat{p}_i)\}.$$

Unlike the procedure presented in Sect. 3.1 which involves $J + K + 1$ calibration constraints, the above calibration procedure involves three constraints only.

3.3 Multiple Imputation Approach

Let $Z_i = (Z_{1i}, Z_{2i}), i = 1, \ldots, n$, with $Z_{1i} = \widehat{m}_i$, $Z_{2i} = \widehat{p}_i$ and let $S_i = (S_{1i}, S_{2i})$ be the vector of standardized scores, where $S_{1i} = \widehat{\sigma}_m^{-1}(\widehat{m}_i - \bar{\widehat{m}}_n)$ and $S_{2i} = \widehat{\sigma}_p^{-1}(\widehat{p}_i - \bar{\widehat{p}}_n)$ with $\bar{\widehat{m}}_n$ and $\bar{\widehat{p}}_n$ denoting respectively the usual sample means of the $\widehat{p}_i$'s and $\widehat{m}_i$'s and $\widehat{\sigma}_m$ and $\widehat{\sigma}_p$ denoting the corresponding sample standard deviations. [7] proposed a multiply robust nonparametric multiple imputation (MRM) procedure, which can be implemented as follows:

(Step1). Calculate $S_i, i = 1, \ldots, n$, from the original sample.

(Step2). To obtain the lth imputation, draw a bootstrap sample of size n with replacement from the original sample, fit the working models in $\mathscr{C}_1$ and $\mathscr{C}_2$ using the bootstrap sample, and calculate $S_i^{(l)}$, the version of S_i corresponding to the lth imputation.

(Step3). Calculate the distance between each missing subject $i \in s_m$ and every respondent $j \in s_r^{(l)}$ as

$$d(i, j) = \left\{\lambda \left(S_{1i} - S_{1j}^{(l)}\right)^2 + (1 - \lambda) \left(S_{2i} - S_{2j}^{(l)}\right)^2\right\}^{1/2}, \tag{20}$$

where $0 \leq \lambda \leq 1$ and $s_r^{(l)}$ denotes the set of respondents corresponding to the lth imputation. The value of λ reflects one's confidence about the different working models. A small value of λ places more weight on the outcome regression models, whereas a large value of λ places more weight on the propensity score models.

(Step4). Define the nearest-H neighborhood $R_H^{(l)}(i)$ for each missing unit $i \in s_m$ as H unit in $s_r^{(l)}$ who have the smallest H distances (d) from unit i.

(Step5). Randomly select one unit from $R_H^{(l)}(i)$ and use its value $Y_i^{*(l)}$ as the imputed value for unit i.

(Step6). Repeat (Step2) to (Step5) L times to obtain L multiply imputed data sets with $\tilde{Y}_i^{(l)} = \left\{R_i Y_i + (1 - R_i) Y_i^{*(l)}\right\}, i = 1, \ldots, n, l = 1, \ldots, L$.

A point estimator is obtained by pooling the L multiply imputed data sets, which leads to

$$\widehat{\theta}_{MRM} = \frac{1}{L} \sum_{l=1}^{L} \widehat{\theta}^{(l)}, \tag{21}$$

where $\widehat{\theta}^{(l)} = n^{-1} \sum_{i=1}^{n} \tilde{Y}_i^{(l)}$. Using Rubin's rule, the variance of (21) is readily estimated by

$$\widehat{V}_{MRM} = \bar{U}_L + \left(1 + \frac{1}{L}\right) B_L, \tag{22}$$

where $\bar{U}_L$ and B_L denote the within and between components given respectively by

$$\bar{U}_L = \frac{1}{L} \sum_{l=1}^{L} U^{(l)}, \tag{23}$$

and

$$B_L = \frac{1}{L-1} \sum_{l=1}^{L} \left(\widehat{\theta}^{(l)} - \widehat{\theta}_{MRM}\right)^2, \tag{24}$$

with $U^{(l)}$ denoting the sampling variance of $\widehat{\theta}_{MRM}$ based on the lth imputed data set.

An $100(1 - \gamma)$-th confidence interval of θ_0 can be constructed as follows:

$$\left(\widehat{\theta}_{MRM} - z_{1-\gamma/2} \widehat{V}_{MRM}^{1/2}, \quad \widehat{\theta}_{MRM} + z_{1-\gamma/2} \widehat{V}_{MRM}^{1/2}\right),$$

where $z_{1-\gamma/2}$ is the $100(1 - \gamma/2)$-th percentile from standard normal distribution. Under certain regularity conditions, [7] showed that $\widehat{\theta}_{MRM}$ is consistent for θ_0 if at least one of the models in $\mathscr{C}_1$ and $\mathscr{C}_2$ is correctly specified. They also derived the asymptotic expansion of $\widehat{\theta}_{MRM}$.

4 Simulation Study

We conducted a simulation study using a setup similar to that of [4, 11, 18] and [5]. We first generated $B = 1000$ Monte Carlo samples from the following model:

$$Y_i = 210 + 27.4X_{1i} + 13.7(X_{2i} + X_{3i} + X_{4i}) + \epsilon_i, \quad i = 1, \cdots, n,$$

where the errors ϵ_i were independent random variables generated from a standard normal distribution and $\mathbf{X}_i = (X_{1i}, X_{2i}, X_{3i}, X_{4i})^\top$ were generated from a standard multivariate normal distribution. The response indicators R_i were generated independently from a Bernoulli distribution with probability

$$p(\mathbf{X}_i; \boldsymbol{\alpha}) = \{1 + \exp(\alpha_0 + \alpha_1 X_{1i} + \alpha_2 X_{2i} + \alpha_3 X_{3i} + \alpha_4 X_{4i})\}^{-1},$$

where the components of $\boldsymbol{\alpha} = (\alpha_0, \alpha_1, \alpha_2, \alpha_3, \alpha_4)^\top$ were chosen so as to produce response rates of 30%, 50%, and 70%. To assess the performance of the multiply robust methods described in Sects. 3.1–3.3 in the presence of model misspecification, we considered the following transformations of the X-variables: $Z_1 = \exp(X_1/2)$, $Z_2 = X_2\{1 + \exp(X_1)\}^{-1} + 10$, $Z_3 = (X_1X_3/25 + 0.6)^3$, and $Z_4 = (X_2 + X_4 + 20)^2$. Let $\mathbf{Z} = (Z_1, Z_2, Z_3, Z_4)^\top$. The correct nonresponse and imputation models were estimated by

$$p^{(1)}(\mathbf{X}; \boldsymbol{\alpha}^{(1)}) = \left\{1 + \exp(\alpha_0^{(1)} + \alpha_1^{(1)} X_1 + \alpha_2^{(1)} X_2 + \alpha_3^{(1)} X_3 + \alpha_4^{(1)} X_4)\right\}^{-1},$$

and

$$m^{(1)}(\mathbf{X}; \boldsymbol{\beta}^{(1)}) = \beta_0^{(1)} + \beta_1^{(1)} X_1 + \beta_2^{(1)} X_2 + \beta_3^{(1)} X_3 + \beta_4^{(1)} X_4.$$

The incorrect nonresponse and imputation models were estimated by replacing variables $\mathbf{X}$ in $p^{(1)}(\mathbf{X}; \boldsymbol{\alpha}^{(1)})$ and $m^{(1)}(\mathbf{X}; \boldsymbol{\beta}^{(1)})$ with $\mathbf{Z}$ and we denote them by $p^{(2)}(\mathbf{Z}; \boldsymbol{\alpha}^{(2)})$ and $m^{(2)}(\mathbf{Z}; \boldsymbol{\beta}^{(2)})$.

We were interested in estimating the population mean of Y: $\theta_0 = E(Y)$. We considered the following methods:

(M1). The benchmark estimator by assuming no missing values: $\hat{\theta}_B = n^{-1}\sum_{i\in s} Y_i$.

(M2). The unadjusted estimator that corresponds to the mean from the respondents: $\hat{\theta}_R = n_r^{-1}\sum_{i\in s_r} Y_i$.

(M3). MR estimators obtained using the calibration approach: $\hat{\theta}_{MRC}(1010)$, $\hat{\theta}_{MRC}(1001)$, $\hat{\theta}_{MRC}(0110)$, $\hat{\theta}_{MRC}(0101)$, $\hat{\theta}_{MRC}(1110)$, $\hat{\theta}_{MRC}(1101)$, $\hat{\theta}_{MRC}(1011)$, $\hat{\theta}_{MRC}(0111)$, and $\hat{\theta}_{MRC}(1111)$, where the four digits indicate which models (correct/incorrect) were used. For instance, the estimator $\hat{\theta}_{MRC}(1110)$ is based on both the correct and incorrect propensity score models and the correct imputation model.

(M4). MR estimators obtained using the projection approach: $\hat{\theta}_{MRP}(1010)$, $\hat{\theta}_{MRP}(1001)$, $\hat{\theta}_{MRP}(0110)$, $\hat{\theta}_{MRP}(0101)$, $\hat{\theta}_{MRP}(1110)$, $\hat{\theta}_{MRP}(1101)$, $\hat{\theta}_{MRP}(1011)$, $\hat{\theta}_{MRP}(0111)$, and $\hat{\theta}_{MRP}(1111)$.

(M5). MR estimators obtained using the multiple imputation approach: $\hat{\theta}_{MRM}(1010)$, $\hat{\theta}_{MRM}(1001)$, $\hat{\theta}_{MRM}(0110)$, $\hat{\theta}_{MRM}(0101)$, $\hat{\theta}_{MRM}(1110)$, $\hat{\theta}_{MRM}(1101)$, $\hat{\theta}_{MRM}(1011)$, $\hat{\theta}_{MRM}(0111)$, and $\hat{\theta}_{MRM}(1111)$.

For each point estimator, we computed the Monte Carlo percent relative bias (RB), the percent relative standard error (RSE), and the percent relative root mean squared error (RRMSE). The results are presented in Table 1. As expected, the benchmark estimator showed negligible RB and small RSE and RRMSE in all the scenarios. The unadjusted estimator was biased with values of absolute RB ranging from 2.8% to 6.6%. The MRC, MRP, and MRM estimators showed negligible bias when at least one model (either the propensity score model or the imputation model) was correctly specified. When all the models were misspecified, all the estimators showed some bias. It is worth pointing out that, unlike the MRC estimators, the MRP estimators performed poorly in terms of RB and RSE when all the models were misspecified. More accurate MRC type estimators may be obtained by using the calibration procedure described in Sect. 3.2.

MRM estimators showed a little larger RBs, RSEs, and RRMSE than MRC and MRP estimators since they were based on a nonparametric procedure and only used partial information from the assumed models, but all the RBs were less than 1% and therefore, may not be significantly different from 0. MRC estimators had best performance in terms of balancing the RBs and RSEs, since they were somewhat robust against near-zero propensity score estimates.

For each estimator, we also computed an estimate of standard error by using the jackknife as described in [5] as well as the corresponding Monte Carlo percent relative bias, coverage probability, and average length of 95% confidence intervals. We only present the case for $n = 800$ and response rate of 50%. Results for the other scenarios were similar. The results are presented in Table 2. The Monte Carlo relative biases of the jackknife standard error estimators were small in all the scenarios except the case when both models were wrong. As a result, the coverage rates were close to 95% when at least one model was correctly specified. MRC method showed the best performance in terms of balancing the coverage rates with average lengths. It also led to the lowest relative biases of standard error estimators.

5 Real Application

In this section, we compare the three approaches considered in Sect. 3 using data from the 2015–2016 National Health and Nutrition Examination Survey (NHANES). The 2015–2016 NHANES is a stratified multi-stage household survey which oversampled certain minority groups including Hispanic or Black and Asian populations. The target population is the noninstitutionalized civilian population

Table 1 The Monte Carlo Relative Bias (RB), Relative Standard Error (RSE), and Relative Root Mean Squared Error (RRMSE) with different response rates

Response rate	30%			50%			70%		
method	RB (%)	RSE (%)	RRMSE (%)	RB (%)	RSE (%)	RRMSE (%)	RB (%)	RSE (%)	RRMSE (%)
$\widehat{\mu}_B$	0.015	0.605	0.605	−0.011	0.592	0.592	0.003	0.589	0.589
$\widehat{\mu}_R$	−6.667	1.045	6.749	−4.775	0.809	4.843	−2.872	0.722	2.962
$\widehat{\mu}_{MRC}(1010)$	0.016	0.605	0.605	−0.010	0.592	0.592	0.002	0.589	0.589
$\widehat{\mu}_{MRC}(1001)$	0.154	0.900	0.913	0.056	0.725	0.727	0.045	0.627	0.628
$\widehat{\mu}_{MRC}(0110)$	0.016	0.605	0.606	−0.011	0.592	0.592	0.002	0.589	0.589
$\widehat{\mu}_{MRC}(0101)$	−1.440	0.947	1.723	−1.200	0.762	1.421	−0.738	0.659	0.990
$\widehat{\mu}_{MRC}(1110)$	0.016	0.605	0.605	−0.010	0.592	0.592	0.002	0.589	0.589
$\widehat{\mu}_{MRC}(1101)$	0.118	0.898	0.905	0.030	0.727	0.728	0.007	0.616	0.616
$\widehat{\mu}_{MRC}(1011)$	0.016	0.605	0.606	−0.010	0.592	0.592	0.002	0.589	0.589
$\widehat{\mu}_{MRC}(0111)$	0.016	0.606	0.606	−0.010	0.592	0.592	0.002	0.589	0.589
$\widehat{\mu}_{MRC}(1111)$	0.016	0.606	0.606	−0.010	0.592	0.592	0.002	0.589	0.589
$\widehat{\mu}_{MRP}(1010)$	0.016	0.605	0.605	−0.011	0.592	0.592	0.002	0.589	0.589
$\widehat{\mu}_{MRP}(1001)$	0.149	1.231	1.240	0.024	0.918	0.918	0.023	0.684	0.685
$\widehat{\mu}_{MRP}(0110)$	0.011	0.688	0.688	−0.012	0.615	0.615	0.002	0.598	0.598
$\widehat{\mu}_{MRP}(0101)$	−8.475	37.568	38.512	−6.074	22.465	23.272	−2.441	6.995	7.408
$\widehat{\mu}_{MRP}(1110)$	0.016	0.605	0.605	−0.011	0.592	0.592	0.002	0.589	0.589
$\widehat{\mu}_{MRP}(1101)$	0.015	1.227	1.227	−0.015	0.918	0.918	−0.008	0.683	0.684
$\widehat{\mu}_{MRP}(1011)$	0.016	0.605	0.605	−0.011	0.592	0.592	0.002	0.589	0.589
$\widehat{\mu}_{MRP}(0111)$	0.011	0.688	0.688	−0.012	0.615	0.615	0.002	0.598	0.598
$\widehat{\mu}_{MRP}(1111)$	0.016	0.605	0.605	−0.011	0.592	0.592	0.002	0.589	0.589
$\widehat{\mu}_{MRM}(1010)$	−0.178	0.654	0.678	−0.121	0.611	0.623	−0.049	0.602	0.604
$\widehat{\mu}_{MRM}(1001)$	−0.224	0.839	0.868	−0.137	0.709	0.722	−0.046	0.622	0.624

(continued)

Table 1 (continued)

Response rate	30%			50%			70%		
method	RB (%)	RSE (%)	RRMSE (%)	RB (%)	RSE (%)	RRMSE (%)	RB (%)	RSE (%)	RRMSE (%)
$\widehat{\mu}_{MRM}(0110)$	−0.229	0.655	0.694	−0.138	0.614	0.630	−0.043	0.602	0.604
$\widehat{\mu}_{MRM}(0101)$	−1.117	0.879	1.421	−0.841	0.724	1.110	−0.420	0.638	0.763
$\widehat{\mu}_{MRM}(1110)$	−0.179	0.656	0.680	−0.120	0.611	0.623	−0.045	0.601	0.603
$\widehat{\mu}_{MRM}(1101)$	−0.301	0.838	0.891	−0.164	0.707	0.726	−0.062	0.620	0.623
$\widehat{\mu}_{MRM}(1011)$	−0.179	0.653	0.677	−0.121	0.611	0.623	−0.044	0.602	0.604
$\widehat{\mu}_{MRM}(0111)$	−0.229	0.654	0.693	−0.138	0.614	0.629	−0.044	0.602	0.604
$\widehat{\mu}_{MRM}(1111)$	−0.181	0.655	0.680	−0.119	0.610	0.622	−0.046	0.601	0.603

Table 2 The 95% Coverage Rates (CR), Average Lengths (AL) of confidence intervals, and Relative Biases of standard errors for different methods with sample size 800 and response rate 50%

Method	CR (%)	AL	RB (%)
$\widehat{\mu}_{MRC}(1010)$	94.9	5.00	−2.12
$\widehat{\mu}_{MRC}(1001)$	94.5	5.80	−1.84
$\widehat{\mu}_{MRC}(0110)$	94.8	5.00	−2.14
$\widehat{\mu}_{MRC}(0101)$	61.0	6.14	−1.63
$\widehat{\mu}_{MRC}(1110)$	95.0	5.00	−2.11
$\widehat{\mu}_{MRC}(1101)$	95.3	5.86	−1.31
$\widehat{\mu}_{MRC}(1011)$	94.9	5.00	−2.12
$\widehat{\mu}_{MRC}(0111)$	94.9	5.01	−2.16
$\widehat{\mu}_{MRC}(1111)$	94.8	5.01	−2.10
$\widehat{\mu}_{MRP}(1010)$	94.9	5.03	−1.61
$\widehat{\mu}_{MRP}(1001)$	95.2	7.16	1.84
$\widehat{\mu}_{MRP}(0110)$	95.1	5.30	9.89
$\widehat{\mu}_{MRP}(0101)$	74.7	67.32	50.91
$\widehat{\mu}_{MRP}(1110)$	94.8	5.03	−1.62
$\widehat{\mu}_{MRP}(1101)$	95.0	7.28	6.82
$\widehat{\mu}_{MRP}(1011)$	94.9	5.03	−1.61
$\widehat{\mu}_{MRP}(0111)$	95.1	5.30	9.89
$\widehat{\mu}_{MRP}(1111)$	94.8	5.03	−1.62
$\widehat{\mu}_{MRM}(1010)$	96.0	5.67	9.02
$\widehat{\mu}_{MRM}(1001)$	95.2	6.31	11.59
$\widehat{\mu}_{MRM}(0110)$	96.1	5.70	9.41
$\widehat{\mu}_{MRM}(0101)$	79.2	6.23	5.88
$\widehat{\mu}_{MRM}(1110)$	96.1	5.67	9.22
$\widehat{\mu}_{MRM}(1101)$	95.1	6.29	10.59
$\widehat{\mu}_{MRM}(1011)$	96.0	5.67	9.10
$\widehat{\mu}_{MRM}(0111)$	95.8	5.70	9.38
$\widehat{\mu}_{MRM}(1111)$	96.3	5.67	9.05

including all people living in households, excluding institutional group quarters and those persons on active duty with the military. The primary objective of NHANES is to produce a broad range of descriptive health and nutrition statistics for sex, race and Hispanic original, and age group of the U.S. population. For more information about the design and objectives of NHANES, please see https://wwwn.cdc.gov/nchs/nhanes/analyticguidelines.aspx#sample-design.

In this application, we first created a subset of the original 2015–2016 NHANES data by keeping only the adults and by removing cases with missing values on the following variables: Education, Marital status, Household income, and Systolic blood pressure. This resulted in a data file of 4811 cases. We considered Systolic blood pressure as the outcome variable and the following variables as predictors: age, gender, race, marital status, education, total number of people in the household, number of children 5 years or younger in the household, number of children 6–17 years old in the household, number of adults 60 years or older in the household, and household income. For each unit on the data file, we simulated response indicators using independent Bernoulli trials with probability defined by the Logistic function with the following predictors: gender, age, education, total number of people in the household, household income and the square of age and household size. The response rate was about 30% and the number of respondents was about 1450. The parameter of interest was the population mean of Systolic blood pressure. We compared all the methods considered in the simulation study. We started by considering a model that incorporated all of the above predictors, as well as all the two-way interaction and quadratic terms. We then performed a backward selection procedure to obtain the final model. For the incorrect model, we only incorporated the following predictors without interaction and quadratic terms: gender, race, education, marital status, and household income. For the incorrect model, no model selection procedure was performed.

We computed point estimates and 95% confidence intervals. The results are presented in Table 3. In terms of point estimation, the naive estimator showed the largest bias since it only used outcome variable information for the respondents. When both models were incorrect, MRC, MRP, and MRM estimators showed large biases. When the nonresponse model was misspecified, MRC, MRP, and MRM showed larger biases compared to other estimators, as expected. MRC, MRP, and MRM estimators had comparable performances for both point estimates and confidence intervals.

6 Discussion

In this paper, we reviewed three existing multiply robust estimation approaches for handling missing data. We also compared the approaches through both a simulation study and a real application. According to the simulation study, all MR estimators enjoyed the multiply robustness and showed negligible bias when at least one of the models was correctly specified. MRM estimators were slightly less efficient compared with MRC and MRP methods, which can be explained by the fact that MRM is a nonparametric procedure. MRC estimators had the best performance in terms of balancing the bias and standard error since they were more robust against near-zero propensity score estimates and one could incorporate auxiliary information more efficiently through the calibration procedure. According to the results in both simulation study and real application, we recommend the researchers to consider more than one outcome regression models or propensity score models to deal with missing data analysis in practice since it can improve the robustness of the estimates. Han [12, 13] discussed Multiply Robust estimation procedure for handling missing data in regression analysis. Han et al. [16] discussed some parametric modeling based approaches for quantile estimation. Han [14] proposed calibration approach by using parametric model for handling data not missing at random. For future research direction, it would be interesting to consider estimating other parameters such as percentiles and distribution functions and handling nonignorable nonresponse with semi-parametric or nonparametric approaches.

Table 3 The Point estimates, 95% Lower Bounds (LB) and 95% Upper Bounds (UB) with different methods by using 2015–2016 NHANES data

Method	Estimate	LB	UB
$\widehat{\mu}_B$	125.41	NA	NA
$\widehat{\mu}_R$	120.86	NA	NA
$\widehat{\mu}_{MRC}(1010)$	125.39	122.45	128.33
$\widehat{\mu}_{MRC}(1001)$	125.91	121.33	130.49
$\widehat{\mu}_{MRC}(0110)$	126.08	123.15	129.02
$\widehat{\mu}_{MRC}(0101)$	121.64	120.43	122.85
$\widehat{\mu}_{MRC}(1110)$	126.14	122.20	130.09
$\widehat{\mu}_{MRC}(1101)$	126.65	120.83	132.47
$\widehat{\mu}_{MRC}(1011)$	125.48	122.51	128.45
$\widehat{\mu}_{MRC}(0111)$	123.99	119.80	128.19
$\widehat{\mu}_{MRC}(1111)$	126.46	123.82	129.09
$\widehat{\mu}_{MRP}(1010)$	125.57	123.08	128.06
$\widehat{\mu}_{MRP}(1001)$	125.97	122.97	128.96
$\widehat{\mu}_{MRP}(0110)$	124.36	123.03	125.70
$\widehat{\mu}_{MRP}(0101)$	121.65	120.43	122.88
$\widehat{\mu}_{MRP}(1110)$	125.57	123.09	128.05
$\widehat{\mu}_{MRP}(1101)$	125.96	122.96	128.96
$\widehat{\mu}_{MRP}(1011)$	125.57	123.08	128.06
$\widehat{\mu}_{MRP}(0111)$	124.34	123.01	125.68
$\widehat{\mu}_{MRP}(1111)$	125.57	123.09	128.05
$\widehat{\mu}_{MRM}(1010)$	125.65	123.62	127.34
$\widehat{\mu}_{MRM}(1001)$	125.39	122.52	130.12
$\widehat{\mu}_{MRM}(0110)$	124.95	123.03	126.70
$\widehat{\mu}_{MRM}(0101)$	121.68	120.69	122.92
$\widehat{\mu}_{MRM}(1110)$	125.64	123.44	127.73
$\widehat{\mu}_{MRM}(1101)$	125.45	122.02	130.11
$\widehat{\mu}_{MRM}(1011)$	125.64	123.71	127.03
$\widehat{\mu}_{MRM}(0111)$	124.96	123.10	126.49
$\widehat{\mu}_{MRM}(1111)$	125.54	123.37	127.39

Acknowledgments We thank Professor Yichuan Zhao for inviting us to contribute to this book. We thank the reviewers for their comments which helped improving the paper substantially. Dr. Sixia Chen is partially supported by National Institutes of Health, National Institute of General Medical Sciences [Grant 5U54GM104938-07, PI Judith James]. The research of Dr. David Haziza is supported by grants from the Natural Sciences and Engineering Research Council of Canada.

References

1. Bang, H., Robins, J.: Doubly robust estimation in missing data and causal inference models. Biometrics **61**, 962–973 (2005)
2. Boistard, H., Chauvet, G., Haziza, D.: Doubly robust inference for the distribution function in the presence of missing survey data. Scand. J. Stat. **43**, 683–699 (2016)

3. Cao, W., Tsiatis, A.A., Davidian, M.: Improving efficiency and robustness of the doubly robust estimator for a population mean with incomplete data. Biometrika **96**, 723–734 (2009)
4. Chan, K.C.G., Yam, S.C.P.: Oracle, multiple robust and multipurpose calibration in a missing response problem. Stat. Sci. **29**, 380–396 (2014)
5. Chen, S., Haziza, D.: Multiply robust imputation procedures for the treatment of item nonresponse in surveys. Biometrika **104**, 439–453 (2017)
6. Chen, S., Haziza, D.: Multiply robust imputation procedures for zero-inflated distributions in surveys. Metron **75**, 333–343 (2017)
7. Chen, S., Haziza, D.: On the nonparametric multiple imputation with multiply robustness. Stat. Sin. **29**, 2035–2053 (2019)
8. Chen, S., Haziza, D., Mashreghi, Z.: Multiply robust bootstrap variance estimation in the presence of singly imputed survey data. Minor revision at J. Survey. Stat. Methodol. (2019). https://doi.org/10.1093/jssam/smaa004
9. Deville, J.C., Särndal, C.E.: Calibration estimators in survey sampling. J. Am. Stat. Assoc. **87**, 376–382 (1992)
10. Duan, X., Yin, G.: Ensemble approached to estimation of the population mean with missing responses. Scand. J. Stat. **44**, 899–917 (2017)
11. Han, P.: A further study of the multiply robust estimator in missing data analysis. J. Stat. Plan. Infer. **148**, 101–110 (2014)
12. Han, P.: Multiply robust estimation in regression analysis with missing data. J. Am. Stat. Assoc. **109**, 1159–1173 (2014)
13. Han, P.: Combining inverse probability weighting and multiple imputation to improve robustness of estimation. Scand. J. Stat. **43**, 246–260 (2016)
14. Han, P.: Calibration and multiple robustness when data are missing not at random. Stat. Sin. **28**, 1725–1740 (2018)
15. Han, P., Wang, L.: Estimation with missing data: Beyond double robustness. Biometrika **100**, 417–430 (2013)
16. Han, P., Kong, L., Zhao, J., Zhou, X.: A general framework for quantile estimation with incomplete data. J. R. Stat. Soc. Ser. B. Stat. Methodol. **81**, 305–333 (2019)
17. Haziza, D., Nambeu, C.O., Chauvet, G.: Doubly robust imputation procedures for finite population means in the presence of a large number of zeroes. Canad. J. Statist. **42**, 650–669 (2014)
18. Kang, J.D.Y., Schafer, J.L.: Demystifying double robustness: A comparison of alternative strategies for estimating a population mean from incomplete data (with discussion). Stat. Sci. **22**, 523–539 (2007)
19. Kim, J.K., Haziza, D.: Doubly robust inference with missing data in survey sampling. Stat. Sin. **24**, 375–394 (2014)
20. Long, Q., Hsu, C.H., Li, Y.: Doubly robust nonparametric multiple imputation for ignorable missing data. Stat. Sin. **22**, 149–172 (2012)
21. Robins, J.M., Rotnitzky, A., Zhao, L.P.: Estimation of regression coefficient when some regressors are not always observed. J. Am. Stat. Assoc. **89**, 846–866 (1994)
22. Rubin, D.B.: Inference and missing data. Biometrika **63**, 581–592 (1976)
23. Rubin, D.B.: Multiple Imputation for Nonresponse in Surveys. Wiley, New York (1987)
24. Rubin, D.B., Van der Laan, M.J.: Empirical efficiency maximization: Improved locally efficient covariate adjustment in randomized experiments and survival analysis. Int. J. Biostatist. **4**, Article 5. (2008)
25. Scharfstein, D.O., Rotnitzky, A., Robins, J.M.: Adjusting for nonignorable drop-out using semiparametric nonresponse models (with discussion and rejoinder). J. Am. Stat. Assoc. **94**, 1096–1146 (1999)
26. Tan, Z.: A distributional approach for causal inference using propensity scores. J. Am. Stat. Assoc. **101**, 1619–1637 (2006)
27. Wu, C., Lu, W.W.: Calibration weighting methods for complex surveys. Int. Stat. Rev. **84**, 79–98 (2016)

Part II
Clinical Trials, FDR, and Applications in Health Science

Approaches to Combining Phase II Proof-of-Concept and Dose-Finding Trials

Yutao Liu, Ying Kuen Cheung, Naitee Ting, and Qiqi Deng

1 Introduction

In a typical clinical development program for a drug treating non-life-threatening disease, there are two questions to be answered in Phase II. The first one is that whether there is a reasonable likelihood that the drug is efficacious, which is often referred to as proof-of-concept (PoC). The second one is what would be the dose(s) to use in large Phase III confirmatory clinical trials (dose-finding). A PoC study and a dose-finding study are traditionally separated as different studies designed to answer these questions separately. In this case, the first Phase II trial will be a PoC trial that typically includes only two treatment groups: a placebo group and a test product treatment group. In order to offer the best opportunity for the test product to demonstrate its efficacy, the dose of test product used in a PoC tends to be the highest possible dose. This dose is usually the maximally tolerable dose (MTD) or a dose that is slightly below MTD. This design allows the project team to make a Go/No-Go decision on the test product after study results read out. After the concept is proven, the second Phase II trial will be a dose-finding trial to explore and recommend the dose(s) to be tested in Phase III. PoC is usually faster and cheaper as it only requires a well-tolerated dose of test therapy plus the placebo (control) group. A dose-finding study, however, needs multiple doses of the test therapy in order to help characterize the dose–response relationship.

Y. Liu · Y. K. Cheung
Department of Biostatistics, Columbia University, New York, NY, USA
e-mail: yl3050@cumc.columbia.edu; yc632@cumc.columbia.edu

N. Ting (✉) · Q. Deng
Boehringer Ingelheim Pharmaceuticals, Inc., Ridgefield, CT, USA
e-mail: Naitee.ting@boehringer-ingelheim.com; qiqi.deng@boehringer-ingelheim.com

Y. Zhao, (Din) D.-G. Chen (eds.), *Modern Statistical Methods for Health Research*, Emerging Topics in Statistics and Biostatistics,
https://doi.org/10.1007/978-3-030-72437-5_6

In recent years, more companies and project teams tend to combine the PoC and dose-finding studies into one single study. The advantage of such a design is to first make a Go/No-Go decision based on PoC. If the decision is Go, then the same study would sequentially provide dose-finding information to help design future studies. There are different ways to implement hypothesis test for PoC in such a study with the two objectives combined. One method is MCP-Mod (Multiple Comparison Procedure and Modeling approach) proposed by Bretz et al. [1], which received a positive Committee for Medical Products for Human Use (CHMP) qualification opinion in January 2014 as an efficient statistical methodology for model-based design and analysis of Phase II dose-finding studies under model uncertainty.

Another useful, yet not as popular, method is ordinal linear contrast test (OLCT). This technique is very simple, and it was referred to as a linear contrast test, or trend test, previously. It has been successfully implemented in designing early Phase II clinical trials [2]. Zhang et al [3] compared these two approaches (MCP-Mod, OLCT) with ANOVA F-test, Dunnett's test, and highest dose against placebo. They pointed out that MCP-Mod, OLCT, and highest dose against placebo are among the most powerful and robust ways for PoC in such combined Phase IIa/b studies. When well designed and analyzed, the combined study saves development time by providing a range of efficacious doses going forward. The disadvantage is more investment before the concept is proven. In case the test drug does not work, this translates into larger sunk costs. One way to mitigate the risk of large sunken cost is to have a two-stage strategy, either in one single trial or in two separate trials, and proceed to the second stage only if there is adequate signal from the first stage.

In this chapter, different strategies for dealing with these Phase II development challenges will be introduced. Some modification will be proposed to improve one of the existing two-stage designs. In addition, the operating characteristics will be illustrated and compared through simulation of a case study. In order to make comparisons, a program-wise error rate is introduced and used as a metric for evaluation. Finally, based on the proposed metric and simulation results, some practical recommendations are provided to help mitigate risks in Phase II clinical development of new drugs.

2 Two Studies—Phase IIa (Proof-of-Concept) and Phase IIb (Dose-Finding)

As indicated earlier, in recent years, many project teams are combining Phase IIa and IIb into a single clinical trial. The objective of this chapter is to compare Phase II development strategies—the two-trial strategy vs. various combined designs. When different designs of a single trial are compared, it is natural to consider that if the Type I and Type II error rates are fixed, then under a fixed clinical treatment effect size (treatment difference divided by standard deviation), the total sample sizes can be used as a criterion for comparison. However, these metrics are usually defined in the trial level and cannot be directly applied to compare development strategies.

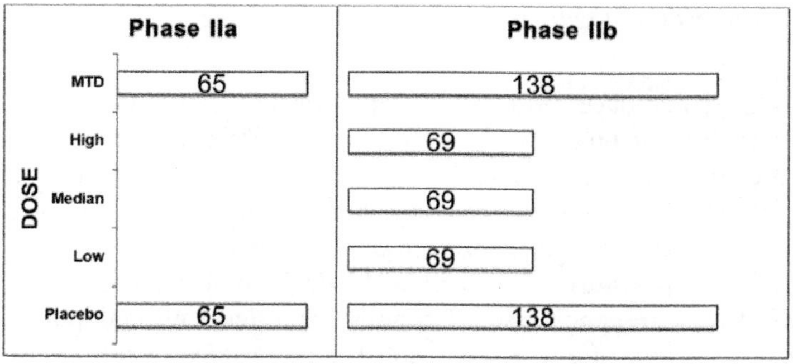

Fig. 1 A hypothetical Phase II program with two studies and program-wise Type I error $\alpha = 0.05$ and power $1 - \beta \approx 90\%$

Under this circumstance, it helps to specify Phase II program-wise (overall) Type I and Type II errors, instead of using the study-wise Type I/II error rates. Given such background, we consider programs with two-sided program-wise Type I error set at 0.05 and a power close to be 90% (one-sided Type II error being about 10%). For a two-study strategy, following the idea of Brown et al. [4], the Type I error of the Phase IIa trial could be set at $\alpha_1 = 0.4$ (two-sided) with desired power being $1 - \beta_1 = 95\%$, and the Phase IIb study is proposed to be with Type I error rate of $\alpha_2 = 0.125$ (two-sided), again with $1 - \beta_2 = 95\%$ power. Based on this setup, assuming independence, the two-study strategy has a program-wise two-sided Type I error of $\alpha_1 \times \alpha_2 = 0.05$ and $(1 - \beta_1) \times (1 - \beta_2) \approx 90\%$ power. Figure 1 displays a hypothetical Phase II program using such strategy. The program starts with a Phase IIa trial with two treatment groups (highest dose versus placebo) and continues with a Phase IIb full dose-ranging trial, only when the Phase IIa trial indicates promising results. Otherwise, the program is terminated at the end of Phase IIa trial. The hypothetical program is designed with normality assumption for a continuous endpoint, with standardized effect size $\delta = 1/3$. For Phase IIa, a two-sample t-test is applied. For Phase IIb, Multiple Comparison Procedure–Modeling Approach (MCP-Mod) procedure can be applied, which will be discussed in Sect. 3.1.

In the comparisons, this strategy having two separate studies is denoted as strategy A. All other designs considered in this chapter are based on the combined Phase IIa/IIb study designs and are discussed in Sect. 3.

3 A Single Study with Combined Objectives (PoC and DF)

In this section, we introduce and compare various approaches to combine proof-of-concept and dose-finding trials.

3.1 Single Fixed Design

Bretz et al. [1] introduced Multiple Comparison Procedure–Modeling Approach (MCP-Mod) that combines the objectives of proof-of-concept and dose-finding. In such a combined Phase IIa/IIb trial, patients are randomized to a wide range of doses of interest with a pre-specified allocation ratio. The combined study is designed with a set of possible parametric dose–response models. Based on each model, an optimal contrast test is obtained, which combines data from all of the test doses. The corresponding set of contrasts is tested with multiple comparison adjustment. The proof-of-concept is established when at least one contrast indicates significant results. For a continuous endpoint, with normality assumption and known variance, each dose–response model and the corresponding optimal contrast vector lead to a normally distributed test statistics, and the Type I error control is based on the multivariate normally distributed test statistics. Once proof-of-concept is established, dose–response estimation is based on the models selected according to certain criteria. Both sets of analysis are accomplished at the end of the trial when all patient data are available and the single trial functions as both a proof-of-concept study and a dose-finding study. If the experimental treatment is efficacious, such combined trial can expedite the clinical development with an overall smaller sample size for Phase II study. However, such trial is associated with large investment of resource when the experimental treatment is futile, if no futility stopping rule is pre-specified.

In order to make comparisons between the two-study strategy (as mentioned in Sect. 2) and the combined Phase IIa/IIb approaches, MCP-Mod is employed in this chapter to construct such a combined design. The first scenario being considered is a one-stage, single-trial, fixed design without interim analysis strategy. Under this setting, a five-group Phase II trial is designed with unbalance randomization. In this trial, four test dose groups of the drug candidate are included vs. a placebo control group. The four test doses are the highest dose, the high dose, the median dose, and the low dose. The unbalanced sample size allocation is in a 2:1:1:1:2 ratio where the highest dose and the placebo group receive more patients than the three middle doses. Advantages of this allocation can be found in Deng and Ting [5]. Again, in order to maintain comparability across various strategies, the two-sided Type I error is set at 0.05, with a power of 90%. In the comparisons, this strategy is denoted as strategy B. Figure 2 displays a hypothetical Phase II program designed using MCP-Mod, and the corresponding dose–response models used for the contrast test will be discussed in Sect. 4.

3.2 Two-Stage Phase IIa/IIb Adaptive Designs

The single fixed design using MCP-Mod specified in Sect. 3.1 can be modified by deploying adaptive strategies, more specifically, an interim analysis for futility

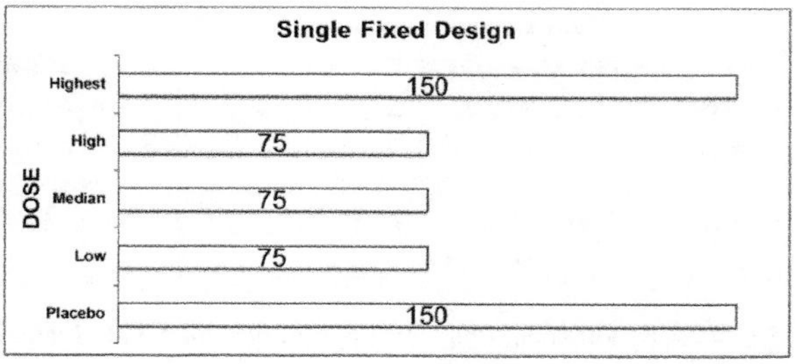

Fig. 2 A hypothetical Phase II program using MCP-Mod with Type I error $\alpha = 0.05$ and power $1 - \beta \approx 90\%$

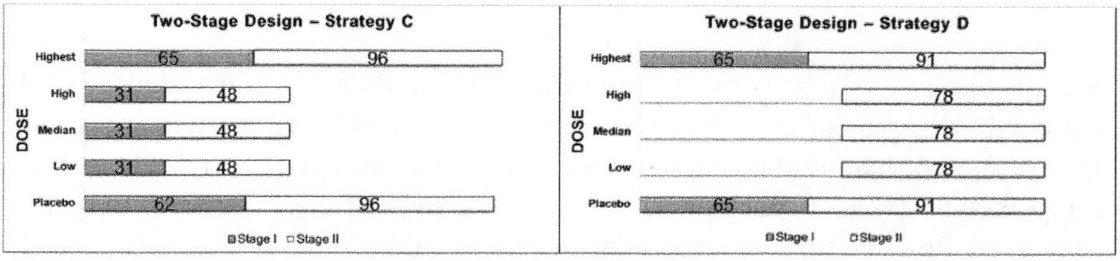

Fig. 3 Hypothetical two-stage Phase IIa/IIb adaptive designs with Type I error $\alpha \approx 0.05$ and power $1 - \beta \approx 90\%$ using strategy C and strategy D

purpose. The following three adaptive strategies were considered, leading to three two-stage adaptive designs.

Strategy C starts with randomizing patients to all five treatment groups with 2:1:1:1:2 randomization ratio, and an interim futility analysis is performed to determine whether the study should be continued or not. If the interim results are not promising, the study is terminated. Strategy D differs from strategy C by starting with patients on only two treatment groups (the highest does versus placebo) instead of all five. If the interim results are positive, then three middle doses are added, and the study continues to recruit. Figure 3 displays two hypothetical clinical programs using the two-stage Phase IIa/IIb adaptive designs. With normality assumption of the continuous endpoint, a multivariate normal distribution can be used to model the joint distribution of the test statistics in both stages and derive the decision boundary.

In practice, results of interim analysis might not be available immediately (depending on time to endpoint), resulting in patient overflow. More specifically, the actual number of enrolled patients can be larger than the stage I sample size even when the program is terminated. If the program continues with promising results from interim analysis, operationally, in strategy D, three middle doses can be added when all arms have the same number of remaining patients to recruit, so that 1:1:1:1:1 randomization ratio can be used.

Strategy E further modifies strategy D using a dynamic strategy with two potential paths of development, borrowing idea from Deng et al. [6] with the intention to utilize data from patient overflow. Strategy E starts with two treatment groups (the highest dose and placebo), and then an interim analysis is performed to decide which of the two potential paths to take. If the interim results are not promising, the study will continue, but with only two treatment groups ("Go Slow"

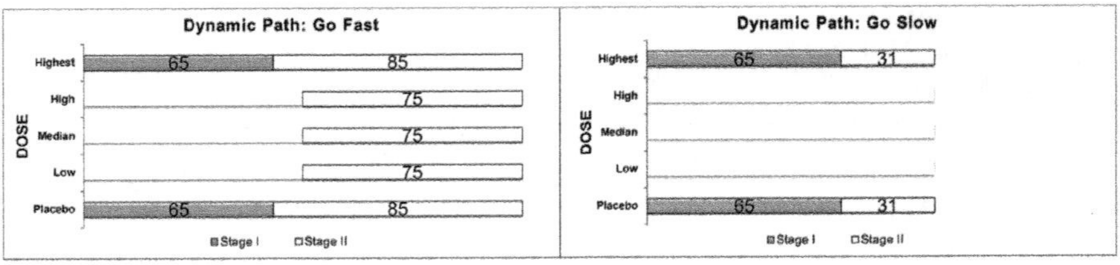

Fig. 4 A hypothetical Phase II program designed with dynamic path with Type I error $\alpha \approx 0.05$ and power $1 - \beta \approx 90\%$

path). If the interim results are positive, then three middle doses are added, and the study will be expanded to a full dose-ranging study ("Go Fast" path), and there will be a total of all five treatment groups when the study completes. Figure 4 displays a hypothetical Phase II program designed using such strategy. In this chapter, we propose to further improve this design by utilizing MCP-Mod for analysis at the end of the study under the "Go Fast" path. And this leads to further increase of the study power from Deng et al. [6]. The sample size is calculated by matching the desired Type I error and power by simulation.

4 Sample Size Comparison and Discussion

We compare the resulting sample sizes of the five strategies in designing a hypothetical Phase II program with a normally distributed continuous endpoint and standardized effect size $\delta = 1/3$. All programs are designed to control Type I errors at $\alpha \approx 0.05$ and achieve power $1-\beta \approx 90\%$. If the design involves two trials/stages, the first trial/stage is designed with $\alpha_1 = 0.4$ and power $1 - \beta_1 = 95\%$. The five dose–response models in Fig. 5 were considered in the design stage. The Type I errors and powers for all the designs were confirmed with simulation studies with 10,000 replicates. In each replicate, patient responses were simulated from the five-candidate dose–response models 5. Data analysis also followed these five models. The power is defined as the average power under the five-candidate set models.

Table 1 summarizes the sample sizes for each strategy, including sample sizes in each stage/trial, minimum and maximum sample sizes, and expected average sample sizes under the null and alternative hypotheses. Figure 6 further illustrates expected average sample size in plots.

When the drug does not work (under H_0), strategy B has the highest average sample size. This reflects the large upfront investment and sunken cost for the combined strategy without any interim analysis. The other designs significantly reduce the average sample size by either separating the development into two studies (strategy A) or adding adaptation rule based on interim analysis (strategies A, C, D, and E).

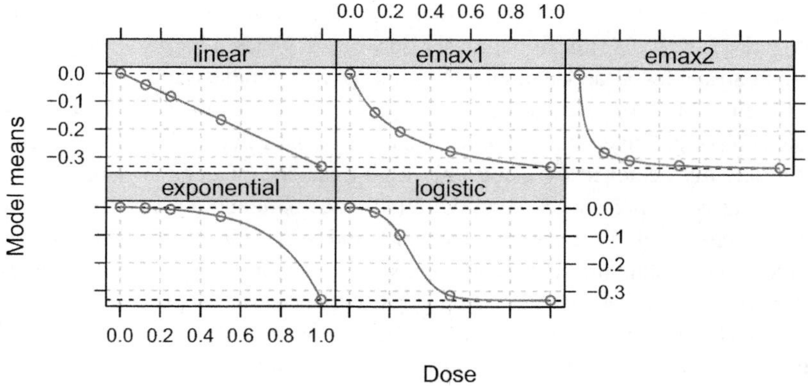

Fig. 5 Dose–response models considered for deriving the optimal contrast tests in the design stage as well as for artificial data generation in the simulation study

Table 1 Sample size summary for strategies A–E, including sample sizes in each stage/trial, minimum and maximum sample sizes, and average sample sizes under the null and alternative hypotheses

Sample size	A	B	C	D	E	
					Fast	Slow
Stage/Trial I	130	–	217	130	130	130
Stage/Trial II	483	–	336	416	395	62
Min	130	525	217	130	192	
Max	613	525	553	546	525	
Average (H_0)	323.2	525	351.4	296.4	325.2	
Average (H_a)	588.85	525	536.2	525.2	508.35	

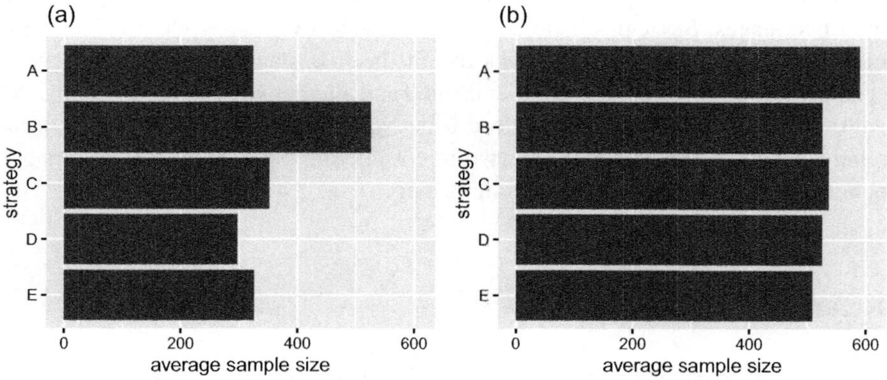

Fig. 6 Average sample sizes under the (**a**) null and (**b**) alternative hypotheses for each strategy

When the drug works (under H_a), strategy A yields a much higher average sample size than all other strategies. It also has a much higher maximum sample size. Generally, combined study with or without interim adaptation (strategies B–E) leads to smaller sample size when the drug works, and they also lead to shorter development timeline that is very attractive in drug development. Out of the three combined designs with interim analysis, strategy C yields a higher average sample size than strategies D and E under the alternative hypothesis. The reason behind it is that the objective in stage I is to detect signal of drug efficacy for Go/No-Go decision-making. Under the monotonic dose–response relationship, this objective is most efficiently achieved by using only high dose and placebo, where the largest treatment effect is present. Strategy C randomizes patients to all treatment groups at the beginning of the program (stage I), and such allocation leads to loss of efficiency in detecting the signal and results in higher sample size. As a comparison, by randomizing patients to only two groups (highest dose versus placebo) in stage I, strategy D improves strategy C in all aspects. However, in practice, there could be patient overflow for strategies C and D when time to endpoint is long, so the average sample sizes under the null hypothesis might be larger than the numbers in the table. In this case, strategy E would be attractive. Strategy E yields a slightly higher average sample size under the null hypothesis, compared to strategy D. However, it lowers the average sample size under the alternative by giving a second chance in the Go Slow path, reducing maximum sample size when achieving similar power. In addition, since additional samples are needed under either path under strategy D, the data from overflow patients can still contribute to analysis.

5 Concluding Remarks

We compare five strategies to combine Phase IIa and Phase IIb clinical programs, including two-study approach, single study with fixed design, and single study with two stages. Strategies using single study with two stages with patient only randomized to highest dose and placebo in the first stage (D and E) achieve a considerable sample size saving under the null and alternative hypotheses, compared with other approaches. We recommend using strategy D when time to endpoint is relatively short, while strategy E is worth considering when there is considerable patient overflow when time to endpoint is long.

References

1. Bretz, F., Pinheiro, J. C., Branson, M.: Combining multiple comparisons and modeling techniques in dose-response studies. Biometrics **61**(3), 738–748 (2005)
2. Ting, N.: Practical and statistical considerations in designing an early phase II osteoarthritis clinical trial: a case study. Commun. Stat. Theory Methods **38**(18), 3282–3296 (2009)
3. Zhang, Y., Deng, Q., Wang, S., Ting, N.: A simple and efficient statistical approach for designing an early phase II clinical trial: ordinal linear contrast test. In: New Advances in Statistics and Data Science, pp. 179–196. Springer, Cham (2017)
4. Brown, M.J., Chuang-Stein, C., Kirby, S.: Designing studies to find early signals of efficacy. J. Biopharm. Stat. 22(6), 1097–1108 (2012). https://doi.org/10.1080/10543406.2011.570466

5. Deng, Q., Ting, N.: Sample size allocation in a dose-ranging trial combined with PoC. In: Statistical Applications from Clinical Trials and Personalized Medicine to Finance and Business Analytics, pp. 77–90. Springer, Cham (2016)
6. Deng, Q., Bai, X., Ting, N.: Dynamic development paths for expanding a proof-of-concept study to explore dose range. Stat. Med. **37**(22), 3244–3253 (2018)

Designs of Early Phase Cancer Trials with Drug Combinations

José L. Jiménez, Márcio Augusto Diniz, André Rogatko, and Mourad Tighiouart

1 Introduction

The primary objective of a phase I oncology trial is to estimate a maximum tolerable dose (MTD) of a new drug or combination of drugs for future efficacy evaluation in phase II/III trials. For the case of combination trials with two drugs, the MTD is any dose combination (x, y) of drugs A and B that produces DLT in a pre-specified proportion of patients θ [16].

$$P(\mathrm{DLT}|x, y) = \theta. \tag{1}$$

The definition of DLT depends on the type of cancer and drugs used in the trial, but it is typically defined as a grade 3 or 4 non-hematologic or grade 4 hematologic toxicity. Different types and grades of toxicity are described in the Common Terminology Criteria for Adverse Events (CTCAE), an observer-rated toxicity grading system used in cancer clinical trials to assess the severity of various organ system toxicities associated with treatment [58]. Depending on the nature and severity of treatment-attributable toxicity, the target probability of DLT θ typically takes values between 0.1 and 0.4.

To model the probability of DLT, we assume a parametric model of the form

$$P(\mathrm{DLT}|x, y) = F(x, y; \boldsymbol{\beta}), \tag{2}$$

J. L. Jiménez
Novartis Pharma A.G., Basel, Switzerland
e-mail: jose_luis.jimenez@novartis.com

M. A. Diniz · A. Rogatko · M. Tighiouart (✉)
Samuel Oschin Comprehensive Cancer Institute, Los Angeles, CA, USA
e-mail: Marcio.Diniz@cshs.org; Andre.Rogatko@cshs.org; mourad.Tighiouart@cshs.org

Y. Zhao, (Din) D.-G. Chen (eds.), *Modern Statistical Methods for Health Research*, Emerging Topics in Statistics and Biostatistics,
https://doi.org/10.1007/978-3-030-72437-5_7

where $F(.)$ is a known link function (e.g., power model or a logistic model), and $\boldsymbol{\beta} \in R^p$ is a $p \times 1$ vector of unknown parameters. Non-parametric designs have also been proposed in the past, both for single agent and drug combination settings, see e.g., [15, 23, 27, 30, 64]. The common assumption in these designs is monotonicity (i.e., the probability of DLT increases with the dose of any one of the agents when the other one is held constant), which is imposed either through the prior distribution, or by choosing only monotonic contours when escalating.

Following [51, 53], the general phase I design for drug combinations can be stated as follows. Let S be the set of all dose combinations available in the trial and C be the set of combinations (x, y) that produce DLT in a proportion of patients that is equal to the target risk of DLT. Hence,

$$C = \{(x, y) \in S : F(x, y; \boldsymbol{\beta}) = \theta\}. \tag{3}$$

An alternative definition of the MTD is the set of dose combinations (x, y) that satisfy $|F(x, y; \boldsymbol{\beta}) - \theta| \leq \delta$, since the set C in (3) may be empty. This can happen, for example, when S is finite and the MTD is not part of the dose combinations available in the trial. The threshold parameter δ, $0 < \delta < 1$, referred to as "$100 \times \delta$-point window" in [5] must be pre-specified by the clinician.

Consecutive cohorts of one to three patients are enrolled in the trial, and the model parameters and estimated probabilities of toxicities are updated sequentially, using dose combinations allocated to all previously treated patients and their DLT outcomes. The next cohort of patients receives doses determined by minimizing the risk of exceeding the target probability of DLT according to some loss function. This general framework of dose finding for drug combinations was studied extensively in the last two decades, see e.g., [5, 12, 23, 27, 38, 42, 45, 50, 51, 53, 61, 62, 65, 67]. These methods are aimed at either identifying a single MTD or recommending more than one MTD combination for future efficacy studies. Approaches where a single MTD is selected may be sub-optimal because important dose combinations with similar acceptable DLT level and possibly with high probability of response may be missed. This could happen for two reasons. First, the discrete set of dose combinations is selected by the investigator based on prior experience with single agents. Therefore, when these agents are combined, the selected set may not include intermediate dose combinations with probability of DLT close to the target probability of DLT and the target probability of treatment response. Second, even if this discrete set includes dose combinations with probability of DLT close to the target, their probability of response may be very different and these approaches may recommend a dose combination with a low probability of response. Hence, approaches that recommend more than one MTD should be used for future efficacy studies using randomized or response-adaptive designs.

The main goal of early phase oncology phase I–II trials is to identify one or many dose combinations that are both safe and efficacious. In single-agent trials, where efficacy is evaluated within a short window of time (e.g., one or two cycles of therapy), one-stage sequential designs are frequently used by updating the joint probability of toxicity and efficacy after each cohort of patients [4, 7, 20, 31, 41,

44, 46]. This methodology has been extended to accommodate drug combinations [6, 19, 26, 39, 60, 67, 68]. However, if efficacy cannot be evaluated in a short time interval, two-stage designs are frequently employed. In the first stage, a set of maximum tolerated dose combinations is selected, and in the second stage, the set is tested for efficacy. The patient population used in the second stage may be different than that from the first stage [8, 24, 40]. For drug combination trials, different methods for two-stage designs have been proposed for binary efficacy endpoints [43, 47, 68, 70] and time-to-event efficacy endpoints [21].

In Sect. 2, we review some designs of drug combination trials focusing on continuous dose levels of both drugs. Estimation of doses to be allocated to the next cohort of patients uses the escalation with overdose control (EWOC) principle [1, 2, 13, 48, 49, 52, 54–56, 69, 71] and the continual reassessment method (CRM) [9, 14, 17, 29, 32–34]. A method that incorporates a covariate with the patients' baseline characteristics and settings where an unknown fraction of attributable DLTs will also be reviewed. In Sect. 3, we describe two-stage phase I/II designs based on the work of [47] and [21]. In each case, stage 1 follows the designs described in Sect. 2.1 to estimate the MTD curve. In stage 2, [21, 47] search for combinations along this MTD curve that maximize the probability of treatment response or median time to an event of interest. We conclude this chapter with a discussion including practical implementation of these designs and related ongoing research.

2 Designs for Phase I Clinical Trials

2.1 Phase I Model-based Designs for Drug Combinations

Model

Tighiouart et al. [51, 53] assumed that the doses (x, y) from a combination of two drugs A and B are continuous and standardized into the interval [0,1], with a dose-toxicity model of the form

$$P(Z = 1|x, y) = F(\beta_0 + \beta_1 x + \beta_2 y + \beta_3 xy), \tag{4}$$

where $\beta_1, \beta_2 > 0$, $\beta_3 \geq 0$, $Z = 1$ if a patient exhibits DLT within one cycle of therapy given the dose combination (x, y) and $Z = 0$ otherwise, and F is a cumulative distribution function (c.d.f). In particular, the logistic function, $F(u) = (1 + e^{-u})^{-1}$, has been used by several authors for single and drug combination trials, and the probit, normal, and complementary log-log link functions were used by Tighiouart et al. [51, 53] and Diniz et al. [12] to assess model misspecification.

Following (1) and (4), the MTD set is defined as

$$C = \left\{(x^*, y^*) \in S : y^* = \frac{F^{-1}(\theta) - \beta_0 - \beta_1 x^*}{\beta_2 + \beta_3 x^*}\right\}, \tag{5}$$

where (x^*, y^*) represents any dose combinations such that $P(Z = 1|x^*, y^*) = \theta$. In this context, the MTD is a hyperbola in the Cartesian plane (or a decreasing line if $\beta_3 = 0$).

Tighiouart et al. [51] reparameterized the model in (4) using the parameters $\rho_{10}, \rho_{01}, \rho_{00}$ corresponding to the probabilities of DLT when the levels of drugs A and B are 1 and 0, 0 and 1, and both 0, respectively. These parameters can be easily interpreted by clinicians, and they facilitate prior specifications since prior information on ρ_{01}, ρ_{10}, and ρ_{00} may be available from the previous trials. Moreover, this parametrization extends the one presented in [53], where it was assumed that the MTD of each drug is within the range of available doses of the corresponding agent. In this case, the MTD of each agent can lie outside the range of available doses in the trial when the other one is held at its minimum value.

The original parametrization can be recovered as follows:

$$\begin{aligned} \beta_0 &= F^{-1}(\rho_{00}), \\ \beta_1 &= F^{-1}(\rho_{10}) - F^{-1}(\rho_{00}), \\ \beta_2 &= F^{-1}(\rho_{01}) - F^{-1}(\rho_{00}), \\ \beta_3 &= \eta, \end{aligned} \tag{6}$$

such that $0 < \rho_{00} < \min(\rho_{01}, \rho_{10})$ since β_1 and β_2 are positive. The MTD set (5) becomes

$$C = \left\{ (x^*, y^*) \in S : y^* = \frac{F^{-1}(\theta) - F^{-1}(\rho_{00}) - (F^{-1}(\rho_{10}) - F^{-1}(\rho_{00}))x^*}{F^{-1}(\rho_{01}) - F^{-1}(\rho_{00}) + \eta x^*} \right\}. \tag{7}$$

Prior and Posterior Distributions

Tighiouart et al. [51] assumed that ρ_{01}, ρ_{10}, and η are independent a priori with $\rho_{01} \sim beta(a_1, b_1)$, $\rho_{10} \sim beta(a_2, b_2)$, and conditional on (ρ_{01}, ρ_{10}), $\frac{\rho_{00}}{min(\rho_{01}, \rho_{10})} \sim beta(a_3, b_3)$. A gamma distribution with mean $E(\eta) = a/b$ and variance $Var(\eta) = a/b^2$ is placed on the interaction term η. Vague $beta$ priors are achieved by taking $a_j = b_j = 1$, for $j = 0, 1, 2, 3$, while a vague gamma prior is chosen with a mean of 21 and a variance of 540.

Let $D_n = \{x_i, y_i\}, i = 1, \ldots, n$, be the data collected after enrolling n patients in the trial. The likelihood function for the model parameters is

$$\begin{aligned} \mathscr{L}(\rho_{00}, \rho_{10}, \rho_{01}, \eta) = \prod_{i=1}^{n} &(H(\rho_{00}, \rho_{10}, \rho_{01}, \eta; x_i, y_i))^{z_i} \\ &\times (1 - H(\rho_{00}, \rho_{10}, \rho_{01}, \eta; x_i, y_i))^{1-z_i}, \end{aligned} \tag{8}$$

where, using Eq. (6),

$$H(\rho_{00}, \rho_{10}, \rho_{01}, \eta; x_i, y_i)$$
$$= F\left(F^{-1}(\rho_{00}) + (F^{-1}(\rho_{10}) - F^{-1}(\rho_{00}))x_i + (F^{-1}(\rho_{01}) - F^{-1}(\rho_{00}))y_i + \eta x_i y_i\right). \quad (9)$$

Therefore, using Bayes rule, the posterior distribution of the model parameters $\rho_{00}, \rho_{01}, \rho_{10}$, and η is proportional to the product of the likelihood and the prior distribution

$$\pi(\rho_{00}, \rho_{01}, \rho_{10}, \eta | D_n) \propto \pi(\rho_{00} | \rho_{01}, \rho_{10}) \times \pi(\rho_{01}) \times \pi(\rho_{10}) \times \pi(\eta) \times \mathscr{L}(\rho_{00}, \rho_{10}, \rho_{01}, \eta), \quad (10)$$

which is analytically intractable. Therefore, Monte Carlo Markov Chain (MCMC) methods are employed such as R [37] and JAGS [35] to estimate the features of the posterior distribution of the model parameters.

Trial Design

Tighiouart et al. [51] use a dose escalation/de-escalation algorithm that treats cohorts of two patients simultaneously based on the EWOC criterion, where at each stage of the trial, one subject receives a new dose of agent *A* for a given dose of agent *B* that was previously assigned and the other patient receives a new dose of agent *B* for a given dose of agent *A* that was previously assigned. Diniz et al. [12] extended this algorithm to the CRM criterion. The dose escalation algorithm is illustrated in Fig. 1.

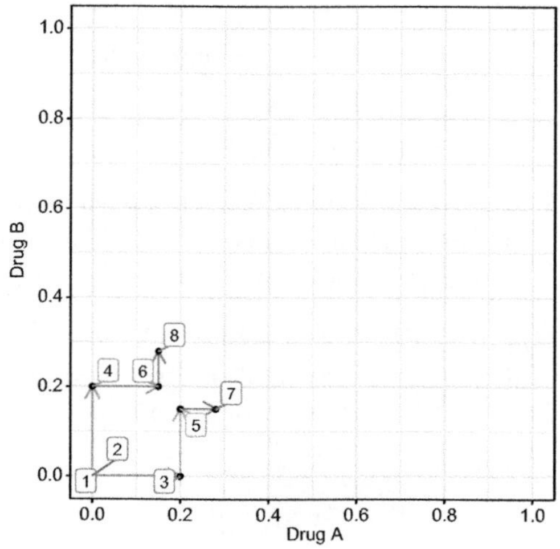

Fig. 1 Illustration of the dose escalation algorithm for the first 8 patients

Specifically, the design proceeds as follows:

1. Each patient in the first cohort of 2 patients receives the same dose combination $(x_i, y_i) = (0, 0)$ for $i = 1, 2$.
2. In the i-th cohort of 2 patients, for $i \geq 2$,

   (a) If i is even, then patient $2i - 1$ receives dose (x_{2i-1}, y_{2i-3}) and patient $2i$ receives dose (x_{2i-2}, y_{2i}), where

$$x_{2i-1} = \Pi^{-1}_{\Gamma_{A|B=y_{2i-3}}}(\alpha|D_{2i-2})$$
$$y_{2i} = \Pi^{-1}_{\Gamma_{B|A=x_{2i-2}}}(\alpha|D_{2i-2})$$

   for EWOC criterion.

$$x_{2i-1} = \underset{x}{\operatorname{argmin}}|H(\hat{\rho}_{00}, \hat{\rho}_{01}, \hat{\rho}_{10}, \hat{\eta}; x, y_{2i-3}) - \theta|$$
$$y_{2i} = \underset{y}{\operatorname{argmin}}|H(\hat{\rho}_{00}, \hat{\rho}_{01}, \hat{\rho}_{10}, \hat{\eta}; x_{2i-2}, y) - \theta|$$

   for CRM criterion.

   (b) If i is odd, then patient $2i - 1$ receives dose (x_{2i-3}, y_{2i-1}) and patient $2i$ receives dose (x_{2i}, y_{2i-2}), where

$$x_{2i} = \Pi^{-1}_{\Gamma_{A|B=y_{2i-2}}}(\alpha|D_{2i-2})$$
$$y_{2i-1} = \Pi^{-1}_{\Gamma_{B|A=x_{2i-3}}}(\alpha|D_{2i-2})$$

   for EWOC criterion.

$$x_{2i} = \underset{x}{\operatorname{argmin}}|H(\hat{\rho}_{00}, \hat{\rho}_{01}, \hat{\rho}_{10}, \hat{\eta}; x, y_{2i-2}) - \theta|$$
$$y_{2i-1} = \underset{y}{\operatorname{argmin}}|H(\hat{\rho}_{00}, \hat{\rho}_{01}, \hat{\rho}_{10}, \hat{\eta}; x_{2i-3}, y) - \theta|$$

   for CRM criterion.

3. Repeat step 2 until n patients are enrolled in the trial subject to a safety stopping rule in which the trial is stopped if the estimated probability of DLT at the lowest dose combination is higher than a pre-specified threshold.

$\Pi^{-1}_{\Gamma_{A|B=y}}(\cdot|D)$ denotes the inverse c.d.f. of the posterior distribution of the MTD of drug A given the level of drug $B = y$, and for the CRM method, $\hat{\rho}_q, \hat{\eta}, q \in \{00, 01, 10\}$ are the posterior medians.

The EWOC criterion consists of finding a dose $x^\star$ such that the posterior probability that the MTD exceeds this dose is bounded by a feasibility bound α. For example, in step 2 of the above algorithm, the dose of drug A is the maximum dose level of A such that the posterior probability that the MTD of A given that the level of drug B is y_{2i-3} exceeds $x^\star$ is bounded by α, i.e., $x^\star = x_{2i-1} = \Pi^{-1}_{\Gamma_{A|B=y_{2i-3}}}(\alpha|D_{i-1})$. Babb et al. [1] suggested a fixed feasibility boundary α equal to 0.25. Babb and Rogatko [2] introduced an increasing feasibility boundary until 0.5 with initial α equal 0.25, while Wheeler et al. [63] suggested a similar strategy, but conditional on the previous patient having no DLT.

The CRM criterion consists of finding a dose $x^\star$ such that it minimizes the absolute value difference between the estimated probabilities of DLT for the target toxicity rate θ. For example, in step 2 of the above algorithm, the dose of drug A is the dose $x^\star$ that minimizes $|H(\hat{\rho}_{00}, \hat{\rho}_{01}, \hat{\rho}_{10}, \hat{\eta}; x^\star, y_{2i-3}) - \theta|$.

At the end of the trial, the MTD (7) is estimated as

$$\widehat{C} = \left\{ (x^*, y^*) \in S : y^* = \frac{F^{-1}(\theta) - F^{-1}(\widehat{\rho}_{00}) - (F^{-1}(\widehat{\rho}_{10}) - F^{-1}(\widehat{\rho}_{00}))x^*}{F^{-1}(\widehat{\rho}_{01}) - F^{-1}(\widehat{\rho}_{00}) + \widehat{\eta}_3 x^*} \right\}. \tag{11}$$

The discussed approach can be easily extended to a discrete grid of doses, i.e., $(x_1, \cdots, x_r)$ and $(y_1, \cdots, y_r)$ be the doses of agents A and B, respectively. Trial design proceeds using the algorithm described in Sect. 2.1 with the continuous doses recommended in step 2 being rounded to the nearest discrete dose level.

At the end of the trial, a discrete set Γ of dose combinations satisfying (i) and (ii) below is selected as MTDs. Let C_i be the estimated MTD curve at the end of the trial and denote by $d((x_j, y_k), C_i)$ the Euclidian distance between the dose combination (x_j, y_k) and C_i as in (14).

(i) Let $\Gamma_A = \bigcup_{t=1}^{r} \left\{ (x, y_t) : x = \underset{x_j}{\text{argmin}}\, d((x_j, y_t), C_i) \right\}$,

$\Gamma_B = \bigcup_{t=1}^{r} \left\{ (x_t, y) : y = \underset{y_j}{\text{argmin}}\, d((x_t, y_j), C_i) \right\}$, and $\Gamma_0 = \Gamma_B \cap \Gamma_A$.

(ii) Let $\Gamma = \Gamma_0 \backslash \{(x*, y*) : P(|P(Z = 1|(x*, y*)) - \theta| > \delta_1 | D_n) > \delta_2\}$.

In (i), dose combinations closest to the MTD are selected by first minimizing the distances across the levels of drug A and then across the levels of drug B. In (ii), we exclude MTDs from (i) that likely to be either too toxic or too low. The design parameter δ_1 is selected after consultation with a clinician, and the parameter δ_2 is selected after exploring a large number of scenarios for a given prospective trial. Following [51], $\delta_1 = 0.1$, $\delta_2 = 0.3$.

Design Operating Characteristics

The performance of trial designs with finite sample size is assessed based on operating characteristics calculated from a Monte Carlo simulation study with m replicates, often with $m = 1000$.

In single agents, there are several operating characteristics such as bias, mean-squared error, average DLT rate, percentage of trials in which DLT rate is within an optimal toxicity interval, the percentage of trials with the estimated MTD within an optimal MTD interval, and the percentage of patients receiving optimal doses defined by those optimal intervals among others [13]. These operating characteristics can be divided in two classes measuring the safety of the trial design and the efficiency to estimate the MTD curve.

However, not all of them can be easily extended when estimating the MTD as a curve instead of a point in the dose space. Tighiouart et al. [53] presented some of these extensions.

Safety

The average percentage of DLT and the percentage of trials that have a DLT rate exceeding $\theta + \delta$ are, respectively, given by

$$\bar{\theta} = \frac{1}{m}\sum_{i=1}^{m}\hat{\theta}_i \tag{12}$$

$$\bar{\theta}_\delta = \frac{1}{m}\sum_{i=1}^{m}\mathbb{1}(\hat{\theta}_i > \theta + \delta) \tag{13}$$

where $\hat{\theta}_i$ is the estimated DLT rate for ith replicate for $i = 1, \ldots, m$. It is expected that $\bar{\theta}$ is close to θ, and the threshold $\delta = 0.1$ is considered to be an indication of an excessive DLT rate.

Efficiency

The pointwise average relative minimum distance from the true MTD curve to the estimated MTD curve can be interpreted as the pointwise average bias when estimating the MTD.

Let C_i be the estimated MTD curve for the ith Monte Carlo replicate and C_{true} be the true MTD curve. For every point $(x, y) \in C_{true}$, the minimum relative distance of the point (x, y) on the true MTD curve to the estimated MTD curve C_i can be calculated as follows:

$$d^{(i)}_{(x,y)} = sign(y' - y) \times min_{\{(x^*,y^*):(x^*,y^*)\in C_i\}}((x - x^*)^2 + (y - y^*)^2)^{1/2}, \tag{14}$$

where y' is such that $(x, y') \in C_i$ for $i = 1, \ldots, m$. If the point (x, y) is below C_i, then $d^{(i)}_{(x,y)}$ is positive. Otherwise, it is negative.

Then, the pointwise average bias is defined as follows:

$$d_{(x,y)} = \frac{1}{m} \sum_{i=1}^{m} d^{(i)}_{(x,y)}. \tag{15}$$

As the magnitude of bias is relative to the true MTD, it is also important to quantify the percentage of trials satisfying a given condition relative to the true MTD value. Let $\Delta(x, y)$ be the Euclidean distance between the minimum dose combination $(0, 0)$ and the point (x, y) on the true MTD curve, such that the minimum distance of the point (x, y) from the true MTD curve to the estimated MTD curve C_i is no more than $(100 \times p)\%$ of the distance of the true MTD from the minimum dose,

$$R_{(x,y)} = \frac{1}{m} \sum_{i=1}^{m} I\left(|d^{(i)}_{(x,y)}| \le p\Delta(x, y)\right), \tag{16}$$

where $0 < p < 1$.

One can interpret (16) as drawing a circle with center (x, y) on the true MTD curve and radius $p\Delta(x, y)$, and then the percent of trials with the MTD curve estimate C_i within this circle is given by $R_{(x,y)}$. Therefore, the statistic (16) measures the percentage of correct recommendations.

Results

The methodology for a phase I trial proposed by Tighiouart et al. [51, 53] and Diniz et al. [12] has also been used by Diniz et al. [10], Tighiouart [47], and Jiménez et al. [21]. Therefore, there are several scenarios available in the literature with different values for ρ_{00}, ρ_{01}, ρ_{10}, and η. For illustration purposes, we present the operating characteristics of one of these multiple scenarios based on 2000 simulated trials. Dose escalation proceeds following EWOC and CRM criteria with the target toxicity rate $\theta = 0.33$. For EWOC, the feasibility boundary α starts at 0.25 with an increment of 0.05 for each new cohort of patients up to 0.5. Cohorts of two patients were accrued with the total sample size of 40 patients.

Assuming $(\rho_{00}, \rho_{10}, \rho_{01}, \eta) = (1, 0.01, 0.6, 10)$ from [51], Table 1 shows safety operating characteristics indicating that the proposed designs rarely surpass the toxicity rate given that one drug has low toxicity. Figure 2A shows the estimated MTD, with Fig. 2B indicating increasing bias at the edges of the MTD curves, varying from −0.06 to 0.06 for EWOC and −0.045 to 0.045 for CRM. The percentage of correct recommendation in Fig. 2C displays high values for both tolerances $p = 0.1, 0.2$ reaching the minimum values on the far left edge of MTD curve, with 63% for EWOC and 74% for CRM. Therefore, the CRM criterion

Table 1 Safety results from the simulated scenario presented in Fig. 2 from [51]

Design	Average % of toxicities	% of trials with DLT rate $> \theta + 0.05$	% of trials with DLT rate $> \theta + 0.10$
CRM	27.21	0.20	0.00
EWOC	25.25	0.05	0.00

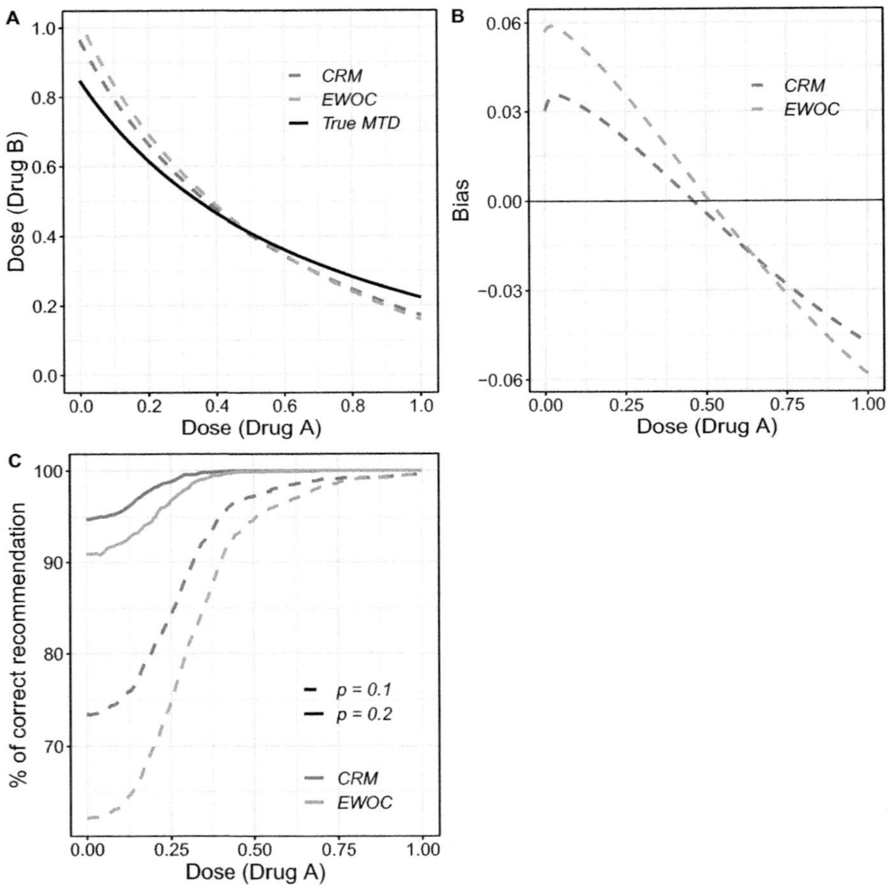

Fig. 2 Simulated scenario taken from [51], $(\rho_{00}, \rho_{10}, \rho_{01}, \eta) = (1, 0.01, 0.6, 10)$. In (A), we show the true and estimated MTD curves as defined in Eq. (7) as well as each final recommended dose combination after simulating 1000 trials. In (B) and (C), we observe the bias and the percentage of correct recommendation, respectively, for each value of dose for drug A contained in the MTD curve

presents superior operating characteristics for this scenario. Overall, both designs have good operating characteristics and are able to estimate the MTD curve while keeping the proportion of DLTs within reasonable boundaries.

2.2 Attributing Dose-Limiting Toxicities

Model

Following [22] and using the same notation as the one defined in Sect. 2.1, the doses of drugs A and B are standardized to be in a desired interval. The marginal probability of DLT of each compound is defined in terms of the power model (i.e., $P(Z = 1|x) = x^\alpha$ and $P(Z = 1|y) = y^\beta$), and we specify the joint probability of DLT using the Gumbel copula model (see [31]) as

$$\begin{aligned} &P(\delta_A, \delta_B|x, y) \\ &\quad = (x^\alpha)^{\delta_A}\left(1 - x^\alpha\right)^{1-\delta_A}(y^\beta)^{\delta_B}\left(1 - y^\beta\right)^{1-\delta_B} + (-1)^{(\delta_A+\delta_B)}\gamma(x, y), \end{aligned} \tag{17}$$

where $\gamma(x, y) = x^\alpha\,(1 - x^\alpha)\,y^\beta\left(1 - y^\beta\right)\frac{e^{-\gamma}-1}{e^{-\gamma}+1}$, δ_A is the binary indicator of DLT attributed to drug A, δ_B is the binary indicator of DLT attributed to drug B, and γ is the interaction parameter. A sufficient condition for the monotonicity assumption to hold is to assume that x^α and y^β are the increasing functions (i.e., $\alpha > 0$ and $\beta > 0$). Using (17), if the DLT is attributed exclusively to drug A, then

$$P(\delta_A = 1, \delta_B = 0|x, y) = \pi^A = x^\alpha(1 - y^\beta) - \gamma(x, y). \tag{18}$$

If the DLT is attributed exclusively to drug B, then

$$P(\delta_A = 0, \delta_B = 1|x, y) = \pi^B = y^\beta(1 - x^\alpha) - \gamma(x, y). \tag{19}$$

If the DLT is attributed to both A and B, then

$$P(\delta_A = 1, \delta_B = 1|x, y) = \pi^{AB} = x^\alpha y^\beta + \gamma(x, y). \tag{20}$$

Equation (18) represents the probability that a DLT is caused only by drug A. This can happen, for example, when a type of DLT of taxotere (A), such as grade 4 neutropenia, is observed. However, this type of DLT can never be observed with metformin (B). This can also happen when the clinician attributes a grade 4 diarrhea to taxotere (A) but not to metformin (B) in the case of a low-dose level of this later even though both drugs have this common type of side effect. The fact that dose level y is present in Eq. (18) is a result of the joint modeling of the two marginals and accounts for the probability that drug B does not cause a DLT. This later case is, of course, based on the clinician's judgment. Equations (19) and (20) can be interpreted similarly.

The overall probability of DLT is calculated following [65] as the sum of (18), (19), and (20), which translates into

$$P(\text{DLT}|x, y) = \pi = x^\alpha + y^\beta - x^\alpha y^\beta - \gamma(x, y). \tag{21}$$

To calculate the MTD, re-write Eq. (1) as a second-degree polynomial in y^{β} and solve for the solutions. This allows us to define the MTD set C as

$$C = \left\{ (x_*, y_*) : y_* = \left[\frac{-(1 - x_*^{\alpha} - \kappa) \pm \sqrt{(1 - x_*^{\alpha} - \kappa)^2 - 4\kappa(x_*^{\alpha} - \theta)}}{2\kappa} \right]^{\frac{1}{\beta}} \right\}, \tag{22}$$

where

$$\kappa = x_*^{\alpha}(1 - x_*^{\alpha}) \frac{e^{-\gamma} - 1}{e^{-\gamma} + 1}.$$

Among patients treated with dose combination (x, y) who exhibit DLT, suppose that an unknown fraction η of these patients have a DLT with known attribution, i.e., the clinician knows if the DLT is caused by drug A only, or drug B only, or both drugs A and B. Let $\mathscr{A}$ be the indicator of DLT attribution when $Z = 1$. It follows that for each patient treated with dose combination (x, y), there are five possible toxicity outcomes. This is illustrated in the chance tree diagram in Fig. 3. Using Eqs. (18), (19), (20), (21), and Fig. 3, we can define the contributions to the likelihood from each of the five observable outcomes as defined in Table 2.

The likelihood function is defined as

$$\mathscr{L}(\alpha, \beta, \gamma, \eta) = \prod_{i=1}^{n} \left[\left(\eta \pi_i^{(\delta_{A_i}, \delta_{B_i})} \right)^{\mathscr{A}_i} (\pi_i \, (1 - \eta))^{1 - \mathscr{A}_i} \right]^{Z_i} (1 - \pi_i)^{1 - Z_i}, \tag{23}$$

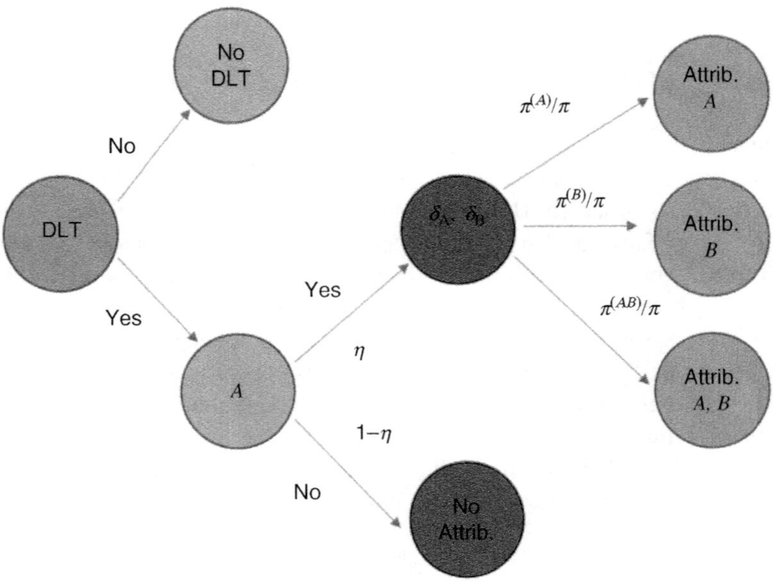

Fig. 3 A chance tree illustrating the 5 possible outcomes we can find in a trial

Table 2 Contributions to the likelihood function based on the observed outcomes: toxicity, attribution, attribution to drug A (δ_A), and attribution to drug B (δ_B) for each patient

Toxicity (Z)	Attribution ($\mathscr{A}$)	δ_A	δ_B	Likelihood
0	–	–	–	$1-\pi = 1-\left[x^{\alpha}+y^{\beta}-x^{\alpha}\times y^{\beta}-\gamma(x,y)\right]$
1	0	–	–	$\pi\times(1-\eta) = \left[x^{\alpha}+y^{\beta}-x^{\alpha}\times y^{\beta}-\gamma(x,y)\right]\times(1-\eta)$
1	1	1	0	$\pi\times\eta\times\frac{\pi^{(1,0)}}{\pi} = \eta\times\left[x^{\alpha}(1-y^{\beta})-\gamma(x,y)\right]$
1	1	0	1	$\pi\times\eta\times\frac{\pi^{(0,1)}}{\pi} = \eta\times\left[y^{\beta}(1-x^{\alpha})-\gamma(x,y)\right]$
1	1	1	1	$\pi\times\eta\times\frac{\pi^{(1,1)}}{\pi} = \eta\times\left[x^{\alpha}y^{\beta}+\gamma(x,y)\right]$

and the joint posterior probability distribution of the model parameters as

$$P(\alpha,\beta,\gamma,\eta|x,y,\delta_A,\delta_B) \propto P(\alpha)P(\beta)P(\gamma)P(\eta)\times\mathscr{L}(\alpha,\beta,\gamma,\eta). \tag{24}$$

Using Eq. (24), we can easily sample and obtain MCMC estimates of α, β, γ, and η.

Trial Design

Dose escalation/de-escalation proceeds using the following modified univariate continual reassessment method (CRM) [32] described in Sect. 2.1:

1. Each patient in the first cohort of 2 patients receives the same dose combination $(x_i, y_i) = (0, 0)$ for $i = 1, 2$.
2. In the i-th cohort of 2 patients, for $i \geq 2$,

   (a) If i is even, then patient $2i-1$ receives dose (x_{2i-1}, y_{2i-3}) and patient $2i$ receives dose (x_{2i-2}, y_{2i}), where

$$x_{2i-1} = \underset{x}{\text{argmin}}\left|\widehat{\text{Prob}}(Z=1|x, y_{2i-3})-\theta\right|,$$

$$y_{2i} = \underset{y}{\text{argmin}}\left|\widehat{\text{Prob}}(Z=1|x_{2i-2}, y)-\theta\right|.$$

   If a DLT was observed in the previous cohort of two patients and was attributable to drug A, then x_{2i-1} is further restricted to be no more than x_{2i-3}. On the other hand, if a DLT was observed in the previous cohort of two patients and was attributable to drug B, then y_{2i} is further restricted to be no more than y_{2i-2}.

   (b) If i is odd, then patient $2i-1$ receives dose (x_{2i-3}, y_{2i-1}) and patient $2i$ receives dose (x_{2i}, y_{2i-2}), where

$$x_{2i} = \underset{x}{\text{argmin}}\left|\widehat{\text{Prob}}(Z=1|x, y_{2i-2})-\theta\right|$$

$$y_{2i-1} = \underset{y}{\text{argmin}}\left|\widehat{\text{Prob}}(Z=1|x_{2i-3}, y)-\theta\right|.$$

If a DLT was observed in the previous cohort of two patients and was attributable to drug A, then x_{2i} is further restricted to be no more than x_{2i-2}. On the other hand, if a DLT was observed in the previous cohort of two patients and was attributable to drug B, then y_{2i-1} is further restricted to be no more than y_{2i-3}.

3. Repeat step 2 until n patients are enrolled in the trial subject to a safety stopping rule in which the trial is stopped if the estimated probability of DLT at the lowest dose combination is higher than a pre-specified threshold.

Results

An extensive simulation study is performed by Jimenez et al. [22]. For illustration purposes, in Fig. 4, we present the results of one scenario that illustrates the main conclusion of this chapter.

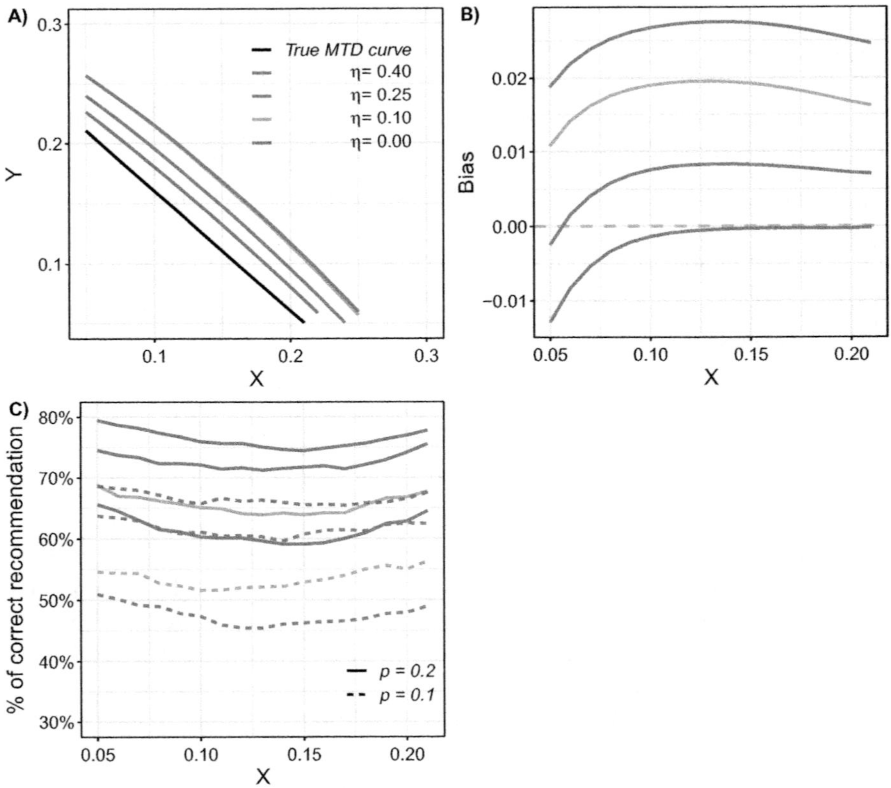

Fig. 4 Simulated scenario taken from [22]. In (A), we show the true and estimated MTD curves as defined in Eq. (22) as well as each final recommended dose combination after simulating 1000 trials for different levels of toxicity attribution. In (B) and (C), we observe the bias and the percentage of correct recommendation, respectively, for each value of X contained in the MTD curve

Table 3 Safety results from the simulated scenario presented in Fig. 4 from [22]

η	Average % of toxicities	% of trials with DLT rate $> \theta + 0.05$	% of trials with DLT rate $> \theta + 0.10$
0.00	33.62	25.90	4.10
0.10	32.67	22.60	4.80
0.25	31.55	17.60	2.70
0.40	30.70	13.30	2.00

Jimenez et al. [22] evaluate the effect of toxicity attribution in several scenarios assuming proportions of attributed DLTs of 0%, 10%, 25% and 40% (i.e., $\eta = \{0, 0.1, 0.25, 0.4\}$). These values are reasonable because higher values of η in practice are very rare. In general, increasing the value of η increases the pointwise percent of MTD recommendation and reduces bias. The approach of partial toxicity attribution generates safe trial designs, as presented in Table 3, and efficient estimation of the MTD. Further details about the approach and computer codes can be found in [22].

2.3 *Adding a Baseline Covariate*

Although chemotherapy and radiotherapy are still the main cancer treatments for tumors after surgical excision, these conventional therapies may be combined with targeted agents to enhance treatment efficacy. Traditional drug combination designs as presented in the previous section assume that the patient population is homogeneous of treatment tolerance. Therefore, a design that specifies the dose-toxicity relationship given a baseline covariate that indicates when a patient is more susceptible to a given targeted agent is desirable for drug combinations.

Model

Diniz et al. [10] proposed a parametric model to identify tolerable dose combinations of two synergistic drugs A and B given a patient with a binary baseline covariate with value w. Assuming the same notation used along this chapter, the proposed model is defined as

$$P(Z = 1|x, y, w) = F(\beta_0 + \beta_1 x + \beta_2 y + \beta_3 xy + \beta_4 w). \qquad (25)$$

The MTD for a patient with covariate value w is defined as the set of combinations (x^*, y^*) such that

$$C = \left\{ (x^*, y^*) \in S : y^* = \frac{F^{-1}(\theta) - \beta_0 - \beta_1 x^* - \beta_4 w}{\beta_2 + \beta_3 x^*} \right\}. \qquad (26)$$

The model (25) is reparameterized to allow a more meaningful prior elicitation defining ρ_{000} as the probability of DLT when the level of drugs A and B is minimum, and $w = 0$; ρ_{100} as the probability of DLT when the level of drug A is maximum, the level of drug Y is minimum and $w = 0$; ρ_{101} as the probability of DLT when the level of drug X is maximum, the level of drug B is minimum and $w = 1$; ρ_{010} as the probability of DLT when the level of drugs A is minimum, the level of drug B is maximum, and $w = 0$. Then, it follows that

$$\begin{aligned} \beta_0 &= F^{-1}(\rho_{000}) \\ \beta_1 &= F^{-1}(\rho_{100}) - F^{-1}(\rho_{000}) \\ \beta_2 &= F^{-1}(\rho_{010}) - F^{-1}(\rho_{000}) \\ \beta_3 &= \eta \\ \beta_4 &= F^{-1}(\rho_{101}) - F^{-1}(\rho_{100}). \end{aligned} \tag{27}$$

The MTD set defined in (26) can be written as

$$C = \left\{ (x^*, y^*) \in S : y^* = \frac{G(\theta, \rho_{000}) - (G(\rho_{100}, \rho_{000}))x^* - (G(\rho_{101}, \rho_{100}))w}{G(\rho_{010}, \rho_{000}) + \eta x^*} \right\}, \tag{28}$$

where $G(a, b) = F^{-1}(a) - F^{-1}(b)$.

Let $D_n = \{(x_i, y_i, z_i, \delta_i), i = 1, \ldots, n\}$ be the data after enrolling n patients in the trial. The likelihood function under the reparameterization is

$$\begin{aligned} \mathscr{L}(\rho_{000}, \rho_{100}, \rho_{101}, \rho_{010}, \eta | D_n) = \prod_{i=1}^{n} &(H(\rho_{000}, \rho_{100}, \rho_{101}, \rho_{010}, \eta; x_i, y_i, w_i))^{\delta_i} \\ &\times (1 - H(\rho_{000}, \rho_{100}, \rho_{101}, \rho_{010}, \eta; x_i, y_i, z_i))^{1-\delta_i}, \end{aligned} \tag{29}$$

where

$$\begin{aligned} &H(\rho_{000}, \rho_{100}, \rho_{101}, \rho_{010}, \eta; x_i, y_i, z_i) \\ &\quad = F(F^{-1}(\rho_{000}) + (F^{-1}(\rho_{100}) - F^{-1}(\rho_{000}))x_i + (F^{-1}(\rho_{010}) - F^{-1}(\rho_{000}))y_i \\ &\qquad + (F^{-1}(\rho_{101}) - F^{-1}(\rho_{100}))w_i + \beta_3 x_i y_i). \end{aligned} \tag{30}$$

Prior and Posterior Distributions

Diniz et al. [10] consider the priors $\rho_{100} \sim \text{beta}(a_1, b_1)$, $\rho_{010} \sim \text{beta}(a_3, b_3)$, $\rho_{101} \sim \text{beta}(a_2, b_2)$, $\rho_{000}/min(\rho_{100}, \rho_{010}) \sim \text{beta}(a_0, b_0)$, and $\eta \sim \text{gamma}(a, b)$

with mean $E(\eta) = a/b$ and variance $Var(\eta) = a/b^2$. See Sect. 2.1 for the definition of the hyperparameter values of each distribution. The posterior distribution is given by

$$\begin{aligned} P(\rho_{000}, \rho_{100}, \rho_{101}, \rho_{010}, \eta | D_n) \propto \prod_{i=1}^{n} & (H(\rho_{000}, \rho_{100}, \rho_{101}, \rho_{010}, \eta; x_i, y_i, w_i))^{Z_i} \\ & \times (1 - H(\rho_{000}, \rho_{100}, \rho_{101}, \rho_{010}, \eta; x_i, y_i, w_i))^{1-Z_i} \\ & \times P(\rho_{000}|\rho_{100}, \rho_{010}) P(\rho_{100}) P(\rho_{101}) P(\rho_{010}) P(\eta). \end{aligned} \quad (31)$$

Trial Design

The algorithm for dose escalation/de-escalation is similar to the one discussed in Sect. 2.1 with the additional binary covariate information. It uses the EWOC principle [1] where at each stage of the trial, we seek a dose of one agent using the current posterior distribution of the MTD of the agent given the current dose of the other agent and the next patient's baseline covariate value. Specifically, for the i-th cohort of two patients, the design proceeds as follows:

1. If i is even, patient $(2i - 1)$ receives dose (x_{2i-3}, y_{2i-1}) and patient $2i$ receives dose (x_{2i}, y_{2i-2}), where $y_{2i-1} = \Pi^{-1}_{\Gamma_{B|A=x_{2i-3}, W=w_{2i-1}}}(\alpha | D_{2i-2})$ and $x_{2i} = \Pi^{-1}_{\Gamma_{A|B=y_{2i-2}, Z=z_{2i}}}(\alpha | D_{2i-2})$. Here, $\Pi^{-1}_{\Gamma_{A|B=y, W=w}}(\alpha | D)$ is the inverse cumulative distribution function of the posterior distribution, $\pi(\Gamma_{A|B=y, Z=z} | D)$.
2. Similarly, if i is odd, patient $(2i - 1)$receives dose (x_{2i-1}, y_{2i-3}) and patient $2i$ receives dose (x_{2i-2}, y_{2i}), where $x_{2i-1} = \Pi^{-1}_{\Gamma_{A|B=y_{2i-3}, W=w_{2i-1}}}(\alpha | D_{2i-2})$ and $y_{2i} = \Pi^{-1}_{\Gamma_{B|A=x_{2i-2}, W=w_{2i}}}(\alpha | D_{2i-2})$.

As described in Sect. 2.1, dose escalation is further restricted to be no more than a pre-specified fraction of the dose range of the corresponding agent as well as stopping rules.

At the completion of the trial, an estimate of the MTD curve for $w = 0, 1$ is obtained using Eq. (28) as

$$\hat{C} = \left\{ (x^*, y^*) \in S : y^* = \frac{G(\theta, \hat{\rho}_{000}) - (G(\hat{\rho}_{100}, \hat{\rho}_{000}))x^* - (G(\hat{\rho}_{101}, \hat{\rho}_{100}))w}{G(\hat{\rho}_{010}, \hat{\rho}_{000}) + \hat{\beta}_3 x^*} \right\}, \quad (32)$$

where $G(a, b) = F^{-1}(a) - F^{-1}(b)$, and $\hat{\rho}_{000}, \hat{\rho}_{100}, \hat{\rho}_{101}, \hat{\rho}_{010}$, and $\hat{\beta}_3$ are the posterior medians given the data D_n.

Table 4 Safety results from the simulated scenario presented in Fig. 5 from [10]

Covariate (W)	Average % of toxicities	% of trials with DLT rate $> \theta + 0.05$	% of trials with DLT rate $> \theta + 0.10$
Overall	30.70	4.80	0.40
0	22.10	0.60	0.10
1	39.40	58.80	32.80

Results

In [10] several scenarios we evaluated, including a comparison between including and not including a baseline covariate in parallel trials. We illustrate the design for drug combination with a baseline covariate using a simulation study with 1000 trials. Dose escalation proceeds following EWOC criterion with the target toxicity rate $\theta = 0.33$, and the feasibility boundary α starts at 0.25 with an increment of 0.05 for each new cohort of patients up to 0.5. Cohorts of two patients were accrued with the total sample size of 40 patients such that two sub-groups of 20 patients randomly accrued over each trial.

Table 4 shows safety operating characteristics indicating that the proposed design is able to control the overall average DLT, with higher overdose for patients with $W = 1$ because they are more susceptible, i.e., their MTD curve is closer to the minimum dose. Figure 5A shows the estimated MTD for both sub-groups, with Fig. 5B indicating increasing bias at the edges of the MTD curves, but still with negligible absolute values. The percentage of correct recommendation in Fig. 5C displays high values for both tolerances $p = 0.1, 0.2$ when $W = 0$ and only $p = 0.2$ when $W = 1$.

3 Designs for Phase I–II Clinical Trials

3.1 *Binary Endpoint*

Let $\widehat{C}$ be the estimated MTD curve obtained in Eq. (11) and suppose it is defined for $(x, y) \in [X_1, X_2] \times [Y_1, Y_2] \subset [X_{\min}, X_{\max}] \times [Y_{\min}, Y_{\max}]$. Let E be the indicator of treatment response, $E = 1$ if we have a positive response, and $E = 0$ otherwise. Let p_0 be the probability of efficacy of the standard-of-care treatment. The goal of the stage II trial is to identify dose combinations $(x, y) \in \widehat{C}$ such that $P(E = 1|(x, y)) > p_0$.

Model

Tighiouart [47] models the probability of response by first mapping dose combinations on $\widehat{C}$ to $[0, 1]$ as follows. For $(x, y) \in \widehat{C}$, let x be the vertical projection of

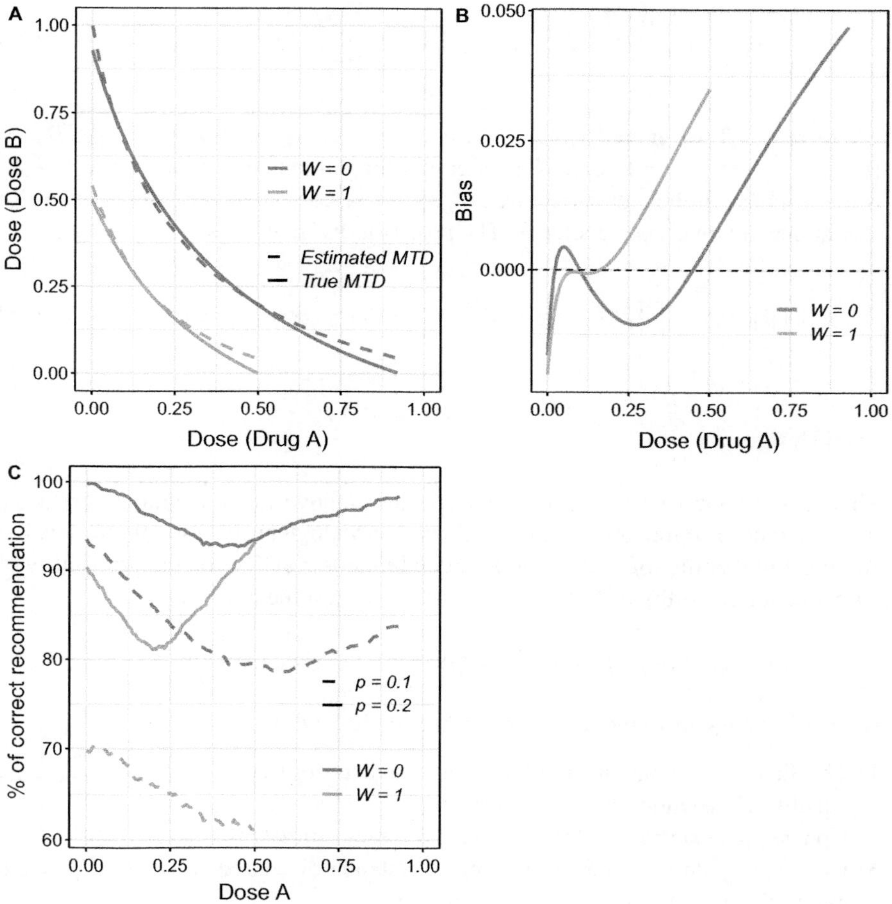

Fig. 5 Simulated scenario taken from [10], $(\rho_{000}, \rho_{100}, \rho_{010}, \rho_{101}, \eta) = (0.01, 0.40, 0.40, 0.80, 10)$. In (A), we show the true and estimated MTD curves as defined in Eq. (28) as well as each final recommended dose combination after simulating 1000 trials. In (B) and (C), we observe the bias and the percentage of correct recommendation, respectively, for each value of drug A contained in the MTD curve

(x, y) on the interval $[X, Y]$ and $z = h(x) = (x - X)/(Y - X)$. z can be considered as a dose combination since there is a one-to-one transformation mapping $z \in [0, 1]$ to $(x, y) \in \widehat{C}$. Let

$$P(E = 1|z, \boldsymbol{\psi}) = F(f(z; \boldsymbol{\psi})) \tag{33}$$

be the probability of efficacy, where F is a known link function, $f(z; \boldsymbol{\psi})$ is unknown, and $\boldsymbol{\psi}$ is an unknown parameter. A flexible way to model the probability of efficacy along the MTD curve is the cubic spline function

$$f(z; \boldsymbol{\psi}) = \beta_0 + \beta_1 z + \beta_2 z^2 + \sum_{j=3}^{k} \beta_j (z - \kappa_j)_+^3, \tag{34}$$

where $\boldsymbol{\psi} = (\boldsymbol{\beta}, \boldsymbol{\kappa})$, $\boldsymbol{\beta} = (\beta_0, \ldots, \beta_k)$, $\boldsymbol{\kappa} = (\kappa_3, \ldots, \kappa_k)$ with $\kappa_3 = 0$. Let $D_m = \{(z_i, E_i), i = 1, \ldots, m\}$ be the data after enrolling m patients in the trial, where E_i is the response of the i-th patient treated with dose combination z_i and let $\pi(\boldsymbol{\psi})$ be a prior density on the parameter $\boldsymbol{\psi}$. The posterior distribution is

$$\pi(\boldsymbol{\psi}|D_m) \propto \prod_{i=1}^{m} [F(f(z_i; \boldsymbol{\psi}))]^{E_i} [1 - F(f(z_i; \boldsymbol{\psi}))]^{1-E_i} \pi(\boldsymbol{\psi}). \tag{35}$$

Trial Design

This stage of the trial makes use of response-adaptive randomization to allocate patients to dose combinations that are likely to have high probability of efficacy. Let p_z be the probability of efficacy at dose combination z and p_0 be the probability of a treatment not worthy of further investigation. To test the hypothesis

$$\text{H}_0 : p_z \leq p_0 \text{ for all } z \text{ versus } \text{H}_1 : p_z > p_0 \text{ for some } z,$$

we enroll n patients in the trial according to the following design:

1. The first n_1 patients are randomly assigned to dose combinations $z_1, \ldots, z_{n_1}$ equally spaced along the MTD curve C_{est}.
2. Update the posterior in (35) and obtain a Bayes estimate $\hat{\boldsymbol{\psi}}$.
3. Generate n_2 dose combinations from the standardized density $F(f(z; \hat{\boldsymbol{\psi}}))$ and assign them to the next cohort of n_2 patients.
4. Repeat steps (2) and (3) until n patients have been enrolled subject to pre-specified stopping rules.

This algorithm can be viewed as an extension of a Bayesian adaptive design to select a superior arm among a finite number of arms [3] to selecting a superior arm from an infinite number of arms.

Decision Rule At the end of the trial, accept H_1 if

$$\text{Max}_z[P(F(f(z; \boldsymbol{\psi})) > p_0|D_n)] > \delta_u, \tag{36}$$

where δ_u is a design parameter.

Stopping Rules For ethical considerations and to avoid exposing patients to sub-therapeutic doses, the trial may be stopped for futility after j patients are evaluable for efficacy if there is strong evidence that none of the dose combinations are promising, i.e., $\text{Max}_z[P(F(f(z; \boldsymbol{\psi})) > p_0|D_j)] < \delta_0$, where δ_0 is a small pre-specified threshold. In cases where the investigator is interested in stopping the trial early for superiority, the trial may be terminated after j patients are evaluable for efficacy if $\text{Max}_z[P(F(f(z;\psi)) > p_0|D_j)] > \delta_1$, where $\delta_1 \geq \delta_u$ is a pre-specified threshold and the corresponding dose combination $z^* = \text{argmax}_u\{P(F(f(u;\psi)) > p_0|D_j)\}$ is selected for future randomized phase II or III studies.

Results

Performance of this design depends on a number of parameters including the sample size n, the probability of a poor treatment efficacy p_0, design parameter δ_u, and desired effect size. Using extensive simulations, [47] showed that this phase 2 response-adaptive design has good operating characteristics using sample sizes and effect sizes comparable to single-arm phase 2 trials with one dose level. For illustration purpose, we provide in Fig. 6 the 6 scenarios presented in [47], where scenarios A–C favor the null hypothesis and scenarios D–F favor the alternative hypothesis (see Sect. 3.1). These were used to derive the operating characteristics of a combination trial cisplatin–cabazitaxel in advanced prostate cancer patients with clinical benefit as the treatment response. The probability of a poor treatment response is $p_0 = 0.15$ and the effect size is 0.25. Thirty patients were enrolled in stage 2 following 30 patients in stage 1. Scenarios A–C have estimated powers of 0.896, 0.921, and 0.81, respectively. Scenarios D–F have estimated type-I error probabilities of 0.1, 0.19, and 0.143, respectively. Additional results such as average bias and percentage of correct recommendation, and safety for stage 1 are presented in [47] as well as in its supplementary material. These results allow to conclude that

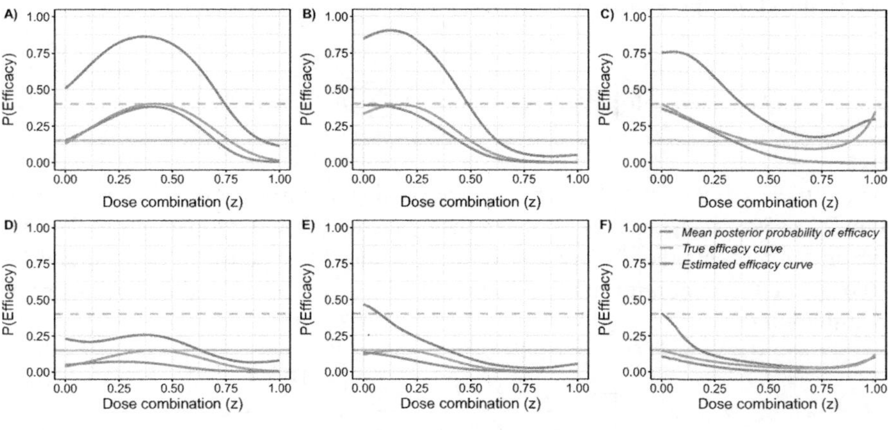

Fig. 6 True efficacy curves, mean posterior probability of efficacy curves, and estimated efficacy curves for different dose combinations (z) in 6 scenarios under H_0 and H_1. The grey-solid lines represent the null probability of efficacy p_0 (i.e., the probability of a poor treatment efficacy) and the grey-dashed lines represent the target probability of efficacy (i.e., the effect size)

this design has, in general, good operating characteristics allowing to identify the dose combination that maximizes the efficacy.

3.2 Survival Endpoint

Introduction

In this section, we review the work of Jiménez et al. [21] that extends the methodology in [47] from binary efficacy endpoint to time-to-event endpoint.

Model

Jiménez et al. [21] model the time to progression as a Weibull distribution with probability density function

$$f(t; z) = \frac{k}{\lambda(z; \boldsymbol{\psi})} \left(\frac{t}{\lambda(z; \boldsymbol{\psi})} \right)^{k-1} \exp\left(-\frac{t}{\lambda(z; \boldsymbol{\psi})} \right)^{k}, \tag{37}$$

where $\lambda > 0$ is the shape parameter and $k > 0$ is the scale parameter.

The median TTP is

$$\mathrm{Med}(z) = \lambda(z; \boldsymbol{\psi})(\log 2)^{\frac{1}{k}}. \tag{38}$$

A flexible way of modeling the median TTP along the MTD curve is through the use of the cubic spline function

$$\lambda(z; \boldsymbol{\psi}) = \exp\left(\beta_0 + \beta_1 z + \beta_2 z^2 + \sum_{j=3}^{5} \beta_j (z - \phi_j)_+^3 \right), \tag{39}$$

where $\boldsymbol{\psi} = (\boldsymbol{\beta}, \boldsymbol{\phi})$, with $\boldsymbol{\beta} = (\beta_0, \ldots, \beta_5)$ and $\boldsymbol{\phi} = (\phi_3, \ldots, \phi_5)$, being $\phi_3 = 0$. Let $D_n = \{(z_i, t_i, \delta_i), i = 1 \ldots, n\}$ be the data after enrolling n patients in the trial where t represents the TTP or last follow-up, and δ the censoring status, and let $\pi(\boldsymbol{\psi}, k)$ be the joint prior density on the parameter vectors $\boldsymbol{\psi}$ and k. The posterior distribution is

$$\pi(\boldsymbol{\psi}, k | D_m) \propto \pi(\boldsymbol{\psi}, k) \prod_{i=1}^{n} \left[\frac{k}{\lambda(z_i; \boldsymbol{\psi})} \left(\frac{t_i}{\lambda(z_i; \boldsymbol{\psi})} \right)^{k-1} \right]^{\delta_i} \times \exp\left(-\frac{t_i}{\lambda(z_i; \boldsymbol{\psi})} \right)^{k}. \tag{40}$$

Let Med_z be the median TTP at dose combination z, and let Med_0 be the median TTP of the standard-of-care treatment. We propose an adaptive design in order to test the hypothesis

$$\begin{aligned} \text{H}_0 &: \text{Med}_z \leq \text{Med}_0 \text{ for all } z \quad \text{vs.} \\ \text{H}_1 &: \text{Med}_z > \text{Med}_0 \text{ for some } z. \end{aligned} \tag{41}$$

It is important to keep in mind that the reason why [21] propose a model with a fairly large number of parameters is because they work in a continuous dose space. In a discrete dose space, it is not common to test so many dose combinations. Also, a model with a large number of parameters would most likely be non-identifiable, even with large sample sizes. The use of continuous dose combinations is not uncommon in dose-finding studies since the drugs are administered intravenously and this allows to administer any drug concentration we desire.

Trial Design

This stage of the trial makes use of response-adaptive randomization to decide in which dose combinations cohorts of patients are allocated. The algorithm is similar to the one discussed in Sect. 3.1 with the difference that in this one [21] work with time-to-event data:

1. We first treat n_1 patients at dose combinations $x_1, \ldots, x_{n_1}$, which are equally spaced along the estimated maximum tolerated dose combination curve C_{est}.
2. Obtain posterior distribution of $\boldsymbol{\psi}$ and k given the data D_{n_1} using Eq. (40). Note that prior to obtaining the posterior distribution of the model parameters, patients who have not progressed are right censored.
3. Generate n_2 dose combinations from the standardized density $\text{Med}(z) = \lambda(z; \boldsymbol{\psi})(\log 2)^{\frac{1}{k}}$, and assign them to the next n_2 patients.
4. Repeat steps 2 and 3 until a total of n patients have been enrolled in the trial subject to pre-specified stopping rules.

Decision Rule: At the end of the trial, we reject the null hypothesis if $\text{Max}_z\{P(\text{Med}(z; \boldsymbol{\psi}_i) > \text{Med}_0 | D_{n,i})\} > \delta_u$, where δ_u is a design parameter.

Stopping Rule (Safety): For a prospective trial, a separate stopping rule for safety using, for example, a Bayesian continuous monitoring for toxicity (see e.g., [66]) should be implemented as discussed in [47].

Stopping Rule (Futility): For ethical reasons and to avoid treating patients at sub-therapeutic dose levels, we will stop the trial for futility if there is strong evidence that none of the dose combinations are promising, i.e., $\text{Max}_z\{P(\text{Med}(z; \boldsymbol{\psi}_i) > \text{Med}_0 | D_{n,i})\} < \delta_0$, where δ_0 is a design parameter.

Stopping Rule (Efficacy): For ethical reasons, if the investigator considers there is enough evidence in favor of one or more dose combinations being tested, and no further patients need to be enrolled, the trial can be terminated if $\text{Max}_z\{P(\text{Med}(z; \boldsymbol{\psi}_i) > \text{Med}_0|D_{n,i})\} > \delta_1$, where $\delta_1 \geq \delta_u$ is a study parameter and the dose combination $z^{\text{opt}} = \arg\max_v\{P(\text{Med}(v; \boldsymbol{\psi}_i) > \text{Med}_0|D_{n,i})\}$ is selected for further randomized phase II or phase III clinical trials.

The rational for this approach is based on the rejection-sampling principle, which can be used to generate observations from a target distribution (in our case (38)). Hence, if we generate data from (38), we will be allocating patients to dose combinations that are more likely to have higher TTP according to the current estimation of (38) (i.e., the shape of (38) will be updated as patients enroll).

Results

An extensive simulation with several scenarios was performed by Jiménez et al. [21]. For illustration purposes, in Fig. 7, we show one scenario that summarizes the main conclusions of this chapter.

In Fig. 7A, we show the dose–efficacy relationship within the MTD curves selected in stage 1. For this particular case, this curve represents a scenario where high levels of drug Y and low levels of X are more efficacious. In Fig. 7B, we observe how the proposed design identifies lower levels of z, which represents high levels of drug Y and low levels of X as the more efficacious dose combinations.

In Table 5, we observe the corresponding Bayesian power, type-I error probability, and type-I + type-II error probability with effect sizes of 1.5 and 2 months and accrual rates of 1 and 2 patients per month. Additional results are presented in the supplementary material of [21] such as average bias and percentage of correct recommendation. These results allow to conclude that this design has, in general, good operating characteristics allowing to identify the dose combination that maximizes the efficacy.

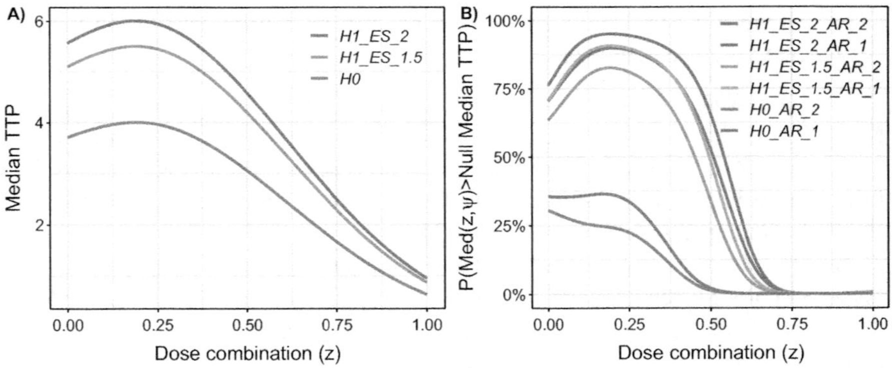

Fig. 7 Median TTP (A) and posterior probability of having $\text{Med}(z, \psi) >$null Median TTP (B) for different dose combinations (z) under H_0 and H_1, with effect sizes (ES) of 1.5 and 2 months and accrual rates (AR) of 1 and 2 patients per month

Table 5 Bayesian power, type-I error probability, and type-I + type-II error probability with effect sizes of 1.5 and 2 months and accrual rates of 1 and 2 patients per month

	Power (effect size of 1.5 months)		Power (effect size of 2 months)		Probability of type-I error		Probability of type-I + type-II errors (effect size of 1.5 months)		Probability of type-I + type-II errors (effect size of 2 months)	
	δ_u		δ_u		δ_u		δ_u		δ_u	
Accrual rate	0.8	0.9	0.8	0.9	0.8	0.9	0.8	0.9	0.8	0.9
1	0.924	0.844	0.971	0.927	0.227	0.121	0.303	0.277	0.256	0.194
2	0.824	0.674	0.920	0.829	0.107	0.048	0.283	0.374	0.187	0.219

4 Discussion

The use of drug combinations in early phase cancer clinical trials has been extensively studied over the last decade. The overall goal of early phase clinical trials in oncology is to find a set of one or more safe dose combinations that maximize efficacy. To achieve this goal, we propose that, in the first step, a phase I trial is designed to identify one or more maximum tolerated doses (MTDs). Following this step, a phase II trial is designed to search for a combination that maximizes efficacy within the set of MTDs. It is worth noting that the main objective of the majority of phase I designs is to identify a single MTD. We recommend the use of designs that select more than one MTD for efficacy trials as this may result in less failed phase II trials.

In this chapter, we focused on dose-finding methods tailored for drug combinations with continuous dose levels. The use of continuous dose levels is very common in clinical oncology research, especially in early phase trials where the existing or first-in-human drugs are delivered as infusions intravenously. In addition, discretizing the dose levels may lead to a recommended phase 2 dose that has either a small or high probability of DLT relative to the target risk of DLT, if the true MTD is not part of the discrete set of doses. As showed by Diniz et al. [13], continuous dose schemes generally have equal or better safety and efficiency results than the discrete dose schemes, although alternative approaches to improve efficiency of discrete dose schemes have been recently published where new doses are added during the trial into the original discrete set [18]. In cases where there is no information about the location of the MTD, a continuous dose scheme would certainly be much more appealing. Furthermore, although the seminal CRM design and several related dose-finding methods are based on regression models, their dose escalation algorithms are based on pre-specified skeletons to incorporate prior information, which cannot be adapted to continuous doses.

In phase I trial designs, consecutive cohorts of two patients were treated simultaneously with different dose combinations to better explore the space of doses. The method was studied extensively by Tighiouart et al. [50, 51, 53] under the EWOC criterion and by Diniz et al. [12] and Jimenez et al. [22] using the

CRM principle via simulations. Comparisons of EWOC and CRM in the settings of dichotomous DLTs and ordinal toxicity grades can be found in [11].

Most drug combination designs assume that the binary DLT is attributable to either one of the drugs or both. This is a reasonable assumption because of the rarity of cancer drugs with non-overlapping toxicities of any grade. However, certain combinations may lead to some non-overlapping toxicities. For instance, when combining taxotere with metformin, an occurrence of a grade 4 neutropenia can only be attributed to taxotere and not to metformin. This event will guide the clinician to hold the current dose of metformin and decrease the taxotere dose for the next cohort of patients, even if the statistical algorithm recommends a dose decrease for both agents. We described the work developed by Jimenez et al. [22], where a clinician can attribute the DLT to one or more drugs in an unknown fraction of attributable DLTs by extending the previous statistical models. This is useful in a situation where the two drugs do not have many overlapping toxicities (see, e.g. [28]). However, it is also important to note that this method relies on clinical judgment regarding DLT attribution.

Another approach reviewed in this chapter is the inclusion of a baseline covariate to estimate patient-specific MTD curves [10]. We found that in the presence of a clinically significant baseline covariate, the design with a covariate had a smaller pointwise average bias and a higher percent of MTD recommendation relative to a design that ignores the covariate. Moreover, we stand to lose little in terms of safety of the trial and efficiency of the estimated MTD curve, if we include a practically not important covariate in the model.

In the second part of this chapter, we described two-stage designs developed by Tighiouart [47] and Jiménez et al. [21] where the estimated MTD curve from a phase I trial is used as input to a phase II efficacy trial using Bayesian adaptive randomization. Two-stage designs are required when it takes several cycles of therapy to resolve treatment efficacy or patient characteristics in phases I and II are clinically different. For instance, efficacy in the cisplatin–cabazitaxel trial that was described in [47] is resolved after three cycles of treatment, and patients in stage I must have metastatic, castration resistant prostate cancer, whereas patients in stage II must have visceral metastasis. As mentioned in these articles, these designs can be viewed as an extension of the Bayesian adaptive design comparing a finite number of arms [3] to that with an infinite number of arms. In particular, when the dose levels of the two agents are discrete, methods such as the ones described in [45, 59, 62] can be used to identify a set of MTDs in stage I, and the trial in stage II can select the most efficacious dose by adaptive randomization. One limitation of these two-stage approaches is that uncertainty of the estimated MTD curve in stage I is not taken into account in stage II of the design, which implies that the MTD curve is not updated as a result of observing DLTs in stage II. However, this problem is also inherent to single-agent two-stage designs where the MTD from the phase I trial is used in phase II studies. In both cases, safety is monitored continuously during the second stage of the design. A potential alternative design would account for first-, second-, and third-cycle DLT in addition to efficacy outcome at each cycle. In addition, the nature of DLT (reversible vs. non-reversible) should be taken into account since patients with a reversible DLT are usually treated for that side effect and kept in the trial with dose reduction in subsequent cycles. These topics are the subject of future research.

Successful implementation of these designs requires active involvement and collaboration between the clinicians and the biostatisticians in many situations. This includes the design stage, prior distribution calibration, specification of scenarios with various locations of the true MTD set of doses or safe and efficacious doses, and computations of sequential posterior probabilities for dose allocation. This process may be challenging since it requires special expertise of biostatisticians who can program MCMC algorithms, adapt the existing computer codes to their trial, and modify them as needed since every trial is unique. The process is also time-consuming at the design stage to derive the operating characteristics. An R package `EWOC2` for designing the trials in [51] can be found in [25], and R codes for deriving the operating characteristics of the trials in [21, 22, 47] can be found in the supplementary material of the corresponding journal web site. An application of the phase I–II design in Sect. 3.1 is described in [47] where the clinician Dr. Posadas worked with Dr. Tighiouart in calibrating the prior distributions of the model parameters of the phase I part using preliminary data from a similar phase I trial, using the same combination of cabazitaxel and cisplatin. Operating characteristics were derived based on scenarios elicited by the clinician regarding the location of the true MTD curve and expected clinical benefit rate. Other recent applications of these methods for single-agent trials were designed by Drs. Tighiouart and Rogatko and published in [36, 57].

References

1. Babb, J., Rogatko, A., Zacks, S.: Cancer phase I clinical trials: efficient dose escalation with overdose control. Stat. Med. **17**(10), 1103–1120 (1998)
2. Babb, J.S., Rogatko, A.: Patient specific dosing in a cancer phase I clinical trial. Stat. Med. **20**(14), 2079–2090 (2001)
3. Berry, S.M., Carlin, B.P., Lee, J.J., Muller, P.: Bayesian Adaptive Methods for Clinical Trials. CRC Press, New York (2010)
4. Braun, T.M.: The bivariate continual reassessment method: extending the CRM to phase I trials of two competing outcomes. Contemp. Clin. Trials **23**(3), 240–256 (2002)
5. Braun, T.M., Wang, S.: A hierarchical Bayesian design for phase I trials of novel combinations of cancer therapeutic agents. Biometrics **66**(3), 805–812 (2010)
6. Cai, C., Yuan, Y., Ji, Y.: A Bayesian dose finding design for oncology clinical trials of combinational biological agents. Appl. Stat. **63**, 159–173 (2014)
7. Chen, Z., Yuan, Y., Li, Z., Kutner, M., Owonikoko, T., Curran, W.J., Khuri, F., Kowalski, J.: Dose escalation with over-dose and under-dose controls in phase I/II clinical trials. Contemp. Clin. Trials **43**, 133–141 (2015)
8. Chen, Z., Zhao, Y., Cui, Y., Kowalski, J.: Methodology and application of adaptive and sequential approaches in contemporary clinical trials. J. Probab. Stat. **2012**, 20 (2012). https://doi.org/10.1155/2012/527351
9. Cheung, Y.K., Chappell, R.: Sequential designs for phase I clinical trials with late-onset toxicities. Biometrics **56**(4), 1177–1182 (2000)

10. Diniz, M.A., Kim, S., Tighiouart, M.: A Bayesian adaptive design in cancer phase I trials using dose combinations in the presence of a baseline covariate. J. Probab. Stat. **2018**, 11 (2018). https://doi.org/10.1155/2018/8654173
11. Diniz, M.A., Kim, S., Tighiouart, M.: A Bayesian adaptive design in cancer phase I trials using dose combinations with ordinal toxicity grades. Stats **3**, 221–238 (2020)
12. Diniz, M.A., Li, Q., Tighiouart, M.: Dose finding for drug combination in early cancer phase I trials using conditional continual reassessment method. J. Biom. Biostat. **8**, 6 (2017)
13. Diniz, M.A., Tighiouart, M., Rogatko, A.: Comparison between continuous and discrete doses for model based designs in cancer dose finding. PloS One **14**, 1 (2019)
14. Faries, D.: Practical modifications of the continual reassessment method for phase I cancer clinical trials. J. Biopharm. Stat. **4**(147), 164 (1994)
15. Gasparini, M., Eisele, J.: A curve-free method for phase I clinical trials. Biometrics **56**(2), 609–615 (2000)
16. Gatsonis, C., Greenhouse, J.B.: Bayesian methods for phase I clinical trials. Stat. Med. **11**(10), 1377–1389 (1992)
17. Goodman, S., Zahurak, M., Piantadosi, S.: Some practical improvements in the continual reassessment method for phase I studies. Stat. Med. **14**, 1149–1161 (1995)
18. Hu, B., Bekele, B.N., Ji, Y.: Adaptive dose insertion in early phase clinical trials. Clinical Trials **10**, 216–224 (2013)
19. Huang, X., Biswas, S., Oki, Y., Issa, J.-P., Berry, D.A.: A parallel phase I/II clinical trial design for combination therapies. Biometrics **63**(2), 429–436 (2007)
20. Ivanova, A.: A new dose-finding design for bivariate outcomes. Biometrics **59**(4), 1001–1007 (2003)
21. Jiménez, J.L., Kim, S., Tighiouart, M.: A Bayesian seamless phase I–II trial design with two stages for cancer clinical trials with drug combinations. Biom. J. **62**(5), 1300–1314 (2020)
22. Jimenez, J.L., Tighiouart, M., Gasparini, M.: Cancer phase I trial design using drug combinations when a fraction of dose limiting toxicities is attributable to one or more agents. Biom. J. **61**(2), 319–332 (2019)
23. Lam, C.K., Lin, R., Yin, G.: Non-parametric overdose control for dose finding in drug combination trials. J. R. Stat. Soc.: Ser. C: Appl. Stat. **68**(4), 1111–1130 (2019)
24. Le Tourneau, C., Lee, J.J., Siu, L.L.: Dose escalation methods in phase I cancer clinical trials. JNCI J. Natl. Cancer Inst. **101**(10), 708–720 (2009)
25. Li, Q., Tighiouart, M.: EWOC2: Escalation with Overdose Control using 2 Drug Combinations (2019). R package version 1.0
26. Lyu, J., Ji, Y., Zhao, N., Catenacci, D.: AAA: Triple-adaptive Bayesian designs for the identification of optimal dose combinations in dual-agent dose-finding trials. J. R. Stat. Soc.: Ser. C: Appl. Stat. **68**(2), 385–410 (2019)
27. Mander, A.P., Sweeting, M.J.: A product of independent beta probabilities dose escalation design for dual-agent phase I trials. Stat. Med. **34**(8), 1261–1276 (2015)
28. Miles, D., von Minckwitz, G., Seidman, A.D., et al.: Combination versus sequential single-agent therapy in metastatic breast cancer. ONCOLOGIST-MIAMISBURG **7**, 13–19 (2002)
29. Moller, S.: An extension of the continual reassessment methods using a preliminary up-and-down design in a dose finding study in cancer patients, in order to investigate a greater range of doses. Stat. Med. **14**, 911–922 (1995)
30. Mozgunov, P., Gasparini, M., Jaki, T.: A surface-free design for phase I dual-agent combination trials. Stat. Methods Med. Res. **29**(10), 3093–3109 (2020). 0962280220919450
31. Murtaugh, P.A., Fisher, L.D.: Bivariate binary models of efficacy and toxicity in dose-ranging trials. Commun. Stat. Theory Methods **19**(6), 2003–2020 (1990)
32. O'Quigley, J., Pepe, M., Fisher, L.: Continual reassessment method: a practical design for phase 1 clinical trials in cancer. Biometrics, 33–48 (1990)
33. O'Quigley, J., Shen, L.Z.: Continual reassessment method: a likelihood approach. Biometrics **52**, 673–684 (1996)
34. Piantadosi, S., Fisher, J.D., Grossman, S.: Practical implementation of a modified continual reassessment method for dose-finding trials. Cancer Chemother. Pharmacol. **41**, 429–436 (1998)

35. Plummer, M., et al.: JAGS: A program for analysis of Bayesian graphical models using Gibbs sampling. In: *Proceedings of the 3rd International Workshop on Distributed Statistical Computing*, vol. 124, pp. 1–10. Vienna, Austria (2003)
36. Qayed, M., Cash, T., Tighiouart, M., MacDonald, T., Goldsmith, K., Tanos, R., Kean, L., Watkins, B.C., Wetmore, C., Katzenstein, H.M.: A phase I study of sirolimus in combination with metronomic therapy (CHOAnome) in children with recurrent or refractory solid and brain tumors. Pediatr. Blood Cancer **67**(4), e28134 (2019)
37. R Core Team. R: A Language and Environment for Statistical Computing. R Foundation for Statistical Computing, Vienna, Austria (2018)
38. Riviere, M., Yuan, Y., Dubois, F., Zohar, S.: A Bayesian dose-finding design for drug combination clinical trials based on the logistic model. Pharm. Stat. **13**, 247–257 (2014)
39. Riviere, M., Yuan, Y., Dubois, F., Zohar, S.: A Bayesian dose-finding design for clinical trials combining a cytotoxic agent with a molecularly targeted agent. J. R. Stat. Soc. Ser. C **64**, 215–229 (2015)
40. Rogatko, A., Ghosh, P., Vidakovic, B., Tighiouart, M.: Patient-specific dose adjustment in the cancer clinical trial setting. Pharm. Medicine **22**(6), 345–350 (2008)
41. Sato, H., Hirakawa, A., Hamada, C.: An adaptive dose-finding method using a change-point model for molecularly targeted agents in phase I trials. Stat. Med. **35**(23), 4093–4109 (2016)
42. Shi, Y., Yin, G.: Escalation with overdose control for phase I drug-combination trials. Stat. Med. **32**(25), 4400–4412 (2013)
43. Shimamura, F., Hamada, C., Matsui, S., Hirakawa, A.: Two-stage approach based on zone and dose findings for two-agent combination phase I/II trials. J. Biopharm. Stat., **28**(6), 1025–1037 (2018)
44. Thall, P.F., Cook, J.D.: Dose-finding based on efficacy-toxicity trade-offs. Biometrics **60**(3), 684–693 (2004)
45. Thall, P.F., Millikan, R.E., Mueller, P., Lee, S.-J.: Dose-finding with two agents in phase I oncology trials. Biometrics **59**(3), 487–496 (2003)
46. Thall, P.F., Russell, K.E.: A strategy for dose-finding and safety monitoring based on efficacy and adverse outcomes in phase I/II clinical trials. Biometrics, 251–264 (1998)
47. Tighiouart, M.: Two-stage design for phase I–II cancer clinical trials using continuous dose combinations of cytotoxic agents. J. R. Stat. Soc.: Ser. C: Appl. Stat. **68**(1), 235–250 (2019)
48. Tighiouart, M., Cook-Wiens, G., Rogatko, A.: Incorporating a patient dichotomous characteristic in cancer phase I clinical trials using escalation with overdose control. Journal of Probab. Stat. **2012**, 10 (2012)
49. Tighiouart, M., Cook-Wiens, G., Rogatko, A.: A Bayesian adaptive design for cancer phase I trials using a flexible range of doses. J. Biopharm. Stat. **28**(3), 562–574 (2018)
50. Tighiouart, M., Li, Q., Piantadosi, S., Rogatko, A.: A Bayesian adaptive design for combination of three drugs in cancer phase I clinical trials. Am. J. Biostat. **6**(1), 1 (2016)
51. Tighiouart, M., Li, Q., Rogatko, A.: A Bayesian adaptive design for estimating the maximum tolerated dose curve using drug combinations in cancer phase I clinical trials. Stat. Med. **36**(2), 280–290 (2017)
52. Tighiouart, M., Liu, Y., Rogatko, A.: Escalation with overdose control using time to toxicity for cancer phase I clinical trials. Plos One **9**, 3 (2014)
53. Tighiouart, M., Piantadosi, S., Rogatko, A.: Dose finding with drug combinations in cancer phase I clinical trials using conditional escalation with overdose control. Stat. Med. **33**(22), 3815–3829 (2014)
54. Tighiouart, M., Rogatko, A.: Dose finding with escalation with overdose control (EWOC) in cancer clinical trials. Stat. Sci. **25**(2), 217–226 (2010)
55. Tighiouart, M., Rogatko, A.: Number of patients per cohort and sample size considerations using dose escalation with overdose control. J. Probab. Stat. **2012**, 16 (2012). https://doi.org/10.1155/2012/692725
56. Tighiouart, M., Rogatko, A., Babb, J.S.: Flexible Bayesian methods for cancer phase I clinical trials. dose escalation with overdose control. Stat. Med. **24**(14), 2183–2196 (2005)

57. Tuli, R., Shiao, S.L., Nissen, N., Tighiouart, M., Kim, S., Osipov, A., Bryant, M., Ristow, L., Placencio-Hickok, V.R., Hoffman, D., Rokhsar, S., Scher, K., Klempner, S.J., Noe, P., Davis, M.J., A, W., Lo, S., Jamil, L., Sandler, H., Piantadosi, S., Hendifar, A.: A phase 1 study of veliparib, a PARP-1/2 inhibitor, with gemcitabine and radiotherapy in locally advanced pancreatic cancer. EBioMedicine **40**, 374–381 (2019)
58. US Department of Health and Human Services. National Cancer Institute: Common Terminology Criteria for Adverse Events (CTCAE) Version 4.0. [internet] National Cancer Institute, Bethesda (2009). [cited 2015 sep 22]
59. Wages, N.A.: Identifying a maximum tolerated contour in two-dimensional dose finding. Stat. Med. **36**(2), 242–253 (2017)
60. Wages, N.A., Conaway, M.R.: Phase I/II adaptive design for drug combination oncology trials. Stat. Med. **33**(12), 1990–2003 (2014)
61. Wages, N.A., Conaway, M.R., O'Quigley, J.: Continual reassessment method for partial ordering. Biometrics **67**(4), 1555–1563 (2011)
62. Wang, K., Ivanova, A.: Two-dimensional dose finding in discrete dose space. Biometrics **61**(1), 217–222 (2005)
63. Wheeler, G.M., Sweeting, M.J., Mander, A.P.: Toxicity-dependent feasibility bounds for the escalation with overdose control approach in phase I cancer trials. Stat. Med. **36**(16), 2499–2513 (2017)
64. Whitehead, J., Thygesen, H., Whitehead, A.: A Bayesian dose-finding procedure for phase I clinical trials based only on the assumption of monotonicity. Stat. Med. **29**(17), 1808–1824 (2010)
65. Yin, G., Yuan, Y.: A latent contingency table approach to dose finding for combinations of two agents. Biometrics **65**(3), 866–875 (2009)
66. Yu, J., Hutson, A.D., Siddiqui, A.H., Kedron, M.A.: Group sequential control of overalltoxicity incidents in clinical trials–non-bayesian and bayesian approaches. Stat. Methods Med. Res. **25**(1), 64–80 (2016)
67. Yuan, Y., Yin, G.: Bayesian dose finding by jointly modelling toxicity and efficacy as time-to-event outcomes. J. R. Stat. Soc.: Ser. C: Appl. Stat. **58**(5), 719–736 (2009)
68. Yuan, Y., Yin, G.: Bayesian phase I/II adaptively randomized oncology trials with combined drugs. Ann. Appl. Stat. **5**(2A), 924 (2011)
69. Zacks, S., Rogatko, A., Babb, J.: Optimal Bayesian-feasible dose escalation for cancer phase I trials. Statist. Probab. Lett. **38**(3), 215–220 (1998)
70. Zhang, L., Yuan, Y.: A practical Bayesian design to identify the maximum tolerated dose contour for drug combination trials. Stat. Med. **35**(27), 4924–4936 (2016)
71. Zhengjia, C., Mourad, T., Jeanne, K.: Dose escalation with overdose control using a quasi-continuous toxicity score in cancer phase I clinical trials. Contemp. Clin. Trials **33**(5), 949–958 (2012)

Controlling the False Discovery Rate of Grouped Hypotheses

Peter W. MacDonald, Nathan Wilson, Kun Liang, and Yingli Qin

1 Introduction

Since the seminal work of Benjamini and Hochberg [2], many procedures have been developed to control the false discovery rate (FDR), the expected proportion of false rejections. Compared to the family-wise error rate (FWER), the FDR can provide a more suitable measure of error when performing exploratory analyses on large modern datasets in many fields such as genetics, neuroimaging, and astrophysics. By incorporating information about the overall proportion of true null hypotheses, many procedures have been proposed to further increase the power of the original linear step-up procedure of Benjamini and Hochberg [2] in the intervening years. For example, see Benjamini and Hochberg [3], Storey [19], Storey et al. [20], and MacDonald et al. [17], among others.

Such procedures are designed under the assumption of exchangeability of hypotheses, which does not always hold in practice. Hypotheses often come from heterogeneous sources and hence have a known group structure. Conventional procedures to control the FDR will identify a single rejection threshold and reject all hypotheses with p-value no greater than this threshold. While the FDR control of these procedures is robust to non-exchangeability, allowing group-wise p-value rejection thresholds could lead to substantial power improvement [4].

The common approach in the grouped setting is to assign weights to the p-values according to their group labels so that they can be pooled and analyzed together. Genovese et al. [7] demonstrate that when p-values are weighted according to some a priori known weights, Benjamini and Hochberg's procedure applied to the weighted p-values maintains control of the FDR. Roquain and Van De Wiel [18]

P. W. MacDonald · N. Wilson · K. Liang (✉) · Y. Qin
University of Waterloo, Waterloo, ON, Canada
e-mail: pwmacdon@uwaterloo.ca; kun.liang@uwaterloo.ca; yingli.qin@uwaterloo.ca

Y. Zhao, (Din) D.-G. Chen (eds.), *Modern Statistical Methods for Health Research*, Emerging Topics in Statistics and Biostatistics,
https://doi.org/10.1007/978-3-030-72437-5_8

derive optimal weights when the distributions of false null p-values are known and the number of rejections is fixed. However, neither of these procedures has data-driven implementations with weights derived from the observed p-values. Hu et al. [10] derive weights based on the group-wise proportions of true null hypotheses and only show asymptotic control of the FDR for their data-driven procedure. Capable of adapting to many structures within the list of hypotheses, Li and Barber [15] can control the FDR in finite samples in the grouped setting with weights similarly based on group-wise true null proportions. Zhao and Zhang [23] and more recently Ignatiadis and Huber [11] and [5] describe methods that attempt to select optimal group-wise weights to maximize power. The authors of Zhao and Zhang [23] and [5] are able to prove that their procedures control the FDR asymptotically, while Ignatiadis and Huber [11] are able to show finite sample control of the FDR (with general covariate information).

The aim of such p-value weighting methods is to construct a ranking of significance for the hypotheses that is superior to the naive pooled ranking of the p-values. Cai and Sun [4] study the grouped multiple testing problem from a Bayesian perspective. They show that under independence and other regularity conditions, the local FDR (Lfdr), the posterior probability that a null hypothesis is true [6], is the optimal ranking of significance to maximize power at a fixed level of the FDR. Their oracle procedure achieves control of the overall FDR, but in the data-driven case, they are able to show only asymptotic control of the marginal FDR (mFDR). Under regularity conditions on the p-value model, the mFDR is asymptotically close to the FDR [8].

Another recent FDR control procedure invoked the idea of *knockoffs*, which was first proposed by Barber and Candès [1] to control the FDR for the selected variables in linear regression. In the context of multiple hypothesis testing with covariate information, Lei and Fithian [13] also create knockoff variables to control the FDR. While the procedure developed in Lei and Fithian [13] is designed for continuous covariates, it can easily be tailored to the grouped setting.

This chapter is organized as follows. In Sect. 2, we introduce notation and describe a general framework for grouped multiple testing procedures. In Sect. 3 we review the procedures in the literature and their theoretical guarantees through this framework. Comparison through simulation and a real data application are presented in Sects. 4 and 5, respectively. A brief conclusion is provided in Sect. 6.

2 Modeling and Sequential Framework

In this section, we introduce notation and assumptions on the p-value models. We then motivate a general sequential approach to multiple testing procedures in the grouped setting. All the grouped multiple testing procedures we compare here can be defined under this sequential framework.

2.1 Notation and Models

Consider testing $m = m_1 + \cdots + m_K$ hypotheses from K fixed and known groups. For $k = 1, \ldots, K$ and $i = 1, \ldots, m_k$, let $\mathcal{H}_{k,i}$ be the ith null hypothesis in the kth group and $H_{k,i}$ be the corresponding false null indicator, i.e., false null hypotheses have $H_{k,i} = 1$ and true null hypotheses have $H_{k,i} = 0$. Suppose $m_{0,k} \leq m_k$ hypotheses from each group are true nulls and denote $m_0 = m_{0,1} + \cdots + m_{0,K}$. For $k = 1, \ldots, K$, we call $\pi_{0,k} = m_{0,k}/m_k$ the *true null proportion* for the kth group. The overall true null proportion is the weighted average

$$\pi_0 = \sum_{k=1}^{K} \left(\frac{m_k}{m}\right)\pi_{0,k} = \frac{m_0}{m}.$$

Denote the p-value from testing $\mathcal{H}_{k,i}$ as $p_{k,i}$, $k = 1, \ldots, K$ and $i = 1, \ldots, m_k$. In general, we shall assume that the true null p-values are independent of each other and independent of the false null p-values. p-values that satisfy this condition will be said to follow the *null independence model*, which is used in Benjamini and Hochberg [2], Storey et al. [20], Liang and Nettleton [16], and many others. It is commonly assumed that true null p-values are either uniformly distributed on (0, 1) or *superuniform* , i.e.,

$$\mathbb{P}(p_{k,i} \leq t) \leq t$$

for all $t \in (0, 1)$, and (k, i) such that $H_{k,i} = 0$.

For an arbitrary multiple testing procedure, define R to be the total number of rejections and V the total number of false rejections across all K groups. Define the *false discovery proportion* (FDP) to be the random variable

$$\text{FDP} = \frac{V}{\max\{R, 1\}},$$

and the *false discovery rate* (FDR) to be its expectation, i.e.,

$$\text{FDR} = \mathbb{E}[\text{FDP}].$$

If this quantity is less than or equal to α, then we say that the multiple testing procedure controls the FDR at level α.

This chapter will primarily focus on procedures designed for the frequentist setting described above; however, we also make reference to the well-known Bayesian *two-group model* [6]. Under the two-group model within each of the K groups, we have

$$\begin{cases} H_{k,i} \sim \text{Bernoulli}(1 - \pi_{0,k}), \\ p_{k,i}|H_{k,i} \sim H_{k,i} f_{1,k} + (1 - H_{k,i}) f_{0,k} \end{cases}$$

for $k = 1, \ldots, K$ and $i = 1, \ldots, m_k$, where the $H_{k,i}$'s are independent, and the $p_{k,i}$'s are conditionally independent given the $H_{k,i}$'s. For each k, $f_{0,k}$ and $f_{1,k}$ are continuous densities supported on (0, 1). Note that we consider the false null indicators $H_{k,i}$'s to be fixed but unknown, while under the two-group model, they are random variables. The two-group model gives rise to a useful Bayesian quantity known as the *local false discovery rate* (Lfdr), defined as

$$\mathrm{Lfdr}_k(p) = \mathbb{P}(H_{k,i} = 0 | p_{k,i} = p) = \frac{\pi_{0,k} f_{0,k}(p)}{\pi_{0,k} f_{0,k}(p) + (1 - \pi_{0,k}) f_{1,k}(p)},$$

which is the posterior probability that $H_{k,i} = 0$ given $p_{k,i} = p$.

2.2 A General Framework for Grouped Multiple Testing Procedures

In this section, we will formally define a sequential multiple testing procedure for the grouped setting that encompasses all of the procedures we will compare later. This sequential framework is an interpretable way of analyzing the operational characteristics of different procedures in the grouped setting.

We note that for all the procedures we compare, the rejection region for group k is either a closed interval $[0, s_k]$ or (equivalently) a half-open interval $[0, s_k)$ for some $s_k \in [0, 1]$ [19]. To simplify the presentation of our sequential framework, we will write rejection regions with half-open intervals. Rejection regions of this form reflect two underlying assumptions made explicit in Cai and Sun [4]: (1) the p-values within each group are exchangeable (see, for instance, the two-group model); (2) the smaller p-values are more likely to be non-null. The authors in Cai and Sun [4] call the second assumption the *monotone ratio condition*. Combining the group-wise rejection regions, the overall rejection set S can be described by a K-dimensional vector $\mathbf{s} = (s_1, \ldots, s_K)^\mathsf{T} \in [0, 1]^K$ as

$$S = \{\mathcal{H}_{k,i} : p_{k,i} < s_k, k = 1, \ldots, K\}.$$

We will refer to $\mathbf{s}$ as a *rejection threshold vector*. Notice that these vectors have a natural element-wise ordering: let $\mathbf{s}' = (s'_1, \ldots, s'_K)^\mathsf{T}$, and if $s'_k \le s_k$ for every $k = 1, \ldots, K$, then $\mathbf{s}$ will reject at least as many hypotheses as $\mathbf{s}'$. This ordering motivates a sequential characterization of a typical multiple testing procedure.

Let t denote the step number. At a given step, the vector $\mathbf{s}^{(t)}$ of rejection thresholds defines a set of hypotheses to reject,

$$S^{(t)} = \{\mathcal{H}_{k,i} : p_{k,i} < s_k^{(t)}, k = 1, \ldots, K\}.$$

The procedure then needs to decide whether to terminate and return the current rejection set or proceed to step $t+1$. If it proceeds to step $t+1$, the procedure will decide how to update $\mathbf{s}^{(t)}$ to $\mathbf{s}^{(t+1)}$, where $\mathbf{s}^{(t+1)} \leq \mathbf{s}^{(t)}$ with respect to the element-wise ordering. Since the vector of rejection thresholds has finite dimension K, there is no loss of generality in assuming that each step of the procedure will strictly lower exactly one element of $\mathbf{s}^{(t)}$.

Any multiple testing procedure with this structure is defined by an initialization point and two decision rules. The *stopping rule* decides whether the procedure will terminate for a given rejection set and thus governs its FDR control. The *threshold-updating rule* decides which group's threshold to lower at each update and by how much, which governs the procedure's power. The following gives a more formal notation for the general stages of any such procedure.

Definition 1 (Sequential Procedure for Grouped Hypotheses)

Stage 1: Initialization

Set the rejection threshold vector $\mathbf{s}^{(0)} = (s_1^{(0)}, \ldots, s_K^{(0)})$ and the step number $t = 0$.

Stage 2: Stopping condition

Apply the stopping rule δ_1 to the p-values and rejection threshold vector $\mathbf{s}^{(t)}$. If δ_1 returns 1, the procedure terminates and returns the current rejection set $S^{(t)} = \{\mathcal{H}_{k,i} : p_{k,i} < s_k^{(t)}, k = 1, \ldots, K\}$. If δ_1 returns 0, then continue to Stage 3. δ_1 should be defined to always return 1 if the current rejection set is empty.

Stage 3: Threshold update

Apply the threshold-updating rule δ_2 to the p-values and $\mathbf{s}^{(t)}$. δ_2 lowers exactly one element of $\mathbf{s}^{(t)}$ and leaves the remaining elements unchanged. Let $\mathbf{s}^{(t+1)} = \delta_2(\mathbf{s}^{(t)})$. Update $t \leftarrow t+1$, and return to Stage 2.

In the examples to follow, the stopping rule δ_1 will estimate the overall FDR of the current rejection set and return 1 if and only if this estimate is no larger than the nominal level α. The threshold-updating rule δ_2 will lower the rejection threshold vector based on some pooled ranking of significance for the hypotheses, removing the least significant hypothesis from the current rejection set. As long as the rejection set is empty for some finite step number, the procedure will always terminate. Although this is not the framework under which most of the procedures in the literature of the grouped setting are defined, many can be written in this way. In the following section, we will briefly review several procedures for multiple testing with groups and review their theoretical properties with respect to FDR control and power optimality. We will provide a more detailed treatment of the group-weighted Benjamini–Hochberg (GBH) procedure of Hu et al. [10] (which is representative of many later weighted procedures), the conditional local FDR (CLfdr) procedure of Cai and Sun [4], and the adaptive p-value thresholding (AdaPT) procedure of Lei and Fithian [13].

3 Procedures for Group Multiple Testing

3.1 Conditional Local FDR (CLfdr)

The conditional local FDR procedure Cai and Sun [4] is a thresholding procedure designed for the two-group model, which rejects hypotheses based on an overall threshold for the local FDR. Although in this chapter we focus on procedures with FDR control guarantees applicable in the frequentist setting with fixed false null indicators $\{H_{k,i}\}_{i=1,k=1}^{m_k,K}$, we describe the procedure here as a basic introduction to the sequential framework defined above. Since the simulation settings in Sect. 4 follow the two-group model, we will use the oracle CLfdr procedure as an upper bound on power performance.

Example 1 (Sequential Version of the CLfdr Procedure) In Stage 1, the rejection threshold vector is initialized as $\mathbf{s}^{(0)} = (1, 1, \ldots, 1)$. Suppose the procedure is at step t. In Stage 2, the stopping rule δ_1 checks whether an estimate of the FDR is below the nominal level α. The FDR estimate is given by

$$\widehat{\mathrm{FDR}}_{\mathrm{CLfdr}}(\mathbf{s}^{(t)}) = \frac{1}{\max\{|S^{(t)}|, 1\}} \sum_{k=1}^{K} \sum_{i=1}^{m_k} \mathrm{Lfdr}_k(p_{k,i}) \cdot I(p_{k,i} < s_k^{(t)});$$

that is, the FDR is estimated as the mean of the Lfdr's of the rejected hypotheses. The stopping rule is given by

$$\delta_1(\mathbf{s}^{(t)}) = I(\widehat{\mathrm{FDR}}_{\mathrm{CLfdr}}(\mathbf{s}^{(t)}) \leq \alpha).$$

In Stage 3, define

$$(k^*, i^*) = \underset{(k,i)}{\mathrm{argmax}}\{\mathrm{Lfdr}_k(p_{k,i}) : p_{k,i} < s_k^{(t)}\}.$$

Then, δ_2 lowers the rejection threshold in group k^* to level p_{k^*,i^*}; that is,

$$\delta_2(\mathbf{s}^{(t)}) = (s_1^{(t)}, s_2^{(t)}, \ldots, p_{k^*,i^*}, \ldots, s_k^{(t)}).$$

The functions $\{\mathrm{Lfdr}_1, \ldots, \mathrm{Lfdr}_K\}$ are assumed to be known in the oracle CLfdr procedure and replaced by estimates in the data-driven procedure.

3.2 Group-Weighted Benjamini–Hochberg (GBH)

GBH [10] was the first of a variety of weighted p-value thresholding approaches for multiple testing with group information. In general, these procedures calculate group-wise weights $\{w_k\}_{k=1}^K$ satisfying some normalization condition and apply the usual Benjamini–Hochberg procedure to the reweighted sample:

$$\{p_{k,i}/w_k\}_{i=1,k=1}^{m_k,K}.$$

The FDR control and power properties of each procedure will depend on the choice of weights and the strictness of the weight normalization condition. GBH chooses weights based only on the group-wise true null proportions, ignoring the distribution of the false null p-values. When the true null proportions are known, the oracle GBH procedure achieves finite sample FDR control under the null independence model with uniform true null p-values. In the same setting, the data-driven GBH procedure achieves asymptotic FDR control, as long as the group-wise true null proportions are estimated conservatively. In the following, we describe GBH in our sequential framework.

Example 2 (Sequential Version of the GBH Procedure) In Stage 1, the rejection threshold vector is initialized as $\mathbf{s}^{(0)} = (1, 1, \ldots, 1)$. Suppose the procedure is at step t. In Stage 2, the stopping rule δ_1 checks whether an estimate of the FDR is below the nominal level α. In this case, the estimate is given by

$$\widehat{\mathrm{FDR}}_{\mathrm{GBH}}(\mathbf{s}^{(t)}) = \frac{m \cdot s_W^{(t)}}{\max\{|S^{(t)}|, 1\}},$$

where $s_W^{(t)}$ is the overall rejection threshold on the weighted scale. This overall threshold can be recovered from the group-wise thresholds via the relationship

$$s_W^{(t)} = \sum_{k=1}^{K} \left\{ \left(\frac{m_k}{m} \right) \pi_{0,k} \cdot \max_i \{p_{k,i} : p_{k,i} < s_k^{(t)}\} \right\},$$

with the convention $\max \emptyset = 0$. The true null proportions are taken as known in the oracle procedure or replaced by their estimates in the data-driven case. The stopping rule is given by

$$\delta_1(\mathbf{s}^{(t)}) = I(\widehat{\mathrm{FDR}}_{\mathrm{GBH}}(\mathbf{s}^{(t)}) \leq \alpha).$$

In Stage 3, define

$$(k^*, i^*) = \underset{(k,i)}{\mathrm{argmax}} \{p_{k,i}/w_k : p_{k,i} < s_k^{(t)}\},$$

where for $k = 1, \ldots, K$,

$$w_k = \frac{1 - \pi_{0,k}}{\pi_{0,k}(1 - \pi_0)}$$

are the group-wise weights, where once again the true null proportions are estimated in the data-driven procedure. In the oracle case, these weights satisfy the normalization condition

$$\sum_{k=1}^{K} \frac{m_k \pi_{0,k}}{m} w_k = 1, \tag{1}$$

while in the data-driven case, the weights satisfy the same normalization with $\{\pi_{0,k}\}_{k=1}^{K}$ replaced by an estimate. Then, δ_2 lowers the rejection threshold in group k^* to level p_{k^*,i^*}; that is,

$$\delta_2(\mathbf{s}^{(t)}) = (s_1^{(t)}, s_2^{(t)}, \ldots, p_{k^*,i^*}, \ldots, s_k^{(t)}).$$

Since the sequential procedure is written to reject all hypotheses with p-values strictly below $\mathbf{s}^{(t)}$, the GBH threshold-updating rule will remove the hypothesis or hypotheses with the greatest group-weighted p-value from the current rejection set. The manner in which the rejection threshold vector is updated implies that at each step of the procedure, at least one p-value is removed from the rejection set, so it will terminate in a finite number of steps.

3.3 Weighting Fixed Cutoff (WFC)

WFC [23] can be viewed as an extension of GBH, which uses information about the group-wise distributions of false null p-values to improve the choice of weights. The weights still satisfy the same normalization condition (1) used in GBH but are now chosen to directly maximize the number of rejected p-values for some initial fixed cutoff c:

$$\widehat{\mathcal{O}}(w, c) = \frac{1}{m} \sum_{k=1}^{K} \sum_{i=1}^{m_k} I(p_{k,i}/w_k \le c).$$

In the oracle case, it is possible to choose w to directly maximize the power, and $\widehat{\mathcal{O}}$ can be viewed as an estimate of power based on the empirical CDF of the p-values in each group. The authors in Zhao and Zhang [23] establish asymptotic control of the FDR for both their oracle and data-driven procedures, assuming that all the p-values are independent and the true null p-values are uniformly distributed. Nonetheless, we will show in Sect. 4 that WFC can substantially exceed the nominal FDR level in some settings.

3.4 Structure-Adaptive Benjamini–Hochberg (SABHA)

SABHA [15] is a flexible weighting procedure for general "structured signals," which can include ordering, grouping, or more general covariate information. They discuss the grouped case in Sect. 4.2 of their paper and note its similarity to GBH, as it only incorporates information about the group-wise proportions of true null hypotheses. Like GBH and WFC, SABHA reduces to a group-weighted Benjamini–Hochberg procedure. In the grouped case, the weight normalization condition required by SABHA reduces to

$$\sum_{k=1}^{K} w_k \hat{\pi}_{0,k}(\tau) \leq 1,$$

for a tuning parameter $\tau \in (0, 1)$, where for $k =, 1 \ldots, K$, $\hat{\pi}_{0,k}(\tau)$ is the usual Storey et al. [20] estimator for the proportion of true null hypotheses in group k. This coincides with (1) when all groups are equal in size. Under the null independence model with superuniform true null p-values, the authors in Li and Barber [15] establish a finite sample bound for the FDR in the grouped setting. When run at level α, SABHA controls the FDR at level

$$\alpha \left(1 + \frac{1}{2m\epsilon(1-\tau)} \sum_{k=1}^{K} \sqrt{m_k} \right), \tag{2}$$

where ϵ and τ are tuning parameters. With this bound, one can control the FDR exactly at level α by running SABHA at a more conservative level $\alpha' < \alpha$, but at a cost of some power. In Sect. 4, we apply SABHA at the nominal level and find that in most settings it does control the FDR at or close to the nominal level. The bound in (2) represents a worst case and is highly dependent on the choice of tuning parameters ϵ and τ, which restrict the complexity of the group weights.

3.5 Independent Hypothesis Weighting (IHWc)

IHWc [11] is another group-weighted procedure, which is designed for general covariate information but can be adapted to the group setting. Similar to WFC, their procedure chooses weights by optimizing the estimated power based on the empirical CDFs of the p-values in each group. By choosing weights based on holdout samples and censoring some p-value information, they establish finite sample control of the FDR under the null independence model with superuniform true null p-values.

3.6 Adaptive p-Value Thresholding (AdaPT)

AdaPT [13] is an alternative procedure that does not reduce to group-weighted Benjamini–Hochberg. The authors in Lei and Fithian [13] establish finite sample control of the FDR under the null independence model with uniform true null p-values (Theorem 1) using a martingale argument similar to Barber and Candèes [1]. The construction of the martingale in proof motivates the masking of information, by mirroring the p-values below a threshold. This limited information is the key to maintaining finite sample FDR control. As it is quite distinct from the previous procedures, we describe it here using our sequential framework.

Example 3 (Sequential Version of the AdaPT Procedure) In this case,

$$\mathbf{s}^{(0)} = (1/2, 1/2, \ldots, 1/2).$$

Suppose the procedure is at step t. The stopping rule δ_1 is given by

$$\delta_1(\mathbf{s}^{(t)}) = I(\widehat{\text{FDR}}(\mathbf{s}^{(t)}) \leq \alpha),$$

where

$$\widehat{\text{FDR}}(\mathbf{s}) = \frac{1 + \sum_{k=1}^{K} \sum_{i=1}^{m_k} I(p_{k,i} > 1 - s_k)}{\max\{\sum_{k=1}^{K} \sum_{i=1}^{m_k} I(p_{k,i} < s_k), 1\}}. \tag{3}$$

As in the CLfdr and GBH procedures, stopping is based on a current estimate of the FDR, but in this case, the estimate of rejected true null hypotheses is based on the mirror of the rejection region, basically treating the p-values greater than $1 - s^{(t)}$ as knockoff variables by the mirror symmetry of the uniform distribution. If the p-values follow the two-group model, the optimality results of Cai and Sun [4] motivate an oracle threshold-updating rule based on the local FDR. Define

$$(k^*, i^*) = \underset{(k,i)}{\text{argmax}}\{\text{Lfdr}_k(q_{k,i}) : q_{k,i} < s_k^{(t)}\},$$

where $q_{k,i} = \min\{p_{k,i}, 1 - p_{k,i}\} \in (0, 1/2]$ is the smaller one of the p-value and its mirror image. Similar as in Lei and Fithian [13], $q_{k,i}$ is used here because it is the potential rejection to acceptation change point. Then,

$$\delta_2(\mathbf{s}^{(t)}) = (s_1^{(t)}, s_2^{(t)}, \ldots, q_{k^*,i^*}, \ldots, s_k^{(t)}).$$

If the local FDR functions are unknown or the p-values do not follow the two-group model, the threshold-updating rule attempts to mimic this oracle rule. In order to preserve the FDR control property, a restriction is made on the information available to estimate δ_2 at each step. In particular, suppose that we are at step t with the rejection threshold vector $\mathbf{s}^{(t)}$, and then in the kth group, let

$$R_{t,k} = |\{i : p_{k,i} < s_k^{(t)}\}| \text{ and } A_{t,k} = |\{i : p_{k,i} > 1 - s_k^{(t)}\}|$$

be the number of p-values below the threshold and above the mirror threshold, respectively. Across all groups, let $R_t = \sum_{k=1}^{K} R_{t,k}$ and $A_t = \sum_{k=1}^{K} A_{t,k}$. Define the partially masked p-values as

$$\tilde{p}_{t,k,i} = \begin{cases} p_{k,i} & \text{if } s_k^{(t)} \le p_{k,i} \le 1 - s_k^{(t)}, \\ \{p_{k,i}, 1 - p_{k,i}\} & \text{otherwise,} \end{cases}$$

for $k = 1, \ldots, K$ and $i = 1, \ldots, m_k$. In the first (unmasked) case, we know the true location of the p-value when it is between the threshold and the mirror threshold. In the second (masked) case, we know the unordered pair of p-value and its mirror image but do not know which one is the true p-value. The AdaPT procedure specifies that the threshold-updating rule δ_2 must be estimated using only the information contained in the σ-algebra

$$\mathcal{F}_t = \sigma\left(\left\{\tilde{p}_{t,k,i}\right\}_{i=1,k=1}^{m_k,K}, A_t, R_t\right);$$

that is, $\mathcal{F}_t$ contains all the information about the partially masked p-values plus A_t and R_t at step t. Notice that the collection $\{\mathcal{F}_t\}_{t\ge 0}$ is a filtration, as progressively more information is made available at each step of the procedure.

In data-driven AdaPT, one needs to estimate group-wise local FDR functions with partially masked information in $\mathcal{F}_t$. More precisely, for estimates $\{\widehat{\text{Lfdr}}_1, \ldots, \widehat{\text{Lfdr}}_K\}$ of the group-wise local FDR functions, define

$$(\hat{k}, \hat{i}) = \underset{(k,i)}{\text{argmax}} \left\{\widehat{\text{Lfdr}}_k(q_{k,i}) : q_{k,i} < s_k^{(t)}\right\},$$

and then the threshold-updating rule for the data-driven AdaPT procedure is

$$\delta_2(\mathbf{s}^{(t)}) = \left(s_1^{(t)}, s_2^{(t)}, \ldots, q_{\hat{k},\hat{i}}, \ldots, s_K^{(t)}\right).$$

Estimation is done separately for each of the K groups, and the authors in Lei and Fithian [13] provide an EM approach to impute the masked p-value information. In the Appendix, we provide a two-parameter variant of their EM algorithm.

Note that in contrast to other procedures, AdaPT requires the quantities in the threshold-updating rule to be reestimated as the procedure progresses, as more information is unmasked at each sequential step.

3.7 Linear and Nonlinear Rankings

Here, we briefly highlight a distinction between the weighted procedures and AdaPT, which we describe as *linearity* of the ranking of significance. Note that all the weighted procedures choose a ranking of significance by ordering $\{p_{k,i}/w_k\}_{i=1,k=1}^{m_k,K}$, which restricts the possible rankings available to the procedure. Suppose

$$2p_{1,i'} = p_{1,i} = p_{2,j} = 2p_{2,j'},$$

and test $(1, i)$ is ranked as more significant than test $(2, j)$. Then, we must also have that test $(1, i')$ is ranked as more significant than test $(2, j')$. This is a nontrivial restriction of possible rankings, as the authors in Cai and Sun [4] establish that under the two-group model, the optimal ranking is based on the local FDR, a nonlinear transformation of the p-values. To our knowledge, AdaPT is currently the only procedure with finite sample FDR control which does not restrict to linear rankings of significance.

4 Simulation

In this section, we compare the performance of the oracle and data-driven versions of the various grouped multiple testing procedures described above. Procedures presented for comparison are the modified Benjamini–Hochberg procedure (`MBH`) described in Storey et al. [20], the group-weighted Benjamini–Hochberg procedure (`GBH`) of Hu et al. [10], the weighted fixed cutoff procedure (`WFC`) of Zhao and Zhang [23], the structure-adaptive Benjamini–Hochberg procedure (`SABHA`) of Li and Barber [15], the independent hypothesis weighting procedure (`IHWc`) of Ignatiadis and Huber [11], and the `AdaPT` procedure of Lei and Fithian [13]. The ADDOW procedure of Durand et al. [5] is very similar to `WFC` and has no readily available implementation, so we do not include it here.

The oracle CLfdr procedure of Cai and Sun [4], which is theoretically optimal in these simulation settings, is used as a benchmark level to assess the power of other procedures. `MBH` can be viewed as a baseline for comparison, as it is designed for the exchangeable case and ignores group labels altogether. Note that Zhao and Zhang [23] define two weighted fixed cutoff procedures, and we utilize their so-called "Pro2," which is more powerful than their "Pro1" both in theory and in their simulation study. `SABHA` is implemented using R code available on the author's website and run at the nominal level. `IHWc` is implemented in the R package `IHW`, available on Bioconductor. `AdaPT` for the normal model is implemented using the two-parameter EM algorithm described in the Appendix and for the beta model is implemented in the R package `adaptMT`. In `IHW`, we specify the parameter `null_proportion = TRUE` to control FDR at the exact level, rather than the default $\pi_0\alpha$ level. In adaptMT, we specify the parameter Mstep_type='weighted', where the recommended default option is 'unweighted'. Lei and Fithian [13] conducted simulation studies with continuous covariates and found that the default option of 'unweighted' leads to consistently good performance, while the 'weighted' option could be unstable. The detail is described in Appendix A.3 of [14]. In our grouped settings, the weighted option provides better power than the unweighted option.

With the exception of IHWc, which does not have an oracle implementation, all of the procedures considered have both oracle and data-driven versions. As noted in the original paper [15], the oracle version of SABHA coincides with the oracle version of GBH, so it is not included here. In the data-driven versions of GBH and WFC, the group-wise true null proportions $\{\pi_{0,k}\}_{k=1}^{K}$ are estimated using the lowest-slope procedure [3], as in Hu et al. [10] and Zhao and Zhang [23]. The data-driven MBH also utilizes the lowest-slope procedure to estimate the overall true null proportion. The lowest-slope procedure leads to conservative estimation of π_0 [16], and MBH with the lowest-slope π_0-estimator controls the FDR at the nominal level in finite samples [17].

In the data-driven AdaPT, rather than estimating new parameters for the Lfdr at every sequential step, the estimates are updated $G = 5$ times for each group as more information becomes available. The sensitivity analysis to the choice of this "refresh rate" G showed that 5 updates are sufficient, and there is no significant power advantage to update the Lfdr parameters more often. This partially mitigates the concerns of Ignatiadis and Huber [11] (Section 5.2) that AdaPT runs slowly since its model parameters need to be reestimated at each iteration. Nonetheless, IHWc is still about 5–10 times faster than AdaPT for the settings described here, and its computation time empirically scales better in m, the total number of tests.

We have 7 simulation settings in total, where settings 1–3 are similar to those in Cai and Sun [4] and Zhao and Zhang [23]. We investigate the effect of the number of groups in setting 4 and a beta model in settings 5–7. In settings 1–4, the p-values are calculated from normal statistics: true null statistics follow standard normal N(0, 1), and false null statistics follow N(μ, 1) for some $\mu > 0$. We refer to μ as the signal strength. The p-values are calculated to test $H_{k,i} : \mu_{k,i} = 0$ against the one-sided alternative $\mu_{k,i} > 0$. In settings 1–4, the data-driven AdaPT estimates the Lfdr from the correct parametric model. In settings 5–7, false null p-values follow a Beta(τ, 1) distribution. We run the two versions of AdaPT, one with the correct parametric model and the other with a misspecified normal model, to investigate the robustness of the data-driven AdaPT to a misspecified parametric model. Note that in the normal case, the large values of μ correspond to strong signals, while in the beta case, the small values of τ correspond to strong signals. In all settings, the nominal significance level is $\alpha = 0.1$ and $J = 1000$ independent replications are performed.

The details of settings are as follows:

1. *Varying true null proportions with normal signals*: $K = 2$ groups of sizes $m_1 = 3000$ and $m_2 = 1500$. Signal strengths are fixed at $\mu_1 = 2$ and $\mu_2 = 4$. The true

null proportion for group 2 is fixed at $\pi_{0,2} = 0.9$, while $\pi_{0,1}$ varies from 0.7 to 1 with increment size of 0.03.

2. *Varying signal strength with normal signals*: $K = 2$ groups of sizes $m_1 = 3000$ and $m_2 = 1500$. The signal strength for group 2 is fixed at $\mu_2 = 4$, while μ_1 varies from 2.5 to 4.9 with increment size of 0.2. True null proportions are fixed at $\pi_{0,1} = 0.8$ and $\pi_{0,2} = 0.9$.
3. *Varying # tests with normal signals*: $K = 2$ groups, with $m_2 = 1500$ fixed, while m_1 varies from 500 to 5000 with increment size of 500. Signal strengths are fixed at $\mu_1 = 2$ and $\mu_2 = 4$, and true null proportions are fixed at $\pi_{0,1} = 0.8$ and $\pi_{0,2} = 0.9$.
4. *Varying # groups with normal signals*: $m = 5000$ and split into K equal-sized groups, where K takes on the values $2, 4, 5, 8, 10, 15$, and 20. The signal strengths μ_k are taken as an equally spaced sequence of length K between 2 and 6, and the true null proportions $\pi_{0,k}$ are taken as an equally spaced sequence of length K between 0.65 and 1.
5. *Varying true null proportions with beta signals*: $K = 2$ groups of sizes $m_1 = 3000$ and $m_2 = 1500$. False null p-values follow a Beta(τ, 1) distribution, with $\tau_1 = 1/5$ and $\tau_2 = 1/12$. The true null proportion for group 2 is fixed at $\pi_{0,2} = 0.9$, while $\pi_{0,1}$ varies from 0.7 to 1 with increment size of 0.03.
6. *Varying signal strength with beta signals*: $K = 2$ groups of sizes $n_1 = 3000$ and $n_2 = 1500$. False null p-values follow a Beta(τ, 1) distribution, with $\tau_2 = 1/12$ fixed, while τ_1^{-1} varies from 5 to 15 with increment size of 1. True null proportions are fixed at $\pi_{0,1} = 0.8$ and $\pi_{0,2} = 0.9$.
7. *Varying # tests with beta signals*: $K = 2$ groups, with $m_2 = 1500$ fixed, while m_1 varies from 500 to 5000 with increment size of 500. Signal strengths are fixed at $\tau_1 = 1/5$ and $\tau_2 = 1/12$, and true null proportions are fixed at $\pi_{0,1} = 0.8$ and $\pi_{0,2} = 0.9$.

4.1 Results

Figure 1 presents the results of the oracle procedures for settings 1–4. In the oracle case, `MBH`, `GBH`, and `AdaPT` have theoretical finite sample control of the FDR, while `WFC` controls the FDR asymptotically. All procedures control the FDR reasonably close to the nominal level $\alpha = 0.1$. The power of oracle procedures relative to the oracle CLfdr of Cai and Sun [4] is shown in the second column of Fig. 1. In setting 1, `MBH` does not achieve the power of the other procedures, especially when the group null proportions are sufficiently different and group labeling becomes highly informative. Although the FDR of `AdaPT` is below the nominal level when $\pi_{0,1}$ is close to 1, it still has near the optimal level of power. In setting 2 and when μ_1 is large, `GBH`, which ignores group signal strength, has the lowest power for large values of μ_1. However, for such strong signals, the false null p-values separate from the true nulls, and all methods achieve near-optimal power. Setting 3 demonstrates

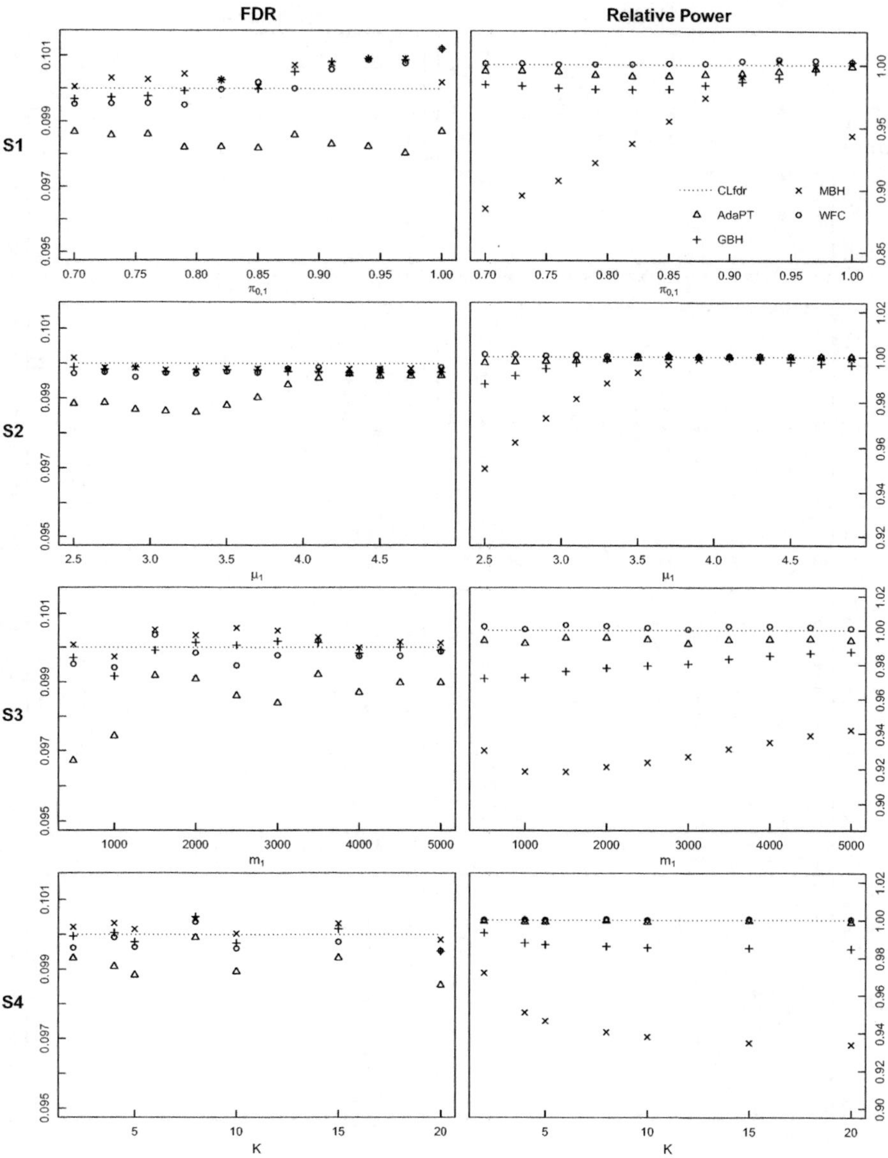

Fig. 1 Realized FDR and relative power, oracle procedures, settings 1–4

relative power performances similar to setting 1. In all oracle cases, only `AdaPT` and `WFC` consistently achieve near the optimal level of power.

Figure 2 presents the results of the data-driven procedures for settings 1–4. In the data-driven case, `MBH`, `IHWc`, and `AdaPT` have theoretical finite sample control of the FDR at the nominal level, while `GBH` and `WFC` control the FDR asymptotically,

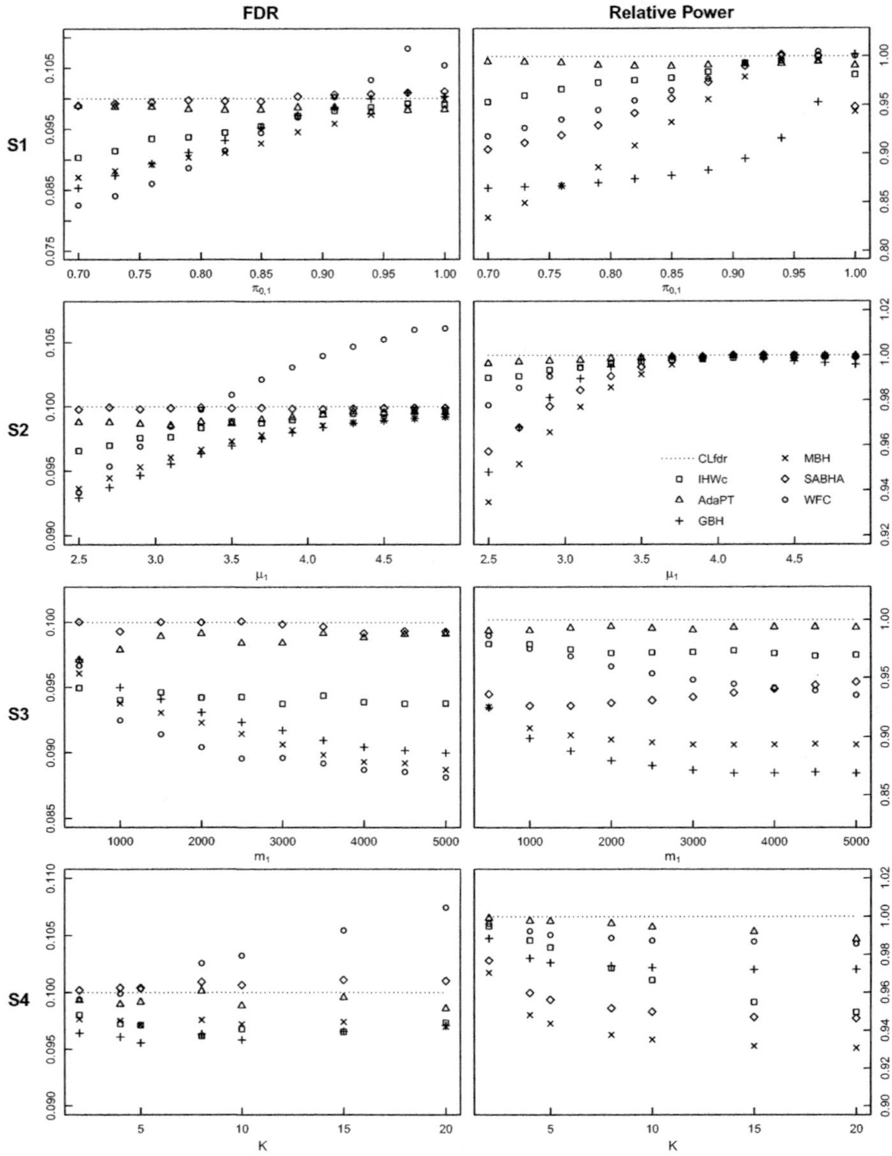

Fig. 2 Realized FDR and relative power, data-driven procedures, settings 1–4

and SABHA has finite sample control of the FDR at an inflated level. In settings 1–3, all procedures except WFC show proper control of the FDR. In setting 4, both WFC and SABHA fail to control the FDR, although the exceedance of WFC is much larger. In particular, the realized FDR levels of WFC exceed the nominal level in setting 1 with high $\pi_{0,1}$ values, in setting 2 with high θ_1 values, and in setting

4 with median and large numbers of groups (K's). In terms of power, AdaPT achieves comparable or significantly better power than competing procedures, in all settings and parameter values. AdaPT, WFC, and SABHA show consistent power improvement over MBH, which does not use group information. Despite their similarity, SABHA is more powerful than GBH, especially in setting 3, when the group sizes become highly imbalanced, and SABHA's weight normalization condition allows it to more aggressively weight p-values from the larger group. For most parameter values in settings 1 and 3, GBH is less powerful than MBH. This is mainly because GBH only considers the group-wise true null proportions and ignores the signal strength differences among groups. The power advantages of AdaPT over WFC is best illustrated in setting 4, where AdaPT outperforms WFC in power despite the fact that the realized FDR levels of WFC are consistently higher than those of AdaPT. Finally, we should point out that the practical performances of WFC and GBH critically depend on the π_0-estimator used. We used the same lowest-slope π_0-estimator [3] as in the simulation studies of Hu et al. [10] and Zhao and Zhang [23]. The lowest-slope estimator has been shown to be one of the most conservative π_0-estimators, see simulation results of Liang and Nettleton [16] and MacDonald et al. [17]. If a less conservative π_0-estimator is used with GBH and WFC, the FDR inflation of WFC is expected to be more pronounced, and it is unclear whether GBH can still control the FDR. On the other hand, AdaPT is theoretically guaranteed to control the FDR in finite samples.

Figure 3 presents the results of the data-driven procedures for settings 5–7, where the alternative p-values are generated from a beta distribution. We did not include oracle results for these settings, although the oracle CLfdr procedure was still run to provide a benchmark level for power. Here, we implement two versions of AdaPT: the two-parameter version described in the Appendix, and a version based on a Beta GLM, implemented in the R package adaptMT. These settings show that AdaPT is robust to model misspecification and achieves the best overall power of all competing procedures. In fact, its performance is nearly indistinguishable between the true and misspecified models. As emphasized by our sequential framework, the power of AdaPT (or any grouped multiple testing procedure) depends primarily on the relative rankings of hypotheses between groups, and the absolute accuracy of the Lfdr functions is not crucial. Even with a misspecified model, it is still able to remove approximately the most likely true null hypothesis from the current rejection set. When $\pi_{0,1}$ is close to 1 in setting 5, WFC can be slightly more powerful than AdaPT, but WFC again loses control of the FDR. When $\pi_{0,1} = 1$ in setting 5, the power of SABHA drops off sharply as the group weights are lower bounded by a tuning parameter $\epsilon = 0.1$, which also appears in the upper bound in (2). Setting 6 again demonstrates the robustness of AdaPT, which is the most powerful procedure. Finally, setting 7 demonstrates that AdaPT achieves the best relative performance in terms of FDR control and power as the group size m_1 grows, while the performances of all other procedures show a decreasing trend. In settings 5–7 with beta signals, all procedures control the FDR more conservatively than in settings 1–4 with normal signals. The *impurity* of the beta distribution [9] leads to identifiability issues in the estimation of $\pi_{0,k}$ and conservatively biased π_0 and FDR estimates.

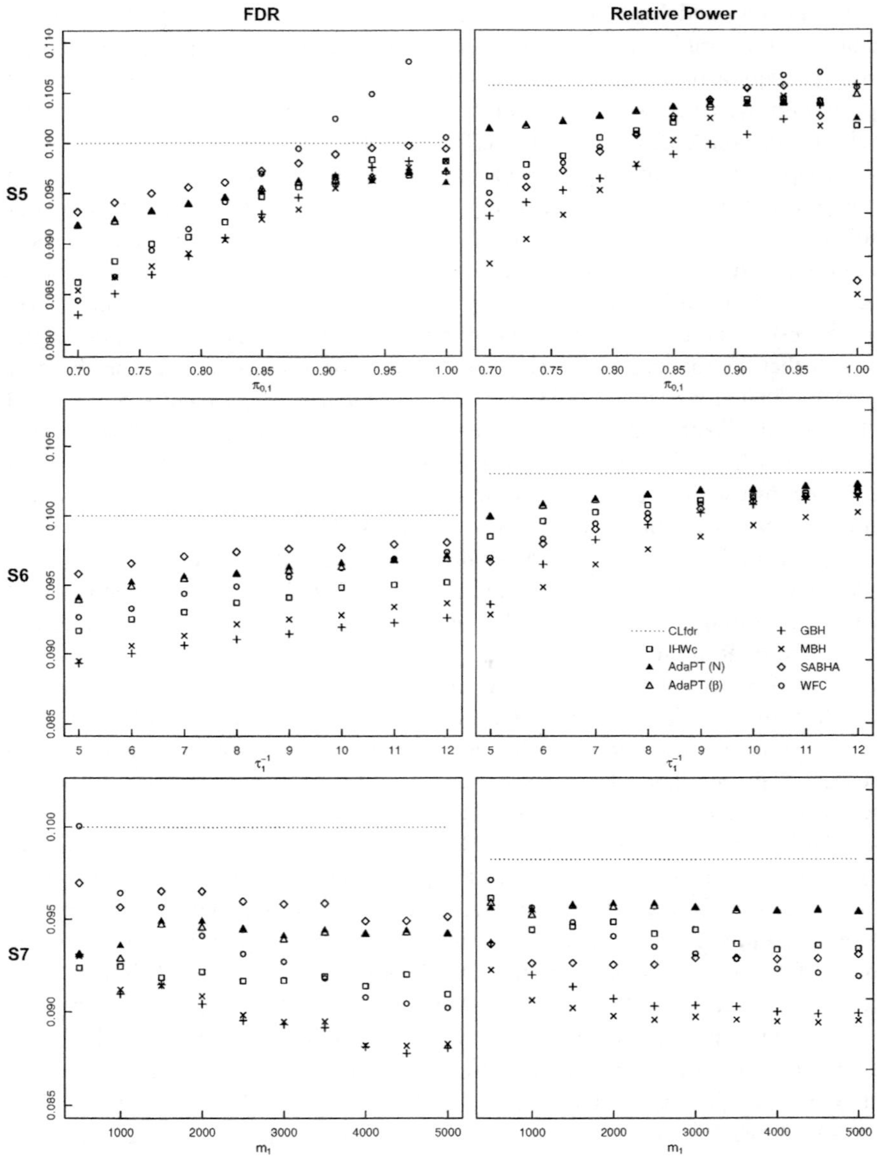

Fig. 3 Realized FDR and relative power, data-driven procedures, settings 5–7

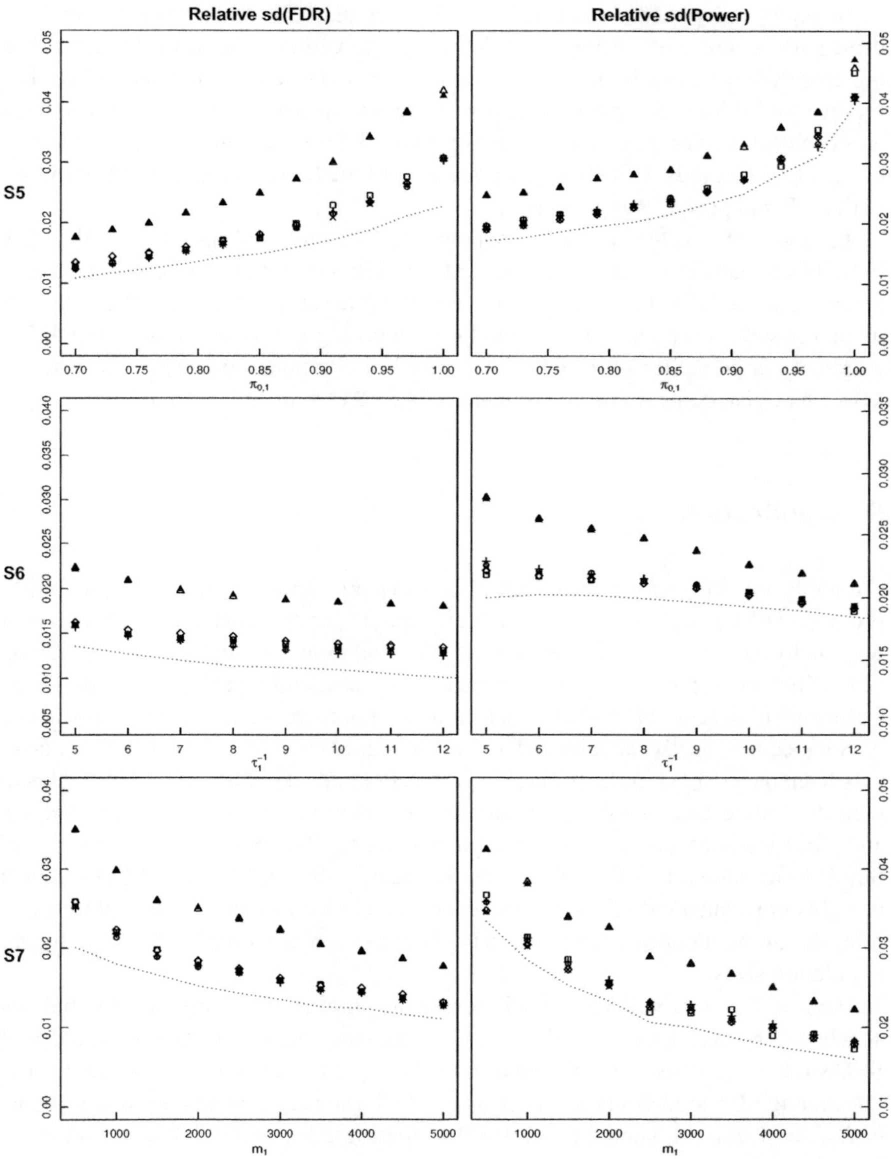

Fig. 4 Standard deviation of realized FDR and relative power, data-driven procedures, settings 5–7

In Fig. 4, we plot the standard deviations of the FDP and power of the data-driven procedures for settings 5–7. While all procedures are more variable than the corresponding oracle, it is clear that AdaPT shows the largest variability. The relative variability of AdaPT's power decreases in setting 6, as all procedures approach full power; however, its variability in FDP remains much higher than that of the other methods. In setting 7, we see that all methods decrease in variability of both FDP and power as m increases.

In summary, AdaPT gives the best power performance and also controls the FDR in finite samples, but it suffers in terms of variability of both power and FDP. IHWc gives the second best performance, again with finite sample control of the FDR, but its power suffers for small m, especially when each group is small in setting 4. For extremely large values of m, where the speed of computation becomes a concern, IHWc will give comparable performance to AdaPT in much less time.

5 Application

We apply the various grouped multiple testing procedures to the adequate yearly progress (AYP) study of California high schools for the year 2007. This dataset was analyzed in a similar fashion by Cai and Sun [4] and Zhao and Zhang [23]. The dataset consists of observations of academic performance for 7867 California high schools. Within each school, we compare the academic performance of socioeconomically advantaged (SEA) students to that of socioeconomically disadvantaged (SED) students in terms of success rate on math exams. The goal is to identify "interesting" schools whose relative performances between SEA students and SED students differ from the typical amount. Previous analysis by Cai and Sun [4] has shown that the relative performance between SEA and SED students is highly correlated with the school size, and a more informative list of "interesting" schools can be identified when the schools are grouped according to their student population sizes.

For $i = 1, \ldots, m$ with $m = 7687$, denote the number of successful SEA students at school i by X_i, out of a total of s_{xi} SEA students and the number of successful SED students at school i by Y_i, out of a total of s_{yi} SED students. Then, the success rate among SEA students is $R_{xi} = X_i/s_{xi}$, and the success rate among SED students is $R_{yi} = Y_i/s_{yi}$. A summary statistic comparing SEA and SED performance at school i can be constructed as

$$Z_i = \frac{R_{xi} - R_{yi} - \gamma}{\sqrt{\frac{R_{xi}(1-R_{xi})}{s_{xi}} + \frac{R_{yi}(1-R_{yi})}{s_{yi}}}},$$

where $\gamma = \text{median}(R_{x1}, \ldots, R_{xm}) - \text{median}(R_{y1}, \ldots, R_{ym})$ is a centering constant. We group the data in the same way as Cai and Sun [4] and Zhao and Zhang [23], into a small group ($s_{xi} + s_{yi} \leq 120$), a medium group ($120 < s_{xi} + s_{yi} < 900$),

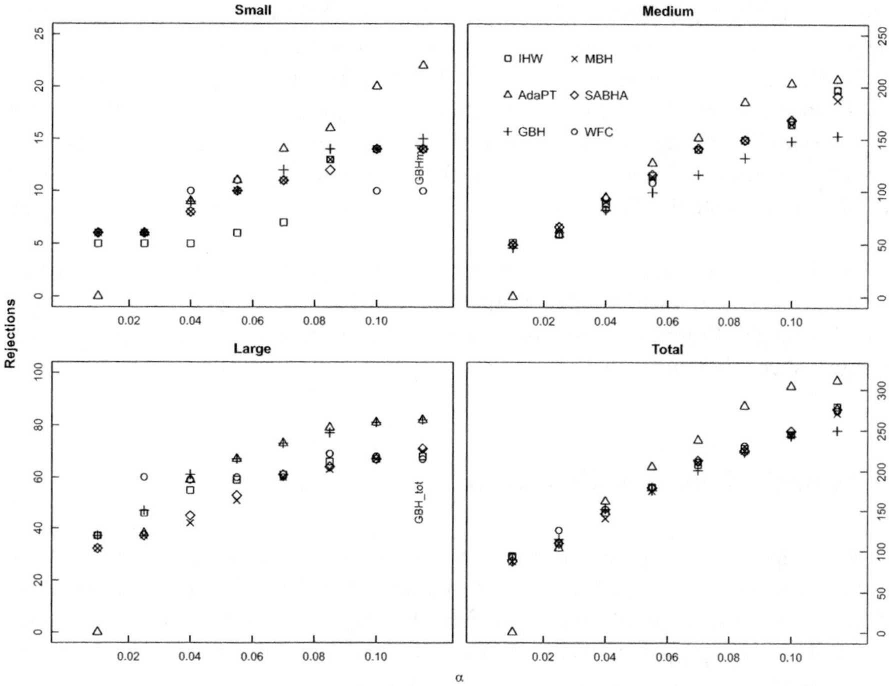

Fig. 5 Group-wise and total rejections, AYP data

and a large group ($s_{xi} + s_{yi} \geq 900$). For each group, the empirical null distribution is estimated using the method of Jin and Cai [12], and the p-values are calculated to test whether each Z_i comes from its group's null distribution. The same four data-driven procedures compared in the simulation study of Sect. 4 are applied to control the FDR at a range of nominal α levels. AdaPT estimates the parameters of the group-wise Lfdr functions using the normal EM algorithm described in the Appendix. GBH, WFC, and MBH estimate their (group-wise) true null proportions using the lowest-slope procedure [3].

Figure 5 plots the numbers of total and group-wise rejections against the nominal FDR levels. As the nominal level α increases, all procedures are able to identify more interesting schools. When the target FDR level α is small, all procedures have similar total numbers of rejections. For sufficiently large α values, more specifically, when $\alpha > 0.04$, AdaPT has the most total number of rejections among all procedures. It can be seen from Fig. 5 that AdaPT achieves the best overall power by focusing on the groups with the best potential of power improvement, namely the medium group, while sacrificing some power in the large group.

The total numbers of rejections of WFC, GBH, SABHA, IHWc, and MBH are close to one another, with no one procedure clearly dominating the others. We also notice that with the exception of WFC, the procedures show a "monotone" property: the number of rejections in each group never decreases with the nominal level α.

However in WFC, the optimization of weights for each specific α-level can lead to a decrease in rejections for a particular group, for example, in the small group.

Notice that the numerator of the AdaPT FDR estimator in (3) is bounded below by 1, so it follows that AdaPT will return zero rejections if there are fewer than $\lceil 1/\alpha \rceil$ possible rejections left during the iteration steps of the sequential procedure, which can limit its effectiveness when the total number of tests m or the target FDR level α is small. This is seen above, as AdaPT returns zero rejections when $\alpha = 0.01$.

As in the simulation results, AdaPT achieves the best power, although this analysis does illuminate another limitation of AdaPT when m or α is small. For small α levels, IHWc is a good alternative, although it too may suffer poor power performance when m is small.

6 Conclusions and Discussions

In this chapter, we compared the operational performance of various multiple testing procedures for the grouped test setting. We introduced a sequential framework to demonstrate how these different procedures leverage group information to improve the ranking of significance. With extensive simulations and a real data application, we show the strengths and weaknesses of different procedures.

While powerful weighted procedures like IHWc and SABHA have finite sample guarantees on control, these guarantees require more strict weighting than WFC, which achieves near-optimal power but often loses control of the FDR. AdaPT achieves the best performance on average, but at the cost of variability, and degeneracy for very small α levels.

Acknowledgments The authors thank the editor and two reviewers for their constructive comments that have led to an improved article. This work is supported by Natural Sciences and Engineering Research Council (NSERC) of Canada grants RGPIN-2020-04739 to Kun Liang and RGPIN-2016-03890 to Yingli Qin. The authors thank Professor Haibing Zhao for sharing his code.

Appendix

A.1 Two-Parameter AdaPT

Here, we describe in detail a multi-parameter implementation of the AdaPT procedure, which is tailored to the grouped test problem. For notational simplicity, the following assumes that we are estimating the local FDR function for a fixed group k and omits the group index.

We assume that the true null p-values are uniformly distributed, and thus f_0 is known. To recover an estimate of the local FDR in the two-group model, for each group, we require estimates of π_0 and f_1, which respect the information restrictions of the AdaPT procedure. Similar to Jin and Cai [12], we model the false null p-values as normally distributed when transformed to the z-scale, that is,

$$z_i = -\Phi^{-1}(p_i) \sim \begin{cases} \mathrm{N}(0, 1), & \text{if } H_i = 0 \\ \mathrm{N}(\mu, \sigma^2), & \text{if } H_i = 1, \end{cases}$$

where Φ^{-1} is the quantile function of the standard normal distribution. This is a one-to-one transformation from p-values to z-values. If the original tests are two-sided, the sign or directional information will be lost when computing the p-values [21]. Recently, the authors in Tian et al. [22] proposed an AdaPT-like procedure that can leverage the sign information to increase power while controlling the FDR. The `adaptMT` R package implements a simplified version of our model. More specifically, if the parameter `dist = inv_gaussian_family()`, `adaptMT` models the alternative z-value distribution as $\mathrm{N}(\mu, 1)$. That is, `adaptMT` restricts $\sigma^2 = 1$ for the normal model. More details can be found in Appendix A.1.2 of Lei and Fithian [13].

If a p-value is masked, then we do not know whether its true value is p_i or $1 - p_i$. After transforming to the z-scale, we do not know whether the true value is z_i or $-z_i$. Hence, we define

$$y_i = |z_i|,$$

and

$$B_i = I(z_i = y_i).$$

When a particular z-value z_i is masked, then we only know the absolute z-value y_i. However, if it is unmasked, then we also know B_i, which gives the sign of z_i, and the true z-value can be recovered. The full data are $\{y_i, B_i, H_i\}_{i=1}^m$, and the full-data likelihood can be written as

$$L(\theta, \pi_0) = \prod_{i=1}^{m} \Big\{ \phi_0(-y_i)^{(1-H_i)(1-B_i)} \cdot \phi_0(y_i)^{(1-H_i)B_i} \cdot \phi_\theta(-y_i)^{H_i(1-B_i)} \cdot \phi_\theta(y_i)^{H_i B_i} \cdot (1-\pi_0)^{H_i} \cdot \pi_0^{(1-H_i)} \Big\}, \tag{A.1}$$

where $\theta = (\mu, \sigma)$ and ϕ_θ denotes the density function of the $\mathrm{N}(\mu, \sigma^2)$ distribution.

H_i is missing for $i = 1, \ldots, m$, and B_i is missing for the masked p_i's. We apply the EM algorithm to estimate π_0 and θ, and the details can be found in the next section.

Based on estimates $\hat{\theta}$ and $\hat{\pi}_0$ of θ and π_0 from the EM algorithm, the Lfdr can be estimated as

$$\widehat{\text{Lfdr}}(p) = \frac{\hat{\pi}_0\phi_0(-\Phi^{-1}(p))}{\hat{\pi}_0\phi_0(-\Phi^{-1}(p)) + (1-\hat{\pi}_0)\phi_{\hat{\theta}}(-\Phi^{-1}(p))}.$$

A.2 EM Steps

From the full-data likelihood $L(\theta, \pi_0)$ in (2), the maximum likelihood estimate for θ can be found by maximizing the partial log-likelihood function,

$$\ell_1(\theta) = \sum_{i=1}^{m} H_i(1-B_i)\log(\phi_\theta(-y_i)) + H_i B_i \log(\phi_\theta(y_i)),$$

and the maximum likelihood estimate for π_0 is found by maximizing the partial log-likelihood function

$$\ell_2(\pi_0) = m\log(\pi_0) + \sum_{i=1}^{m} H_i \log\left(\frac{1-\pi_0}{\pi_0}\right).$$

The EM algorithm produces sequences of estimates $\hat{\theta}^{(1)}, \hat{\theta}^{(2)}, \ldots$ and $\hat{\pi}_0^{(1)}, \hat{\pi}_0^{(2)}, \ldots$ by alternating two steps, an E-step and an M-step, until some stopping criterion is met. For an arbitrary iteration $r+1$ of the EM algorithm, the E-step is derived by calculating the expected log-likelihood for each observation given the observed data and estimates $\hat{\theta}^{(r)}$ and $\hat{\pi}_0^{(r)}$ from the previous iteration of the algorithm. Denote the set of indices of masked p-values by $M^{(t)}$ at step t. For $i \notin M^{(t)}$, B_i is known, and the expected partial log-likelihood functions require the quantity

$$\begin{aligned}\mathbb{E}[H_i|z_i; \hat{\theta}^{(r)}, \hat{\pi}_0^{(r)}] &= \mathbb{P}(H_i = 1|z_i; \hat{\theta}^{(r)}, \hat{\pi}_0^{(r)}) \\ &= \frac{(1-\hat{\pi}_0^{(r)})\phi_{\hat{\theta}^{(r)}}(z_i)}{(1-\hat{\pi}_0^{(r)})\phi_{\hat{\theta}^{(r)}}(z_i) + \hat{\pi}_0^{(r)}\phi_0(z_i)}.\end{aligned}$$

For $i \in M^{(t)}$, B_i is unknown, and the expected partial log-likelihood function requires the quantities

$$\mathbb{E}[H_i B_i | y_i; \hat{\theta}^{(r)}, \hat{\pi}_0^{(r)}],$$

and

$$\mathbb{E}[H_i(1-B_i)|y_i; \hat{\theta}^{(r)}, \hat{\pi}_0^{(r)}].$$

To calculate these two expectations, note that

$$\mathbb{P}(B_i = 1|y_i, H_i = 1; \hat{\theta}^{(r)}, \hat{\pi}_0^{(r)}) = \frac{\phi_{\hat{\theta}^{(r)}}(y_i)}{\phi_{\hat{\theta}^{(r)}}(y_i) + \phi_{\hat{\theta}^{(r)}}(-y_i)},$$

$$\mathbb{P}(B_i = 0|y_i, H_i = 1; \hat{\theta}^{(r)}, \hat{\pi}_0^{(r)}) = \frac{\phi_{\hat{\theta}^{(r)}}(-y_i)}{\phi_{\hat{\theta}^{(r)}}(y_i) + \phi_{\hat{\theta}^{(r)}}(-y_i)},$$

$$\mathbb{P}(H_i = 1|y_i; \hat{\theta}^{(r)}, \hat{\pi}_0^{(r)}) = \frac{(\phi_{\hat{\theta}^{(r)}}(y_i) + \phi_{\hat{\theta}^{(r)}}(-y_i))(1 - \hat{\pi}_0^{(r)})}{(\phi_{\hat{\theta}^{(r)}}(y_i) + \phi_{\hat{\theta}^{(r)}}(-y_i))(1 - \hat{\pi}_0^{(r)}) + 2\phi_0(y_i)\hat{\pi}_0^{(r)}}.$$

So that

$$\begin{aligned}\mathbb{E}[H_i B_i|y_i; \hat{\theta}^{(r)}, \hat{\pi}_0^{(r)}] &= \mathbb{P}(B_i = 1|y_i, H_i = 1; \hat{\theta}^{(r)}, \hat{\pi}_0^{(r)}) \cdot \mathbb{P}(H_i = 1|y_i; \hat{\theta}^{(r)}, \hat{\pi}_0^{(r)}) \\ &= \frac{\phi_{\hat{\theta}^{(r)}}(y_i)(1 - \hat{\pi}_0^{(r)})}{(\phi_{\hat{\theta}^{(r)}}(y_i) + \phi_{\hat{\theta}^{(r)}}(-y_i))(1 - \hat{\pi}_0^{(r)}) + 2 \cdot \phi_0(y_i)\hat{\pi}_0^{(r)}},\end{aligned}$$

$$\begin{aligned}\mathbb{E}[H_i(1 - B_i)|y_i; \hat{\theta}^{(r)}, \hat{\pi}_0^{(r)}] &= \mathbb{P}(B_i = 0|y_i, H_i = 1; \hat{\theta}^{(r)}, \hat{\pi}_0^{(r)}) \cdot \mathbb{P}(H_i = 1|y_i; \hat{\theta}^{(r)}, \hat{\pi}_0^{(r)}) \\ &= \frac{\phi_{\hat{\theta}^{(r)}}(-y_i)(1 - \hat{\pi}_0^{(r)})}{(\phi_{\hat{\theta}^{(r)}}(y_i) + \phi_{\hat{\theta}^{(r)}}(-y_i))(1 - \hat{\pi}_0^{(r)}) + 2 \cdot \phi_0(y_i)\hat{\pi}_0^{(r)}}.\end{aligned}$$

Denote $\mathbb{E}[H_i|z_i; \hat{\theta}^{(r)}, \hat{\pi}_0^{(r)}]$ by $w_i^{(r)}$, $\mathbb{E}[H_i B_i|y_i; \hat{\theta}^{(r)}, \hat{\pi}_0^{(r)}]$ by $w_{i+}^{(r)}$, and $\mathbb{E}[H_i(1 - B_i)|y_i; \hat{\theta}^{(r)}, \hat{\pi}_0^{(r)}]$ by $w_{i-}^{(r)}$. Then, the expected partial log-likelihood for θ is

$$\begin{aligned}Q_1(\theta, \hat{\theta}^{(r)}, \hat{\pi}_0^{(r)}) = &\sum_{i \notin M^{(t)}} w_i^{(r)} \log(\phi_\theta(z_i)) \\ &+ \sum_{i \in M^{(t)}} (w_{i+}^{(r)} \log(\phi_\theta(y_i)) + w_{i-}^{(r)} \log(\phi_\theta(-y_i))),\end{aligned}$$

and the expected partial log-likelihood for π_0 is

$$\begin{aligned}Q_2(\pi_0, \hat{\theta}^{(r)}, \hat{\pi}_0^{(r)}) = m \log(\pi_0) + &\sum_{i \notin M^{(t)}} w_i^{(r)} \log\left(\frac{1 - \pi_0}{\pi_0}\right) \\ &+ \sum_{i \in M^{(t)}} (w_{i+}^{(r)} + w_{i-}^{(r)}) \log\left(\frac{1 - \pi_0}{\pi_0}\right).\end{aligned}$$

The M-step updates the estimates of θ and π_0 by maximizing Q_1 and Q_2, respectively. Q_1 resembles weighted least squares, and the optimal θ has the following closed-form solutions for its components:

$$\hat{\mu}^{(r+1)} = \frac{\sum_{i \notin M^{(t)}} w_i^{(r)} z_i + \sum_{i \in M^{(t)}} (w_{i+}^{(r)} y_i + w_{i-}^{(r)}(-y_i))}{\sum_{i \notin M^{(t)}} w_i^{(r)} + \sum_{i \in M^{(t)}} (w_{i+}^{(r)} + w_{i-}^{(r)})},$$

$$(\hat{\sigma}^{(r+1)})^2 = \frac{1}{\sum_{i \notin M^{(t)}} w_i^{(r)} + \sum_{i \in M^{(t)}} (w_{i+}^{(r)} + w_{i-}^{(r)})} \left\{ \sum_{i \notin M^{(t)}} w_i^{(r)} (z_i - \hat{\mu}^{(r+1)})^2 \right.$$
$$\left. + \sum_{i \in M^{(t)}} (w_{i+}^{(r)} (y_i - \hat{\mu}^{(r+1)})^2 + w_{i-}^{(r)} (-y_i - \hat{\mu}^{(r+1)})^2) \right\}.$$

By differentiating, it is straightforward to show that the optimal π_0 that maximizes Q_2 is

$$\hat{\pi}_0^{(r+1)} = 1 - \frac{1}{m} \left(\sum_{i \notin M^{(t)}} w_i^{(r)} + \sum_{i \in M^{(t)}} (w_{i+}^{(r)} + w_{i-}^{(r)}) \right).$$

Thus, all three parameters of the Lfdr have closed-form updating equations. After initialization, this update step is repeated until the sequence of estimates meets a given stopping criterion. In our implementation of this EM algorithm, we iterated until consecutive estimates satisfied

$$\|(\hat{\theta}^{(r+1)}, \hat{\pi}_0^{(r+1)})^\mathsf{T} - (\hat{\theta}^{(r)}, \hat{\pi}_0^{(r)})^\mathsf{T}\|_\infty < \epsilon = 10^{-4},$$

up to a maximum of 20 iterations.

A.3 Initialization

To initialize the estimates, we note that even when all p-values are masked, we can count the number of p-values in an interval symmetric about 1/2. Hence, we define

$$\hat{\pi}_0^{(0)}(\lambda, \delta) = \min \left\{ \frac{\sum_{i=1}^m I(\lambda \le p_i \le 1 - \lambda)}{m(1 - 2\lambda)}, 1 - \delta \right\}$$

for tuning parameters $\lambda \in (0, 1/2)$ and $\delta > 0$. This is similar to the estimator defined by Storey [19], except that instead of counting the number of p-values in the upper tail region $(\lambda, 1]$, we count the number in the symmetric central region $[\lambda, 1 - \lambda]$. Our estimator is also bounded away from 1 by using $1 - \delta$. If $\hat{\pi}_0^{(0)}$ were initialized at exactly 1, its EM updating equation will always return 1, and the other parameters will also not be updated. Hence, when $\pi_0 \approx 1$, this bounded estimator will give improved estimation accuracy. We observed through simulation that when $\pi_0 = 1$, the effects of bounding are negligible and the EM algorithm appears to still converge to the true parameter values. We set the tuning parameters $\lambda = 0.3$ and $\delta = 0.01$, although λ could also be chosen dynamically using a modified version of the right-boundary procedure [16].

To initialize $\hat{\theta}^{(0)}$, we first estimate $\hat{m}_a = \lfloor m(1 - \hat{\pi}_0^{(0)}(\lambda, \delta)) \rfloor$, and then

$$\hat{\mu}^{(0)} = \frac{1}{\hat{m}_a} \cdot \sum_{i=m-\hat{m}_a+1}^{m} y_{(i)},$$

where $y_{(1)} \leq \cdots \leq y_{(m)}$ denote the order statistics of the absolute z-values. Finally, we initialize $\hat{\sigma}^{(0)} = 1$.

References

1. Barber, R., Candès, E.: Controlling the false discovery rate via knockoffs. Ann. Stat. **43**(5), 2055–2085 (2015)
2. Benjamini, Y., Hochberg, Y.: Controlling the false discovery rate: a practical and powerful approach to multiple testing. J. R. Stat. Soc. Ser. B **57**(1), 289–300 (1995)
3. Benjamini, Y., Hochberg, Y.: On the adaptive control of the false discovery rate in multiple testing with independent statistics. J. Educ. Behav. Stat. **25**(1), 60–83 (2000)
4. Cai, T., Sun, W.: Simultaneous testing of grouped hypotheses: finding needles in multiple haystacks. J. Am. Stat. Assoc. **104**(488), 1467–1481 (2009)
5. Durand, G., et al.: Adaptive p-value weighting with power optimality. Electron. J. Stat. **13**(2), 3336–3385 (2019)
6. Efron, B., Tibshirani, R., Storey, J., Tusher, V.: Empirical Bayes analysis of a microarray experiment. J. Am. Stat. Assoc. **96**(456), 1151–1160 (2001)
7. Genovese, C., Roeder, K., Wasserman, L.: False discovery control with p-value weighting. Biometrika **93**(3), 509–524 (2006)
8. Genovese, C., Wasserman, L.: Operating characteristics and extensions of the false discovery rate procedure. J. R. Stat. Soc. Ser. B **64**(3), 499–517 (2002)
9. Genovese, C., Wasserman, L.: A stochastic process approach to false discovery control. Ann. Stat. **32**(3), 1035–1061 (2004)
10. Hu, J., Zhao, H., Zhou, H.: False discovery rate control with groups. J. Am. Stat. Assoc. **105**(491), 1215–1227 (2010)
11. Ignatiadis, N., Huber, W.: Covariate-powered weighted multiple testing with false discovery rate control (2017). arXiv preprint arXiv:1701.05179
12. Jin, J., Cai, T.: Estimating the null and the proportion of non-null effects in large-scale multiple comparisons. J. Am. Stat. Assoc. **102**(478), 495–506 (2007)
13. Lei, L., Fithian, W.: AdaPT: an interactive procedure for multiple testing with side information. J. R. Stat. Soc. Ser. B **80**, 649–679 (2018)
14. Lei, L., Fithian, W.: AdaPT: an interactive procedure for multiple testing with side information (2018). arXiv preprint arXiv:1609.06035
15. Li, A., Barber, R.: Multiple testing with the structure-adaptive Benjamini–Hochberg algorithm. J. R. Stat. Soc. Ser. B Stat Methodol. **81**(1), 45–74 (2019)
16. Liang, K., Nettleton, D.: Adaptive and dynamic adaptive procedures for false discovery rate control and estimation. J. R. Stat. Soc. Ser. B **74**(1), 163–182 (2012)
17. MacDonald, P., Liang, K., Janssen, A.: Dynamic adaptive procedures that control the false discovery rate. Electron. J. Stat. **13**(2), 3009–3024 (2019)

18. Roquain, E., Van De Wiel, M.: Optimal weighting for false discovery rate control. Electron. J. Stat. **3**, 678–711 (2009)
19. Storey, J.: A direct approach to false discovery rates. J. R. Stat. Soc. Ser. B **64**(3), 479–498 (2002)
20. Storey, J., Taylor, J., Siegmund, D.: Strong control, conservative point estimation and simultaneous conservative consistency of false discovery rates: a unified approach. J. R. Stat. Soc. Ser. B **66**(1), 187–205 (2004)
21. Sun, W., Cai, T.: Oracle and adaptive compound decision rules for false discovery rate control. J. Am. Stat. Assoc. **102**(479), 901–912 (2007)
22. Tian, Z., Liang, K., Li, P.: A powerful procedure that controls the false discovery rate with directional information. Biometrics **77**(1), 212–222 (2021)
23. Zhao, H., Zhang, J.: Weighted p-value procedures for controlling FDR of grouped hypotheses. J. Stat. Plan. Inference **151**, 90–106 (2014)

Classic Linear Mediation Analysis of Complex Survey Data Using Balanced Repeated Replication

Yujiao Mai and Hui Zhang

1 Introduction

Mediation analysis is used to investigate the role of a third variable (also called a mediator) as a transmitter in the relationship between the exposure and the outcome [2, 14, 21, 27]. Although studies in psychology [9, 25], marketing [8, 10, 17], biomedicine [13, 16], and other sciences (e.g., [1, 12, 20]) have widely employed the framework of mediation analysis, only a few studies (e.g., [15]) have recently paid attention to its application to complex survey data from stratified multistage sampling.

Classic linear mediation analysis within structural equation modeling (SEM) framework assumes simple random sampling [4, 27]; while complex surveys usually involve stratified multistage sampling and required adjustments in estimation of parameters [32]. Common variance estimation methods for complex surveys include Jackknife repeated replication (JRR), balanced repeated replication (BRR), bootstrap (replication), and Taylor series linear approximation (paired with one of the other methods). Studies found that, among BRR, JRR, and Taylor series linear approximation, BRR is generally the least expensive regarding computation load and has the highest confidence interval coverage probability; while Taylor series linear approximation and JRR tend to have smaller bias than BRR [32]. It is hard to claim which one of these methods is universally the best choice in research practice.

Y. Mai (✉)
St. Jude Children's Research Hospital, Memphis, TN, USA
e-mail: yujiao.mai@stjude.org

H. Zhang
Northwestern University, Chicago, IL, USA
e-mail: hzhang@northwestern.edu

Y. Zhao, (Din) D.-G. Chen (eds.), *Modern Statistical Methods for Health Research*, Emerging Topics in Statistics and Biostatistics,
https://doi.org/10.1007/978-3-030-72437-5_9

Recently, researchers [15] have proposed an algorithm for classic linear mediation analysis adjusted for complex sampling designs using BRR. In practice, SAS is the dominant computer software for analyzing these national or international survey data. To facilitate the application of mediation analysis with complex survey data employing the proposed algorithm, we will develop a SAS macro named $MediationBRR$.

In the rest of the chapter, we will firstly review the technical details of the algorithm being implemented, then introduce the SAS macro $\%MediationBRR$ followed by application examples with data from Current Population Survey (CPS; [31]) and Program for International Student Assessment (PISA; [19]), and finally discuss the limitations of the present study and directions for future studies.

2 Technical Details

This section reviews the statistical model and algorithms used in the developed SAS macro for linear (multi)mediation analysis for complex surveys suing BRR.

2.1 Mediation Model

Let X be the exposure (continuous or zero-one variable), Y be the response, and $Z_1, \ldots, Z_L$ be the covariates (continuous or zero-one variables). Suppose multiple mediators $M_1, M_2, \cdots, M_K$ (all of the K mediators denoted as $M's$) are to be evaluated. When Y and $M's$ are continuous variables, we have the classic mediation model denoted by the $1+K$ equations as follows:

$$\begin{aligned}
Y|(X, M's) =& \tau_0 + \gamma_0 X + \beta_1 M_1 + \cdots + \beta_K M_K + \gamma_1 Z_1 + \cdots + \gamma_L Z_L + \varepsilon_0 \\
M_1|X =& \tau_1 + \alpha_1 X + \lambda_{11} Z_1 + \cdots + \lambda_{1L} Z_L + \varepsilon_1 \\
M_2|X =& \tau_2 + \alpha_2 X + \lambda_{21} Z_1 + \cdots + \lambda_{2L} Z_L + \varepsilon_2 \\
&\vdots \\
M_K|X =& \tau_K + \alpha_K X + \lambda_{K1} Z_1 + \cdots + \lambda_{KL} Z_L + \varepsilon_K
\end{aligned} \tag{1}$$

where τ_0 and $\tau_1, \tau_2, \cdots, \tau_K$ are intercepts, $\gamma_0, \gamma_1, \ldots, \gamma_L$, $\lambda_{k1}, \lambda_{k2}, \ldots, \lambda_{kL}(k = 1, 2, \ldots, K)$, $\alpha_1, \alpha_2, \cdots, \alpha_K$, and $\beta_1, \beta_2, \cdots, \beta_K$ are structural coefficients (regression coefficients), and ε_0 and $\varepsilon_1, \varepsilon_2, \cdots, \varepsilon_K$ are residuals (disturbances). The model satisfies these general assumptions for structural equation models (SEM; [4]): (a) Residuals are independent of variables on the right-hand side of the equation; (b) Residuals in equations of $M_1, M_2, \cdots, M_K$ are independent of residual in equation of Y; (c) ε_0 and $\varepsilon_1, \varepsilon_2, \cdots, \varepsilon_K$ follow a multivariate normal distribution with the mean vector $\mathbf{0}$ and the covariance matrix $\boldsymbol{\Psi}$, where

$$\boldsymbol{\Psi} = \begin{bmatrix} \sigma^2_{\varepsilon_0} & & & & \\ 0 & \sigma^2_{\varepsilon_1} & & & \\ 0 & \sigma_{\varepsilon_1,\varepsilon_2} & \sigma^2_{\varepsilon_2} & & \\ \vdots & \vdots & \vdots & \ddots & \\ 0 & \sigma_{\varepsilon_1,\varepsilon_K} & \sigma_{\varepsilon_2,\varepsilon_K} & \cdots & \sigma^2_{\varepsilon_K} \end{bmatrix}$$

The product of coefficients, $\alpha_k \beta_k$, is defined as the mediation (indirect) effect [6, 22, 27] via the k-th mediator, $M_k (k = 1, 2, \ldots, K)$, whereas the path, γ_0, from X to Y represents the direct effect. The estimator of the product of coefficients asymptotically follows a normal distribution when using a large-sample-based estimator such as maximum-likelihood estimator [3, 24, 27]:

$$\hat{\alpha_k}\hat{\beta_k} \sim N(\mu_{\hat{\alpha}_k\hat{\beta}_k}, \sigma^2_{\hat{\alpha}_k\hat{\beta}_k}) \text{ as sample size } n \to \infty \text{ for } k = 1, 2, \ldots, K$$

Let $\boldsymbol{S}_n$ denote the sample covariance matrix and $\boldsymbol{\Sigma}(\boldsymbol{\theta})$ denote the model-based covariance matrix, where

$$\begin{aligned} \boldsymbol{\theta} =& (\tau_0, \tau_1, \ldots, \tau_K, \gamma_0, \gamma_1, \ldots, \gamma_L, \lambda_{k1}, \ldots, \lambda_{kL}, \alpha_1, \ldots, \alpha_K, \beta_1, \ldots, \beta_K, \\ & \sigma^2_{\varepsilon_0}, \sigma^2_{\varepsilon_1}, \ldots, \sigma^2_{\varepsilon_K}, \sigma_{\varepsilon_1,\varepsilon_2}, \sigma_{\varepsilon_1,\varepsilon_3}, \ldots, \sigma_{\varepsilon_{K-1},\varepsilon_K}) \end{aligned}$$

with $k = 1, 2, \ldots, K$ is the vector of free parameters specified in the model. Let p denote the number of parameters to estimate (the length of the vector $\boldsymbol{\theta}$). Then the log likelihood function[1] is a function of $\boldsymbol{S}_n$ and $\boldsymbol{\theta}$, denoted as

$$\ell(\boldsymbol{S}_n; \boldsymbol{\theta}) = log|\boldsymbol{\Sigma}(\boldsymbol{\theta})| + trace[\boldsymbol{S}_n\boldsymbol{\Sigma}(\boldsymbol{\theta})^{-1}] - log|\boldsymbol{S}_n| - p \quad (2)$$

2.2 *Complex Surveys Using BRR*

To apply balanced repeated replication (BRR) for variance estimation, the survey must be of a certain type of stratified designs with two primary units sampled per stratum (see Chapter 3 of the book by Wolter [32]). Figure 1 illustrates this type of sampling designs through an example.

[1]The log likelihood function is a function of the sample covariance matrix (or second-order moment matrix) and the model-based covariance matrix (or second-order moment matrix) even in the case of fixed - X. More details can be found in Bollen's book [4].

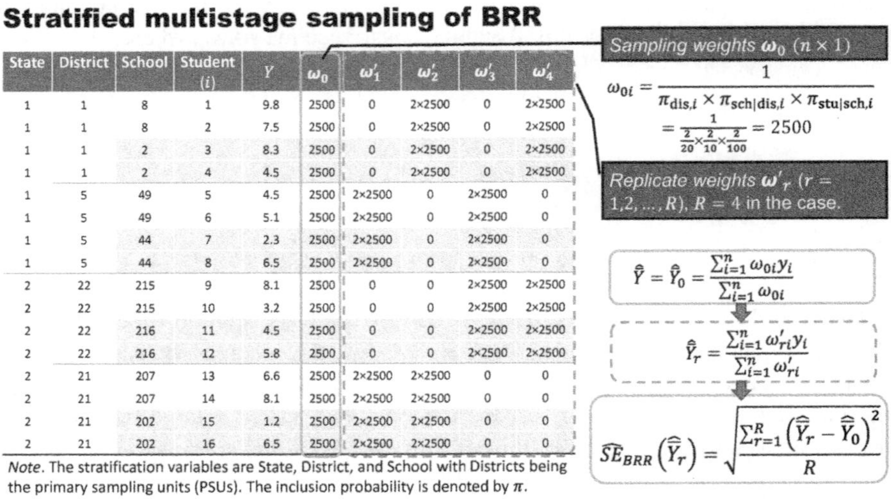

Stratified multistage sampling of BRR

State	District	School	Student (i)	Y	ω_0	ω'_1	ω'_2	ω'_3	ω'_4
1	1	8	1	9.8	2500	0	2×2500	0	2×2500
1	1	8	2	7.5	2500	0	2×2500	0	2×2500
1	1	2	3	8.3	2500	0	2×2500	0	2×2500
1	1	2	4	4.5	2500	0	2×2500	0	2×2500
1	5	49	5	4.5	2500	2×2500	0	2×2500	0
1	5	49	6	5.1	2500	2×2500	0	2×2500	0
1	5	44	7	2.3	2500	2×2500	0	2×2500	0
1	5	44	8	6.5	2500	2×2500	0	2×2500	0
2	22	215	9	8.1	2500	0	0	2×2500	2×2500
2	22	215	10	3.2	2500	0	0	2×2500	2×2500
2	22	216	11	4.5	2500	0	0	2×2500	2×2500
2	22	216	12	5.8	2500	0	0	2×2500	2×2500
2	21	207	13	6.6	2500	2×2500	2×2500	0	0
2	21	207	14	8.1	2500	2×2500	2×2500	0	0
2	21	202	15	1.2	2500	2×2500	2×2500	0	0
2	21	202	16	6.5	2500	2×2500	2×2500	0	0

Note. The stratification variables are State, District, and School with Districts being the primary sampling units (PSUs). The inclusion probability is denoted by π.

Fig. 1 An example using balanced repeated replication

In this example, the finite population ($N = 40{,}000$ students) locate in two ($H = 2$) states. Each state has $G = 20$ districts. Each district has $J = 10$ schools. Each school has $I = 100$ students. We sample two ($n_G = 2$) districts within each state, two ($n_J = 2$) schools within each of the districts, and two ($n_I = 2$) students from each of the schools. In total, we sample $n = 16$ students from the population. Math score, Y, is the outcome we are interested in. $\boldsymbol{\omega}_0(n \times 1)$ is the column of sampling weights. For instance, the sampling weight of student #1 is 2500, which means that the student #1 represents 2500 students in the population. The sampling weight equals the inverse of the probability of being sampled for a specific student #i ($i = 1, 2, \cdots, n$), see formula (3).

$$\omega_{0i} = \frac{1}{\pi_{\text{dis},i} \times \pi_{\text{sch|dis},i} \times \pi_{\text{stu|sch},i}} \tag{3}$$

where $\pi_{\text{dis},i}$, $\pi_{\text{sch|dis},i}$, and $\pi_{\text{stu|sch},i}$ ($i = 1, 2, \cdots, n$) are the inclusion probabilities in the sampling stages of district, school, and student, respectively. In this example, the inclusion probabilities at each sampling stage are the same[2] for all sampled students, that is, $\pi_{\text{dis},i} = n_G/G = 2/20$, $\pi_{\text{sch|dis},i} = n_J/J = 2/10$, $\pi_{\text{stu|sch},i} = n_I/I = 2/100$.

[2]In practice, the number of districts within each state, the number of schools within each district, and the number of students within each school are usually not equal. Therefore, the inclusion probabilities vary across districts, schools, and students; the sampling weights differ across students.

Suppose a problem is to estimate the population mean of Y (denoted as $\bar{Y}$), with sample data y_i $(i = 1, 2, \cdots, n)$. The point estimate is consistent when including the sampling weights using the below formula.

$$\widehat{\bar{Y}} = \widehat{\bar{Y}}_0 = \frac{\sum_{i=1}^{n} \omega_{0i} y_i}{\sum_{i=1}^{n} \omega_{0i}} \tag{4}$$

To estimate the standard errors (or variance of the estimator), the basic idea is to generate a series of replicates (re-samples) by creating $R = 2^H$ columns of replicate weights ($\boldsymbol{\omega}'_r$, an $n \times 1$ vector, $r = 1, 2, \cdots, R$) and to mimic the bootstrap process. For BRR, the replicates must be in full orthogonal balance.[3] In this example, $R = 4$, there are four columns of replicate weights, $\boldsymbol{\omega}'_1 - \boldsymbol{\omega}'_4$. To obtain the first column of replicate weights $\boldsymbol{\omega}'_1$, we drop one district within each state and set the replicate weights at zero for the corresponding students; for the remaining students, the replicate weights equal twice the sampling weights. Similarly, we remove one different district within each state and get the other columns of replicate weights: $\boldsymbol{\omega}'_2$, $\boldsymbol{\omega}'_3$, and $\boldsymbol{\omega}'_4$. Using each column of replicate weights, we can get a replicate estimate of the mean of Y, as follows:

$$\widehat{\bar{Y}}_r = \frac{\sum_{i=1}^{n} \omega'_{ri} y_i}{\sum_{i=1}^{n} \omega'_{ri}} \tag{5}$$

In total, we get four replicate estimates, then we can use the standard formula to calculate the BRR standard error.

$$\widehat{SE}_{BRR}(\widehat{\bar{Y}}) = \sqrt{\frac{\sum_{r=1}^{R} (\widehat{\bar{Y}}_r - \widehat{\bar{Y}}_0)^2}{R}} \tag{6}$$

2.3 *Mediation Incorporating BRR*

As described in the Sect. 2.2 about complex surveys using BRR, the point estimates are obtained by incorporating the sampling weights, while the standard errors estimates are calculated by incorporating a set of replicate weights [32]. This strategy is adapted for analyzing the mediation effects [15] as follows.

[3] To achieve full orthogonal balance, Hadamard matrices are employed to form the replicates (See pp. 112–113; [32]).

Point Estimate

Applying the mediation model to complex survey data with sampling weights $\boldsymbol{\omega}_0$, we replace the sample covariance matrix $\boldsymbol{S}_n$ in formula (2) with the weighted sample covariance matrix $\boldsymbol{S}_{n,w}$ to get the bias-adjusted point estimate of the parameters, which was mentioned in literature (e.g., [5, 18, 29]). With this estimator, we also get the bias-adjusted point estimate of the mediation effect $\hat{\alpha}_{k,0}\hat{\beta}_{k,0}(k = 1, 2, \ldots, K)$. Note that, each element of $\boldsymbol{S}_{n,w}$ can be obtained using the following formula (7) of weighted covariance (see equation A2 in article by Price [23]). For variables Q_1 and Q_2 with sample data $\boldsymbol{q}_1$ ($n \times 1$) and $\boldsymbol{q}_2$ ($n \times 1$), respectively, the weighted covariance is

$$\text{cov}_{\omega_0}(Q_1, Q_2) = \frac{\sum_{i=1}^{n} \omega_{0i}(q_{1i} - \widehat{\bar{Q}}_{10})(q_{2i} - \widehat{\bar{Q}}_{20})}{\sum_{i=1}^{n} \omega_{0i}} \tag{7}$$

where $\widehat{\bar{Q}}_{10}$ and $\widehat{\bar{Q}}_{20}$ are weighted means of Q_1 and Q_2, respectively, calculated with Eq. (4).

Standard Error Estimate

Applying the mediation model to complex survey data using BRR replicate weights $\boldsymbol{\omega}'_r(r = 1, 2, \ldots, R)$, we replace the sample covariance $\boldsymbol{S}_n$ with each of the replicate weighted sample covariance matrix $\boldsymbol{S}_{n,rw}$ to obtain R replicate estimates of the product of coefficients $\hat{\alpha}_{k,r}\hat{\beta}_{k,r}$, where $k = 1, 2, \ldots, K$, $r = 1, 2, \ldots, R$. Similarly, each element of $\boldsymbol{S}_{n,rw}$ can be obtained using the following formula (see equation A2 in article by [23]):

$$\text{cov}_{\omega'_r}(Q_1, Q_2) = \frac{\sum_{i=1}^{n} \omega'_{ri}(q_{1i} - \widehat{\bar{Q}}_{1r})(q_{2i} - \widehat{\bar{Q}}_{2r})}{\sum_{i=1}^{n} \omega'_{ri}} \tag{8}$$

where $\widehat{\bar{Q}}_{1r}$ and $\widehat{\bar{Q}}_{2r}$ are calculated with Eq. (5). We then can use the following formula to calculate the standard errors adjusted for the complex survey design:

$$\widehat{SE}_{BRR}(\hat{\alpha}_k\hat{\beta}_k) = \sqrt{\frac{\sum_{r=1}^{R} (\hat{\alpha}_{k,r}\hat{\beta}_{k,r} - \hat{\alpha}_{k,0}\hat{\beta}_{k,0})^2}{R(1 - f^2)}} \text{for} k = 1, 2, \ldots, K \tag{9}$$

where $f \in [0, 1)$ is the Fay's factor [7, 11]. Including Fay's factor is a compromise between BRR and the jackknife [7, 11]. When $f = 0$, the formula is equivalent to the standard BRR formula of standard errors. We can find the suggested value of Fay's factor from the technical documentation of a survey, the common value is 0.5.

Significance Test

As mentioned before, the product of coefficients follows an asymptotic normal distribution, with the BRR standard errors, we can obtain the test statistic as

$$T_{BRR} = \frac{\hat{\alpha}_{k,0}\hat{\beta}_{k,0}}{\widehat{SE}_{BRR}(\hat{\alpha}_k\hat{\beta}_k)} \tag{10}$$

where $T_{BRR} \sim N(0, 1)$ as $n \to \infty$, under $H_0 : \alpha_k\beta_k = 0$. With this test statistic, we can calculate the p values based on a standard normal distribution. Note that when there are multiple mediation effects to be tested in the model, adjustments for multiplicities are encouraged [15].

The method is suitable for mediation analysis within a general structural equation model, such as a latent mediation model where mediators, the exposure, or the outcome are latent variables. Please check papers by Sobel [27, 28] for detailed model notations about mediation within a structural equation model and Bollen's [4] book for basics about structural equation models.

3 SAS Macro and Illustration

This section briefly introduces the major components of $MediationBRR$, and then provides one example from PISA and one from TUS-CPS for illustrating the usage of the SAS macro.

3.1 Components of %MediationBRR

Table 1 lists the components of the SAS macro: $rma()$, $rvo()$, $fitmodel()$, $fitmodels()$, $parmtests()$, $medtests()$, and $MediationBRR()$. Specifically, the main function is $MediationBRR()$. Table 2 explains its arguments. To perform the analysis, users only need to call the main function and get the results. For the purpose of illustration, the SAS codes of $medtests()$ and $MediationBRR()$ are attached in the Appendix.[4] Technical details about the statistical model and methods of the SAS macros can be found in Sect. 2.

[4]The complete SAS macros can be downloaded from https://github.com/YujiaoMai/MedSurvey/MediationBRR_Mai&Zhang2019.sas.

Table 1 Components of *%MediationBRR*

Name	Short description
rma()	Remove a series of data tables
rvo()	Remove a data table
fitmodel()	Fit the input model with the data once
fitmodels()	Fit the input model with the data and each replicate weight of the series
parmtests()	Calculate the estimation with BRR standard errors for the coefficients
medtests()	Estimate the mediation effects with BRR standard errors
MediationBRR()	The main function (interface) to call

Notes. The *fitmodel*() was developed based on the PROC CALIS [26]

Table 2 Arguments of the function *MediationBRR*()

Argument	Short description
xvar	The exposure (required)
yvar	The outcome (required)
mvars	The mediator (s) (required)
zvars	The covariates (optional)
delim	The symbol to separate the variable names in a list. It is "/" by default
rwname	The general part of the names of weights/replicate weights (required)
Fay	The suggested inverse of Fay's factor. It is 4 by default
RR	Survey design information: the number of replicates (required)
datain	The dataset to be analyzed (required)
adjmethod	The method (s) adjusting for multiplicities (optional). It is HOLM by default

Notes. Following the SAS routine, *Fay* is the inverse of the Fay's factor
PROC Multtest [26] is employed to adjust the p values from multiple tests

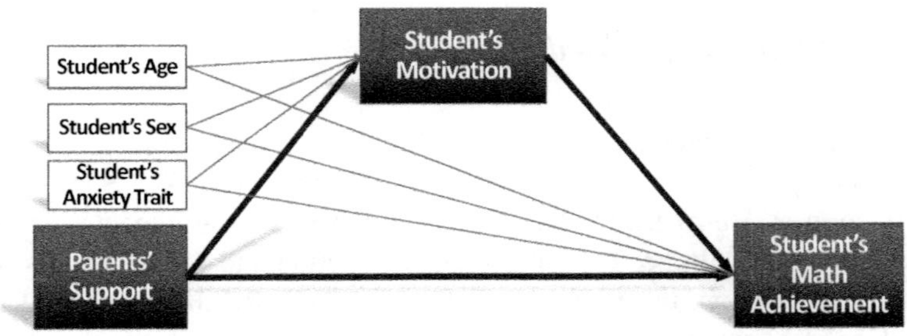

Fig. 2 Student motivation as the mediator between parental support and math achievement

3.2 Application to PISA: A Single-Mediator Model

Figure 2 depicts a single-mediator model: Parental support (*ParenSpt*) influences student's motivation (*StuMtv*) and then influences student's math achievement (*Math*), when controlling for the covariates: student age (*AGE*), sex (*SEX*),

Tests for Mediation Effects												
Mediator	a	SE_BRR (a)	Z (a)	*p* Value (a)	b	SE_BRR (b)	Z (b)	*p* Value (b)	ab	SE_BRR (ab)	Z (ab)	*p* Value (ab)
StuMtv	0.3060	0.0167	18.2864	0.00000	0.5721	0.0496	11.5450	0.00000	0.1751	0.0184	9.4965	0.00000

Fig. 3 Estimation and test results of model in Fig. 2

and anxiety personality ($StuAnxt$); meanwhile, parental support has direct effects on student's math achievement. Data $PisaMed$ (sample size $n = 16{,}058$) are obtained from the 2015 survey of Program for International Student Assessment [PISA; 19]. The main sample weight is *W_FSTURWT0* and the replicate weights are *W_FSTURWT1* $\sim$ *W_FSTURWT80*. The suggested Fay's factor[5] for PISA is 0.5.

To perform the analysis, we call the main function $MediationBRR()$. With all the components (SAS macros) run in advance, we run the below SAS codes.[6]

```
%MediationBRR(xvar='ParenSpt', yvar='Math', mvars='StuMtv'
   zvars='AGE/SEX/StuAnxt',delim='/', datain='PisaMed',
   rwname='W_FSTURWT', RR=80, Fay=4);
```

Figure 3 displays the SAS output of the analysis. The results showed that parental support had positive effects on student's math achievement through strengthening student's motivation (p value < 0.001). Note that "a" and "b" in the SAS output stand for the estimates of α and β, respectively, in the mediation models denoted in Eqs. (1); "ab" stands for the estimate of the mediation effect (product of coefficients $\alpha\beta$); and "Z" is the corresponding test statistic.

3.3 Application to TUS-CPS: A Multi-Mediator Model

Figure 4 presents a classic linear multi-mediator model (with three mediators). Correlation between two mediators is allowed by default. The model was fit with the data $TUSMed$ (sample size $n = 6439$) from the Tobacco Use Supplement (TUS) to the CPS [31]. The data are limited to current smokers. Variables involved in the analysis include the number of cigarettes smoked per day ($numcg$), the

[5]Technical details can be found in Sect. 2 as well as related publications (e.g., [11, 15, 32]).

[6]Data file $PisaMed.sas7bdat$ and the SAS codes can be downloaded from https://github.com/YujiaoMai/MedSurvey/.

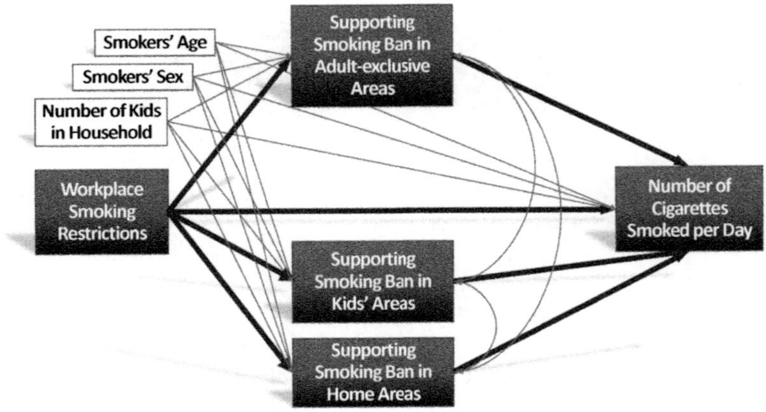

Fig. 4 Supporting smoking bans as the mediators between workplace smoking restrictions and number of cigarettes smoked per day

score of smoking restriction at workplace (*workban*), supporting smoking ban in adult-exclusive areas (e.g., casinos, bars) (*sp_adltban*), supporting smoking ban in children's areas (e.g., children's playground) (*sp_kidsban*), supporting smoking ban in home areas (e.g., apartments building) (*sp_homeban*), age ($PRTAGE$), sex ($PESEX$), number of kids in household ($NumKid$), the sampling (main) weight (*repwgt0*), and the 160 replicate weights ($repwgt1 \sim repwgt160$). The Fay's factor suggested in the technical report of CPS is 0.5 [30]. Please check Mai, Ha, and Soulakova's [15] study for more details about the dataset.

To perform the analysis, we call the main function $MediationBRR()$ of the SAS macros. Note that there are more than one mediator in the model; we have selected three adjustment methods $adjmethod{=}HOLM\ HOMMEL\ FDR$ and got the corresponding adjusted p values for the mediation effects via each mediator. With all the SAS macros run in advance, we finally run the below SAS codes.[7]

```
%MediationBRR(xvar='workban', yvar='numcg', mvars='sp_adltban/sp_
kidsban
  /sp_homeban',zvars='PRTAGE/PESEX/NumKid',delim='/',
datain='TUSMed',
  rwname='repwgt', RR=160, Fay=4, adjmethod=HOLM HOMMEL
FDR);
```

[7]Data file $TUSMed.sas7bdat$ and the SAS codes can be downloaded from https://github.com/YujiaoMai/MedSurvey/.

Tests for Mediation Effects												
Mediator	a	SE_BRR (a)	Z (a)	*p* Value (a)	b	SE_BRR (b)	Z (b)	*p* Value (b)	ab	SE_BRR (ab)	Z (ab)	*p* Value (ab)
sp_adltban	0.0554	0.0142	3.8966	0.00010	-0.2141	0.0413	-5.1897	0.00000	-0.0119	0.0039	-3.0105	0.00261
sp_kidsban	0.0227	0.0132	1.7178	0.08583	-0.2583	0.0401	-6.4473	0.00000	-0.0059	0.0035	-1.6773	0.09348
sp_homeban	0.0176	0.0163	1.0808	0.27978	-0.1424	0.0337	-4.2305	0.00002	-0.0025	0.0024	-1.0398	0.29845

Adjusted p-values				
Mediator	Raw	Holm (Stepdown Bonferroni)	Hommel	False Discovery Rate
sp_adltban	0.00261	0.00780	0.00780	0.00780
sp_kidsban	0.09348	0.18700	0.18700	0.14020
sp_homeban	0.29845	0.29840	0.29840	0.29840

Fig. 5 Estimation and test results of model in Fig. 4

Figure 5 displays the SAS output of the analysis. The mediator supporting smoking ban in adult-exclusive areas (*sp_adltban*) resulted in a significant (Adj. p value $= 0.00780$) mediation effect between smoking ban at workplace and number of cigarettes smoked per day.

4 Discussion

This study has implemented the recently published method for mediation analysis of complex survey data using balanced repeated replication in the SAS macro $\%MediationBRR$. The SAS macro allows users to analyze regular multi-mediator models. The application examples have illustrated the usage of this macro by applying a single-mediator model to the international survey PISA and a three-mediator model to the national survey TUS-CPS.

Two main limitations remained for this study. First, the SAS macro can handle only complex surveys using balanced repeated replication method for variance estimation. The surveys should have two primary sampling units in each stratum. Otherwise, it may not be appropriate to use this tool. Second, the SAS macro currently does not support more complex models such as mediation models involving latent variables.

For future directions, we will (1) develop methods incorporating classic linear mediation analysis with other common variance estimation methods for complex surveys, such as jackknife repeated replication, bootstrap replication, and Taylor series linear approximation; (2) conduct Monte Carlo simulation to compare the performance of different methods; (3) add additional SAS macros implementing the other to-be-developed methods; and (4) extend the functions of the SAS macros for more complex mediation models such as models with latent variables.

Acknowledgments The research was sponsored by American Lebanese Syrian Associated Charities (ALSAC). We also thank the Academic Programs at the SJCRH for training opportunities on writing and thank the University of Notre Dame for the library resources. HZ would thank the Quantitative Data Sciences Core of Robert H. Lurie Comprehensive Cancer Center with an NCI

Cancer Center Support Grant #P30CA060553, and the Data Management and Statistics Core of Mesulam Center for Cognitive Neurology and Alzheimer's Disease with a National Institute of Aging Grant #P30AG013854, both at the Northwestern University Feinberg School of Medicine.

Appendix

```
%macro medtests(estparm=,anames='a1/a2',bnames='b1/b2',
   mednames='sp_adltban/sp_kidban', Fay=4,RR=160,adjmethod=holm);
   Proc iml;
   use &estparm; read all var _ALL_ into estall[colname=varNames];
   names=varNames;close &estparm;
   parmas=scan(&anames, 1:( 1 + countc(&anames, '/')));
   parmbs=scan(&bnames, 1:( 1 + countc(&bnames, '/')));
   mednames=scan(&mednames, 1:( 1 + countc(&mednames, '/')));
   as=estall[,parmas];bs=estall[,parmbs];
   nas=ncol(parmas);nbs=ncol(parmbs);
   R=&RR;Fay=&Fay;
   IF nas=nbs THEN
   abs=as#bs;
   ests=as||bs||abs;
   estbar=ests[1,];estrps=ests[2:R+1,];
   estds=estrps-estbar;
   temp1=(estds#estds);
   sds=SQRT(FAY*MEAN(temp1));
   zs=estbar/sds;
   ps=(1-probnorm(abs(zs)))*2;
   idxa=1:nas; idxb=nas+1:nas+nbs; idxab=nas+nbs+1:nas+nbs+nbs;
   estas=estbar[,idxa];estbs=estbar[,idxb]; estabs=estbar[,idxab];
   sdas=sds[,idxa];sdbs=sds[,idxb];sdabs=sds[,idxab];
   zas=zs[,idxa];zbs=zs[,idxb];zabs=zs[,idxab];
   pas=ps[,idxa];pbs=ps[,idxb];pabs=ps[,idxab];
   sdSB=SQRT((estas##2)#(sdbs##2)+(estbs##2)#(sdas##2));
   zSB=estabs/sdSB;pSB=(1-probnorm(abs(zSB)))*2;
   tests=estas′||sdas′||zas′||pas′||estbs′||sdbs′||zbs′||pbs′||estabs′
   ||sdabs′||zabs′||pabs′;
   mattrib tests colname={'a' 'SD_BRR(a)' 'Z(a)' 'p-value(a)' 'b'
'SD_BRR(b)'
   'Z(b)' 'p-value(b)' 'ab' 'SD_BRR(ab)' 'Z(ab)' 'p-value(ab)'}
   rowname=mednames; medvars = mednames′;
   mattrib medvars colname='mediator' 'test';
```

(continued)

```
create medtable from tests;append from tests;close medtable;
create mediator from medvars[colname='mediator'];
append from medvars;close mediator;
QUIT;
data abpvalues(rename=(COL12=RAW_P)); set medtable; keep
COL12;run;
Data medtable(rename=(COL1=a COL2=SD_BRR_a COL3=Z_a
COL4=pValue_a
COL5=b COL6=SD_BRR_b COL7=Z_b COL8=pValue_b COL9=ab
COL10=SD_BRR_ab COL11=Z_ab COL12=pValue_ab));
set mediator;set medtable;
label COL1="a" COL2="SE_BRR(a)" COL3="Z(a)" COL4="p-value(a)"
COL5="b" COL6="SE_BRR(b)" COL7="Z(b)" COL8="p-value(b)"
COL9="ab"
COL10="SE_BRR(ab)" COL11="Z(ab)" COL12="p-value(ab)";
run;
ODS LISTING CLOSE;ODS HTML CLOSE;
proc multtest inpvalues=abpvalues &adjmethod;ods output pValues=
adjps;run;
data adjpValues(rename=(RAW_P=pValueRaw));
set mediator; set abpvalues; set adjps; drop Raw test;
run;
ODS html file='medtest.html';
title "Tests for Mediation Effects";
proc print data=medtable;run;
title "Adjusted p-values";
proc print data=adjpValues;run;
%rvo(di=Mediator);%rvo(di=abpvalues);%rvo(di=Adjps);
%mend;
%macro MediationBRR(xvar=, yvar=, mvars=,zvars=,delim='/',datain=,
rwname=,
RR=10,Fay=4,adjmethod=holm);
ODS LISTING CLOSE;ods html close;
%fitmodels(xvar=&xvar, yvar=&yvar, mvars=&mvars,zvars=&zvars,delim=
&delim, datain=&datain,rwname=&rwname,RR=&RR, tableout=ESTSpa
ram);
%rma(ina=Ests,RR=&RR);
proc iml;
mnames=scan(&mvars, 1:( 1 + countc(&mvars, &delim)));
nm = prod(dimension(mnames));
anames=BlankStr(200);bnames=BlankStr(200);medeffs = BlankStr(200);
```

(continued)

```
    anames=cat("'",'a',1);   bnames=cat("'",'b',1);   medeffs=cat("'",'a',1,
'b',1);
    if nm >=2 then do;
    do  i=2  to  nm;  anames=cat(anames,'/','a',i);  bnames=cat(bnames,
'/','b',i);
    medeffs=cat(medeffs,'/','a',i,'b',i); end;
    end;
    anames=cat(anames,"'"); bnames=cat(bnames,"'"); medeffs=cat (med-
effs,"'");
    call symputx("as", anames);
    call symputx("bs", bnames);
    call symputx("abs", medeffs);
    quit;
    %medtests(estparm=Estsparam,anames=&as,bnames=&bs,mednames=&
mvars,
    Fay=&Fay,RR=&RR,adjmethod=&adjmethod);
%mend;
```

References

1. Aryee, S., Budhwar, P.S., Chen, Z.X.: Trust as a mediator of the relationship between organizational justice and work outcomes: Test of a social exchange model. J. Organ. Behav. **23**(3), 267–285 (2002). https://doi.org/10.1002/job.138
2. Baron, R.M., Kenny, D.A.: The moderator-mediator variable distinction in social psychological research: Conceptual, strategic, and statistical considerations. J. Pers. Soc. Psychol. **51**(6), 1173–1182 (1986). https://doi.org/10.1037/0022-3514.51.6.1173
3. Bishop, Y.M.M., Fienberg, S.E., Holland, P.W.: Discrete Multivariate Analysis: Theory and Practice. MIT Press, Cambridge, Massachusetts (1975)
4. Bollen, K.A.: Structural Equations with Latent Variables. Wiley, Chapel Hill, NC (1989)
5. Bollen, K.A., Tueller, S.J., Oberski, D.: Issues in the structural equation modeling of complex survey data. In: Proceedings of the 59th World Statistics Congress (2013)
6. Briggs, N.E.: Estimation of the standard error and confidence interval of the indirect effect in multiple mediator models (Doctoral dissertation, PhD dissertation, Department of Psychology, The Ohio State University, Columbus, OH). Retrieved 2018-12-01, from http://citeseerx.ist.psu.edu/viewdoc/download?doi=10.1.1.1004.6088&rep=rep1&type=pdf (2006)
7. Dippo, C.S., Fay, R.E., Morganstein, D.H.: Computing variances from complex samples with replicate weights. In: Proceedings of the Survey Research Methods Section, pp. 489–494 (1984)
8. Doaei, H., Rezaei, A., Khajei, R.: The impact of relationship marketing tactics on customer loyalty: The mediation role of relationship quality. Int. J. Bus. Adm. **2**(3), 83–93 (2011). https://doi.org/10.5430/ijba.v2n3p83
9. Fairchild, A.J., McQuillin, S.D.: Evaluating mediation and moderation effects in school psychology: A presentation of methods and review of current practice. J. Sch. Psychol. **48**(1), 53–84 (2010). https://doi.org/10.1016/j.jsp.2009.09.001

10. Ismail, A.R.: The influence of perceived social media marketing activities on brand loyalty: The mediation effect of brand and value consciousness. Asia Pac. J. Mark. Logist. **29**(1), 129–144 (2017). https://doi.org/10.1108/APJML-10-2015-0154
11. Judkins, D.R.: Fay's method for variance estimation. J. Off. Stat. **6**(3), 223–239 (1990)
12. Lin, S.-C., Huang, Y.-M.: The role of social capital in the relationship between human capital and career mobility: Moderator or mediator? J. Intellect. Cap. **6**(2), 191–205 (2005). https://doi.org/10.1108/14691930510592799
13. Lockhart, G., MacKinnon, D.P., Ohlrich, V.: Mediation analysis in psychosomatic medicine research. Psychosom. Med. **73**(1), 29–43 (2011). https://doi.org/10.1097/PSY.0b013e318200a54b
14. MacKinnon, D.P. (2008). Introduction to Statistical Mediation Analysis. Erlbaum, Mahwah, NJ
15. Mai, Y., Ha, T., Soulakova, J.N.: Multimediation method with balanced repeated replications for analysis of complex surveys. Struct. Equ. Model. Multidiscip. J. **26**(5), 678–684 (2019). https://doi.org/10.1080/10705511.2018.1559065
16. Mooney, M., O'Brien, B., Cormack, S., Coutts, A., Berry, J., Young, W.: The relationship between physical capacity and match performance in elite Australian football: A mediation approach. J. Sci. Med. Sport **14**(5), 447–452 (2011). https://doi.org/10.1016/j.jsams.2011.03.010
17. Moutinho, L., Smith, A.: Modelling bank customer satisfaction through mediation of attitudes towards human and automated banking. Int. J. Bank Mark. **18**(3), 124–134 (2000). https://doi.org/10.1108/02652320010339699
18. Muthen, B., Satorra, A.: Complex sample data in structural equation modeling. Sociol. Methodol. **25**, 267–316 (1995)
19. OECD: PISA 2015 technical report (Tech. Rep.). Author, Paris. Retrieved from https://www.oecd.org/pisa/sitedocument/PISA-2015-technicalreport-final.pdf (2017)
20. Petchsawang, P., Duchon, D.: Workplace spirituality, meditation, and work performance. J. Manag. Spiritual. Religion **9**(2), 189–208 (2012). https://doi.org/10.1080/14766086.2012.688623
21. Preacher, K.J. (2015). Advances in mediation analysis: A survey and synthesis of new developments. Annu. Rev. Psychol. **66**, 825–852. https://doi.org/10.1146/annurev-psych-010814-015258
22. Preacher, K.J., & Hayes, A.F.: Asymptotic and resampling strategies for assessing and comparing indirect effects in multiple mediator models. Behav. Res. Methods **40**(3), 879–891 (2008). https://doi.org/10.3758/BRM.40.3.879
23. Price, G.R.: Extension of covariance selection mathematics. Ann. Hum. Genet. **35**(4), 485–490 (1972)
24. Rao, C.R.: Linear Statistical Inference and Its Applications, 2nd edn., vol. 2. Wiley, New York, NY (1973)
25. Rucker, D.D., Preacher, K.J., Tormala, Z.L., Petty, R.E.: Mediation analysis in social psychology: Current practices and new recommendations. Soc. Personal. Psychol. Compass **5**(6), 359–371 (2011). https://doi.org/10.1111/j.1751-9004.2011.00355.x
26. SAS Institute Inc.: SAS/STAT®9.4 User's Guide–The CALIS procedure (Tech. Rep.). SAS Institute Inc. Retrieved from https://support.sas.com/documentation/onlinedoc/stat/131/calis.pdf (2013)
27. Sobel, M.E.: Asymptotic confidence intervals for indirect effects in structural equation models. Sociol. Methodol. **13**, 290–312 (1982). https://doi.org/10.2307/270723
28. Sobel, M.E.: Some new results on indirect effects and their standard errors in covariance structure models. Sociol. Methodol. **16**, 159–186 (1986). Retrieved from http://www.jstor.org/stable/270922
29. Stapleton, L.M.: An assessment of practical solutions for structural equation modeling with complex sample data. Struct. Equ. Model. **13**(1), 28–58 (2006)

30. U.S. Bureau of Labor Statistics, U.S. Census Bureau: Current Population survey: Design and methodology (technical paper 66) (Tech. Rep. No. October). Retrieved from https://www.census.gov/prod/2006pubs/tp-66.pdf (2006)
31. U.S. Department of Commerce, U.S. Census Bureau: National Cancer Institute and Food and Drug Administration co-sponsored Tobacco Use Supplement to the Current Population Survey. 2014–15. Retrieved 2018-06-01, from http://thedataweb.rm.census.gov/ftp/cps_ftp.html#cpssupps. Technical Documentation https://www.census.gov/programs-surveys/cps/technicaldocumentation/complete.html (2016)
32. Wolter, K.: Introduction to Variance Estimation. Springer, New York, NY (2007)

A Review of Bayesian Optimal Experimental Design on Different Models

Hongyan Jiang and Yichuan Zhao

1 Introduction

When starting an experiment, decisions must be made before the data collection, which is known as the design of the experiment. The design of an experiment should provide as much information as possible, when the observations are collected from restricted resources. The basic aim of the experimental design is to improve the statistical inference by arranging the allocations of design points appropriately. The purposes of the experiment generate different design criteria. The three focuses of experimental design are: estimation of parameters, prediction of the outcomes and model selection, and discrimination. The alphabetic optimality criteria are generated in terms of some convex functions of the Fisher information matrix, such as D-, A-, G-, and T-optimality. For example, in estimation problems, the D-optimal design criterion is considered when estimators with small variances are desirable. If more than one quantity of interest is considered at the same time, then the compound design criterion is applied. According to the different ways that incorporate parameter uncertainties and prior information into the design process, the Bayesian optimal design can be divided into two groups: pseudo-Bayesian optimal design and fully Bayesian optimal design. The pseudo-Bayesian design is obtained by averaging the classical design criteria over the parameter space with the prior as a weight, while the fully Bayesian design is obtained by maximizing the expected utility function, which is a function of the posterior.

H. Jiang
Department of Mathematics and Physics, Huaiyin Institute of Technology, Huaian, China
e-mail: hyitjhy@hyit.edu.cn

Y. Zhao (✉)
Department of Mathematics & Statistics, Georgia State University, Atlanta, GA, USA
e-mail: yichuan@gsu.edu

Y. Zhao, (Din) D.-G. Chen (eds.), *Modern Statistical Methods for Health Research*, Emerging Topics in Statistics and Biostatistics,
https://doi.org/10.1007/978-3-030-72437-5_10

1.1 Pseudo-Bayesian Optimal Design

Classical optimal experimental designs have been widely developed for linear models in both theory and practice. The optimal designs are usually derived using optimality criteria that are based on the Fisher information matrix. Hence, Fisher information matrix is the basis of optimal designs. While for nonlinear models, the designs are usually "locally optimal" because the Fisher information matrix usually depends on the values of the model parameters, misspecification of the parameters may lead to unsatisfactory experimental results. Moreover, if the parameters are well known, there is no need for the experimentation. Hence, a more realistic idea is to obtain designs by giving the prior information of the unknown parameters, which allows for the uncertainty in the parameter values. Bayesian design criteria, which incorporate the prior information of the parameters into the designs of the experiment, have been considered by many researchers, see Atkinson et al. [3], Chaloner and Verdinelli [8], Ryan et al. [51, 53]. This Bayesian approach takes expectation of the "locally" designed criteria over the prior distribution of the unknown parameters, and the corresponding design criteria are termed as "pseudo-Bayesian" alphabetic optimal design criteria [3]. For example, defining ξ as the design, the Bayesian D-optimal design can be found to minimize

$$\Phi^D(\xi) = \int_\Theta |M^{-1}(\xi, \theta)| p(\theta) d\theta, \tag{1}$$

where $p(\theta)$ is the prior of the unknown parameters, and $M(\xi, \theta)$ is the Fisher information matrix.

The Bayesian A-optimal design can be found to minimize the expected total variance of the parameter estimates $\Phi^A(\xi)$

$$\Phi^A(\xi) = \int_\Theta tr(M(\xi, \theta)) p(\theta) d\theta. \tag{2}$$

If we are interested in estimating the linear combination of the parameters $\mathbf{c}^T\theta$ with minimal variance, then the Bayesian c-optimal design can be found to minimize the expected variance of the linear contrasts

$$\Phi^c(\xi) = \int_\Theta c^T M^{-1}(\xi, \theta) c p(\theta) d\theta, \tag{3}$$

where c is a known vector of constants.

All of the integrals are usually performed analytically or numerically by Monte Carlo method.

1.2 Fully Bayesian Optimal Design

The fully Bayesian design uses the posterior distribution $p(\theta, y|\xi)$ directly and maximizes the expected utility function that is chosen according to the aim of an experiment. It is defined in Chaloner and Verdinelli [8] as follows:

$$\begin{aligned} \xi^* &= argmax_{\xi \in \chi^n} \int_Y \int_\Theta U(\xi, y, \theta) p(\theta, y|\xi) d\theta dy \\ &= argmax_{\xi \in \chi^n} \int_Y \int_\Theta U(\xi, y, \theta) p(y|\xi, \theta) p(\theta) d\theta dy, \end{aligned} \tag{4}$$

where $U(\xi, y, \theta)$ is the utility function for design, and $\xi \in \chi^n$, χ^n is the design space. Let $y = (y_1, y_2, \ldots, y_n)^T \in Y$ be the observed response variable and Y be the set of responses. $p(\theta, y|\xi)$ is the posterior, which is derived from the likelihood $p(y|\xi, \theta)$ and the prior distribution $p(\theta)$, and Θ is the set of θ. The commonly used Bayesian utility functions for parameter estimation are information-based utilities, scalar functions of the posterior covariance matrix, and quadratic loss. In the review paper of Bayesian optimal design, Chaloner and Verdinelli [8] have reviewed these commonly used utility functions.

When the aim of the experiment is to obtain a good estimate of $g(\theta)$, which is a function of θ, one of the most commonly used Bayesian design criteria is the mutual information. The mutual information aims to gain the largest information on parameter estimation and is given by

$$\begin{aligned} &U_I(d) \\ &= \int_\Theta \int_Y p(g(\theta), y \mid \xi)[logp(g(\theta), y \mid \xi) - logp(y \mid \xi) - logp(g(\theta))] dy d\theta, \end{aligned} \tag{5}$$

where $p(g(\theta), y \mid \xi)$ is the posterior, which is derived from the likelihood $p(y|\xi, g(\theta))$ and the prior distribution $p(g(\theta))$, and $p(y \mid \xi)$ is the marginal likelihood.

Another commonly used Bayesian design criterion is the Kullback–Leibler divergence (KLD) between the prior and posterior distributions,

$$U_{KLD}(d) = \int_\Theta p(g(\theta) \mid y, \xi) logp(y \mid \xi, g(\theta)) d\theta - logp(y \mid \xi). \tag{6}$$

In fact, the mutual information $U_I(d)$ is the KLD between the joint distribution $logp(g(\theta), y \mid \xi)$ and the product of marginal distributions of $g(\theta)$ and y. Since the prior distribution does not depend on the optimal designs, maximizing the expected gain in KLD is equivalent to maximizing the expected gain in Shannon information.

When one is interested in maximizing the joint posterior precision of all or a subset of the model parameters, the inverse of the determinant of the posterior covariance matrix (IDPCM) is used as the utility function, which is also named Bayesian D-posterior precision,

$$U_{IDPCM}(d) = \frac{1}{\mid cov(g(\theta) \mid \xi, y) \mid}. \tag{7}$$

This utility is estimated by finding the minimal reciprocal of the determinant of the variance–covariance matrix of $g(\theta)$, which is sampled from its posterior distribution.

When the focus is to obtain point estimates of the parameters or linear combinations of the parameters, a quadratic loss utility function is applied.

$$U_{QL}(d) = -\int_{\Theta} (g(\theta) - \hat{g}(\theta))^T A(g(\theta) - \hat{g}(\theta))p(g(\theta) \mid \xi, y)d\theta, \tag{8}$$

where A is a symmetric non-negative definite matrix, and $p(g(\theta) \mid \xi, y)$ is the posterior distribution.

Mutual information is also used as the utility function to find optimal designs for model discrimination. Masoumi et al. [35] and McGree et al. [37] used the total separation utility for model discrimination. A model discrimination utility was proposed in Vanlier et al. [59], which was based on a k-nearest neighbor estimate of the Jensen–Shannon divergence between the multivariate predictive densities of several alternative models. However, optimal designs for the aim of an experiment may not be suitable for other aims of the experiment. Utilities for prediction of future observations were discussed by Diggle and Lophaven [15], Ryan et al. [52], and Solonen et al. [56].

When researchers have more than one single aim in an experiment, for these compound design problems, different design targets can be incorporated into one or several corresponding utility functions. McGree et al. [38] and Drovandi and Pettitt [17] considered the compound utility functions for dose-finding studies.

However, Eq. (4) does not usually have a closed-form solution, in addition to the posterior $p(\theta, y|\xi)$ distribution. Numerical approximations are often used to solve this optimization problem, and then thousands of posterior distributions will be required to obtain the Bayesian design, which is a computationally intensive work. Hence, fully Bayesian experimental designs for these models with non-analytic posterior distribution, such as nonlinear mixed-effects models, are largely unexplored.

This chapter aims to review those papers that discussed optimal experimental design under Bayesian-decision theoretic approach for different models. Although there are many review papers on Bayesian optimal design [8, 52, 53], such an investigation is necessary in order to reflect the recent applications of the Bayesian optimal experimental design literature on various models. We do not focus on the development of Bayesian theory on the optimal design, but on the Bayesian optimal design of various models. In fact, the ability to deal with more complex models is the reflection of new development on the Bayesian optimal design theory.

The rest of this chapter is organized as follows. Section 2 devotes to designs for linear models. In Sect. 3, we consider the generalized linear models, and Sect. 4 examines the nonlinear models, including designs in clinical trials and industrial applications. The concluding remarks are given in Sect. 5.

2 Bayesian Designs for Linear Models

Early Bayesian theory of optimal experimental design for linear models includes Chaloner [6], DasGupta and Studden [12], Dette [14], El-Krunz and Studden [20], and Lindley [31, 32]. Suppose a classical normal theory linear model

$$y = f^T(x)\beta + \varepsilon, \varepsilon \sim N(0, \sigma^2), \tag{9}$$

where the regression functions $f^T(x) = (f_1(x), f_2(x), \ldots, f_k(x))$ are independent, real-valued linear functions, and β is the k-dimensional vector of unknown parameters.

When σ^2 is known, under conjugate normal prior $\pi(\beta \mid \sigma^2)$ with mean β_0 and variance matrix $\sigma^2 R^{-1}$ on β, the posterior distribution for β is also normal with covariance matrix $\sigma^2(f \cdot f^T + R)$. Many authors proposed optimal design criteria as a function of the posterior covariance matrix, see Owen [43] and Pilz [46], etc. In particular, a group of criteria that is defined as Bayesian alphabetical optimal design criteria is discussed, such as Bayesian D-optimality (Eq. (1)), Bayesian A-optimality (Eq. (2)), Bayesian c-optimality (Eq. (3)), Bayesian E-optimality, and Bayesian G-optimality [3]. El-Krunz and Studden [20] described the Elfving's theorem in the context of Bayesian designs to check if the design found is optimal for the aim of the experiment. Pilz [46] dealt with Bayesian experimental designs for linear models in a more general approach, with no assumption of the model or of the prior, and defined the Bayesian optimal design as an extension of non-Bayesian, although the D- and E-optimalities are not included. Chaloner and Verdinelli [8] provided a review of these pseudo-Bayesian design criteria under different utility functions. The main similarity for normal regression models is that design criteria do not depend on the unknown parameters β but depend on a covariance matrix of the least squares estimate or the posterior covariance matrix of β. To show how to apply Bayesian framework to optimal design, a linear regression model with one design variable is discussed [50].

Example 1 Consider a linear regression model with one design variable, which was discussed in Ryan et al. [50]:

$$y = \theta_0 + \theta_1 x + \varepsilon, \varepsilon \sim N\left(0, \sigma^2\right), \tag{10}$$

where the prior of $\theta = (\theta_0, \theta_1)'$ is assumed to be normal $N(\bar{\theta}, \sigma^2 R^{-1})$, and R is a known 2×2 matrix. When using the KLD (Eq. (6)) as the utility function, a closed-form expression of the expected utility function is available: $U(d) = |X^T X + R|$. The design space is the interval [0, 1], and the quasi-Newton algorithm is used to find the optimal design. When the number of design points is 11, the optimal design consists of 2 different support points, which is just the two end points of design space, with 5 replications on 0 and 6 replications on 1. In this simple example, the fully Bayesian optimal design can be obtained smoothly. For higher dimensions of unknown parameters or nonlinear models, this may not be the case.

When σ^2 is unknown with prior density $p(\sigma^2)$, the prior distribution for β conditioned on σ^2 can still be assumed to belong to a conjugate family $\beta \mid \sigma^2 \sim N(\beta_0, \sigma^2 R^{-1})$. A simple solution to this problem is to substitute the value of σ^2 with its prior mean, see Brooks [5] and Pukelsheim [48]. There is no difficulty in extending the Bayesian optimal design to the case where σ^2 is unknown; however, Chaloner and Verdinelli [8] pointed out that the integrals of some utilities may be intractable (see Eq. (4)), and no closed-form expression can be derived. Then, numerical approaches or approximations can be used to find the Bayesian designs [60].

Most studies of Bayesian optimal designs for canonical linear models mainly focus on the conjugate priors of β. DasGupta and Studden [12] considered a prior that was induced by a metric on the space of non-negative measures. The resulting optimal design was still kept optimal for different utilities, and although it was derived with known error variance, the result was also valid with unknown σ^2.

Whether or not σ^2 is known, special attention should be paid to the aim of the experiment, which decides the design criteria [11] we should use. Many of the Bayesian optimal designs focus on parameter estimation or linear combinations of them. For normal linear models, when one is interested in point estimates of the parameters, the classical D-optimal or A-optimal criteria could be used as the utility. When one is interested in linear combinations of the parameters, the classical c-optimal criterion is used as the utility function. To the authors' knowledge, the earliest paper on prediction under Bayesian-decision framework was in Lindley [31], and then followed by the articles from Brooks [4, 5]. However, these designs may perform poorly on the model discrimination. Analytical expressions for Eq. (4) can be obtained for many Bayesian utilities, only if the model dimension and decision space are small in normal linear models. Ng and Chick [40] pointed out that mutual information had commonly been used as the utility function in the Bayesian design literature to design for the model discrimination. Recently, Leonard and Edwards [28] proposed a Bayesian modification to the DP-criterion, which provided some safeguards against misspecification of the model for the construction of optimal designs, and they also obtained a model-independent estimate of σ^2. So far, Bayesian optimal design for testing problems has remained unexploited. In conclusion, the field of Bayesian optimal designs still has some open problems, even for normal linear models.

3 Bayesian Designs for Generalized Linear Models

The family of generalized linear models (GLMs) extends the normal regression models to any distributions belonging to the exponential family, including the gamma, Poisson, and binomial distributions. These models are important in scientific and industrial experiments whose responses are binary, binomial, or count data because the classical normal linear models fail to describe these data well [36]. The model can be written as

$$E(y) = \mu = \eta = f^T(x)\theta. \tag{11}$$

There are three components in this generalized linear model:

1. A distribution for the univariate response y with mean μ.
2. A linear predictor $\eta = f^T(x)\theta$, where $f(x)$ is a p vector of known functions of the explanatory variable x, and θ is a p vector of unknown model parameters.
3. A link function $g(\mu) = \eta$, relating x to the mean μ.

The distribution of y determines the relationship between the mean and variance of the responses. The variance of y is $var(y) = \phi V(\mu)$, where ϕ is a "dispersion parameter," equal to σ^2 for the normal distribution and equal to one for the binomial and Poisson distributions. For a generalized linear model, y obeys a distribution in the exponential family:

$$f(y|\theta, \phi) = exp\left\{\frac{y\theta - b(\theta)}{a(\phi)} + c(y, \phi)\right\}, \tag{12}$$

where a, b, c are some known functions.

The key difference between the design of experiments for linear and generalized linear models is that for GLMs, the Fisher information matrix is a weighted form, which includes the unknown parameters. Hence, initial estimates of the model parameters must be available. Only under this condition, the optimal design can be constructed. Robust designs for GLMs were investigated by Li and Wiens [30] and Woods et al. [61]. The Bayesian method to find the robust designs is described in Chaloner and Larntz [7], Chaloner and Verdinelli [8], and Firth and Hinde [21]. Atkinson and Woods [2] reviewed the development of design methodology for GLMs. In Woods et al. [62], the authors described the combination of Gaussian processes with cyclic descent optimization algorithms, to find Bayesian optimal designs for generalized linear models. When some prior information is known, most of the work on Bayesian optimal design for GLMs focuses on D-optimality, and the design criterion is named Bayesian D-optimal, see Eq. (1). McGree et al. [38] and Atkinson and Woods [2] derived an analytical expression for pseudo-Bayesian design for the first-order Poisson regression model. Their method allowed robust designs to be quickly derived with uncertainties in the parameter space and linear predictor and suggested putting replications at design points for higher-order regression models. Zhang and Ye [63] considered the Bayesian D-optimal design for a Poisson regression model and used the equivalence theorem to verify whether the design is optimal or not. For fully Bayesian, Lewi et al. [29] presented a sequential design framework that searched for the optimal design for a generalized linear model in neurophysiology, in which the mutual information between the prior and posterior distributions is maximized.

Although there are many significant studies in the statistical inference for generalized linear models (GLMs) [36], more research needs to be done on its optimal design under Bayesian framework. Bayesian design is a powerful tool for design problems with discrete responses; however, methodology has been restricted to simple generalized linear models and pseudo-Bayesian optimal designs [53]. Until now, the majority of the literature on Bayesian optimal designs for GLMs focus on parameter estimation, and little work has been done on model-robust designs for GLMs. To our knowledge, Woods et al. [62] provided the first investigation of design for screening variables under the generalized linear model and pointed out that an efficient approach to Bayesian design is still in urgent demand. More discussion of the analytical equations and computational approximations to the expected utility functions defined in Eqs. (5)–(8) can be found in Chaloner and Verdinelli [8], Ryan et al. [50], and Woods et al. [62].

For generalized linear models with mixed effects (GLMMs), the situation is more complicated because it is hard to get an analytical likelihood for GLMMs. Linearization of the GLMMs is commonly used, and the quasi-likelihood can be obtained by using the marginal quasi-likelihood (MQL) method and the penalized quasi-likelihood (PQL). The linearizations of GLMMs using the PQL and MQL methods lead to linear mixed models. For the design problem in mixed-effects logistic models, we refer to Abebe et al. [1] and Maram and Jafari [34]. Abebe et al. [1] considered Bayesian D-optimal design for binary longitudinal responses in a mixed logistic regression model and found the optimal number and the allocations of time points for different priors, cost constraint, and covariance structures of the random effects. Maram and Jafari [34] discussed the Bayesian D-optimal design for a logistic regression model with exponential distribution for the random intercept. Most recently, Singh and Mukhopadhyay [55] discussed the exact D-optimal Bayesian designs for time-series experiments, where the conditional distribution of the count responses given a weakly stationary latent process was assumed to follow a log-linear model and had a correlated structure over time points. Jiang et al. [26] considered the optimal design problem for multivariate mixed-effects logistic models with longitudinal data. Jiang and Yue [25] concerned the pseudo-Bayesian D-optimal design for the first-order Poisson mixed model with time-dependent correlated errors, when considering the experimental cost. The Poisson mixed-effects model with correlated errors considered in Jiang and Yue [25] is more complicated than the ordinary Poisson regression model. By using the MQL method, an approximation of the Fisher information matrix can be obtained, and the pseudo-Bayesian optimal design can be obtained by the "fmincon" function in MATLAB.

Example 2 Consider a Poisson mixed-effects model with correlated errors [25]:

$$\begin{aligned} y_{ij} \mid b_i &\sim Poisson(\lambda_{ij}), \quad i = 1, \ldots, N, \quad j = 1, \ldots, m_i, \\ \log\left(\lambda_{ij}\right) &= x_{ij}^T \beta + z_{ij}^T b_i. \end{aligned} \tag{13}$$

Here, x_{ij} is a $p \times 1$ vector of covariates associated with the responses, and β is the corresponding vector of unknown fixed-effects parameters. z_{ij} is a $q \times 1$ vector that is usually a subset of vector x_{ij} $(q \leq p)$, and b_i is the corresponding vector of random effects, which is assumed to be a normal distribution with zero mean and covariance matrix G. $R_i(\rho) = (\rho^{|t_{ij}-t_{ij'}|})_{j,j'=1,\ldots,m_i}$ is the correlation structure among different responses measured at design points. Based on the quasi-information matrix deduced by using the MQL method, the optimal number of design points among different Bayesian designs is discussed when the experimental cost is considered. The results show that the optimal number and allocations of design points depend on the cost ratio and interclass autoregressive coefficient ρ. The locations of the optimal design points are moderately affected by the autocorrelation coefficient ρ, especially for small ρ. However, fully Bayesian optimal design has not been solved for this model. In fact, the development and application of Bayesian design for GLMs and GLMMs have been restricted to simple models mainly because of the complex calculation.

4 Bayesian Designs for Nonlinear Models

In a nonlinear regression model, the response y is related to explanatory variable x through a nonlinear function $f(x, \theta)$, and the classical nonlinear model can be written as

$$y = f^T(x, \theta) + \varepsilon, \varepsilon \sim N(0, \sigma^2). \tag{14}$$

In the classical optimal design theory, designs are locally dependent on the values of the parameters in these nonlinear models, and only locally optimal designs can be obtained. To overcome the dependence of the designs on the initial values of the parameters, the Bayesian approach for constructing experimental designs for nonlinear models has been applied by many researchers [8]. Extensions of Bayesian optimal design criteria to nonlinear models are commonly based on linearization of the model and Gaussian approximations of the posterior distribution. These papers [3, 10, 18, 19, 41] considered the pseudo-Bayesian optimal designs that incorporated prior information of the unknown parameters and average local design criteria over the prior distributions, so that the obtained designs may be robust to the uncertainty of these unknown parameters. The pseudo-Bayesian design criteria are much more computationally intensive than the classical design criteria, and Monte Carlo integration is commonly proposed to solve the integration problems.

Pseudo-Bayesian designs are robust to the uncertainty of the unknown parameters, while the Bayesian utility function (Eqs. (5)–(8)) describes the utility of choosing the design ξ. However, it is much more computationally intensive to integrate the Bayesian utility function (Eq. (4)) for nonlinear models. Cook et al. [9] used Bayesian simulation-based strategies to determine optimal designs for botanical epidemic experiments that were modeled by nonlinear stochastic processes. Under the assumption of different priors, Han and Chaloner [22] analyzed the optimal design for a nonlinear mixed-effects model.

To give an idea of the role that prior distribution plays in the Bayesian optimal design for nonlinear models, a compartment model arising from chemical kinetics is given in Example 3.

Example 3 Consider a simple model,

$$y = \theta_3 \left(e^{-\theta_1 t} - e^{-\theta_2 t}\right) + \varepsilon, \varepsilon \sim N\left(0, \sigma^2\right), \tag{15}$$

where the unknown parameters $(\theta_1, \theta_2, \theta_3)$ are such that $\theta_2 > \theta_1$. Atkinson et al. [3] discussed the locally optimal design by giving the prior estimates of the three unknown parameters. They also considered designs to estimate functions such as the area under the curve (AUC) and the time to the maximum concentration, with the minimum variance. The effects of different priors on the optimal designs are discussed. An optimal design obtained under one prior distribution may be inefficient for the other. Bayesian design using precise prior information can improve the design considerably. Hence, the prior information needs to be chosen carefully before the experiment.

4.1 Bayesian Optimal Designs for PKPD Models

Compartment models (Eq. (15)) are commonly used to model the mean of a pharmacokinetics (PK) or pharmacodynamics (PD) model, and the relating optimal design problem has attracted the interest of many researchers. Pharmacokinetics (PK) models describe the time course of drug concentrations in the body, while pharmacodynamics (PD) models describe the effects of the drug on the body. Pharmacokinetics–pharmacodynamics models are nonlinear in the parameters, and the design variables of interest are the times, where the samples are collected.

In the case of fixed-effects pharmacokinetics–pharmacodynamics (PKPD) model, an individual design is considered. Atkinson et al. [3] found designs that minimized the variance of the AUC, the maximum concentration (C_{max}), and the time to maximum concentration (t_{max}) estimates for the one-compartmental pharmacokinetics model with first-order absorption input and a constant variance term by incorporating the prior information. Dokoumetzidis and Aarons [16] used the standard Monte Carlo sampling to perform the numerical integration (see Eq. (1)) and used the sequential quadratic programming optimization algorithm that is implemented in the routine "fmincon" in the MATLAB optimization toolbox to provide a fast solution. The designs found by Atkinson et al. [3] and Dokoumetzidis and Aarons [16] are both pseudo-Bayesian designs. Recently, Duffull et al. [19], McGree et al. [37], Ryan et al. [50, 51] obtained the optimal Bayesian experimental designs for pharmacokinetic models, when the design space was small. Ryan et al. [52] considered the fully Bayesian optimal designs for different measures of interest by using four Bayesian utility functions. In their paper, three methods for calculating Bayesian utility functions were compared and contrasted, including importance sampling using the prior as the importance distribution, Laplace approximations, and importance sampling using the Laplace approximation to the posterior as the importance distribution. The results showed that different utility functions brought great differences between their corresponding optimal designs, but different methods used for calculating the utility functions almost had no effect on the designs. However, the computational burden of searching over a large number of design points is heavy for high-dimensional parameters. Recently, Price et al. [47] proposed an efficient search heuristic algorithm suitable for optimal Bayesian experimental design problems, by considering a Markov death model, a one-compartment pharmacokinetics model, and a four-factor logistic regression model. This new algorithm was computationally efficient for moderately large design problems (up to approximately 40 dimensions).

For the mixed-effects pharmacokinetics–pharmacodynamics (PKPD) models, the number of parameters is higher, including the inter-individual variability parameters. The nonlinear mixed-effects model (NLME) models the fixed and random effects simultaneously, and a population design is considered. The parameters of interest include the fixed-effects parameters, variances of the random-effects parameters, and variances of the random errors. Since the likelihood function of a nonlinear mixed-effects model (NLME) is analytically intractable, the Fisher information matrix, which includes both the parameters of fixed effects and the variances of the random effects, cannot be expressed explicitly. Thus, Mentré et al. [39] proposed an approximation of the model using a first-order Taylor series expansion around the random effects, and the optimal design for a NLME model could be obtained. This approach was applied to a single-response model and was further developed by Retout and Mentré [49] to include covariates and inter-occasion variability. Stroud and Rosner [57] discussed optimal sampling times in these pharmacokinetics studies by exploring the Bayesian-decision theoretic solutions. Their methods are simulation-based and therefore can be applied to a wide variety of probability models and utility functions. Dokoumetzidis and Aarons [16] also considered the pseudo-Bayesian D-optimal population design for the pharmacokinetics model, where the simulated annealing algorithm was used for optimization. The fully Bayesian optimal design for a horse population pharmacokinetics study was presented in Ryan et al. [52], when the experimental cost was considered. The design problem was to determine the optimal urine sampling times and the number of subjects and samples per subject to obtain precise posterior distributions of the population parameters.

There are a number of aspects in Bayesian framework for optimal design, such as the prior distribution, utilities, and the algorithm. However, the difficulties in the selection of prior and utility functions and the computational difficulty in optimizing the expected utility function make the application of fully Bayesian designs for complex models limited.

4.2 Bayesian Optimal Designs for Biological and Chemical Models

Although many of the existing papers on applying Bayesian for optimal designs are related to pharmaceuticals, Bayesian optimal designs are also commonly used in the fields of biological applications and chemical engineering systems. Most of these models are nonlinear, and some are even modeled by differential equations. While the early work on Bayesian optimal designs for simple models focused on evaluating the expected utility function over small design space, recent studies on Bayesian optimal designs for more complicated models take advantage of recent advancements in methods for approximating the Bayesian utility functions faster [53].

In biological experiments, a simulation-based approach was used in Huang et al. [24] to deal with design problems in Bayesian hierarchical nonlinear (mixed-effects) models, which characterized long-term viral dynamics. To the best of our knowledge, the first study on Bayesian optimal experimental designs for nonlinear dynamic systems was proposed in Paulson et al. [45], which considered the Bayesian optimal experiment designs for parameter inference in dynamic nonlinear models with constraint under incomplete and indirect measurements. The asymptotic approximations for the multi-dimensional integrals arising in the expected utility function was proposed in Papadimitriou and Argyris [44], and analytical expressions to find the effects of the variances of Bayesian Gaussian priors on the optimal design were also developed. The results are valid with a large number of data with small prediction errors, and the method can be applied to complex linear and nonlinear dynamical models. When the motivation of the experiment was to estimate the parameters precisely, Overstall et al. [42] studied the Bayesian optimal design for a model where the response distribution depended on the solution to a system of nonlinear ordinary differential equations, which described the transport of amino acids through cell membranes in human placentas. A method to derive Bayesian experimental design for discriminating between rival epidemiological models with computationally intractable likelihood was proposed in Dehideniya et al. [13].

In chemical engineering experiments, Terejanu et al. [58] applied model-based Bayesian optimal design to estimate the reaction kinetics using maximum entropy sampling. Huan and Marzouk [23] used polynomial chaos approximations and nested Monte Carlo integration to estimate the KLD (see Eq. (6)) between the prior and posterior distributions to find optimal designs, which enabled us to make inferences of the parameters in chemical kinetic models about the combustion. The Bayesian optimal designs were also applied to polymerization systems using a factorial lumped model in order to reduce the computational cost in Scott et al. [54]. Luna and Martinez [33] applied Bayesian designs to determine the conditions to run the reactor in order to maximize the probability of their polymer product and polystyrene and meet the specifications. The latest paper [27] considered the Bayesian optimal design in the system of carbon dioxide sorption on UiO-66 sorbents and used the design to get the estimates of the Langmuir adsorption isotherm parameters. This modified Langmuir adsorption isotherm model is given by

$$q_{eq} = q_m \frac{bp_{co_2}}{1 + bp_{co_2}}, \tag{16}$$

where q_m is the maximum saturation capacity at a given temperature and b is the adsorption affinity constant. Equation (16) is also a nonlinear model.

5 Conclusions

Bayesian optimal design is a promising and fast developing research area. The optimizations of design criteria are based on the posterior distribution, which takes the prior information into consideration. Recently, there are many exciting developments on Bayesian designs for different models, such as clinical trials, cognitive science, natural science, etc. In this chapter, we have reviewed Bayesian experimental designs for various models that reflected the application of Bayesian experimental design. Since Chaloner [6] published the paper on Bayesian optimality for linear regression models, the ability of incorporating parameters and prior information into the optimal design makes Bayesian design widely applied to nonlinear models, such as chemical models, dynamic differential equation models, etc.

The computational development for approximating the Bayesian utility functions plays an important role in Bayesian optimal designs. Most of the references listed in this chapter have already involved a number of algorithms, such as Markov chain Monte Carlo, sequential Monte Carlo, and approximate Bayes methods. Ryan et al. [53] reviewed the commonly used Bayesian utility functions and different algorithms that have been used to perform Bayesian optimal designs.

The future of Bayesian experimental designs lies in finding solutions to complex or non-standard models, such as nonlinear mixed-effects models and error-in-variable models, in which the likelihood has a non-analytic expression or the posterior distribution is computationally intensive, or models with high dimension of design variables. Algorithm developments and the utilization of parallel computing technology may be two effective solutions to these challenging problems, especially for the fully Bayesian optimal designs [53].

Acknowledgments The authors would like to thank the two reviewers for their insightful suggestions and helpful comments that improve the quality and presentation of this chapter substantively. Dr. Yichuan Zhao acknowledges the research support from the Simons Foundation.

References

1. Abebe, H.T., Tan, F.E.S., Breukelen, G.J.P.V., Berger, M.P.F.: Bayesian *D*-optimal designs for the two-parameter logistic mixed effects model. Comput. Stat. Data Anal. **71**, 1066–1076 (2014)
2. Atkinson, A.C., Woods, D.C.: Designs for generalized linear models. In: Handbook of Design and Analysis of Experiments. Chapman and Hall/CRC, Boca Raton (2015)
3. Atkinson, A.C., Donev, A.N., Tobias, R.D.: Optimal Experimental Designs, With SAS. Oxford University Press, Oxford (2007)
4. Brooks, R.J.: On the choice of an experiment for prediction in linear regression. Biometrika **61**, 303–311 (1974)
5. Brooks, R.J.: Optimal regression designs for prediction when prior knowledge is available. Metrika **23**, 217–221 (1976)
6. Chaloner, K.: Optimal Bayesian experimental designs for linear models. Ann. Stat. **12**, 283–300 (1984)
7. Chaloner, K., Larntz, K.: Optimal Bayesian designs applied to logistic regression experiments. J. Stat. Plann. Inference **21**, 191–208 (1989)
8. Chaloner, K., Verdinelli, I.: Bayesian experimental design: a review. Stat. Sci. **10**, 273–304 (1995)
9. Cook, A.R., Gibson, G.J., Gilligan, C.A.: Optimal observation times in experimental epidemic processes. Biometrics **64**, 860–868 (2008)
10. D'Argenio, D.Z.: Incorporating prior parameter uncertainty in the design of sampling schedules for pharmacokinetic parameter estimation experiments. Math. Biosci. **99**, 105–118 (1990)
11. DasGupta, A.: Review of Optimal Bayes Designs, Technical report. Purdue University, West Lafayette (1995)
12. DasGupta, A., Studden, W.: Robust Bayes designs in normal linear models. Ann. Stat. **19**, 1244–1256 (1991)
13. Dehideniya, M.B., Drovandi, C.C., Mcgree, J.M.: Optimal Bayesian design for discriminating between models with intractable likelihoods in epidemiology. Comput. Stats Data Anal. **124**, 277–297 (2018)
14. Dette, H.: Bayesian D-optimal and model robust designs in linear regression models. Statistics **25**, 27–46 (1993)
15. Diggle, P., Lophaven, S.: Bayesian geostatistical design. Scand. J. Stat. **33**(1), 53–64 (2006)
16. Dokoumetzidis, A., Aarons, L.: Bayesian optimal designs for pharmacokinetic models: sensitivity to uncertainty. J. Biopharm. Stat. **4**(18), 851–867 (2007)
17. Drovandi, C.C., Pettitt, A.N.: Bayesian experimental design for models with intractable likelihoods. Bio-metrics **69**(4), 937–948 (2013)
18. Duffull, S., Waterhouse, T., Eccleston, J.: Some considerations on the design of population pharmacokinetic studies. J. Pharmacokinet. Pharmacodynamics **32**, 441–457 (2005)
19. Duffull, S.B., Graham, G., Mengersen, K., Eccleston, J.: Evaluation of the pre-posterior distribution of optimized sampling times for the design of pharmacokinetic studies. J. Biopharm. Stat. **22**, 16–29 (2012)

20. El-Krunz, S., Studden, W.: Bayesian optimal designs for linear regression models. Ann. Stat. **19**, 2183–2208, 1991.
21. Firth, D., Hinde, J.P.: On Bayesian D-optimum criteria and the equivalence theorem in non-linear models. J. R. Stat. Soc. Ser. B **59**(4), 793–797 (1997)
22. Han, C., Chaloner, K.: Bayesian experimental design for nonlinear mixed-effects models with application to HIV dynamics. Biometrics **60**, 25–33 (2004)
23. Huan, X., Marzouk, Y.M.: Simulation-based optimal Bayesian experimental design for nonlinear systems. J. Comput. Phys. **232**(1), 288–317 (2013)
24. Huang, Y., Wu, H., Acosta, E.P.: Hierarchical Bayesian inference for HIV dynamic differential equation models incorporating multiple treatment factors. Biom. J. **52**(4), 470–486 (2010)
25. Jiang, H.Y., Yue, R.X.: Pseudo-Bayesian D-optimal designs for longitudinal Poisson mixed models with correlated errors. Comput. Stat. **34**, 71–87 (2019b)
26. Jiang, H.Y., Yue R.X., Zhou X.D.: Optimal designs for multivariate logistic mixed models with longitudinal data. Commun. Stat Theory Methods **48**, 850–864 (2019a)
27. Kalyanaraman, J., Kawajiri, Y., Realff, M.J.: Bayesian design of experiments for adsorption isotherm modeling. Comput. Chem. Eng. **135**, article 106774 (2020)
28. Leonard, R.D., Edwards, D.J.: Bayesian D-optimal screening experiments with partial replication. Comput. Stats Data Anal. **115**, 79–90 (2017)
29. Lewi, J., Butera, R., Paninski, L.: Sequential optimal design of neurophysiology experiments. Neural Comput. **21**, 619–687 (2009)
30. Li, P., Wiens, D.P.: Robustness of design in dose-response studies. J. R. Stat. Soc. **73**(2), 215–238 (2011)
31. Lindley, D.: The choice of variables in multiple regression. J. R. Stat. Soc. Ser. B **30**, 31–53 (1968)
32. Lindley, D.: Bayesian Statistics—A Review. SIAM, Philadelphia (1972)
33. Luna, M.F., Martinez, E.C.: Sequential Bayesian experimental design for process optimization with stochastic binary outcomes. Comput. Aided Chem. Eng. **43**, 943–948 (2018)
34. Maram, P.P., Jafari, H.: Bayesian D-optimal design for logistic regression model with exponential distribution for random intercept. J. Commun. Stat. Theory Methods **43**, 1234–1247 (2016)
35. Masoumi, S., Duever, T.A., Reilly, P.M.: Sequential Markov Chain Monte Carlo (MCMC) model discrimination. Can. J. Chem. Eng. **91**(5), 862–869 (2013)
36. McCullaghand, P., Nelder, J.A.: Generalized Linear Models. Chapman and Hall, London (1989)
37. McGree, J., Drovandi, C.C., Pettitt, A.N.: A Sequential Monte Carlo Approach to the Sequential Design for Discriminating between Rival Continuous Data Models. Technical report. Queensland University of Technology, Queensland (2012)
38. McGree, J., Drovandi, C.C., Thompson, H., Eccleston, J., Duffull, S., Mengersen, K., Pettitt, A.N., Goggin, T.: Adaptive Bayesian compound designs for dose finding studies. J. Statist. Plann. Inference **142**(6), 1480–1492 (2012b)
39. Mentré, M., Mallet, A., Baccar, D.: Optimal design in random effect regression models. Biometrika **84**, 429–442 (1997)
40. Ng, S.H., Chick, S.E.: Design of follow-up experiments for improving model discrimination and parameter estimation. Nav. Res. Logist. **51**, 1129–1148 (2004)
41. Ogungbenro, K., Aarons, L.: Design of population pharmacokinetic experiments using prior information. Xenobiotica **37**, 1311–1330 (2007)
42. Overstall, A., Woods, D., Parker, B.: Bayesian optimal design for ordinary differential equation models with application in biological science. Statistics **115**, 583–598 (2019)
43. Owen, R.J.: The optimum design of a two-factor experiment using prior information. Ann. Math. Stat. **41**, 1917–1934 (1970)
44. Papadimitriou, C., Argyris, C.: Bayesian optimal experimental design for parameter estimation and response predictions in complex dynamical systems. Procedia Eng. **199**, 972–977 (2017)
45. Paulson, J.A., Martin-Casas, M., Mesbah, A.: Optimal Bayesian experiment design for nonlinear dynamic systems with chance constraints. J. Process Control **77**, 155–171 (2019)

46. Pilz, J.: Bayesian Estimation and Experimental Design in Linear Regression Models (2nd ed). Wiley, New York (1991)
47. Price, D.J., Bean, N.G., Ross, J.V., Tuke, J.: An induced natural selection heuristic for finding optimal Bayesian experimental designs. Comput. Stat. Data Anal. **126**, 112–124 (2018)
48. Pukelsheim, F.: Optimal Design of Experiments. Wiley, NewYork (1993)
49. Retout, S., Mentr, F.: Further developments of the Fisher information matrix in nonlinear mixed effects models with evaluation in population pharmacokinetics. J. Biopharm. Stat. **13**, 209–227 (2003)
50. Ryan, E.G., Drovandi, C.C., Thompson, M., Pettitt, A.N.: Towards Bayesian experimental design for nonlinear models that require a large number of sampling times. Comput. Stat. Data Anal. **70**, 45–60 (2014)
51. Ryan, E.G., Drovandi, C.C., Pettitt, A.N.: Fully Bayesian experimental design for pharmacokinetic studies. Entropy **17**, 1063–1089 (2015a)
52. Ryan, E.G., Drovandi, C.C., Pettitt, A.N.: Simulation-based fully Bayesian experimental design for mixed effects models. Comput. Stat. Data Anal. **92**(C), 26–39 (2015b)
53. Ryan, E.G., Drovandi, C.C., McGree, J.M., Pettitt, A.N.: A review of modern computational algorithms for Bayesian optimal design. Int. Stat. Rev. **84**(1), 128–154 (2016)
54. Scott, A.J., Nabifar, A., Madhuranthakam, CMR., Penlidi, A.: Bayesian design of experiments applied to a complex polymerization system: Nitrile Butadiene Rubber production in a train of CSTRs. Macromol. Theory Simul. **24**(1), 13–27 (2014)
55. Singh, R., Mukhopadhyay, S.: Exact Bayesian designs for count time series. Comput. Stat. Data Anal. **134**, 157–170 (2018)
56. Solonen, A., Haario, H., Laine, M.: Simulation-based optimal design using a response variance criterion. J. Comput. Graph. Stat. **21**(1), 234–252 (2012)
57. Stroud, J.R., Rosner, M.G.L.: Optimal sampling times in population pharmacokinetic studies. J. R. Stat. Soc. **50**(3), 345–359 (2001)
58. Terejanu, G., Upadhyay, R.R., Miki, K.: Bayesian experimental design for the active nitridation of graphite by atomic nitrogen. Exp. Thermal Fluid Sci. **36**, 178–193 (2012)
59. Vanlier, J., Tiemann, C., Hilbers, P., van Riel, N.: Optimal experimental design for model selection in biochemical networks. BMC Syst. Biol. **8**, 8–20 (2014)
60. Verdinelli, I.: Bayesian design for the normal linear model with unknown error variance. Biometrika **87**, 222–227 (2000)
61. Woods, D.C., Lewis, S.M., Eccleston, J.A., Russell, K.G.: Designs for generalised linear models with several variables and model uncertainty. Technometrics **48**, 284–292 (2006)
62. Woods, D.C., Overstall, A.M., Adamou, M., Waite, T.W.: Bayesian design of experiments for generalized linear models and dimensional analysis with industrial and scientific application. Qual. Eng. **29**, 91–103 (2017)
63. Zhang, Y., Ye, K.: Bayesian D-optimal designs for Poisson regression models. Commun. Stat. Theory Methods **43**, 1234–1247 (2014)

Part III
Big Data Analytics and Its Applications

A Selective Review on Statistical Techniques for Big Data

Yaqiong Yao and HaiYing Wang

1 Introduction

As the collection and storage of data are becoming much cheaper than before, volumes of available data are increasing exponentially and big data problems attract a wide range of attentions from scientists [13]. In many disciplines, a lot of data with extraordinary sizes emerge and need more advanced technologies and approaches to analyze them, because traditional methods may fail due to large data volumes. For big data, the size is not the only concern. The difficulty of analyzing big data can be evaluated in three aspects: volume, velocity, and variety. Here, volume is the size related to both the dimension and the number of observations, velocity is the interaction speed with the data, and variety means various data structures [20].

In this review, we mainly discuss the case that the number of observations far exceeds the data dimension and consider two challenges caused by big data. The one is that analyzing the entire dataset is time-consuming and the other is that the data are too large to be held in the computer's random access memory (RAM). To deal with these two problems, a bunch of statistical methods have been developed: some methods target at one of the challenges and some methods are useful to meet both challenges.

To speed up the calculation for the first challenge, one may project the massive dataset to a lower dimensional space using some randomized transforms. This procedure is called random projection, and existing methods often rely on the Hadamard transform or the Johnson–Lindenstrauss transform [10, 26].

Another intuitive solution is to select a subset of the full data to analyze. This approach can be implemented through a random subsampling procedure or a

Y. Yao · H. Y. Wang (✉)
University of Connecticut, Storrs, CT, USA
e-mail: yaqiong.yao@uconn.edu; haiying.wang@uconn.edu

Y. Zhao, (Din) D.-G. Chen (eds.), *Modern Statistical Methods for Health Research*, Emerging Topics in Statistics and Biostatistics,
https://doi.org/10.1007/978-3-030-72437-5_11

deterministic selection method. For random subsampling, nonuniform subsampling probabilities are often used for spotting more informative data points (e.g., [9]). Algorithmic leveraging is an example of this procedure, which uses statistical leverage scores to define subsampling probabilities for linear regression models [24]. Another example is the local case–control subsampling that is designed for logistic regression with imbalanced data [14]. Optimal subsampling is a recently developed technique that derives the optimal subsampling probabilities by minimizing the asymptotic mean squared error of the resulting subsample estimator. This method typically needs to be implemented in an adaptive way because the optimal subsampling probabilities contain unknown parameters [38]. The information-based optimal subdata selection is a novel deterministic selection method designed for linear regression models [39]. This method has the advantage that the relevant information contained in the resulting subsample is not restricted by the subsample size.

When the data volume is so large that the whole data cannot be analyzed in the available RAM, one solution is to process the data piece by piece. The divide-and-conquer method is a typical example of this approach. With this method, one divides the entire dataset into small blocks, analyzes data in each block, and then aggregates results from all blocks to form a final estimator (e.g., [22]). Stochastic gradient descent is another example of processing the data piece by piece. This method reads the observations one by one or batch by batch; and it updates the estimator step by step, so there is no need to store the data that have been used.

Besides the approaches that we are going to discuss in this chapter, there are a bunch of other methods focusing on a particular model when responses could be correlated, such as resampling-based stochastic approximation method [21] and multi-resolution approximation method [18] for Gaussian processes, online asynchronous decentralized leverage score sampling for vector autoregressive model [41].

The rest of the chapter is organized as follows. Section 2 discusses the randomized numerical linear algebra including methods based on random projection and random subsampling. Section 3 presents the information-based optimal subdata selection methods. Section 4 is devoted to informative subsampling methods including the optimal subsampling methods and local case–control subsampling methods. Section 5 presents divide-and-conquer methods, online updating methods, and stochastic gradient descent methods. Section 6 gives brief summary and discussions.

2 Randomized Numerical Linear Algebra

Suppose that $\{\boldsymbol{x}_i, y_i\}_{i=1}^n$ are n observations with $\boldsymbol{x}_i \in \mathbb{R}^d$ being the covariate and y_i being the response. Assume that they follow a linear regression model with the following form:

$$y_i = \boldsymbol{x}_i^{\mathrm{T}} \boldsymbol{\beta} + \epsilon_i, \quad i = 1, \ldots, n, \tag{1}$$

where $\boldsymbol{\beta} \in \mathbb{R}^d$ is the unknown regression coefficient and $\{\epsilon_i\}_{i=1}^n$ are uncorrelated error terms with $\mathbb{E}(\epsilon_i) = 0$ and $\mathbb{V}(\epsilon_i) = \sigma^2$. This model can also be written as

$$\boldsymbol{y} = \boldsymbol{X}\boldsymbol{\beta} + \boldsymbol{\epsilon}, \tag{2}$$

where $\boldsymbol{X} = (\boldsymbol{x}_1, \boldsymbol{x}_2, \ldots, \boldsymbol{x}_n)^{\mathrm{T}} \in \mathbb{R}^{n \times d}$ is the covariate matrix or design matrix, $\boldsymbol{y} = (y_1, y_2, \ldots, y_n)^{\mathrm{T}}$ is the n-dimensional vector of responses, and $\boldsymbol{\epsilon} = (\epsilon_1, \epsilon_2, \ldots, \epsilon_n)^{\mathrm{T}}$ is the n-dimensional vector of model errors.

The ordinary least-squares (OLS) estimator is commonly used to estimate $\boldsymbol{\beta}$, and it has a form of

$$\hat{\boldsymbol{\beta}} = \arg\min_{\boldsymbol{\beta} \in \mathbb{R}^d} \|\boldsymbol{X}\boldsymbol{\beta} - \boldsymbol{y}\|^2 = \boldsymbol{X}^+ \boldsymbol{y}, \tag{3}$$

where $\|\cdot\|$ represents the Euclidean norm and $\boldsymbol{X}^+$ is the Moore–Penrose inverse of $\boldsymbol{X}$. If $\boldsymbol{X}$ is a full-rank matrix, $\hat{\boldsymbol{\beta}}$ has an expression of

$$\hat{\boldsymbol{\beta}} = (\boldsymbol{X}^{\mathrm{T}}\boldsymbol{X})^{-1}\boldsymbol{X}^{\mathrm{T}}\boldsymbol{y} = \left(\sum_{i=1}^n \boldsymbol{x}_i \boldsymbol{x}_i^{\mathrm{T}}\right)^{-1} \sum_{i=1}^n \boldsymbol{x}_i y_i. \tag{4}$$

Under the setting of $n > d$, both (3) and (4) can be computed in $O(nd^2)$ time. However, for extremely large n and potentially large d, obtaining the OLS estimator is not trivial. One reason is that the $O(nd^2)$ computational time may not be affordable, and another reason is that the size of the dataset may exceed the capacity of the available RAM. In the following, we discuss two methods proposed to fast approximate the OLS estimator: one is based on random projection after the Hadamard transform and the other is based on the nonuniform subsampling according to leverage scores of the design matrix. For other investigations on randomized numerical linear algebra, the readers can refer to [26, 27] and the references therein.

2.1 *Random Projection*

Random projection is a widely used method, which reduces the dimension of a matrix by mapping it to a comparatively low-dimensional space with a relatively small error [16, 26]. A random projection method for solving the least-squares problem was introduced in [10], which combines random projection (and uniform sampling) with the randomized Hadamard transform (also known as the Walsh–Hadamard transform).

Before presenting this method, we need to introduce the Hadamard transform, which is defined recursively through the Hadamard matrix. Suppose that $\boldsymbol{H}_n$ represents the $n \times n$ Hadamard matrix in which $n = 2^a$ for some positive integer a. When $n = 2$ ($a = 1$), define

$$\boldsymbol{H}_2 = \begin{pmatrix} +1 & +1 \\ +1 & -1 \end{pmatrix}.$$

The Hadamard matrix $\boldsymbol{H}_n$ is defined as

$$\boldsymbol{H}_n = \boldsymbol{H}_2 \otimes \boldsymbol{H}_{n/2},$$

where $\otimes$ is the kronecker product. A computational advantage of the Hadamard transform is that it takes $O(n \log_2 n)$ time to obtain $\boldsymbol{H}_n \boldsymbol{x}$ for any $\boldsymbol{x} \in \mathbb{R}^n$. For example, this can be achieved by using Algorithm 1. However, a disadvantage of the Hadamard transform is that n has to be a power of 2.

Algorithm 1 Fast Walsh-Hadamard transform (FWHT)

Input: $\boldsymbol{x} \in \mathbb{R}^n$ with $n = 2^a$
Output: $\eta = \boldsymbol{H}_n \boldsymbol{x} = \text{FWHT}(\boldsymbol{x})$
1: **if** $n = 2$ **then**
2: $\quad \eta = \begin{pmatrix} x_1 + x_2 \\ x_1 - x_2 \end{pmatrix}$ where $\boldsymbol{x} = (x_1, x_2)^{\mathrm{T}}$,
3: **else**
4: $\quad$ partition $\boldsymbol{x}$ into $\boldsymbol{x} = \binom{\boldsymbol{x}^1}{\boldsymbol{x}^2}$, where $\boldsymbol{x}^1$ and $\boldsymbol{x}^2$ are of the same dimension, and calculate $\eta^1 \leftarrow \text{FWHT}(\boldsymbol{x}^1)$, $\eta^2 \leftarrow \text{FWHT}(\boldsymbol{x}^2)$, and $\eta = \begin{pmatrix} \eta^1 + \eta^2 \\ \eta^1 - \eta^2 \end{pmatrix}$,
5: **end if**

The basic idea of the proposed algorithm in [10] is to first average the information of observations by using the Hadamard transform on both the response vector and the design matrix and then randomly project the transformed data into a lower dimensional space or uniformly draw data points from the transformed data. The final estimator, say $\tilde{\boldsymbol{\beta}}^{S}$, is calculated based on the projected data or the selected subsample from the transformed data. The algorithm based on random projection is described in Algorithm 2.

Algorithm 2 Random projection after randomized Hadamard transform

Input: X, y, r, q

Output: $\tilde{\boldsymbol{\beta}}^{S}$

1: Let $\S \in \mathbb{R}^{r\times n}$ be a sparse projection matrix such that for $i = 1, 2, \ldots, r$ and $j = 1, 2, \ldots, n$,

$$\S_{ij} = \begin{cases} +\sqrt{\frac{1}{rq}}, & \text{with probability } \frac{q}{2}, \\ -\sqrt{\frac{1}{rq}}, & \text{with probability } \frac{q}{2}, \\ 0, & \text{with probability } 1-q, \end{cases} \qquad \text{independently.}$$

2: Let $\boldsymbol{R} \in \mathbb{R}^{n\times n}$ be a diagonal matrix whose diagonal elements are $+1$ or -1 with equal probability.

3: The estimator $\tilde{\boldsymbol{\beta}}^{S}$ is obtained as

$$\tilde{\boldsymbol{\beta}}^{S} = (\S \boldsymbol{H}_n \boldsymbol{R}\boldsymbol{X})^{+} \S \boldsymbol{H}_n \boldsymbol{R} \boldsymbol{y}.$$

Using Algorithm 1, the term $\boldsymbol{H}_n\boldsymbol{R}\boldsymbol{X}$, in Algorithm 2, can be calculated in $O(nd \log_2 n)$ time, which is the major computational cost in the algorithm if $\S$ is sparse enough. Theorem 3 of [10] provides formulas for determining the values of r and q based on a desired level of relative approximation error.

In [10], the authors also considered the case that $\S$ is a subsampling matrix defined in this way: for $i = 1, 2, \ldots, r$, randomly choose j from $\{1, 2, \ldots, n\}$, and set $\S_{ij} = 1$ and $\S_{ij'} = 0$ for $j' \neq j$. This is just to take a subsample from the transformed data using uniform subsampling with replacement. There is a computational benefit of using this approach. We actually only keep r rows of $\boldsymbol{H}_n\boldsymbol{R}\boldsymbol{X}$ after multiplying the sampling matrix $\S$, and the time complexity of $\S\boldsymbol{H}_n\boldsymbol{R}\boldsymbol{X}$ is $O(nd \log_2 r)$ according to [4]. The authors also proved, in Theorem 2 of [10], that the value of r should be

$$r = \max\left(48^2 d \ln(40nd) \ln\left\{100^2 d \ln(40nd)\right\}, 40d \ln(40nd)/\alpha\right),$$

in order to achieve the $(1+\alpha)$ relative error approximation with high probability, where $\alpha \in (0, 1)$. The overall time complexity of the proposed algorithm is $O(nd \ln d)$ if $d \leq n \leq \exp(d)$. The full data need to be read in one time to conduct the randomized Hadamard transform. Based on the approach in [10], a least-squares solver `BLENDENPIK` is developed in [5].

Note that $\boldsymbol{H}_n\boldsymbol{H}_n = n\boldsymbol{I}$ and $\boldsymbol{R}\boldsymbol{R} = \boldsymbol{I}$, where $\boldsymbol{I}$ is the identity matrix. Thus, the randomized Hadamard transform does not change the full data OLS estimator, because for the OLS estimator based on the transformed data,

$$\hat{\boldsymbol{\beta}}_{\boldsymbol{H}_n} = \{(\boldsymbol{H}_n\boldsymbol{R}\boldsymbol{X})^{\mathrm{T}}\boldsymbol{H}_n\boldsymbol{R}\boldsymbol{X}\}^{-1}(\boldsymbol{H}_n\boldsymbol{R}\boldsymbol{X})^{\mathrm{T}}\boldsymbol{H}_n\boldsymbol{R}\boldsymbol{y} = (\boldsymbol{X}^{\mathrm{T}}\boldsymbol{X})^{-1}\boldsymbol{X}^{\mathrm{T}}\boldsymbol{y} = \hat{\boldsymbol{\beta}}.$$

However, the randomized Hadamard transform makes the data points more similar, so a uniform subsampling will not miss any very informative data points. This also indicates that if the data have light-tailed distributions, the randomized Hadamard transform may not be very effective. For example, if $(\boldsymbol{x}_i, y_i)$ are independent and identically distributed (i.i.d.) with a multivariate normal distribution, then the randomized Hadamard transformed data follow the same distribution.

2.2 Nonuniform Random Sampling

Instead of transforming the data to be more uniform and then using uniform sampling, another idea is to use nonuniform subsampling and assign higher probabilities to more informative data points. We obtain the least-squares or weighted least-squares estimator based on the sample drawn according to those nonuniform subsampling probabilities.

A general approach of nonuniform subsampling for the overconstrained linear regression problem was proposed in [9], which only needs to process the full data by one pass. Leverage scores are commonly used to construct nonuniform subsampling probabilities, and this kind of algorithms is summarized in [24] and is named as algorithmic leveraging.

Suppose that $\boldsymbol{X}$ is full rank with singular value decomposition (SVD),

$$\boldsymbol{X} = \boldsymbol{U}\boldsymbol{\Sigma}\boldsymbol{V}^{\mathrm{T}}, \tag{5}$$

where $\boldsymbol{U}$ is a $n \times d$ orthonormal matrix, $\boldsymbol{V}$ is a $d \times d$ orthonormal matrix, and $\boldsymbol{\Sigma} \in \mathbb{R}^{d\times d}$ is a diagonal matrix with diagonal elements being the singular values. Denote each row of $\boldsymbol{U}$ as $\boldsymbol{u}_1, \boldsymbol{u}_2, \ldots, \boldsymbol{u}_n$. The leverage scores are

$$h_i = \|\boldsymbol{u}_i\|^2, \quad i = 1, 2, \ldots, n,$$

which are equivalent to

$$h_i = \boldsymbol{x}_i^{\mathrm{T}}(\boldsymbol{X}^{\mathrm{T}}\boldsymbol{X})^{-1}\boldsymbol{x}_i, \quad i = 1, 2, \ldots, n,$$

and they satisfy that $\sum_{i=1}^{n} h_i = d$.

The algorithmic leveraging is to use normalized leverage scores, $d^{-1}h_i$, $i = 1, \ldots, n$, to define a subsampling distribution. Algorithm 3 describes how to obtain the algorithmic leveraging estimator $\tilde{\boldsymbol{\beta}}^{\mathrm{AL}}$.

The authors of [24] investigated the properties of $\tilde{\boldsymbol{\beta}}^{\mathrm{AL}}$ and proposed the shrinkage leveraging (SLEV) method that uses

$$\left\{\pi_i = \rho\frac{h_i}{d} + (1-\rho)\frac{1}{n}\right\}_{i=1}^{n},$$

Algorithm 3 Algorithmic leveraging

Input: $\{\boldsymbol{x}_i, y_i\}_{i=1}^n, r$

Output: $\tilde{\boldsymbol{\beta}}^{\mathrm{AL}}$

1: Sample with replacement for a subsample of size r from the full data, using the sampling distribution

$$\left\{\pi_i = \frac{h_i}{d}\right\}_{i=1}^n.$$

2: Denote the selected subsample and the corresponding subsampling probabilities as $\{\boldsymbol{x}_i^*, y_i^*, \pi_i^*\}_{i=1}^r$. The estimator $\tilde{\boldsymbol{\beta}}^{\mathrm{AL}}$ is

$$\tilde{\boldsymbol{\beta}}^{\mathrm{AL}} = \left(\sum_{i=1}^r \frac{\boldsymbol{x}_i^* \boldsymbol{x}_i^{*\mathrm{T}}}{\pi_i^*}\right)^{-1} \sum_{i=1}^r \frac{\boldsymbol{x}_i^* y_i^*}{\pi_i^*}.$$

---

where $\rho \in (0, 1)$ is a tuning parameter. They showed that the SLEV estimator often has a smaller variance. In addition, the asymptotic normality and unbiasedness of $\tilde{\boldsymbol{\beta}}^{\mathrm{AL}}$ have been examined in [25] under some regularity conditions.

Another issue of algorithmic leveraging is that the leverage scores need $O(nd^2)$ time to compute. To alleviate the computational burden, the authors in [11] proposed to fast approximate leverage scores h_i's by using

$$\tilde{h}_i = \|(\boldsymbol{X}(\Pi_1 \boldsymbol{X})^+ \Pi_2)_{i*}\|^2, \quad i = 1, \ldots, n,$$

where $\Pi_1 =\in \mathbb{R}^{r_1 \times n}$ is the subsampled randomized Hadamard transform (e.g., $\S \boldsymbol{H}_n \boldsymbol{R}$ in Algorithm 2) and $\Pi_2 \in \mathbb{R}^{r_1 \times r_2}$ is the Johnson–Lindenstrauss transform (JLT) [2, 3]. To obtain the JLT, each entry of Π_2 is generated independently as

$$\Pi_{2(i,j)} = \begin{cases} +\sqrt{3/r_2} & \text{with probability } \frac{1}{6} \\ -\sqrt{3/r_2} & \text{with probability } \frac{1}{6} \\ 0 & \text{with probability } \frac{2}{3}. \end{cases}$$

The values of r_1 and r_2 are discussed in Lemma 6 and Lemma 4 of [11], respectively. This algorithm runs in $O(nd \ln n)$ time if $d \leq n$ and $n = o(e^d)$.

Instead of solving a subsample OLS problem, [8] suggested to use the following estimator to estimate the true parameter:

$$\tilde{\boldsymbol{\beta}}^{\mathrm{NS}} = \left(\sum_{i=1}^n \boldsymbol{x}_i \boldsymbol{x}_i^{\mathrm{T}}\right)^{-1} \sum_{i=1}^r \frac{\boldsymbol{x}_i^* y_i^*}{\pi_i^*},$$

for the situation with measurement constraints. This is a scenario that all $\boldsymbol{x}_i$'s are available, but the number of responses that can be measured is limited, and the goal is to sample $\boldsymbol{x}_i$'s and then measure the corresponding values of y_i's to estimate $\boldsymbol{\beta}$. This is a typical problem of interest in the field of survey sampling and design of experiments in statistics. The estimator $\tilde{\boldsymbol{\beta}}^{\mathrm{NS}}$ does not improve the computational efficiency compared with the full data OLS. However, there is an explicit formula for the mean squared error (MSE) of $\tilde{\boldsymbol{\beta}}^{\mathrm{NS}}$, and the authors obtained the optimal subsampling probabilities under the A-optimality criteria in optimal design.

Linear regression with measurement constraints is further discussed in [36]. Let r be the number of y_i's can be measured. They proposed to first obtain a computationally tractable relaxed A-optimal design,

$$\boldsymbol{\zeta}^0 = \arg\min_{\boldsymbol{\zeta}=\{\zeta_i\}_{i=1}^n} \operatorname{tr}\left\{\left(\sum_{i=1}^n \zeta_i \boldsymbol{x}_i^{\mathrm{T}} \boldsymbol{x}_i\right)^{-1}\right\}, \quad \text{subject to} \quad 0 \le \zeta_i \text{ and } \sum_{i=1}^n \zeta_i \le r.$$

Additionally, for Poisson subsampling, it is required that $\max(\zeta_i) \le 1$. With $\boldsymbol{\zeta}^0 = \{\zeta_i^0\}_{i=1}^n$, they assign the subsampling probabilities as

$$\left\{\pi_i^{(1)} = \frac{\zeta_i^0 \boldsymbol{x}_i^{\mathrm{T}} (\sum_{j=1}^n \zeta_j^0 \boldsymbol{x}_j^{\mathrm{T}} \boldsymbol{x}_j)^{-1} \boldsymbol{x}_i}{d}\right\}_{i=1}^n \quad \text{for subsampling with replacement; and}$$

$$\left\{\pi_i^{(2)} = \frac{\zeta_i^0}{r}\right\}_{i=1}^n \quad \text{for Poisson subsampling.}$$

3 Information-Based Optimal Subdata Selection

The methods discussed in the previous sections are based on random subsampling or random projection. The asymptotic variances of the resulting estimators are typically at the orders of the inverse subsample sizes. This means that if the subsample size r does not go to infinity, then the subsample estimator does not converge to the true parameter, no matter how fast the full data sample size n goes to infinity. In other words, the subsample estimator is not consistent if r does not go to infinity. The information-based optimal subdata selection (IBOSS) aims to solve this issue.

The IBOSS method was proposed in [39] for the linear regression model (1) or (2). Here, the linear regression model contains an intercept parameter, and we emphasize this fact by writing $\boldsymbol{x}_i = (1, x_{i,1}, \ldots, x_{i,d-1})^{\mathrm{T}}$ for $i = 1, \ldots, n$ and $\boldsymbol{\beta} = (\beta_0, \beta_1, \ldots, \beta_{d-1})^{\mathrm{T}}$.

Unlike the random sampling approaches we have discussed, the IBOSS deterministically selects data points according to some optimality criterion on the information matrix. Suppose that $\mathcal{D} = \{\boldsymbol{x}_i^*, y_i^*\}_{i=1}^r$ is a deterministic subset of the full dataset and that the selection rule depends on $\boldsymbol{X} = (\boldsymbol{x}_1^{\mathrm{T}}, \ldots, \boldsymbol{x}_n^{\mathrm{T}})^{\mathrm{T}}$ only.

Since the selection rule does not depend on $\boldsymbol{y} = (y_1, y_2, \ldots, y_n)^{\mathrm{T}}$, based on the subsample, the least-squares estimator

$$\tilde{\boldsymbol{\beta}} = \left\{ \sum_{i=1}^{r} \boldsymbol{x}_i^* \boldsymbol{x}_i^{*\mathrm{T}} \right\}^{-1} \sum_{i=1}^{r} \boldsymbol{x}_i^* y_i^* \tag{6}$$

is still the best linear unbiased estimator of $\boldsymbol{\beta}$. The information matrix of the subsample corresponding to the least-squares estimator for $\boldsymbol{\beta}$ is

$$I(\mathcal{D}) = \frac{1}{\sigma^2} \sum_{i=1}^{r} \boldsymbol{x}_i^* \boldsymbol{x}_i^{*\mathrm{T}}.$$

The IBOSS aims to select a subsample that, under some optimality criterion, maximizes $I(\mathcal{D})$, which is equivalent to minimize the covariance matrix of $\tilde{\boldsymbol{\beta}}$. Under the D-optimality criterion, one needs to find the subsample that maximizes $|\sum_{i=1}^{n} \boldsymbol{x}_i^* \boldsymbol{x}_i^{*\mathrm{T}}|$. Since there are $\binom{n}{r}$ different subsamples, the exact solution is computational infeasible due to the combinatorial time complexity. The authors derived an upper bound of $|\sum_{i=1}^{n} \boldsymbol{x}_i^* \boldsymbol{x}_i^{*\mathrm{T}}|$, which indicates that the D-optimal subsample is related to the extremes of the covariates. Based on this observation, they proposed to select $k = [\frac{r}{2(d-1)}]$ observations corresponding to the smallest and largest values of each covariate variable, where $[\cdot]$ means rounding to the nearest integer. The procedure of IBOSS is summarized in Algorithm 4.

Algorithm 4 IBOSS

Input: $\{\boldsymbol{x}_i, y_i\}_{i=1}^n$, $k = [\frac{r}{2(d-1)}]$

Output: $\tilde{\boldsymbol{\beta}}^{\mathrm{IBOSS}}$

Initializing: $\mathcal{D} \leftarrow \varnothing$, $\mathcal{D}^c \leftarrow \{\boldsymbol{x}_i, y_i\}_{i=1}^n$,

1: **for** $j \in \{1, 2, 3, \ldots, d-1\}$ **do**

2: with a partition-based selection algorithm, choose the observations in $\mathcal{D}^c$ with the k smallest values of $x_{i,j}$ and the k largest values of $x_{i,j}$; record these $2k$ observations as $\mathcal{D}_j$;

3: update $\mathcal{D}^c \leftarrow \mathcal{D}^c \setminus \mathcal{D}_j$ and $\mathcal{D} \leftarrow \mathcal{D} \cup \mathcal{D}_j$;

4: **end for**

5: Calculate $\tilde{\boldsymbol{\beta}}^{\mathrm{IBOSS}}$ defined in (6) using the observations in $\mathcal{D}$.

The IBOSS procedure in Algorithm 4 has a time complexity of $O(nd)$, which is a linear time in terms of the full data and is faster than the algorithms described in Sect. 2. The authors investigated the variance of the resulting estimator $\tilde{\boldsymbol{\beta}}^{\mathrm{IBOSS}}$ in various settings. One key conclusion is that the variance for a slope estimator may converge to zero at a rate related to both r and n. Theorem 5 of [39] shows that the variance of a slope estimator satisfies

$$\mathbb{V}(\tilde{\boldsymbol{\beta}}_j^{\text{IBOSS}}|\boldsymbol{X}) = O_P\left(\frac{d-1}{r\{x_{(n-k+1),j} - x_{(k),j}\}^2}\right), \quad j = 1, 2, \ldots, d-1,$$

where $x_{(i),j}$ is the i-th order statistics of $x_{1,j}, \ldots, x_{n,j}$. This result indicates that even if r is fixed, the variance of a slope estimator can still go to 0 as n increases if the support of the covariate distribution is not bounded. For example, if the covariate follows a t distribution with degrees of freedom ν, then the corresponding slope estimator has a variance of order $\mathbb{V}(\tilde{\boldsymbol{\beta}}_j^{\text{IBOSS}}|\boldsymbol{X}) = O_P(r^{-1}n^{-2/\nu})$. In addition, every covariate should be read into memory in one time to select the subdata. Since the data are stored in hard disk by row, the IBOSS fails when full data volume exceeds the capacity of the available RAM. To solve this, the IBOSS was combined with the divide-and-conquer approach in [32]. Another benefit of this investigation is to utilize the distributed and parallel computing facilities.

4 Informative Subsampling

In Sects. 2 and 3, the subsampling approaches do not depend on the responses, and our discussion has focused on linear regression models. In this section, we will introduce some informative subsampling methods that are applicable to nonlinear models. By informative subsampling, we mean that the subsampling depends on the responses.

4.1 Optimal Subsampling

Optimal subsampling is an informative subsampling approach that aims to maximize the estimation efficiency. The basic strategy is to find subsampling probabilities that minimize the asymptotic variance of the subsample estimator.

The optimal subsampling method under the A-optimality criterion (OSMAC) was first introduced for logistic regression in [38], where the authors derived subsampling probabilities that minimize the asymptotic MSE of the subsample approximation error.

Consider a logistic regression model,

$$P(y_i = 1|\boldsymbol{x}_i) = p(\boldsymbol{x}_i, \boldsymbol{\beta}) = \frac{\exp(\boldsymbol{x}_i^{\mathrm{T}}\boldsymbol{\beta})}{1 + \exp(\boldsymbol{x}_i^{\mathrm{T}}\boldsymbol{\beta})}, \quad i = 1, 2, \ldots, n, \tag{7}$$

where $y_i \in \{0, 1\}$ is the response, $\boldsymbol{x}_i \in \mathbb{R}^d$ is the covariate, and $\boldsymbol{\beta}$ is the unknown regression coefficient. Let $\{\boldsymbol{x}_i^*, y_i^*, \pi_i^*\}_{i=1}^r$ be a subsample taken according to subsampling probabilities $\{\pi_i\}_{i=1}^n$ such that $\sum_{i=1}^n \pi_i = 1$. A general subsample estimator is

$$\tilde{\boldsymbol{\beta}}^{\text{gen}} = \arg\max_{\boldsymbol{\beta}} \sum_{i=1}^{r} \frac{y_i^* \boldsymbol{\beta}^{\text{T}} \boldsymbol{x}_i^* - \log\left(1 + e^{\boldsymbol{\beta}^{\text{T}} \boldsymbol{x}_i^*}\right)}{\pi_i^*}, \tag{8}$$

which aims to approximate the full data maximum likelihood estimator (MLE), denoted as $\hat{\boldsymbol{\beta}}_{\text{MLE}}$. The authors of [38] derived the following optimal subsampling probabilities that minimize the asymptotic MSE of the approximation error $\tilde{\boldsymbol{\beta}}^{\text{gen}} - \hat{\boldsymbol{\beta}}_{\text{MLE}}$,

$$\pi_i = \frac{|y_i - p(\boldsymbol{x}_i, \hat{\boldsymbol{\beta}}_{\text{MLE}})| \|\boldsymbol{M}_x^{-1} \boldsymbol{x}_i\|}{\sum_{j=1}^{n} |y_j - p(\boldsymbol{x}_j, \hat{\boldsymbol{\beta}}_{\text{MLE}})| \|\boldsymbol{M}_x^{-1} \boldsymbol{x}_j\|}, \quad i = 1, \ldots, n, \tag{9}$$

where $\boldsymbol{M}_x = \frac{1}{n} \sum_{i=1}^{n} p(\boldsymbol{x}_i, \hat{\boldsymbol{\beta}}_{\text{MLE}})\{1 - p(\boldsymbol{x}_i, \hat{\boldsymbol{\beta}}_{\text{MLE}})\} \boldsymbol{x}_i \boldsymbol{x}_i^{\text{T}}$. Since (9) contains $\hat{\boldsymbol{\beta}}_{\text{MLE}}$, the full data MLE, the author proposed an adaptive algorithm stated in Algorithm 5. Note that, to reduce the computational burden, $\boldsymbol{M}_x$ can be approximated by pilot sample. Using this way, the approximated optimal subsampling probabilities can be computed by going through the full data once. After sampling the index of the subsample from 1 to n under the approximated optimal subsampling probabilities, the subsample is obtained by reading in the full data in one pass.

Algorithm 5 Two-stage adaptive subsampling

Input: $\{\boldsymbol{x}_i, y_i\}_{i=1}^{n}$, r_0, r

Output: $\tilde{\boldsymbol{\beta}}^{\text{OS}}$

1: **Pilot sampling:** Sample with replacement for a subsample of size r_0, $\{\boldsymbol{x}_i^{*0}, y_i^{*0}, \pi_i^{*0}\}_{i=1}^{r_0}$, using uniform sampling $\{\pi_i^0 = n^{-1}\}_{i=1}^{n}$ or case–control sampling $\{\pi_i^0 = (2n_0)^{-y_i+1}(2n_1)^{-y_i}\}_{i=1}^{n}$, where n_0 and n_1 are the number of 0's and 1's, respectively, in the responses. Obtain the pilot estimator $\tilde{\boldsymbol{\beta}}^{*0}$ and substitute $\hat{\boldsymbol{\beta}}_{\text{MLE}}$ in (9) with $\tilde{\boldsymbol{\beta}}^{*0}$ to calculate the approximated optimal probabilities $\tilde{\pi}_i$.

2: **Second stage sampling:** Sample with replacement based on $\{\tilde{\pi}_i\}_{i=1}^{n}$ for a subsample of size r, $\{\boldsymbol{x}_i^*, y_i^*, \tilde{\pi}_i^*\}_{i=1}^{r}$.

3: **Estimation:** The final estimator $\tilde{\boldsymbol{\beta}}^{\text{OS}}$ is obtained by combing the two state samples

$$\tilde{\boldsymbol{\beta}}^{\text{OS}} = \arg\max_{\boldsymbol{\beta}} \left\{ \sum_{i=1}^{r_0} \frac{y_i^{*0} \boldsymbol{\beta}^{\text{T}} \boldsymbol{x}_i^{*0} - \log\left(1 + e^{\boldsymbol{\beta}^{\text{T}} \boldsymbol{x}_i^{*0}}\right)}{\pi_i^{*0}} + \sum_{i=1}^{r} \frac{y_i^* \boldsymbol{\beta}^{\text{T}} \boldsymbol{x}_i^* - \log\left(1 + e^{\boldsymbol{\beta}^{\text{T}} \boldsymbol{x}_i^*}\right)}{\tilde{\pi}_i^*} \right\}. \tag{10}$$

The authors of [38] also proved the consistency of the resultant estimator to $\hat{\boldsymbol{\beta}}_{\text{MLE}}$ given the full data and derived its asymptotic distribution. This method was improved in [33] in terms of the estimation efficiency by using an unweighted target function. Specially, instead of using (10), the author suggested to obtain

$$\tilde{\boldsymbol{\beta}}^{\mathrm{uw}} = \arg\max_{\boldsymbol{\beta}} \sum_{i=1}^{r} \left\{ y_i^* \boldsymbol{\beta}^{\mathrm{T}} \boldsymbol{x}_i^* - \log\left(1 + e^{\boldsymbol{\beta}^{\mathrm{T}} \boldsymbol{x}_i^*}\right) \right\}, \tag{11}$$

correct the bias of $\tilde{\boldsymbol{\beta}}^{\mathrm{uw}}$ to have $\tilde{\boldsymbol{\beta}}^{\mathrm{bs}} = \tilde{\boldsymbol{\beta}}^{\mathrm{uw}} + \tilde{\boldsymbol{\beta}}^{*0}$, and then aggregate $\tilde{\boldsymbol{\beta}}^{\mathrm{bs}}$ and $\tilde{\boldsymbol{\beta}}^{*0}$ instead of combining the two-stage subsamples. Here, the bias correction procedure is similar to that proposed for the local case–control subsampling method [14] to be discussed in the next section. The author of [33] also investigated the Poisson subsampling procedure and showed that it has a higher estimation efficiency in addition to its computational benefits.

Although the OSMAC was proposed in the context of logistic regression, it is applicable to other statistical models. It has been generalized in [42] to softmax regression, in which the response y_i has $B + 1$ possible values, $0, 1, 2, \ldots, B$, with the following probabilities:

$$\begin{aligned} P(y_i = 0|\boldsymbol{x}_i) &= p_i(0, \boldsymbol{\beta}) = \frac{1}{1+\sum_{j=1}^{B} \exp(\boldsymbol{x}_i^{\mathrm{T}} \boldsymbol{\beta}_j)}, \quad \text{and} \\ P(y_i = b|\boldsymbol{x}_i) &= p_i(b, \boldsymbol{\beta}) = \frac{\exp(\boldsymbol{x}_i^{\mathrm{T}} \boldsymbol{\beta}_b)}{1+\sum_{j=1}^{B} \exp(\boldsymbol{x}_i^{\mathrm{T}} \boldsymbol{\beta}_j)}, \quad m = 1, 2, \ldots, B. \end{aligned} \tag{12}$$

Here, $\boldsymbol{\beta}_b \in \mathbb{R}^d$ is the regression coefficient for the b-th category, and we set $\boldsymbol{\beta}_0 = \mathbf{0}$ for model identifiability. The whole unknown parameter vector is $\boldsymbol{\beta} = \{\boldsymbol{\beta}_1^{\mathrm{T}}, \boldsymbol{\beta}_2^{\mathrm{T}}, \ldots, \boldsymbol{\beta}_B^{\mathrm{T}}\}^{\mathrm{T}}$. The optimal subsampling probabilities under the A-optimality criterion used to draw subsamples for approximating the full data MLE $\hat{\boldsymbol{\beta}}_{\mathrm{MLE}}$ are

$$\pi_i = \frac{\|\boldsymbol{M}_S^{-1}\{\boldsymbol{s}_i(\hat{\boldsymbol{\beta}}_{\mathrm{MLE}}) \otimes \boldsymbol{x}_i\}\|}{\sum_{j=1}^{n} \|\boldsymbol{M}_S^{-1}\{\boldsymbol{s}_j(\hat{\boldsymbol{\beta}}_{\mathrm{MLE}}) \otimes \boldsymbol{x}_j\}\|}, \quad i = 1, \ldots, n,$$

where $\boldsymbol{M}_S = n^{-1} \sum_{i=1}^{n} \Upsilon_i(\hat{\boldsymbol{\beta}}_{\mathrm{MLE}}) \otimes (\boldsymbol{x}_i \boldsymbol{x}_i^{\mathrm{T}})$; $\Upsilon_i(\boldsymbol{\beta})$ is a $B \times B$ matrix whose b-th diagonal element is $\Upsilon_{i,(b,b)}(\boldsymbol{\beta}) = p_i(b, \boldsymbol{\beta}) - p_i^2(b, \boldsymbol{\beta})$ and $b_1 b_2$-th off-diagonal element is $\Upsilon_{i,(b_1,b_2)}(\boldsymbol{\beta}) = -p_i(b_1, \boldsymbol{\beta}) p_i(b_2, \boldsymbol{\beta})$; and $s_i(\boldsymbol{\beta}) \in \mathbb{R}^B$ with b-th element being $s_{i,b}(\boldsymbol{\beta}) = I(y_i = b) - p_i(b, \boldsymbol{\beta})$.

In [1], the OSMAC was generalized to include generalized linear models (GLMs) with the following form:

$$f(y_i, |\boldsymbol{x}_i, \boldsymbol{\beta}) = h(y_i) \exp\left[y_i g(\boldsymbol{x}_i^{\mathrm{T}} \boldsymbol{\beta}) - c\{g(\boldsymbol{x}_i^{\mathrm{T}} \boldsymbol{\beta})\} \right], \tag{13}$$

where $h(\cdot)$, $g(\cdot)$, and $c(\cdot)$ are known functions. The optimal subsampling probabilities under A-optimality for approximating the full data MLE $\hat{\boldsymbol{\beta}}_{\mathrm{MLE}}$ are

$$\pi_i = \frac{|y_i - \dot{c}\{g(\boldsymbol{x}_i^{\mathrm{T}} \hat{\boldsymbol{\beta}}_{\mathrm{MLE}})\}| \|\boldsymbol{M}_G^{-1} \dot{g}(\boldsymbol{x}_i^{\mathrm{T}} \hat{\boldsymbol{\beta}}_{\mathrm{MLE}}) \boldsymbol{x}_i\|}{\sum_{j=1}^{n} |y_j - \dot{c}\{g(\boldsymbol{x}_j^{\mathrm{T}} \hat{\boldsymbol{\beta}}_{\mathrm{MLE}})\}| \|\boldsymbol{M}_G^{-1} \dot{g}(\boldsymbol{x}_j^{\mathrm{T}} \hat{\boldsymbol{\beta}}_{\mathrm{MLE}}) \boldsymbol{x}_j\|}, \quad i = 1, \ldots, n,$$

where $\dot{c}(\cdot)$ and $\dot{g}(\cdot)$ are the first-order derivatives of $c(\cdot)$ and $g(\cdot)$, respectively; and

$$\boldsymbol{M}_G = \frac{1}{n}\sum_{i=1}^{n}\{\ddot{g}(\boldsymbol{x}_i^{\mathrm{T}}\hat{\boldsymbol{\beta}}_{\mathrm{MLE}})\boldsymbol{x}_i\boldsymbol{x}_i^{\mathrm{T}}[\dot{c}\{g(\boldsymbol{x}_i^{\mathrm{T}}\hat{\boldsymbol{\beta}}_{\mathrm{MLE}})\} - y_i]$$
$$+ \ddot{c}\{g(\boldsymbol{x}_i^{\mathrm{T}}\hat{\boldsymbol{\beta}}_{\mathrm{MLE}})\}\dot{g}^2(\boldsymbol{x}_i^{\mathrm{T}}\hat{\boldsymbol{\beta}}_{\mathrm{MLE}})\boldsymbol{x}_i\boldsymbol{x}_i^{\mathrm{T}}\},$$

with $\ddot{c}(\cdot)$ and $\ddot{g}(\cdot)$ being the second-order derivatives of $c(\cdot)$ and $g(\cdot)$, respectively.

The OSMAC was extended to quantile regression in [34], which assumes that the τ-th quantile ($0 < \tau < 1$) of the response y_i at the give value $\boldsymbol{x}_i$ satisfies

$$q_\tau(y_i|\boldsymbol{x}_i) = \boldsymbol{x}_i^{\mathrm{T}}\boldsymbol{\beta}.$$

The regression coefficient $\boldsymbol{\beta}$ is estimated through minimizing

$$Q_N(\boldsymbol{\beta}) = \frac{1}{n}\sum_{i=1}^{n}(y_i - \boldsymbol{\beta}^{\mathrm{T}}\boldsymbol{x}_i)\{\tau - I(y_i < \boldsymbol{\beta}^{\mathrm{T}}\boldsymbol{x}_i)\}, \tag{14}$$

and the L-optimal subsampling probabilities used to draw subsamples for approximating the full data estimator are

$$\pi_i = \frac{|\tau - I(y_i - \boldsymbol{x}_i^{\mathrm{T}}\boldsymbol{\beta} < 0)|\,\|\boldsymbol{x}_i\|}{\sum_{j=1}^{n}|\tau - I(y_j - \boldsymbol{x}_j^{\mathrm{T}}\boldsymbol{\beta} < 0)|\,\|\boldsymbol{x}_j\|}, \quad i = 1, \ldots, n. \tag{15}$$

To obtain the A-optimal subsampling probabilities, one just replaces $\|\boldsymbol{x}_i\|$ in (15) with $\|\boldsymbol{M}_Q^{-1}\boldsymbol{x}_j\|$, where $\boldsymbol{M}_Q = n^{-1}\sum_{i=1}^{n} f_{\boldsymbol{x}_i}(0)\boldsymbol{x}\boldsymbol{x}_i^{\mathrm{T}}$, and $f_{\boldsymbol{x}_i}(0)$ is the density function of $y_i - \boldsymbol{x}_i^{\mathrm{T}}\boldsymbol{\beta}$ evaluated at 0 for a given $\boldsymbol{x}_i$. For quantile regression, the authors recommended the L-optimality over the A-optimality because $f_{\boldsymbol{x}_i}(0)$'s in $\boldsymbol{M}_Q$ are typically infeasible to obtain. In addition, the L-optimal subsampling probabilities take $O(nd)$ time to calculate, while the A-optimal subsampling probabilities take $O(nd^2)$ time to calculate even if $\boldsymbol{M}_Q$ is available. To perform statistical inference without estimating $f_{\boldsymbol{x}_i}(0)$'s, the authors proposed an iterative subsampling procedure based on the L-optimal probabilities.

Using the similar idea of OSMAC to approximate full data maximum quasi-likelihood estimator $\hat{\boldsymbol{\beta}}_{\mathrm{QLE}}$ by Poisson subsampling was discussed in [43]. A distributed sampling system based on the divide-and-conquer method was also introduced.

4.2 *Local Case–Control Subsampling*

Local case–control (LCC) sampling was proposed by Fithian and Hastie [14] for the logistic regression model (7) with imbalanced datasets. Unlike the case–control sampling in which the subsampling probabilities only depend on the responses $\{y_i\}_{i=1}^n$, the LCC subsampling probabilities depend on both the responses and the covariates. Specifically, the LCC subsampling probabilities for estimating the parameter $\boldsymbol{\beta}$ in the logistic regression model (7) are

$$\pi_i^{\mathrm{LCC}} = |y_i - p(\boldsymbol{x}_i, \tilde{\boldsymbol{\beta}}^p)|, \quad i = 1, \ldots, n, \tag{16}$$

where $\tilde{\boldsymbol{\beta}}^p$ is a pilot estimator. The LCC subsampling is based on Poisson sampling. A detailed algorithm for estimating the regression parameter $\boldsymbol{\beta}$ is presented in Algorithm 6. Given a pilot estimator, the subsample is obtained by reading the full data once because we can calculate π_i^{LCC} based on i-th observation and determine whether to include i-th observation in the sample or not immediately after knowing π_i^{LCC}.

Algorithm 6 Local case–control subsampling

Input: $\{\boldsymbol{x}_i, y\}_{i=1}^n$, $\tilde{\boldsymbol{\beta}}^p$ (a pilot estimator)
Output: $\tilde{\boldsymbol{\beta}}^{\mathrm{LCC}}$
Initializing: $\mathcal{D} \leftarrow \varnothing$
for i in $\{1, 2, \ldots, n\}$ **do**
  generate $u_i \sim \mathrm{Uniform}(0, 1)$ and calculate $\pi_i^{\mathrm{LCC}} = |y_i - p(\boldsymbol{x}_i, \tilde{\boldsymbol{\beta}}^p)|$
  if $u_i < \pi_i^{\mathrm{LCC}}$ **then**
    $\mathcal{D} \leftarrow \mathcal{D} \cup \{(\boldsymbol{x}_i, y_i)\}$
  end if
end for
Estimation: Denote the obtained subsample as $\mathcal{D} = \{\boldsymbol{x}_i^*, y_i^*\}_{i=1}^r$. Calculate $\tilde{\boldsymbol{\beta}}^{\mathrm{uw}}$ according to (11) and the final LCC estimator is $\tilde{\boldsymbol{\beta}}^{\mathrm{LCC}} = \tilde{\boldsymbol{\beta}}^{\mathrm{uw}} + \tilde{\boldsymbol{\beta}}^p$.

From Algorithm 6, the actual subsample size is random, and with a consistent pilot estimator, the expected subsample size is asymptotically $n\mathbb{E}|y - p(\boldsymbol{x}, \boldsymbol{\beta})| = 2n[p(\boldsymbol{x}, \boldsymbol{\beta})\{1 - p(\boldsymbol{x}, \boldsymbol{\beta})\}] \le n/2$. Although this expected subsample size is at the same order of the full data sample size n, it can be much smaller than half of the full sample size for very imbalanced data. The authors derived the asymptotic distribution of $\tilde{\boldsymbol{\beta}}^{\mathrm{LCC}}$ unconditionally on the full data. The asymptotic variance of $\tilde{\boldsymbol{\beta}}^{\mathrm{LCC}}$ is twice as large as that of the full data MLE, if the logistic regression model is correct.

The idea of LCC sampling is extended to the softmax regression model (12) in [15], and the method is named as local uncertainty sampling (LUS). Given a pilot estimator $\tilde{\boldsymbol{\beta}}^p$, the authors proposed the following subsampling probabilities:

$$\pi(\boldsymbol{x}_i, y_i) = \begin{cases} \frac{1-q_i}{\theta - \max(q_i, 0.5\theta)} & \text{if } p_i(y_i, \tilde{\boldsymbol{\beta}}^p) = q_i \\ \min(1, 2q_i/\theta) & \text{otherwise,} \end{cases},$$

where $\theta \geq 1$ is a prespecified number so that the expected subsample size is no more than n/θ; and $q_i = \max\{0.5, p_i(0, \tilde{\boldsymbol{\beta}}^p), p_i(1, \tilde{\boldsymbol{\beta}}^p), p_i(2, \tilde{\boldsymbol{\beta}}^p), ..., p_i(B, \tilde{\boldsymbol{\beta}}^p)\}$. Denote the obtained subsample as $\mathcal{D} = \{\boldsymbol{x}_i^*, y_i^*\}_{i=1}^r$. The authors of [15] derived the conditional distribution of y_i^* given $\boldsymbol{x}_i^*$ as follows:

$$
\begin{aligned}
P(y_i^* = 0|\boldsymbol{x}_i^*) &= \frac{1}{1+\sum_{j=1}^B \exp\left\{\boldsymbol{\beta}_j^{\mathrm{T}}\boldsymbol{x}_i^* + \log\frac{\pi(\boldsymbol{x}_i^*, j)}{\pi(\boldsymbol{x}_i^*, 0)}\right\}}, \\
P(y_i^* = b|\boldsymbol{x}_i^*) &= \frac{\exp\left\{\boldsymbol{\beta}_b^{\mathrm{T}}\boldsymbol{x}_i^* + \log\frac{\pi(\boldsymbol{x}_i^*, b)}{\pi(\boldsymbol{x}_i^*, 0)}\right\}}{1+\sum_{j=1}^B \exp\left\{\boldsymbol{\beta}_j^{\mathrm{T}}\boldsymbol{x}_i^* + \log\frac{\pi(\boldsymbol{x}_i^*, j)}{\pi(\boldsymbol{x}_i^*, 0)}\right\}}, \quad b = 1, 2, \ldots, B.
\end{aligned}
\tag{17}
$$

Note that the Poisson subsampling is used, so $\{\boldsymbol{x}_i^*, y_i^*\}_{i=1}^r$ are i.i.d. conditional on $\tilde{\boldsymbol{\beta}}^p$. Thus, for a given $\tilde{\boldsymbol{\beta}}^p$, (17) can be used to construct the likelihood function for the subsample, and the final estimator $\tilde{\boldsymbol{\beta}}^{\mathrm{LUC}}$ is the MLE based on the sampled data.

5 Divide-and-Conquer and Updating Methods

This section introduces the divide-and-conquer method, which partitions the full data into smaller pieces, performs calculations on them separately, and then combines these calculation results to obtain a final estimator. Most updating methods also process data piece by piece, but in a sequential manner, so we will discuss several updating methods in this section as well.

5.1 *Divide-and-Conquer Methods*

Unlike the methods we have discussed in the previous sections that use part of the original full data or transformed full data to perform the final analysis, the divide-and-conquer approach provides another scheme to deal with massive data. This method partitions the whole dataset into K pieces, processes these K pieces separately to obtain relevant subdata statistics, and then aggregates these subdata statistics to obtain the final estimator. Note that although divide-and-conquer method can take the advantage of distributed and parallel computing facility, it may not save computing time if we have a single computer. Furthermore, there is no general approach to do the aggregation. One way is to use the simple average of the subdata estimators as the final estimator, but this may not have the highest estimation efficient. In the following, we will discuss how to aggregate subdata estimators for estimation equation [22] and how to determine the sparsity pattern for high-dimensional case [7].

A divide-and-conquer method was investigated by Lin and Xie [22] in terms of estimation equation. Let the independent full dataset be $\{z_i\}_{i=1}^n$, which satisfies that $\sum_{i=1}^{n} \mathbb{E}\{\psi(z_i, \boldsymbol{\beta}_t)\} = 0$ for some smooth function ψ, where $\boldsymbol{\beta}_t$ is the true parameter. The estimating equation estimator $\hat{\boldsymbol{\beta}}^{\mathrm{EE}}$ is the solution to

$$\sum_{i=1}^{n} \psi(z_i, \boldsymbol{\beta}) = 0. \tag{18}$$

Here, the model setup is quite general and it includes regression models if we let $z_i = (\boldsymbol{x}_i, y_i)$. If the full data volume is too large to be loaded in one machine, the authors of [22] proposed the aggregated estimating equation (AEE) estimator as presented in Algorithm 7. The divide-and-conquer method has an obvious benefit on memory efficiency because the full data are processed block by block, and we only record $\{\boldsymbol{C}_{\tilde{\boldsymbol{\beta}}_k}, \tilde{\boldsymbol{\beta}}_k\}$ for each block.

Algorithm 7 Divide-and-conquer method for estimation equation

Input: $\{z_i\}_{i=1}^{n}$

Output: $\tilde{\boldsymbol{\beta}}^{\mathrm{AEE}}$

1: Partition the full dataset into K blocks, $\{z_i^k\}_{i=1}^{n_k}$, where $n_1, \ldots, n_K$ ($\sum_{k=1}^{K} n_k = n$) are the number of observations in each block, respectively, and z_i^k is the i-th observation in the k-th block.

2: **for** $k \in \{1, 2, \ldots K\}$ **do**

3: obtain the k-th block estimator $\tilde{\boldsymbol{\beta}}_k$ by solving

$$\sum_{i=1}^{n_k} \psi(z_i^k, \boldsymbol{\beta}) = 0;$$

4: calculate

$$\boldsymbol{C}_{\tilde{\boldsymbol{\beta}}_k} = -\sum_{i=1}^{n_k} \dot{\psi}(z_i^k, \tilde{\boldsymbol{\beta}}_k),$$

where $\dot{\psi}(\cdot)$ is the gradient of $\psi(\cdot)$ with respect to $\boldsymbol{\beta}$.

5: Record $\{\boldsymbol{C}_{\tilde{\boldsymbol{\beta}}_k}, \tilde{\boldsymbol{\beta}}_k\}$.

6: **end for**

7: Obtain the aggregated estimating equation estimator as

$$\tilde{\boldsymbol{\beta}}^{\mathrm{AEE}} = \left\{\sum_{k=1}^{K} \boldsymbol{C}_{\tilde{\boldsymbol{\beta}}_k}\right\}^{-1} \sum_{k=1}^{K} \boldsymbol{C}_{\tilde{\boldsymbol{\beta}}_k} \tilde{\boldsymbol{\beta}}_k.$$

It was proved that $\tilde{\boldsymbol{\beta}}^{\mathrm{AEE}}$ is consistent to the original full data estimation equation estimator $\hat{\boldsymbol{\beta}}^{\mathrm{EE}}$ under some regularity conditions [22].

The divide-and-conquer approach is applied to the generalized linear model (13) with high-dimensional data in [7]. A penalty term is added to the log-likelihood in this setting to ensure sparsity, and the estimator is named as split-and-conquer estimator. The full data penalized estimator $\hat{\boldsymbol{\beta}}^{\mathrm{PL}}$ is defined as

$$\hat{\boldsymbol{\beta}}^{\mathrm{PL}} = \arg\max_{\boldsymbol{\beta}} \left\{ \sum_{i=1}^{n} \frac{\log f(y_i|\boldsymbol{x}_i, \boldsymbol{\beta})}{n} - \lambda(\boldsymbol{\beta}, b) \right\},$$

where $\lambda(\cdot)$ is the penalty function to ensure sparsity (some components of $\hat{\boldsymbol{\beta}}^{\mathrm{PL}}$ are 0), and b is the tuning parameter. The full dataset is partitioned into K blocks, and within each block, a coefficient estimator $\tilde{\boldsymbol{\beta}}_k^{\mathrm{PL}}$ is obtained for $k = 1, 2, \ldots, K$. Since $\tilde{\boldsymbol{\beta}}_k^{\mathrm{PL}}$'s are calculated from different data blocks, their sparsity patterns are typically different, and this complicates the aggregation step. The authors of [7] proposed the majority voting method to specify the sparsity pattern of the split-and-conquer estimator, denoted as $\tilde{\boldsymbol{\beta}}^{\mathrm{SC}} = (\tilde{\beta}_1^{\mathrm{SC}}, \ldots, \tilde{\beta}_d^{\mathrm{SC}})^{\mathrm{T}}$. The majority voting method sets

$$\tilde{\beta}_j^{\mathrm{SC}} = 0 \quad \text{if} \sum_{k=1}^{K} I(\tilde{\beta}_{k,j}^{\mathrm{PL}} \neq 0) \leq \omega, \quad j = 1, 2, \ldots, d,$$

where $\omega \in [0, K)$ controls the number of zeros in the final estimator. If $\omega = 0$, then $\tilde{\beta}_j^{\mathrm{SC}} = 0$ only if all $\tilde{\beta}_{k,j}^{\mathrm{PL}}$'s are 0; if $\omega \in [K-1, K)$, then $\tilde{\beta}_j^{\mathrm{SC}} = 0$ if any of $\tilde{\beta}_{k,j}^{\mathrm{PL}}$ is 0. The nonzero elements of $\tilde{\boldsymbol{\beta}}^{\mathrm{SC}}$ are obtained by aggregating the corresponding elements of $\tilde{\boldsymbol{\beta}}_k^{\mathrm{PL}}$, $k = 1, 2, \ldots, K$. The author proved that $\tilde{\boldsymbol{\beta}}^{\mathrm{SC}}$ and the full data estimator $\hat{\boldsymbol{\beta}}^{\mathrm{PL}}$ are asymptotically equivalent by showing that these two estimators have the same asymptotic variances. This method reduces the computational burden from $O(n^2 d)$ to $O(n^2 d)/K$ given that $d \gg n$, if the LARS algorithm proposed by Efron et al. [12] is used for linear regression.

Some other related investigations on the divide-and-conquer approach include [6, 30, 40, 44], among others. Note that K cannot grow too fast as N goes to infinity in order to obtain a good final estimator [22]. The choice of K is discussed in [30] in the smoothing spline setting, and the authors stated that the rate of K should be no faster than the sharp upper bound $O(n^{2s/(2s+1)})$ in order for the aggregated smooth spline estimator to attain the minimax optimal convergence rate, where s is the degree of smoothness of the true regression function. The authors of [6] studied statistical inferences with the divide-and-conquer approach for high-dimensional linear and generalized linear models. They obtained the order of K under which the error caused by the divide-and-conquer method is negligible compared with the statistical error. In [40], the adaptive LASSO estimator for the sparse Cox regression model is approximated through a three-step divide-and-conquer algorithm. The divide-and-conquer method was introduced to kernel ridge regression in [44] in which the final estimator could achieve a minimax optimal convergence rate.

5.2 Updating Methods

The aforementioned divide-and-conquer methods assume that all blocks of data are accessible simultaneously. For streaming data, one does not have access to all the data at a time and may not be able to store all the historical data. Thus, one needs to update the estimator as new data come in. The online updating method was introduced to deal with this situation. Stochastic gradient descent is a popular optimization method, which uses new data or sampled data to approximate the gradient of the objective function in each iterative step. This is essentially to update the estimator with new pieces of data, so we categorize it as an updating method here.

Online Updating Methods

Under the simple linear regression model, the online updating method for streaming data was investigated in [19], where the updating formulas for estimators of the intercept, the slope, and the model error variance are derived.

An online updating method based on the divide-and-conquer technique for estimating equation (18) is proposed in [29], and a novel cumulatively updated estimating equation (CUEE) estimator is developed. Suppose that in Algorithm 7, data blocks are coming sequentially, and each block of data is accessible only once. The CUEE estimator up to block k, $\tilde{\boldsymbol{\beta}}_k^{\text{CUEE}}$, is defined as

$$\tilde{\boldsymbol{\beta}}_k^{\text{CUEE}} = \left\{\sum_{i=1}^{k} \boldsymbol{C}_{\check{\boldsymbol{\beta}}_i}\right\}^{-1} \left\{\sum_{i=1}^{k} \boldsymbol{C}_{\check{\boldsymbol{\beta}}_i}\check{\boldsymbol{\beta}}_i + \sum_{i=1}^{k} \boldsymbol{u}_i(\check{\boldsymbol{\beta}}_i)\right\},$$

where

$$\check{\boldsymbol{\beta}}_k = \left(\sum_{i=1}^{k-1} \boldsymbol{C}_{\check{\boldsymbol{\beta}}_i} + \boldsymbol{C}_{\tilde{\boldsymbol{\beta}}_k}\right)^{-1} \left(\sum_{i=1}^{k-1} \boldsymbol{C}_{\check{\boldsymbol{\beta}}_i}\check{\boldsymbol{\beta}}_i + \boldsymbol{C}_{\tilde{\boldsymbol{\beta}}_k}\tilde{\boldsymbol{\beta}}_k\right),$$

$\boldsymbol{u}_k(\boldsymbol{\beta}) = \sum_{i=1}^{n_k} \psi(z_i^k, \boldsymbol{\beta})$, $\boldsymbol{C}_{\check{\boldsymbol{\beta}}_0} = \boldsymbol{0}_{d\times d}$ and $\check{\boldsymbol{\beta}}_0 = \boldsymbol{0}_d$. For the CUEE estimator, there is no need to store the raw data, and one only needs to store the following statistics for updating: $\sum_{i=1}^{k-1} \boldsymbol{C}_{\check{\boldsymbol{\beta}}_i}$, $\sum_{i=1}^{k-1} \boldsymbol{C}_{\check{\boldsymbol{\beta}}_i}\check{\boldsymbol{\beta}}_i$, and $\sum_{i=1}^{k-1} \boldsymbol{u}_i(\check{\boldsymbol{\beta}}_i)$. When the k-th data block arrives, these statistics are updated and $\tilde{\boldsymbol{\beta}}_k^{\text{CUEE}}$ is calculated. The author proved that the CUEE estimator is consistent to $\hat{\boldsymbol{\beta}}^{\text{EE}}$ under some regularity conditions. Another interesting problem studied by Wang et al. [37] is how to update the estimator when new covariate variables are introduced into the model at some time point k.

A method to approximate the MLE for GLMs with streaming data is proposed in [23], in which they focus on GLMs with a dispersion parameter in addition to the mean parameter $\boldsymbol{\beta}$ as shown in model (13). Let $\boldsymbol{U}_k(\boldsymbol{\beta})$ be the score function (the gradient of the log-likelihood function) and $\boldsymbol{J}_k(\boldsymbol{\beta})$ be the negative observed information matrix (the negative Hessian matrix of the log-likelihood function), for the mean parameter based on the k-th block of data, $k = 1, \ldots, K$. The proposed incremental updating algorithm obtains the updated estimator $\tilde{\boldsymbol{\beta}}_k^{\mathrm{RN}}$ when the k-th data block arrives by solving

$$\sum_{i=1}^{k-1} \boldsymbol{J}_i(\tilde{\boldsymbol{\beta}}_i^{\mathrm{RN}})(\tilde{\boldsymbol{\beta}}_{k-1}^{\mathrm{RN}} - \tilde{\boldsymbol{\beta}}_k^{\mathrm{RN}}) + \boldsymbol{U}_k(\tilde{\boldsymbol{\beta}}_{k-1}^{\mathrm{RN}}) = \mathbf{0}.$$

This chapter also provides the updating formula for estimating the dispersion parameter enabling one to perform real-time statistical inference. The resultant estimator is consistent to the true parameter and is asymptotically normal, and these asymptotic properties are true without imposing the condition that $K = O(n_k^{\nu})$ for some $\nu < \frac{1}{3}$ and any k which is needed in [22, 29].

Stochastic Gradient Descent

Stochastic gradient descent (SGD) is a popular optimization technique for massive data, which recursively updates estimators and discards the involving raw data in each step to improve the memory efficiency. Here we focus on a case of parameter estimation through the log-likelihood function which is presented as an optimization problem. Let $\{(\boldsymbol{x}_i, y_i)\}_{i=1}^n$ be i.i.d. data, and denote the log-likelihood for each data point as $\ell(y_i; \boldsymbol{x}_i, \boldsymbol{\beta})$. In this setting, the MLE $\hat{\boldsymbol{\beta}}_{\mathrm{MLE}}$ maximizes the log-likelihood function of the full data $\sum_{i=1}^n \ell(y_i; \boldsymbol{x}_i, \boldsymbol{\beta})$, and SGD is a commonly used maximization algorithm to approximate $\hat{\boldsymbol{\beta}}_{\mathrm{MLE}}$.

A popular classic SGD algorithm is defined as

$$\tilde{\boldsymbol{\beta}}_i^{\mathrm{sgd}} = \tilde{\boldsymbol{\beta}}_{i-1}^{\mathrm{sgd}} + \gamma_i \boldsymbol{D}_i \dot{\ell}(y_i; \boldsymbol{x}_i, \tilde{\boldsymbol{\beta}}_{i-1}^{\mathrm{sgd}}), \quad i = 1, 2, \ldots, n, \tag{19}$$

where $\dot{\ell}(y_i; \boldsymbol{x}_i, \boldsymbol{\beta}) = \partial \log \ell(y_i; \boldsymbol{x}_i, \boldsymbol{\beta}) / \partial \boldsymbol{\beta}$ is the gradient of the log-likelihood, $\gamma_i = O(n^{-c})$ is the learning rate, $c \in (0.5, 1]$, and $\boldsymbol{D}_i$ is a positive definite matrix which is often chosen to be the identity matrix or a diagonal matrix for computational efficiency. The learning rate is critical for the performance of an SGD algorithm. If γ_i's are too large, then the SGD procedure in (19) may not converge. To alleviate this problem, the authors of [31] proposed an implicit SGD algorithm that updates the parameter estimate $\tilde{\boldsymbol{\beta}}_i^{\mathrm{im}}$ in each step by solving

$$\tilde{\boldsymbol{\beta}}_i^{\mathrm{im}} = \tilde{\boldsymbol{\beta}}_{i-1}^{\mathrm{im}} + \gamma_i \boldsymbol{D}_i \dot{\ell}(y_i; \boldsymbol{x}_i, \tilde{\boldsymbol{\beta}}_i^{\mathrm{im}}).$$

The implicit SGD differs from the classic SGD in that the stochastic gradient in the i-th step is evaluated at the i-th estimate instead of previous estimate in the $(t-1)$-th step. The implicit SGD converges for a larger range of the learning rate, and the resulting estimator is consistent to the true parameter and shares the same asymptotic variance as that for the classic SGD estimator under mild conditions.

Another problem of the SGD is that only one data point $(\boldsymbol{x}_i, y_i)$ is used, so the gradient may have a large variance, resulting in a slow convergence rate of the algorithm. Mini-batch SGD alleviates this issue to some extent, but the computation burden can be high for a large batch size. Several methods have been proposed to reduce the variation of the gradient. Stochastic variance reduced gradient (SVRG) proposed by Johnson and Zhang [17] introduces an average gradient term, and the resulting algorithm has been proved to converge in a linear rate for a smooth and strong convex optimization target function.

The gradient variance can also be reduced by nonuniform sampling, which assigns different probabilities for different observations to be selected. This approach was discussed in [28, 45]. The nonuniform probabilities can be obtained by minimizing the variance of the gradient, which are proportional to the norms of the gradients. Calculating gradient norms for all observations in each step is computationally expensive. The authors of [45] constructed upper bounds of gradient norms that do not depend on $\boldsymbol{\beta}$ and use them to construct nonuniform sampling probabilities. Furthermore, a weighted SGD is used to ensure the unbiasedness, such as

$$\tilde{\boldsymbol{\beta}}_t^{\mathrm{sgd}} = \tilde{\boldsymbol{\beta}}_{t-1}^{\mathrm{sgd}} + \gamma_t \frac{\dot{\ell}(y_t; \boldsymbol{x}_t, \tilde{\boldsymbol{\beta}}_{t-1}^{\mathrm{sgd}})}{\pi_t^{\mathrm{IS}}}, \quad t = 1, 2, 3, \ldots,$$

where $(\boldsymbol{x}_t, y_t)$ is a random sample from the full data according to the sampling distribution $\{\pi_t^{\mathrm{IS}}\}_{t=1}^n$.

Using control variate is another way to reduce the variation of the stochastic gradient [35]. One uses a vector $\tilde{\dot{\ell}}(y_i; \boldsymbol{x}_i, \boldsymbol{\beta})$, which has the same expectation as $\dot{\ell}(y_i; \boldsymbol{x}_i, \boldsymbol{\beta})$ but has a smaller variance, to substitute the gradient $\dot{\ell}(y_i; \boldsymbol{x}_i, \boldsymbol{\beta})$. Here, $\tilde{\dot{\ell}}(y_i; \boldsymbol{x}_i, \boldsymbol{\beta})$ can be constructed as

$$\tilde{\dot{\ell}}(y_i; \boldsymbol{x}_i, \boldsymbol{\beta}) = \dot{\ell}(y_i; \boldsymbol{x}_i, \boldsymbol{\beta}) - \boldsymbol{A}^{\mathrm{T}}\{\kappa(y_i; \boldsymbol{x}_i, \boldsymbol{\beta}) - \kappa_e(\boldsymbol{\beta})\},$$

where $\kappa(y_i; \boldsymbol{x}_i, \boldsymbol{\beta})$ is the control variate with $\mathbb{E}\{\kappa(y_i; \boldsymbol{x}_i, \boldsymbol{\beta})\} = \kappa_e(\boldsymbol{\beta})$ and $\boldsymbol{A}$ is a $d \times d$ matrix obtained by minimizing $\mathbb{V}\{\tilde{\dot{\ell}}(y_i; \boldsymbol{x}_i, \boldsymbol{\beta})\}$. The control variate $\kappa(y_i; \boldsymbol{x}_i, \boldsymbol{\beta})$ is expected to be highly correlated with $\dot{\ell}(y_i; \boldsymbol{x}_i, \boldsymbol{\beta})$ to achieve the desired effect of variance reduction. Different optimization problems have different control variates, and a useful way is to construct the control variate is by using low-order moments. The author also discussed that $\boldsymbol{A}$ can be a diagonal matrix or even a single number to attain faster computational speed.

6 Summary and Discussion

We have selectively introduced several statistical methods aiming at reducing computational burden for massive datasets, including randomized numerical linear algebra, IBOSS, informative subsampling, and divide-and-conquer and updating methods. All of these methods exhibit excellent estimation efficiency and computation efficiency. Meanwhile, they all have their limitations. Based on different datasets and situations, we need to know how to choose an appropriate method.

Even though we have so many elegant methods to deal with big data problems, there are still many research problems remaining to be solved. Most of the methods require that the model is correctly specified. However, sometimes, it is hard to build a model accurately due to the complexity and diversity of the data. How to improve the robustness of existing methods is an important topic for future investigation. In addition, real data can have various complex structures and may contain a lot of noises, measurement errors, and censoring, which increase the difficulty to perform data analysis. More advanced methods and complex models are required to fulfill this need.

References

1. Ai, M., Yu, J., Zhang, H., Wang, H.Y.: Optimal subsampling algorithms for big data regressions. Stat. Sin. (2019). https://doi.org/10.5705/ss.202018.0439
2. Ailon, N., Chazelle, B.: Approximate nearest neighbors and the fast Johnson-Lindenstrauss transform. In: Proceedings of the Thirty-eighth Annual ACM Symposium on Theory of Computing, pp. 557–563 (2006)
3. Ailon, N., Chazelle, B.: The fast Johnson–Lindenstrauss transform and approximate nearest neighbors. SIAM J. Comput. **39**(1), 302–322 (2009)
4. Ailon, N., Liberty, E.: Fast dimension reduction using Rademacher series on dual BCH codes. Discrete Comput. Geom. **42**(4), 615 (2009)
5. Avron, H., Maymounkov, P., Toledo, S.: Blendenpik: Supercharging LAPACK's least-squares solver. SIAM J. Sci. Comput. **32**, 1217–1236 (2010)
6. Battey, H., Fan, J., Liu, H., Lu, J., Zhu, Z.: Distributed testing and estimation under sparse high dimensional models. Ann. Stat. **46**(3), 1352 (2018)
7. Chen, X., Xie, M.-g.: A split-and-conquer approach for analysis of extraordinarily large data. Stat. Sin. **24**, 1655–1684 (2014)
8. Chen, S., Varma, R., Singh, A., Kovačcević, J.: A statistical perspective of sampling scores for linear regression. In: 2016 IEEE International Symposium on Information Theory (ISIT), pp. 1556–1560. IEEE, Piscataway (2016)
9. Drineas, P., Mahoney, M.W., Muthukrishnan, S.: Sampling algorithms for l_2 regression and applications. In: Proceedings of the Seventeenth Annual ACM-SIAM Symposium on Discrete Algorithm, pp. 1127–1136. Society for Industrial and Applied Mathematics, Philadelphia (2006)
10. Drineas, P., Mahoney, M.W., Muthukrishnan, S., Sarlos, T.: Faster least squares approximation. Numer. Math. **117**, 219–249 (2011)
11. Drineas, P., Magdon-Ismail, M., Mahoney, M.W., Woodruff, D.P.: Faster approximation of matrix coherence and statistical leverage. J. Mach. Learn. Res. **13**, 3475–3506 (2012)

12. Efron, B., Hastie, T., Johnstone, I., Tibshirani, R., et al.: Least angle regression. Ann. Stat. **32**(2), 407–499 (2004)
13. Fan, J., Han, F., Liu, H.: Challenges of big data analysis. Natl. Sci. Rev. **1**(2), 293–314 (2014)
14. Fithian, W., Hastie, T.: Local case-control sampling: Efficient subsampling in imbalanced data sets. Ann. Stat. **42**(5), 1693 (2014)
15. Han, L., Tan, K.M., Yang, T., Zhang, T.: Local uncertainty sampling for large-scale multiclass logistic regression. Ann. Stat. **48**(3),1770–1788 (2020)
16. Johnson, W.B., Lindenstrauss, J.: Extensions of Lipschitz mappings into a Hilbert space. Contemp. Math. **26**, 189–206 (1984)
17. Johnson, R., Zhang, T.: Accelerating stochastic gradient descent using predictive variance reduction. In Advances in Neural Information Processing Systems, pp. 315–323 (2013)
18. Katzfuss, M.: A multi-resolution approximation for massive spatial datasets. J. Am. Stat. Assoc. **112**(517), 201–214 (2017)
19. Klotz, J.H.: Updating simple linear regression. Stat. Sin., **15**, 399–403 (1995)
20. Laney, D.: 3d data management: Controlling data volume, velocity and variety. META Group Res. Note **6**(70), 1 (2001)
21. Liang, F., Cheng, Y., Song, Q., Park, J., Yang, P.: A resampling-based stochastic approximation method for analysis of large geostatistical data. J. Am. Stat. Assoc. **108**(501), 325–339 (2013)
22. Lin, N., Xie, R.: Aggregated estimating equation estimation. Stat. Interface **4**, 73–83 (2011)
23. Luo, L., Song, P.X.-K.: Renewable estimation and incremental inference in generalized linear models with streaming data sets. J. R. Stat. Soc. B (Stat. Methodol.) **82**(1), 69–97 (2020)
24. Ma, P., Mahoney, M.W., Yu, B.: A statistical perspective on algorithmic leveraging. J. Mach. Learn. Res. **16**(1), 861–911 (2015)
25. Ma, P., Zhang, X., Xing, X., Ma, J., Mahoney, M.: Asymptotic analysis of sampling estimators for randomized numerical linear algebra algorithms. In International Conference on Artificial Intelligence and Statistics, pp. 1026–1035 (2020)
26. Mahoney, M.W.: Randomized algorithms for matrices and data. Found. Trends Mach. Learn. **3**(2), 123–224 (2011)
27. Martinsson, P.-G., Tropp. J.: Randomized numerical linear algebra: Foundations & algorithms (2020). Preprint. arXiv:2002.01387
28. Needell, D., Ward, R., Srebro, N.: Stochastic gradient descent, weighted sampling, and the randomized Kaczmarz algorithm. In: Advances in Neural Information Processing Systems, pp. 1017–1025 (2014)
29. Schifano, E.D., Wu, J., Wang, C., Yan, J., Chen, M.-H.: Online updating of statistical inference in the big data setting. Technometrics **58**(3), 393–403 (2016)
30. Shang, Z., Cheng, G.: Computational limits of a distributed algorithm for smoothing spline. J. Mach. Learn. Res. **18**(1), 3809–3845 (2017)
31. Toulis, P., Airoldi, E.M., et al.: Asymptotic and finite-sample properties of estimators based on stochastic gradients. Ann. Stat. **45**(4), 1694–1727 (2017)
32. Wang, H.Y.: Divide-and-conquer information-based optimal subdata selection algorithm. J. Stat. Theory Pract. **13**(3), 46 (2019)
33. Wang, H.Y.: More efficient estimation for logistic regression with optimal subsamples. J. Mach. Learn. Res. **20**(132), 1–59 (2019)
34. Wang, H., Ma, Y.: Optimal subsampling for quantile regression in big data. Biometrika, **108**(1), 99–112 (2021)
35. Wang, C., Chen, X., Smola, A.J., Xing, E.P.: Variance reduction for stochastic gradient optimization. In: Advances in Neural Information Processing Systems, pp. 181–189 (2013)
36. Wang, Y., Yu, A.W., Singh, A.: On computationally tractable selection of experiments in measurement-constrained regression models. J. Mach. Learn. Res. **18**(1), 5238–5278 (2017)
37. Wang, C., Chen, M.-H., Wu, J., Yan, J., Zhang, Y., Schifano, E.: Online updating method with new variables for big data streams. Canad. J. Stat. **46**(1), 123–146 (2018)
38. Wang, H.Y., Zhu, R., Ma, P.: Optimal subsampling for large sample logistic regression. J. Am. Stat. Assoc. **113**(522), 829–844 (2018)

39. Wang, H.Y., Yang, M., Stufken, J.: Information-based optimal subdata selection for big data linear regression. J. Am. Stat. Assoc. **114**(525), 393–405 (2019)
40. Wang, Y., Hong, C., Palmer, N., Di, Q., Schwartz, J., Kohane, I., Cai, T.: A fast divide-and-conquer sparse Cox regression. Biostatistics. **22**(2), 381–401 (2021)
41. Xie, R., Wang, Z., Bai, S., Ma, P., Zhong, W.: Online decentralized leverage score sampling for streaming multidimensional time series. Proc. Mach. Learn. Res. **89**, 2301 (2019)
42. Yao, Y., Wang, H.Y.: Optimal subsampling for softmax regression. Stat. Papers **60**, 585–599 (2018)
43. Yu, J., Wang, H., Ai, M., Zhang, H.: Optimal distributed subsampling for maximum quasi-likelihood estimators with massive data. J. Am. Stat. Assoc., 1–12 (2020). https://doi.org/10.1080/01621459.2020.1773832s
44. Zhang, Y., Duchi, J., Wainwright, M.: Divide and conquer kernel ridge regression: A distributed algorithm with minimax optimal rates. J. Mach. Learn. Res. **16**(1), 3299–3340 (2015)
45. Zhao, P., Zhang, T.: Stochastic optimization with importance sampling for regularized loss minimization. In International Conference on Machine Learning, pp. 1–9 (2015)

A Selective Overview of Recent Advances in Spectral Clustering and Their Applications

Yang Xu, Arun Srinivasan, and Lingzhou Xue

1 Introduction

In contrast to supervised learning, unsupervised learning provides a suite of techniques for the analysis of unlabeled data [28, 31], including principal components [14, 62, 78, 100, 101], graphical or network models [1, 10, 29, 34, 40, 42–44, 53, 87, 91, 93], and clustering. Grouping observations into clusters by similarity is a fundamental task in data mining. With the explosive growth of computing power and technological innovations, the amount of available data has increased astronomically. In many domains such as bioinformatics [60], geology [73], and economics [32], these data are considered *unlabeled*, that is, lacking group identifying information for each sample. Unlike classification algorithms that require each training data point to be *labeled*, clustering provides a powerful avenue to infer group memberships even when the latent group structure is completely unknown. For example, in bioinformatics, we may wish to use clustering methods to aid in Alzheimer's disease diagnosis or analyze complex gene expression data [3, 63]. In economics, these data may consist of many consumer response surveys that we wish to group for market analysis [36]. In these cases, unsupervised clustering algorithms are a powerful tool to group similar individuals into different classes.

Clustering techniques are extensively studied in the statistics and machine learning literature. Methods such as *k-means* and *hierarchical* clustering are among the most commonly used in day-to-day analysis. These methods are straightforward

Y. Xu
Department of Statistics, North Carolina State University, Raleigh, NC, USA
e-mail: yxu63@ncsu.edu.

A. Srinivasan · L. Xue (✉)
Department of Statistics, Pennsylvania State University, University Park, PA, USA
e-mail: uus91@psu.edu; lzxue@psu.edu

Y. Zhao, (Din) D.-G. Chen (eds.), *Modern Statistical Methods for Health Research*, Emerging Topics in Statistics and Biostatistics,
https://doi.org/10.1007/978-3-030-72437-5_12

Table 1 Notation for spectral clustering

Notation	Description
$G = (V, E)$	Undirected similarity graph
S, W, and A	Similarity, adjacency, and affinity matrix, respectively
$D = diag(d_1, \ldots, d_n)$	Degree matrix, where $d_i = \sum_{j=1}^{n} w_{ij}$
$L = D - S$	Laplacian matrix
$L_{sym} = D^{-\frac{1}{2}} L D^{-\frac{1}{2}}$	Normalized Laplacian matrix from a graph cut point of view
$L_{rw} = D^{-1} L$	Normalized Laplacian matrix from a random walk point of view
$\lambda_1 \leq \ldots \leq \lambda_n$	Eigenvalues of L
$u_1, \ldots, u_n$	Eigenvectors corresponding to $\lambda_1, \ldots, \lambda_n$
U	The embedding matrix
$w(A, B)$	Sum of weights between any pair of nodes in sets A and B
$\|A\|$	The number of vertices in A
$P = D^{-1} W$	Transition matrix from a random walk point of view
$\pi = (\pi_1, \ldots, \pi_n)'$	The stationary distribution of P

and computationally efficient to compute. In cases where clusters are separated by convex boundaries, these algorithms are often extremely accurate. However, when the boundary is non-convex, these simpler methods may fail to recover any sense of the underlying group structure. To assuage the effects of this limitation, *spectral clustering* methods were developed and quickly found much practical success.

In this selective overview, we delve into the expansive array of work on spectral clustering from its basic inception to modern developments. We explore the benefits of employing spectral clustering techniques as opposed to commonly used methods such as k-means and hierarchical clustering. First, we introduce the basic formulation of spectral clustering and its inception from graph-based algorithms. We explore the concept of the similarity matrix which will prove vital for further understanding the method. Next, we will explore both the unnormalized and normalized versions of spectral clustering as well as their relatedness to the kernel k-means algorithm. Moreover, we will study conventional methods to determine the number of clusters k, including general metrics and those specifically tailored to spectral clustering. We will then explore many modern innovations and extensions of spectral clustering before concluding with a brief discussion on important open questions within spectral clustering.

Before proceeding, we summarize the technical notation for spectral clustering and its extensions in Table 1.

2 Spectral Clustering

Spectral clustering is a well-known graph-based method to segment samples into different clusters [19]. In Shi and Malik [68], the term *normalized cut* was firstly proposed from graph cut point of view, in which we aim to minimize

$$Ncut\,(A, B) = \frac{cut(A, B)}{vol(A)} + \frac{cut(A, B)}{vol(B)}. \tag{1}$$

This formulation can maximize in-group weights and minimize between-group weights simultaneously, and we explain the notation and interpretation in a later section. Since finding the optimum of (1.1) is NP-complete, they relaxed the feasible domain to real values and transformed the Ncut problem to a generalized eigenvalue problem, i.e.

$$\min_x Ncut(x) = \min_y \frac{y^T(D - W)y}{y^T Dy},$$

which is equivalent to solving the eigen-decomposition of $D^{-\frac{1}{2}} W D^{-\frac{1}{2}}$.

This work is quite fundamental and forms the most commonly used normalized version of spectral clustering. Many advances were extended based on this framework. Motivated by its good empirical performance on real datasets, Ng et al. [56] enriched the theory of spectral clustering in both ideal case and general case. In the ideal case, i.e. any similarity between any two points from different clusters is zero, they guaranteed the availability of spectral clustering. In the general case when we cannot distinguish clearly k clusters among n points, they proved the robustness of spectral clustering under reasonable assumptions.

If we define $Y \in \mathbb{R}^{n\times k}$ as the first k eigenvectors and $y_j^{(i)}$ as the jth row of cluster i, where $i = 1, \ldots, k$, $j = 1, \ldots, n_i$, and $n = n_1, \ldots, n_k$, then we have the following theorem, whose proof can be found in Ng et al. [56].

Theorem 1 *We assume several mild assumptions as in Ng et al. [56]. Let*

$$\epsilon = \sqrt{k(k-1)\epsilon_1 + k\epsilon_2^2}.$$

If $\delta > (2 + \sqrt{2})\epsilon$, then there exist k orthogonal vectors $r_1, \ldots, r_k$ so that Y's rows satisfy

$$\frac{1}{n}\sum_{i=1}^{k}\sum_{j=1}^{n_i}\left\|y_j^{(i)} - r_i\right\|_2^2 \leq 4C\left(4 + 2\sqrt{k}\right)^2 \frac{\epsilon^2}{(\delta - \sqrt{2}\epsilon)},$$

for all $i = 1, \ldots, k$ and $j = 1, \ldots, n_i$.

Therefore, spectral clustering is a robust algorithm in which perturbations of the data do not yield clusters far different from the ideal setting under reasonable assumptions. Based on their works and contributions, spectral clustering gradually gained popularity with many extensions and applications in various fields.

2.1 The Similarity Matrix

Before running any spectral clustering algorithm, we must construct the similarity matrix that measures the pairwise similarity between any two samples. The construction of a similarity matrix relies on two key decisions. Firstly, we must choose a proper pairwise similarity function. Secondly, we must decide what structure of similarity graph to use. As to the former, the Gaussian kernel function is most commonly used, i.e.

$$A_{ij} = \exp\{- \left\| x_i - x_j \right\|^2 / 2\sigma^2\}.$$

On the other hand, there are a wide range of options to compute the similarity matrix. The three popular methods to construct the similarity matrix are a σ-neighborhood graph, k-nearest neighbor graph (kNN), and a fully connected graph, which we will explore in turn.

In a σ-neighborhood graph, we connect the edge in similarity graph G if and only if $w_{ij} > \sigma$. However, if graph G contains clusters with different scales, it is hard to find a single σ to present the true grouping relationship of samples.

In a k-nearest neighbor graph (kNN), for any node i, we only connect it to the k nearest nodes. Thus, we obtain a directed graph with an asymmetric similarity matrix. The asymmetric nature is challenging for analysis, and thus there are multiple ways to enforce symmetry. The first way is through enforcing an undirected graph structure, also denoted as a kNN graph. In this framework, edge e_{ij} between node i and node j exists if any one of them is among the k nearest neighbor of the other. Another way is through a mutual kNN graph. In this setting, e_{ij} exists if and only if both node i and node j are among the k nearest neighbor of each other. From the perspective of handling samples in different scales, this type of graph is generally better than σ-neighborhood graph. On the one hand, the kNN graph often connects vertices in low-density regions[1] with those in high-density regions. Furthermore, some dense clusters may be separated into several parts due to the limitation of k neighbors. On the other hand, a mutual kNN graph is inclined to connect vertices in regions with constant density. This is because an edge between two vertices in different density regions is more likely to be a directed edge, which will be neglected when constructing the mutual kNN graph.

The third and most commonly used graph structure is the fully connected graph. In this setting, we must decide the value of σ. One straightforward way is to run the algorithm repeatedly for a number of values of σ to choose the one with the smallest distortion [56]. However, this method significantly increases the computational complexity of the algorithm. When dealing with a dataset with different groups of samples in comparatively different density regions, using only one σ to measure

[1]Density regions: a subgraph of G with many interconnected nodes is a *density region*. Usually, the higher the pairwise similarity between nodes is, the denser the region is.

the degree of variance inside samples is obviously not enough. Thus, a local scaling method is proposed to handle this situation [94]. That is, we can calculate a local σ_i for each sample x_i as $\sigma_i = d\left(x_i, x_q\right)$, where x_q is the qth neighbor of point x_i and $d(\cdot, \cdot)$ denotes a distance function. Then,

$$\hat{A}_{ij} = \exp\left\{\frac{-d\left(x_i, x_j\right)}{\sigma_i \sigma_j}\right\}.$$

2.2 *Unnormalized Spectral Clustering*

Suppose that we have data matrix $X = (x_1, \ldots, x_n) \in \mathbb{R}^{m \times n}$ with n samples to be grouped into k clusters. Given a similarity matrix, the goal is to find a reasonable grouping to divide samples with low similarity into different clusters and assign samples with high similarity into the same cluster. If we regard every sample as a node in a graph and the pairwise similarity between x_i and x_j as the weight between nodes i and j in graph G, then we can transform a clustering problem to a graph partitioning problem in similarity graph $G = (V, E)$.

In the original spectral clustering, we construct a Laplacian matrix $L = D - S$, where S denotes the similarity matrix between samples, and D is a diagonal matrix whose diagonal element satisfies $D_{ii} = \sum_j S_{ij}$. We denote the pairwise similarity between nodes i and j as w_{ij} and define $\lambda_1, \ldots, \lambda_n$ as n increasing eigenvalues of L with their corresponding eigenvectors $u_1, \ldots, u_n$.

Some basic properties of L are summarized as follows:

1. L is a symmetric and positive semidefinite matrix.
2. $\forall f \in \mathbb{R}^n,\ f^T L f = \frac{1}{2}\sum_{i,j=1}^{n} w_{ij}(f_i - f_j)^2$.
3. $0 = \lambda_1 \leqslant \lambda_1 \leqslant \ldots \leqslant \lambda_n,\ u_1 = \mathbf{1}_n$.
4. The multiplicity k of eigenvalue 0 of L equals the number of connected components $A_1, \ldots, A_k$ in graph G.

The derivation of these properties can be found in [77].

Thus, in the ideal case when graph G has k completely separated connected components, both similarity matrix S and Laplacian matrix L will have a blockwise structure after rearranging the order of nodes:

$$L = \begin{pmatrix} L_1 & & & \\ & L_2 & & \\ & & \cdots & \\ & & & L_k \end{pmatrix},$$

where the samples in L_i are the same as the ones in A_i. The first k eigenvectors $u_1, \ldots, u_k$, the eigenvectors corresponding to the smallest k eigenvalues (which are all 0 in the ideal case), are called indicator vectors. Define

$$U = (u_1, \dots, u_k) = \left(u_{(1)}, \dots, u_{(n)}\right)^T \in \mathbb{R}^{n\times k},$$

as the embedding matrix. U can be regarded as an embedding of samples from $\mathbb{R}^m$ to $\mathbb{R}^k$. Note every column $u_{(i)}$ contains only one nonzero component implying its grouping information.

However, in general cases, samples are not clearly clustered into their true groups due to errors in real data. Thus, the pairwise similarity between two nodes from different clusters is always nonzero, which means that we should add a small perturbation matrix H on the ideal similarity matrix S. Define $\widetilde{S} := S + H$, then the first k eigenvalues of $\tilde{L} = \tilde{D} - \tilde{A}$ are not all 0, and the elements in embedding matrix $\tilde{U}$ are not all 0 or 1. But in perturbation theory [70], the bias between $\tilde{U}$ and U can be bounded according to the Davis–Kahan theorem [21, 70]. Thus, in most real settings where there is only one connected component in graph G, our goal is to minimize the following objective function:

$$\min_{A_1,\dots,A_k} \sum_{l=1}^{k} \sum_{i\in A_l} (u_{(i)} - \mu_l)^2,$$

where $\mu_l = \frac{1}{|A_l|}\sum_{i\in A_l} u_{(i)}$. This objective is equivalent to the objective function of the k-means algorithm. Thus, after obtaining the embedding matrix U based on the spectral decomposition of Laplacian matrix L, the only thing left to derive the desired grouping structure is to implement k-means algorithm on the rows of U.

Algorithm 1 Unnormalized spectral clustering

Require: S: similarity matrix; k: the number of clusters;
Ensure: Segmentation for n samples
Calculate the Laplacian matrix $L = D - S$;
Compute the first k eigenvectors of L, and note it as embedding matrix $U = (u_1, \dots, u_k)$;
Let $U = \left(u_{(1)}, \dots, u_{(n)}\right)^T$, and regard $u_{(i)}$ as a projection of node i on $\mathbb{R}^k$;
Implement k-means algorithm on $\{u_{(i)}\}_{i=1}^n$.

Unnormalized spectral clustering has its interpretation in graph cut point of view:

Proposition 1 *Unnormalized spectral clustering with L is equivalent to a relaxed Ratiocut problem, which aims to minimize*

$$Ratiocut(A_1, \dots, A_k) = \frac{1}{2}\sum_{i=1}^{k} \frac{w(A_i, \overline{A_i})}{|A_i|},$$

where A_i contains samples belonging to cluster i, and $\overline{A_i}$ is the complementary set of A_i.

Proof Define k indicator vectors $u_j = (u_{1j}, \ldots, u_{nj})^T$ by

$$u_{ij} = \begin{cases} 1/\sqrt{|A_j|} & if v_i \in A_j \\ 0 & otherwise. \end{cases} \quad (2)$$

Let $U = (u_1, \ldots, u_k)$, which satisfies $U^T U = I$. Then,

$$Ratiocut(A_1, \ldots, A_k) = \sum_{j=1}^{k} u_j^T L u_j = tr(U^T LU),$$

$$\min Ratiocut(A_1, \ldots, A_k) \Leftrightarrow \min_{A_1,\ldots,A_k} tr(U^T LU), \text{ s.t. } U^T U = I.$$

If we relax the ratio cut problem by neglecting (2), the question is transformed to the spectral decomposition of L, which is equivalent to unnormalized spectral clustering. The proof of Proposition 1 is complete.

Thus, as a nonlinear graph-based partition method, spectral clustering aims to find a cut that can minimize between-group weights and maximize in-group weights. Furthermore, the algorithm makes a trade-off for sample size, aiming to obtain a partition with averagely separated clusters. Since k-means can only linearly segment samples, grouping results of spectral clustering are always better than normal methods like k-means and hierarchical clustering especially in detecting connections of complicated datasets.

2.3 *Normalized Spectral Clustering*

With the development of unnormalized spectral clustering, there are two natural modifications of the Laplacian matrix: L_{sym} and L_{rw}. These modifications arise from the graph cut and random walk points of view, respectively.

Proposition 2 *Normalized spectral clustering with L_{sym} is equivalent to a relaxed Ncut (normalized cut) problem, which minimizes*

$$Ncut(A_1, \ldots, A_k) = \frac{1}{2} \sum_{i=1}^{k} \frac{w(A_i, \overline{A_i})}{vol(A_i)}.$$

That is to say, we have the following equivalence relationship:

$$\min Ncut(A_1, \ldots, A_k) \Leftrightarrow \min_{A_1,\ldots,A_k} tr(U^T L_{sym} U), \text{ s.t. } U^T U = I.$$

Proposition 3 *Suppose that we run the random walk $(X_t)_{t\in\mathbb{R}}$ with transition matrix P. Define*

$$P(B|A) = P(X_1 \in B|X_0 \in A),$$

in which A and B are two disjoint subsets of V. Then,

$$Ncut(A, \overline{A}) = P(A|\overline{A}) + P(\overline{A}|A).$$

To prove the two propositions above, see [4, 48, 77] for more details.

One thing to note is that after obtaining the embedding matrix of L_{sym}, a normalization step on every row of U is needed before applying k-means. If we denote u_{sym} and u_{rw}, respectively, as the eigenvectors of L_{sym} and L_{rw} corresponding to eigenvalue λ, then we have $u_{sym} = D^{\frac{1}{2}}u_{rw}$. In real settings, L_{sym} is commonly used in spectral clustering, since

$$Ncut = \frac{1}{2}\sum_{i=1}^{k}\frac{w(A_i, \overline{A_i})}{vol(A_i)} = \frac{1}{2}\sum_{i=1}^{k}\left(1 - \frac{w(A_i, A_i)}{vol(A_i)}\right).$$

Thus, normalized spectral clustering not only minimizes the weights between groups but also maximizes the weights inside every group simultaneously. However, there is no such property for unnormalized spectral clustering due to the difference of denominator.

Algorithm 2 Normalized spectral clustering

Require: S: similarity matrix; k: the number of clusters;
Ensure: Segmentation for n samples

1: Calculate normalized Laplacian matrix $L_{sym} = I - D^{-\frac{1}{2}}SD^{-\frac{1}{2}}$;
2: Compute the first k eigenvectors of L_{sym} and note it as $U = (u_1, \ldots, u_k)$;
3: Calculate $\widetilde{U} = D^{-\frac{1}{2}}U$;
4: Let $\widetilde{U} = \left(u_{(1)}, \ldots, u_{(n)}\right)^T$, and regard $u_{(i)}$ as a projection of node i on $\mathbb{R}^k$;
5: Implement k-means algorithm on $\{u_{(i)}\}_{i=1}^n$.

2.4 Equivalence to Weighted Kernel k-Means

Kernel k-means and spectral clustering both are nonlinearly separable methods in sample space. Both methods, however, are closely related. Dhillon et al. [24] proved that normalized spectral clustering, normalized cuts, and a specific weighted kernel k-means are all equivalent. This is an important finding for spectral clustering, since it provides an easier and more efficient way to calculate the embedding matrix instead of implementing time-consuming eigenvector-based algorithms.

Proposition 4 *Normalized spectral clustering, normalized cuts, and weighted kernel k-means are all equivalent algorithms.*

Proof First, we begin by presenting the following equivalence statements for normalized spectral clustering. By manipulating the optimization target, we can therefore translate normalized spectral clustering into the framework of weighted kernel k-means.

$$\begin{aligned}&\text{Normalized Spectral Clustering}\\ &\Leftrightarrow \text{relaxed } \min Ncut(A_1, \ldots, A_k)\\ &\Leftrightarrow \min_{U\in\mathbb{R}^{n\times k}} tr(U^T LU), \text{ s.t. } U^T DU = I \\ &\Leftrightarrow \max_{Z\in\mathbb{R}^{n\times k}} tr(Z^T D^{-\frac{1}{2}} AD^{-\frac{1}{2}} Z), \text{ s.t. } Z^T Z = I.\end{aligned} \tag{3}$$

After some manipulation, weighted kernel k-means is equivalent to the following formulation:

$$\min D(\{\pi_j\}_{j=1}^k) := \sum_{j=1}^{k} \sum_{\alpha\in\pi_j} w(\alpha) \left\|\phi(\alpha) - m_j\right\|^2, \tag{4}$$

where ϕ is a nonlinear projection, and

$$m_j = \frac{\sum_{b\in\pi_j} w(b)\phi(b)}{\sum_{b\in\pi_j} \phi(b)}.$$

This optimization problem can be further expressed as

$$\begin{aligned}&\min_{W_1,\ldots,W_k} tr(W^{\frac{1}{2}}\phi^T\phi W^{\frac{1}{2}}) - tr(Y^T W^{\frac{1}{2}}\phi^T\phi W^{\frac{1}{2}}Y)\\ \Leftrightarrow &\max_{W_1,\ldots,W_k} tr(Y^T W^{\frac{1}{2}} K W^{\frac{1}{2}} Y),\end{aligned} \tag{5}$$

where W is a diagonal matrix of all the w weights, and W_i is the diagonal matrix of the weights in π_i. We also note that

$$Y = \begin{bmatrix} W_1^{\frac{1}{2}}\mathbf{1}/\sqrt{s_1} & & \\ & \cdots & \\ & & W_k^{\frac{1}{2}}\mathbf{1}/\sqrt{s_k}\end{bmatrix},$$

$Y^T Y = I$, and $s = \sum_{\alpha\in\pi_j} w(\alpha)$.

If we let $W = D$ and $K = D^{-1}AD^{-1}$, then we can obtain the equivalence between spectral clustering and weighted kernel k-means. Therefore, the proof of Proposition 4 is complete.

This equivalence between spectral clustering and weighted kernel k-means provides two key takeaways:

1. When the number of vertices n is large, it is often time consuming to compute the eigenvectors of Laplacian matrix L_{sym}. Therefore, the iteration algorithm of k-means can be used to solve the spectral clustering problem quickly.
2. When using k-means for clustering, we can use the indicator vectors calculated by spectral clustering to initialize k-means algorithm. It is conceivable that this initialization can avoid local minimum issues in k-means to some extent.

2.5 *Selecting the Total Number of Clusters*

Choosing the number of clusters is a widely discussed question in clustering. Recently, a variety of methods have been proposed to choose k, which can be divided into the model-dependent and model-independent paradigms. Previous work has established a criterion to choose k under certain assumptions of data [27], but in a broader sense, it is challenging to decide a well-justified method that is applicable on any dataset. We will firstly summarize popular criteria that are not limited to clustering methods and then present two approaches that are only applicable to spectral clustering.

General Clustering-Independent Criteria

In Milligan et al. [55], thirty procedures to determine the number of clusters are summarized and examined with a Monte Carlo simulation. Later in Celeux et al. [8], the authors decomposed the log-likelihood of the mixture problem into two parts and constructed a criterion NEC(K) based on the entropy of the decomposition. Sugar et al. [72] proposed a *jumping method* by revising the distortion term d_K to present a jumping of distortion around the true number of clusters, which is also a popular approach based on information theory. Tibshirani et al. [74] focused on the difference between the pairwise distances in all clusters. By selecting an appropriate null distribution for the distances, they select the number of clusters by maximizing the gap statistic defined by the pairwise distances. In [25], Evanno et al. revised the model based on the work of Pritchard et al. [65], in which a Bayesian posterior probability $Pr(X|K)$ is estimated to determine the number of clusters. We refer to the original manuscripts for notation details and statistical properties.

Cluster Selection Criteria Specific to Spectral Clustering

There are two methods for assessing the number of desired clusters in the framework of spectral clustering. Broadly, these methods rely on statistics derived from the underlying set of eigenvalues and eigenvectors. We summarize the two methods as follows:

1. Calculate the largest eigengap $\lambda_{i+1} - \lambda_i$ and then set the cluster number $k = i$.
2. Define $X \in \mathbb{R}^{n \times K}$ as the eigenvectors obtained by the solution to the associated eigen problem and $Z \in \mathbb{R}^{n \times K}$ as the standard eigenvectors with only one nonzero constant 1 in each row. Then, there must exist a rotation matrix $R \in \mathbb{R}^{k \times k}$ such that $Z = XR$. The objective is to find a cluster number k and a rotation matrix R that minimizes

$$\min_R J = \sum_{i=1}^{n} \sum_{j=1}^{k} \frac{Z_{ij}^2}{M_i^2}, \tag{6}$$

where $M_i = \max_j Z_{ij}$ [94].

Method 1 is more commonly used and is more efficient than Method 2, which only relies on the information of eigenvalues. Method 2 can obtain more information from eigenvectors but is time consuming in practice. Often, a trade-off between both methods is used to obtain a reasonable assessment of cluster number.

Based on the developments of choosing K and local scaling, a modified algorithm is proposed in normalized spectral clustering [94], which self-tunes the number of clusters.

Algorithm 3 Self-tuning normalized spectral clustering

Require: $X = (x_1, \ldots, x_n) \in \mathbb{R}^{m \times n}$: n data samples in $\mathbb{R}^m$
Ensure: Segmentation for n samples
1: Calculate local scale σ_i for each data point x_i.
2: Construct similarity matrix $\hat{A}$ and its Laplacian matrix L or L_{sym}.
3: Choose the largest cluster number k that minimized J in Formula (1.6), and denote it as k_{best}.
4: Take the alignment result Z of the first k_{best} eigenvectors (In normalized case, the eigenvectors should be normalized by row first) and assign x_i to cluster c if and only if $max_j \left(Z_{ij}^2\right) = Z_{ic}^2$.
5: In highly noisy datasets, regard the previous step result as the initialization of k-means or EM algorithm and implement them for more precise clustering.

3 New Developments of Spectral Clustering

In order to extend the applications of spectral clustering, much progress has been made in recent years to solve open questions in various fields. In this section, we will describe Spectral Biclustering, Multi-view Spectral Clustering, High-Order,

Constrained, Evolutionary, Incremental, and Sparse Spectral Clustering in detail. For each, we will study their theory, methods, algorithms, and applications primarily in bioinformatics and image processing.

3.1 Spectral Biclustering

Spectral co-clustering, or spectral biclustering, is a method to co-cluster two indices at the same time. Spectral biclustering was first proposed by Dhillon et al. [23] to solve the problem of matching specific words to documents. It was soon extended by Kluger et al. [35] to analyze genetic microarray data. Cano et al. proposed the Possibilistic Spectral Biclustering (PSB) algorithm based on Fuzzy Technology [7]. We will briefly summarize Dhillon's work and the extension explored by Kluger. For more details and other works related to biclustering, we recommend [16, 64].

In microarray data analysis, we study the expression level of genes under certain experimental conditions. This can be represented as a gene-by-condition matrix with rows and columns representing genes and conditions, respectively. If we define this data matrix as $A = \left(A_{ij}\right) \in \mathbb{R}^{m\times n}$, then our goal is to find the relationship between the subset of m genes and n experimental conditions.

Let $G = (M, N, E)$ denote the bipartite graph. In this framework, we can align genes and conditions together and construct a $(m+n)$ by $(m+n)$ similarity matrix as below:

$$\tilde{A} := \begin{pmatrix} 0 & A \\ A^T & 0 \end{pmatrix}.$$

Since relationship between different genes or different conditions is not of interest for clustering, it is reasonable to set the block-diagonal elements of A as zero. The new diagonal matrix and the Laplacian matrix can be constructed in the identical way as ordinary spectral clustering:

$$D = \begin{pmatrix} D_1 & 0 \\ 0 & D_2 \end{pmatrix}, \quad L = D - \tilde{A} = \begin{pmatrix} D_1 & -A \\ -A^T & D_2 \end{pmatrix},$$

where $D_1\left(i,i\right) = \sum_{j=1}^{n} A_{ij}$, $D_2\left(j,j\right) = \sum_{i=m}^{n} A_{ij}$. By implementing normalized spectral clustering on L, the objective function can be expressed as

$$\min_{U\in\mathbb{R}^{(m+n)\times k}} tr\left(U^T\overline{L}U\right), \text{ s.t. } U^TU = I, \tag{7}$$

in which $\overline{L} = D^{-\frac{1}{2}}LD^{-\frac{1}{2}}$.

Owing to the high dimensionality of L, solving this optimization problem directly is extremely time consuming. Fortunately, the optimal solution of (7) can be calculated by

$$U = \begin{pmatrix} D_1^{-\frac{1}{2}} V_1 \\ D_2^{-\frac{1}{2}} V_2 \end{pmatrix},$$

where V_1 and V_2 are the left and right eigenvectors of $D_1^{-\frac{1}{2}} A D_2^{-\frac{1}{2}}$, respectively.

The derivation of this optimum can be easily obtained via expanding the expression of $\overline{L}$. Thus, we have transformed the original optimization to a $m \times n$ dimensional Singular Value Decomposition (SVD) problem, which can be more easily handled computationally. After obtaining H, the embedding matrix, the procedure implements the k-means algorithm to find the groupings in which certain subsets of genes and conditions are assigned to the same cluster.

However, this method contains a critical drawback: the number of gene clusters must be the same as the number of experimental conditions. This is often unnecessary in practical settings. Therefore, Kluger et al. [35] developed another interpretation to the structure of gene-by-condition matrix A. The authors assumed that the data matrix will have a checkerboard structure after rearranging its entries. It can be proved that for matrices $A^T A$ and AA^T, there must exist stepwise constant eigenvectors u and v that correspond to the same eigenvalue λ. Thus, after the normalization of A, they proposed three methods: independent scaling, bistochastization, and log interactions. We can calculate the first several left and right eigenvectors of the corresponding matrix. Therefore, we can decide the cluster number of genes and conditions by considering the result of fitting the eigenvectors to a step-like structure.

Application of spectral biclustering is not limited to microarray data analysis. Any expression data with two different indices waiting to be clustered can be expressed as a biclustering problem. By looking for the relationship between different conditions and expression profiles, we may find more detailed meanings of gene expression, which helps to make progress in our understanding of the underlying biological mechanism.

3.2 *Multi-View Spectral Clustering*

In practical clustering analysis, we may obtain multiple views of the same samples. For instance, in order to explore brain networks, various methods, such as MRI, diffusion tensor imaging (DTI), and diffusion spectrum imaging (DSI), were proposed to analyze and obtain the same structural clusters. Therefore, there exist several similarity matrices regarding different informative representations of the data. How to integrate the similarity matrices, i.e. the results of spectral clustering in different views, is of vital importance in obtaining a more accurate and consistent clustering. There have been many different methods proposed to solve this problem. Chaudhuri et al. used the Canonical Correlation Analysis (CCA)-based method to project the data in each view to a lower dimensional subspace, making it possible to process multi-view objects at the same time [12]. Zhou et al. used mixtures of Markov chains on multiple graphs to combine multiple view results [96]. Kumar and Daume implemented the co-training idea in semi-supervised learning to spectral clustering, which merges the results of different views by iteration [38]. However, the use of this method is practically prohibitive due to the computation time spent in iteration, which increases with the number of views. Li et al. proposed an iteration-based algorithm on bipartite graphs to obtain a weighted model for multi-view objects [45]. In Kumar et al., two co-regularization schemes are proposed which are commonly used in bioinformatics [39].

Assume that the true underlying clustering will assign corresponding points in each view to the same cluster. Then, there exist corresponding Laplacian matrices $L^{(1)}, \ldots, L^{(p)}$ in each of the p views. Define a measure of disagreement between clustering schemes between any pair of views as follows:

$$D(U^{(v)}, U^{(w)}) := \left\| \frac{KU^{(v)}}{\left\|U^{(v)}\right\|_F^2} - \frac{KU^{(w)}}{\left\|U^{(w)}\right\|_F^2} \right\|_F^2 .$$

If K is a linear kernel, i.e. $KU^{(v)} = U^{(v)}U^{(v)T}$, then

$$D(U^{(v)}, U^{(w)}) = -tr(U^{(v)}U^{(v)^T}U^{(w)}U^{(w)^T}).$$

A natural innovation is to add a penalty term to the objective function of the original spectral clustering and combine the results of multiple views. In doing so, the procedure makes a trade-off between the clustering schemes under different views:

$$\min_{U^{(1)},\ldots,U^{(p)}\in\mathbb{R}^{n\times k}} \sum_{v=1}^{p} tr\left(U^{(v)^T}L^{(v)}U^{(v)}\right) + \lambda \sum_{1\le v,w\le p, v\ne w} tr\left(U^{(v)}U^{(v)^T}U^{(w)}U^{(w)^T}\right)$$

$$\text{s.t. } U^{(v)^T}U^{(v)} = I,\ \forall 1 \le v \le p,$$

which is equivalent to

$$\min_{U^{(v)}} tr\left\{U^{(v)^T}(L^{(v)} + \lambda \sum_{1\le w\le p, w\ne v} U^{(w)}U^{(w)^T})U^{(v)}\right\},\ \text{s.t. } U^{(v)^T}U^{(v)} = I. \tag{8}$$

The following iteration algorithm can be employed to the target (8):

1. With all $U^{(w)}, w \in \{1, \ldots, p\}$ but $U^{(v)}$ fixed, implement traditional spectral clustering to solve formula (8), in which the new Laplacian matrix is

$$L = L^{(v)} + \lambda \sum_{1\leqslant w\leqslant p, w\ne v} U^{(w)}U^{(w)T}.$$

2. Update to the next v, and repeat step 1.
3. Repeat the process until convergence.

Another one is a centroid-based co-regularization approach, which added a consensus embedding matrix U^* to the optimization function. Then, we have

$$\min_{U^{(1)},\ldots,U^{(p)},U^*\in\mathbb{R}^{n\times k}} \sum_{v=1}^{p} tr\left(U^{(v)^T} L^{(v)} U^{(v)}\right) + \sum_{v} \lambda_v tr\left(U^{(v)} U^{(v)^T} U^* U^{*T}\right) \tag{9}$$

$$\text{s.t. } U^{(v)^T} U^{(v)} = I, \forall 1 \leq v \leq p,\ U^{*T} U^* = I.$$

A similar alternate minimization algorithm can be implemented here in centroid framework (9):

1. With consensus eigenvectors U^* and all $U^{(w)}$, $w \in \{1, \ldots, p\}$ but $U^{(v)}$ fixed,

$$\min_{U^{(v)}\in \boldsymbol{R}^{n\times k}} tr(U^{(v)T} L^{(v)} U^{(v)}) + \lambda_v tr(U^{(v)} U^{(v)T} U^* U^{*T}),\ \text{s.t. } U^{(v)^T} U^{(v)} = I.$$

That is, regard this problem as traditional spectral clustering with a modified Laplacian matrix $L = L^{(v)} + \lambda_v U^* U^{*T}$;

2. With all $U^{(w)}$, $w \in \{1, \ldots, p\}$ fixed,

$$\max_{U^*\in \boldsymbol{R}^{n\times k}} \sum_{v} \lambda_v tr(U^{(v)} U^{(v)T} U^* U^{*T}) = \max_{U^*\in \boldsymbol{R}^{n\times k}} tr\left\{U^{*T}\left(\sum_{v} \lambda_v (U^{(v)} U^{(v)T})\right) U^*\right\}.$$

Similarly, regard this problem as traditional spectral clustering with a modified Laplacian matrix $L = \sum_v \lambda_v (U^{(v)} U^{(v)T})$;

3. Update to the next v and repeat (1) and (2);
4. Repeat the process until convergence.

Note that centroid-based method is less computationally intensive than the former approach. We can simply use U^* as the final embedding matrix representing all the views.

Recently, new methods were proposed based on separating the similarity matrix into two parts: a latent matrix with low dimensions and a noise matrix. The LRR model proposed by Xia [83] aims to solve

$$\min_{Z,E_i} \|Z\|_* + \lambda \sum_{i\in V} \|E_i\|_1,\ \text{s.t. } X_i = X_i Z + E_i, i = 1, \ldots, V, \tag{10}$$

where $X_i \in \mathbb{R}^{d_i\times n}$ denotes the data feature presentation for the ith view and E_i is the noise matrix of ith view. Later, Wang et al. improved this method by solving

$$\min_{Z_i,E_i} \sum_{i \in V} [\|Z_i\|_* + \lambda_1 \|E_i\|_1 + \lambda_2 \|Z_i\|_1 + \lambda_3 tr\left(Z_i^T L_i Z_i\right) + \frac{\beta}{2} \sum_{j \in V, j \neq i} \|Z_i - Z_j\|_2^2] \tag{11}$$

$$\text{s.t. } X_i = X_i Z + E_i,\ Z_i \geq 0,\ i = 1, \ldots, V,$$

and further extended his work in [81]. These methods all perform better than previous work, like co-training multi-view spectral clustering in [38] and [39].

As an effective tool to combine different views, multi-view spectral clustering can be broadly used in many fields such as multi-lingual information retrieval, webpage data and image processing, etc. In Chen et al.'s work [13], multi-view spectral clustering was used to integrate diffusion tensor imaging (DTI) and functional MRI (fMRI) data. Diffusion tensor imaging (DTI) and diffusion spectrum imaging (DSI) are used to analyze the brain structural networks in the posterior medial and parietal cerebral cortex. From the fMRI, the functional regions can be revealed by different brain modules. Multi-view spectral clustering makes it possible to integrate the functional and structural networks of human brain, which is helpful to infer groupwise consistent multimodal brain networks. Chen et al. implemented a groupwise co-training process as the combination of the results of two affinity matrices. This achieves balance between two views by repeatedly projecting the affinity matrix of one view to the eigenspace of the other view until convergence. The result of multi-view clustering method significantly increases the efficiency of finding functionally meaningful clusters based on structural connection matrices and paints a clearer picture about brain structures based on the functional clusters. In conclusion, using multi-view spectral clustering enables us to obtain consistent results between structure and function of brain networks, which will aid in further elucidating the function of brain.

3.3 High-Order Spectral Clustering

As an extension of spectral clustering, high-order spectral clustering extended traditional graph cut problem to hypergraph setting. Compared with an ordinary affinity matrix, high-order spectral clustering employs an affinity tensor to represent the relationship between samples, which can grab more information inside datasets. Thus, finding a general method for tensor eigen-decomposition is critical.

There are two major ways to solve a hypergraph partitioning problem. The first one is to transform the information in Laplacian tensor to a normal Laplacian matrix and solve it with traditional spectral clustering algorithms. The second approach is to eigen-decompose the Laplacian tensor directly to find the best partition. It has been proved in Agarwal et al. [2] that almost all the existing methods, such as clique graph Laplacian, star graph Laplacian [99], Rodriguez's Laplacian [66, 67] and Zhou's generalization of normalized Laplacian to hypergraph Ncut interpretation [97], are all equivalent to specific clique graph expansions. Therefore, in most cases, it is sufficient to solve this problem by changing the hypergraph partitioning problem to a graph partitioning problem. We will focus on the segmentation of an undirected weighted k-uniform hypergraph by projecting the hypergraph to an ordinary graph. The k-uniform framework enforces that the degree of every hyperedge is k.

First, we define a hypergraph, $\mathcal{H} = (\mathcal{V}, \varepsilon)$, in which $\mathcal{V}$ denotes vertices and ε represents the hyperedge. Let the weight of each hyperedge be $w_{\mathcal{H}}(e) \in \mathbb{R}_0^+$, and denote $\delta_{\mathcal{H}}(e) = |e| = k$ as the degree of hyperedge. When $k = 2$, the hypergraph is equivalent to a normal graph with a similarity matrix $S \in \mathbb{R}^{|V|^2} = \mathbb{R}^{|V|\times|V|}$. In real hypergraph cases, we note, $k \geq 3$, $S \in \mathbb{R}^{|V|^k}$, is a k-dimensional affinity tensor. Defining the projection as $\pi^w_{\mathcal{H}} : V \times V \mapsto \mathbb{R}_0^+$, this is equivalent to assigning hyperedge weights reasonably to any pair of nodes. Two types of projections are commonly used: the sum-operator and the max-operator.

The sum-operator is defined as

$$\pi^w_{\mathcal{H}}(u, v) = \sum_{e\in\varepsilon} \frac{w_{\mathcal{H}}(e)}{\delta_{\mathcal{H}}(e)} h(u, e)\, h(v, e),$$

where $H := (h(u, e))_{u\in\mathcal{V}, e\in\varepsilon}$, and $h(u, e) = \begin{cases} 1 & u \in e \\ 0 & else \end{cases}$.

It means that for any pairwise nodes u and v, we define $\pi^w_{\mathcal{H}}(u, v)$ as the sum all the weights of hyperedges, which includes both u and v. This is a common way to project the high-order data, which is equivalent to a regularized clique expansion used in [2, 98].

However, the sum projection always yields average weights among all hyperedges. These results are routinely insensitive in detecting the affinity between vertices. Thus, this yields the development of an alternate projection method: the max-operator [59]. The max-operator is defined as

$$\pi^w_{\mathcal{H}}(u, v) = \arg\min_{e\in\varepsilon} w_{\mathcal{H}}(e)\, h(u, e)\, h(v, e). \tag{12}$$

The authors extend this thought to the application of dynamic image segmentation, in which we can segment moving objects by long-time video analysis:

$$\pi^w_{\mathcal{H}}(u, v) = \arg\min_{w_{\mathcal{H}}(e).w, v\in e\in\varepsilon} w_{\mathcal{H}}(e)\, l(e), \tag{13}$$

where $l(e)$ is the number of common frames of all trajectories in e.

In real cases, k is often fixed to three for the following reasons. First, the time and space complexity will increase rapidly with higher affinity tensors. Second, information represented in pictures cannot completely capture the structure of 3D objects. Therefore, using a fourth-order tensor may not helpful to improve clustering results.

The application of high-order clustering is not restricted to motion segmentation. The complexity of networks and multiscale structure of biological data pushed the development of the hypergraph processing technique in bioinformatics. Recently, work has been completed to extend this idea to biological hypergraph clustering and classification [52, 54]. Michoel et al. [54] represented the local and global alignment of protein–protein interaction networks between multiple species by high-order spectral clustering. They proposed a hypergraph partition method based on generalization of the Perron–Frobenius theorem and applied it to the network alignment problem between yeast and human samples. By defining a bipartite hypergraph with 4-uniform hyperedges that denote the degree of alignment between two regions, the algorithm successfully finds a high-density interlog mapping between these two species. A set of one-to-one mapping between proteins has been shown conserved among all eukaryotes due to their function in DNA replication. These results greatly advance our understanding toward the relationship of proteins in different species.

3.4 Constrained Spectral Clustering

It is widely known that clustering is an unsupervised method. In some cases, however, we may have partial grouping information from samples such as must-link or cannot-link constraints. This casts the clustering problem into the semi-supervised setting. To combine a priori information into traditional spectral clustering, two categories of methods are proposed. The first type of method, as in [33, 51, 85], aims to directly add constraints to the Laplacian matrix itself, which transforms constrained spectral clustering to an ordinary spectral clustering problem and makes it possible to implement the traditional algorithm of SC. For example, in Craddock et al. [20], spatial constraints are directly added to the similarity matrix; in Kamvar et al. [33], the authors assign $A_{ij} = A_{ji} = 1$ for must-link samples and assign zero to cannot-link ones. The second kind of method focuses on restricting the feasible solution of the original optimization and trying to solve it efficiently. In Yu and Shi [92], a generalized Rayleigh–Ritz theorem was proposed to project matrices to their subspace based on partial information. Li et al. [46] developed a method by adapting the embedding matrix toward an ideal matrix as consistent with the constraints as possible through an optimization formulation. It is paramount to implement the second type of method, since there is no well-justified way to decide the weights of constraints if one simply modifies the Laplacian matrix.

Next, we will introduce a relatively principled method based on the works of Wang et al. [79, 80] and briefly summarize its applications in image segmentation.

As mentioned above, the partial information can be divided into two parts: must-link and cannot-link constraints. From this, we can define a side information matrix $Q = \left(Q_{ij}\right)_{n\times n}$, where

$$Q_{ij} \begin{cases} > 0 & \text{node } i \text{ and node } j \text{ are more likely to be linked} \\ < 0 & \text{node } i \text{ and node } j \text{ are more likely to be separated} \\ = 0 & \text{no side information.} \end{cases}$$

Let $\boldsymbol{u} \in \{1, -1\}^n$ be a cluster embedding vector, where $\boldsymbol{u}_i = 1$ or -1 is determined by whether node i belongs to a cluster or not. Then,

$$\boldsymbol{u}^T Q\boldsymbol{u} = \sum_{i=1}^{n}\sum_{j=1}^{n} \boldsymbol{u}_i \boldsymbol{u}_j Q_{ij}$$

can be regarded as a measure of how well the clustering result satisfies the target constraints. Specifically, if the value of $\boldsymbol{u}_i$ and $\boldsymbol{u}_j$ is the same (1 or -1) and $Q_{ij} > 0$, this corresponds to the fact that the clustering result is consistent with the side information we obtained and vice versa. Thus, the higher the value of $\boldsymbol{u}^T Q\boldsymbol{u}$ is, the higher clustering satisfaction.

Another strength of this method is that it does not require all constraints to be satisfied but transforms the problem to a soft constraint by setting the value of a threshold α in advance. Define $\overline{Q} = D^{-\frac{1}{2}} Q D^{-\frac{1}{2}}$, and then the objective function of constrained spectral clustering can be expressed as

$$\arg\min_{v\in\mathbb{R}^n} v^T \overline{L} v, \ \text{s.t. } v^T \overline{Q} v \geqslant \alpha, v^T v = vol, v \neq D^{\frac{1}{2}}\mathbf{1}. \tag{14}$$

The Lagrange function can be expressed as

$$\Lambda(v, \lambda, \mu) = v^T \overline{L} v - \lambda(v^T \overline{Q} v - \alpha) - \mu(v^T v - vol).$$

To solve this problem, one can use the Karush–Kuhn–Tucker theorem to transform it into two cases:

1. If $\lambda = 0$, this problem is transformed to unconstrained spectral clustering.
2. When $\lambda > 0$, $v^T \overline{Q} v = \alpha$. If we define $\beta := -\frac{\mu}{\lambda} vol$, we can obtain a prerequisite of the optimal of the objective function:

$$\overline{L} v = \lambda(\overline{Q} - \frac{\beta}{vol} I)v,$$

which is solvable as the Singular Value Decomposition (SVD) can be efficiently computed.

By taking the constraints into consideration, we can handle various situations in many fields especially biomedicine and image segmentation, such as clustering samples collected from hepatitis, breast cancer, etc. In Craddock et al. [20], spectral clustering with spatial constraints was used to specify regions of interests (ROIs) among fMRI data. Also, by processing the color information of pixels, constrained spectral clustering can yield good results in image segmentation [79, 80].

3.5 Evolutionary Spectral Clustering

To cluster data streams on a dynamic web or analyze time series data of genes collected from biological experiments, a new method that can integrate the partition results at multiple time points is essential. This problem was first conceptualized in Chakrabarti et al. [9]. In this setting, the data we obtain before spectral clustering are a time series of similarity matrices. Denote the similarity matrices at different time points as $W_t, t = 1, \ldots, T$. The goals in this setting are twofold:

1. After fixing a time point, static spectral clustering yields an indicator matrix.
2. The clustering results in adjacent time points do not vary greatly.

Inspired by the works of Chakrabarti et al. [9] in which an evolutionary hierarchical clustering algorithm and an evolutionary k-means clustering algorithm are proposed, Chi et al. proposed two formulations of objective function: Preserving Cluster Quality (PCQ) and Preserving Cluster Membership (PCM) to incorporate temporal smoothness in original optimization problem [17, 18]. These methods both focus on giving reasonable penalties to the difference of indicator matrices between adjacent time points, as well as jointly analyzing the clustering results across all time points.

We define the two following costs: cost of snapshot (CS) and cost of temporal (CT) in objective function. The aim is to minimize the integrated cost function:

$$cost = \alpha CS + \beta CT, \alpha + \beta = 1,$$

where $0 \leq \alpha, \beta \leq 1$ are weight parameters that reflect the user's emphasis on the snapshot cost and temporal cost, respectively. For different formulations, there is a different temporal cost. We will explore these formulations and their interpretations in k-means in the following subsections.

PCQ

The first framework, PCQ, aims to minimize the cost with a penalty term of applying the clustering result from time $t-1$ to time t.

1. In normalized cut interpretation,

$$\begin{aligned} Cost_{NC} &= \alpha CS_{NC} + \beta CT_{NC} = \alpha NC_t|_{U_t} + \beta NC_{t-1}|_{U_t} \\ &= \alpha k - \alpha tr\left[U_t^T (D_t^{-\frac{1}{2}} W_t D_t^{-\frac{1}{2}}) U_t\right] + \beta k - \beta tr\left[U_t^T (D_{t-1}^{-\frac{1}{2}} W_{t-1} D_{t-1}^{-\frac{1}{2}}) U_t\right] \end{aligned}$$

$$= k - tr\left[U_t^T\left(\alpha D_t^{-\frac{1}{2}}W_tD_t^{-\frac{1}{2}} + \beta D_{t-1}^{-\frac{1}{2}}W_{t-1}D_{t-1}^{-\frac{1}{2}}\right)U_t\right], \tag{15}$$

where $|_{U_t}$ corresponds to using the partition result U_t at time t to evaluate its consistency with that at time $t-1$.

2. In k-means interpretation,

$$Cost_{KM} = \alpha CS_{KM} + \beta CT_{KM} = \alpha KM_t|_{U_t} + \beta KM_{t-1}|_{U_t}$$
$$= \alpha \sum_{l=1}^{k}\sum_{i\in V_{l,t}} \left\|v_{i,t} - \mu_{l,t}\right\|^2 + \beta \sum_{l=1}^{k}\sum_{i\in V_{l,t}} \left\|v_{i,t-1} - \mu_{l,t-1}\right\|^2, \tag{16}$$

where $\mu_{l,t-1} = \sum_{j\in V_{l,t}} v_{j,t-1}/|V_{l,t}|$ is the average of vertices that belong to cluster l at time t.

According to the definition of k-means, one can easily obtain that the two aforementioned interpretations are equivalent. Thus, the objective function of PCQ is

$$\max_{U_t\in\mathbb{R}^{n\times p}} tr\left[U_t^T\left(\alpha D_t^{-\frac{1}{2}}W_tD_t^{-\frac{1}{2}} + \beta D_{t-1}^{-\frac{1}{2}}W_{t-1}D_{t-1}^{-\frac{1}{2}}\right)U_t\right]$$
$$\text{s.t. } U_t^TU_t = I.$$

PCM

The second framework, PCM, aims to directly minimize the difference between the current and the previous partitions. We will evaluate two interpretations of it and demonstrate their consistency.

1. In normalized cut interpretation, the penalty term CT_{NC} is defined as

$$CT_{NC} = dist\left(U_t, U_{t-1}\right) := \frac{1}{2}\left\|U_tU_t^T - U_{t-1}U_{t-1}^T\right\|^2.$$

Thus,

$$Cost_{NC} = \alpha CS_{NC} + \beta CT_{NC}$$
$$= \alpha k - \alpha tr\left[U_t^T(D_t^{-\frac{1}{2}}W_tD_t^{-\frac{1}{2}})U_t\right] + \frac{\beta}{2}\left\|U_tU_t^T - U_{t-1}U_{t-1}^T\right\|^2$$
$$= k - tr\left[U_t^T\left(\alpha D_t^{-\frac{1}{2}}W_tD_t^{-\frac{1}{2}} + \beta U_{t-1}U_{t-1}^T\right)U_t\right]. \tag{17}$$

2. In k-means interpretation, define

$$\begin{aligned} Cost_{KM} &= \alpha CS_{KM} + \beta CT_{KM} \\ &= \alpha \sum_{l=1}^{k} \sum_{i \in V_{l,t}} \left\| v_{i,t} - \mu_{l,t} \right\|^2 - \beta \sum_{i=1}^{k} \sum_{j=1}^{k} \frac{\left|V_{ij}\right|^2}{\left|V_{i,t}\right| \left|V_{j,t-1}\right|}, \end{aligned} \tag{18}$$

where the second term CT_{KM} comes from χ^2-statistic

$$\chi^2 \left(U_t, U_{t-1}\right) = n \left(\sum_{i=1}^{k} \sum_{j=1}^{k} \frac{\left|V_{ij}\right|^2}{\left|V_{i,t}\right| \left|V_{j,t-1}\right|} - 1 \right),$$

and V_{ij} is the number of vertices in both $V_{i,t}$ and $V_{j,t-1}$.

These two interpretations are equivalent, since it can be shown that

$$k - \sum_{i=1}^{k} \sum_{j=1}^{k} \frac{\left|V_{ij}\right|^2}{\left|V_{i,t}\right| \left|V_{j,t-1}\right|} = \frac{1}{2} \left\| U_t U_t^T - U_{t-1} U_{t-1}^T \right\|^2.$$

We refer to Bach et al. [5] for the complete derivation.

One common application of PCQ and PCM is processing blog data. The content interactions of blogs are constantly changing over time. PCM and PCQ can cluster samples from a global perspective and handle the change of the number of clusters across times.

Determining the Weight Parameter α

We have introduced two major frameworks of evolutionary spectral clustering and interpretations in k-means and graph cut frameworks. In order to ensure computational feasibility, it is common to use the k-means-based formulation as this method is scalable on huge datasets.

However, there is one core challenge remaining. The weight α cannot be determined in a well-justified way. To resolve this issue, Xu et al. [84] defined α as a *forgetting factor* to the past affinities between pairwise data points. The authors define a risk function $\mathscr{R}(\alpha)$ as the expectation of $L(\alpha)$, which is the squared Forbenius norm of the difference between the true affinity matrix and the estimated affinity matrix:

$$L(\alpha) = \left\| \alpha \overline{W}^{t-1} + (1-\alpha) W^t - \Psi^t \right\|_F^2.$$

By minimizing the expectation of $L(\alpha)$, the optimal forgetting factor α^* is therefore

$$\alpha^* = \frac{\sum_{i=1}^{n}\sum_{j=1}^{n} \mathrm{var}(w_{ij}^t)}{\sum_{i=1}^{n}\sum_{j=1}^{n}\{(w_{ij}^{t-1} - \psi_{ij}^t)^2 + \mathrm{var}(w_{ij}^t)\}}.$$

The function $L(\alpha)$ shares a similar philosophy with the shrinkage estimation or regularized estimation of covariance matrices [6, 41, 86, 88–90].

Evolutionary spectral clustering can be applied to various dynamic datasets in bioinformatics. For example, Liu et al. [47] proposed an iteration algorithm based on PCM with good convergence properties to global optimal. In order to explore how the genetic community of monkeys develops over space and time (over cortical layers in the medial prefrontal cortex and age), the authors used their model *PisCES* to process the gene expression data collected from rhesus monkey brains and successfully revealed various development periods of different communities. For instance, their results revealed enrichment for neural projection guidance (NPG) were consistent with existing knowledge, as well as gleaned further knowledge in understanding autism spectrum disorder-based gene interactions. Thus, when dealing with complex datasets changing over spatial and temporal periods, evolutionary spectral clustering can provide us with a more dynamic insight.

3.6 Incremental Spectral Clustering

Similar to evolutionary spectral clustering, incremental spectral clustering also focuses on analysis of dynamic datasets. The difference between them is that evolutionary spectral clustering aims to handle this problem from a more methodological perspective. This method integrates partition results at different time points; however, the goal of incremental spectral clustering is to obtain partition results of time $t + 1$ based on that of time t. This avoids to calculate the new Laplacian matrix L_{t+1} directly, which is computationally efficient especially when the change of Laplacian matrix is small compared with the whole dataset. Recently, many algorithms have been proposed to process incremental data [11, 30], some of which are based on spectral clustering.

There still exist key drawbacks to this method. In Valgren et al. [76] and Kong et al. [37], incremental algorithms can only handle insertion and deletion manipulations of data points over time. Moreover, these algorithms update the clustering result without considering the change of eigenvectors, making it challenging to justify any theoretical properties. However, to assuage this issue, Ning et al. [57, 58] follow the results laid out by [68], updating the eigenvectors incrementally.

First, Ning et al. defined the incidence matrix R, with each column denoted by $r_{ij}(w)$, of which only two elements are nonzero (i.e. the ith row is $\sqrt{w}$ and the jth row is $-\sqrt{w}$). One thing to note is that every column of R is a split part of pairwise weight w_{ij}. That is, two columns of R can be denoted by $r_{ij}w_{ij}^{(1)}$ and $r_{ij}w_{ij}^{(2)}$, if only $w_{ij} = w_{ij}^{(1)} + w_{ij}^{(2)}$. Some key properties of R include:

1. $\forall L = D - W, L = RR^T$.
2. For any kind of similarity change Δw_{ij}, the new incidence matrix can be denoted as $\tilde{R} = [R, r_{ij}(\Delta w_{ij})]$.

The intention of extending the definition of incidence matrix is clearly demonstrated through Property 2. Not limited to nodes insertion and deletion, any kind of similarity change can be processed by adding another column of R. Let $\tilde{L}$ and $\tilde{D}$ be the incremental Laplacian matrix and degree matrix, respectively; then, define $\Delta L = \tilde{L} - L$, $\Delta D = \Delta w_{ij} diag(v_{ij})$ to measure the difference between adjacent time, where v_{ij} is a constant 0 except 1 on row i and row j. Our goal is to estimate $\tilde{q}$ efficiently without directly calculating $\tilde{L}$ via the following equation:

$$Lq = \lambda Dq. \tag{19}$$

Thus, the question is equivalent to computing $\Delta\lambda$ and Δq. The authors in [57, 58] proposed an iterative algorithm by updating $\Delta\lambda$ and Δq until convergence, in which the formula of $\Delta\lambda$ and Δq is generated by differentiating equation (19). For more computational details and associated proofs, we refer to [58].

One crucial problem in the work of [57, 58] is that the time complexity of updating eigenvectors is restrictively high when accounting for complex incremental cases with many pairwise similarity changes. This thereby motivated Dhanjal et al. [22] to develop a more efficient method that can be used in a wider range of occasions with a perturbation bound.

In some cases when the data is too huge to be processed in one go, or it is collected and updated gradually like in the case of streaming data, incremental spectral clustering is well-equipped to handle these situations. handle these situations. The authors in [57, 58] used the continuously updated blog data crawled from webpages and found three stable blog communities in which some correlated topics are mainly discussed. When analyzing complicated biological factors such as proteins, metabolic reactions, and so forth, incremental spectral clustering can provide a good trade-off between accuracy and efficiency. For example, it was used to model the evolution of the HIV epidemic [22] from a dataset collected from HIV+ individuals. The weight matrix denotes the sexual contact between individuals and is updated gradually over time. The authors proposed the *IASC* algorithm to handle various situations of the change of similarity matrix, including adding or removing rows and columns, as well as the addition of a low-rank symmetric matrix. It is interesting to find that the results on this HIV dataset matched or even improved the exact clustering results obtained by computing eigenvectors directly after changing the similarity matrix. Moreover, the proposed algorithm is computationally efficient compared with the state-of-the-art methods as the authors only used at most 5% of the eigenvectors to yield the clustering results.

3.7 Sparse Spectral Clustering

In traditional spectral clustering, the optimization target we want to solve is

$$\min_{U\in\mathbb{R}^{n\times k}} \left\langle L, UU^T \right\rangle, \text{ s.t. } U^T U = I,$$

where $L = D - A$ in unnormalized spectral clustering or $L = I - D^{-\frac{1}{2}} A D^{-\frac{1}{2}}$ in normalized spectral clustering. In the ideal case when similarity graph G contains just k connected components, the embedding matrix U obtained from any eigen-solver can be expressed as

$$U = ZR,$$

where Z is the standard indicator matrix with only one constant element 1 on every row of Z, and $R \in \mathbb{R}^{k\times k}$ is an orthogonal rotation matrix. Thus, it is easy to see that UU^T is a block-diagonal matrix, and every nonzero block is constant one block, corresponding to a connected component to a cluster of graph G.

In practical settings when similarity matrix is perturbed by a small amount of noise, if we simply use traditional spectral clustering, almost all the elements in final embedding matrix are not 0. Thus, the clustering result after implementing k-means algorithm may be negatively affected due to the noise. From this perspective, adding a penalty term to retain the sparsity property of UU^T is needed. Thus, the optimization problem is transformed to

$$\min_{U\in\mathbb{R}^{n\times k}} \left\langle L, UU^T \right\rangle + \mu \left\| UU^T \right\|_0, \text{ s.t. } U^T U = I. \tag{20}$$

However, solving this problem is challenging, as this optimization on a Stiefel manifold with L_0 norm is NP-hard and non-convex [49]. To solve this challenging question, one transforms the L_0 norm in objective function to L_1 norm, as the L_1 norm is the optimal convex approximation of L_0. This yields the following optimization problem [50]:

$$\min_{U\in\mathbb{R}^{n\times k}} \left\langle L, UU^T \right\rangle + \mu \left\| UU^T \right\|_1, \text{ s.t. } U^T U = I. \tag{21}$$

This problem is still complex as $\left\| UU^T \right\|_1$ is a non-smooth, non-convex penalty term, and the feasible domain formed by a Stiefel manifold is also non-convex. Many optimization frameworks attempt to further relax the feasible domain to a convex set and compute the final result by implementing convex optimization algorithms such as ADMM.

For example, in Lu et al. [49, 50], the relaxed convex formulation of sparse spectral clustering is

$$\min_{P \in \mathbb{R}^{n \times n}} \langle P, L \rangle + \mu \|P\|_1, \text{ s.t. } 0 \preceq P \preceq I, Tr(P) = k. \tag{22}$$

Park and Zhao [61] added a convex term $\|P\|_F^2$ to the objective function:

$$\min_{P \in \mathbb{R}^{n \times n}} c \|P\|_F^2 - \langle P, \overline{S} \rangle + \mu \|P\|_1, \text{ s.t. } 0 \preceq P \preceq I, Tr(P) = k. \tag{23}$$

After obtaining $\hat{P}$, Park and Zhao [61] implemented the k-means algorithm to the first k eigenvectors of $\hat{X}$, where $\hat{X}$ is the shrunk target matrix of $\hat{P}$ found by solving:

$$\min_X \left\| X - \hat{P} \right\|_F^2 + \beta \sum_{j<k} \frac{\|X_{j,\cdot} - X_{k,\cdot}\|_2}{\left\| \hat{P}_{j,\cdot} - \hat{P}_{k,\cdot} \right\|_2}, \text{ s.t. } tr(X) = k, 0 \preceq P \preceq I.$$

The recent work by Wang et al. [82] proposed a new manifold proximal linear algorithm to exactly solve the non-convex sparse spectral clustering with provable guarantees.

Sparse spectral clustering can outperform ordinary spectral clustering. The authors in [61] evaluated the performance of sparse spectral clustering on various scRNA-seq data collected from embryonic stem cells, mouse embryos, somatosensory cortex and hippocampal CA1 region, etc. On the Ting cohort [75], the results of sparse spectral clustering outperformed other state-of-the-art methods such as traditional spectral clustering, t-SNE, k-means, and PCA due to a higher value of NMI,[2] as well as the lowest computational time. Although sparse spectral clustering achieves better results in many cases, it is difficult to implement the algorithm to larger datasets with millions of samples due to computational challenges. This yields an interesting open question for future exploration.

4 Discussion

In this chapter, we presented the basic theory, relationship with graph cut and kernel k-means, and three formulations of spectral clustering. We then summarized current extensions of spectral clustering and some of their applications in bioinformatics and image processing. While spectral clustering is a powerful tool for unsupervised learning, there exist core challenges that remain to be solved.

1. Choosing the cluster number k remains a vital open question. Although we have presented some popular methods that can help to decide the number of groups, it is challenging to robustly justify a criterion that is general to multiple datasets.

[2] NMI: Normalized Mutual Information, a commonly used method to measure the goodness of clustering [71].

2. Spectral clustering always groups samples based on the similarity matrix constructed from data, which means at least $O(n^2)$ time complexity. For small datasets, it is feasible to directly use spectral clustering. However, for larger datasets with millions of samples, like single-cell RNA-seq data, it is computationally prohibitive to use this graph-based clustering method. There is current work being explored on employing matrix approximation [26, 69] or landmark-based sparse coding [15] to make spectral clustering scalable. In Fowlkes et al. [26], the authors propose a method to approximate similarity matrix without computing all the pairwise similarities based on Nystrom extension. However, there exists an underlying bias between the embedding matrix calculated from this approximation and true embedding matrix. Another potential avenue is by noting that spectral clustering is also a kernel PCA problem. Therefore, methods such as stochastic optimization methods, which make kernel PCA scalable [95], can also be used to accelerate spectral clustering. In general, more study is needed to overcome the application of spectral clustering to large datasets.
3. Sparse spectral clustering often yields better results than ordinary spectral clustering [50, 83]. Some works combine sparse spectral clustering to other extensions, such as multi-view spectral clustering, to propose a solvable algorithm that can satisfy the analytical need of real data problems. However, as illustrated in the extension of sparse spectral clustering, how to solve this optimization problem accurately and with good convergence properties maintained is an open question.

Although the usage of spectral clustering is still limited due computational complexity, spectral clustering attains excellent performance on real datasets. Furthermore, there is a wide array of literature ensuring rigorous theoretical backing. This ensures that the algorithm can be flexibly applied to biological problems such as medical image segmentation, complex expression data and microarray data analysis.

References

1. Agarwal, A., Xue, L.: Model-based clustering of nonparametric weighted networks with application to water pollution analysis. Technometrics **62**(2), 161–172 (2020)
2. Agarwal, S., Branson, K., Belongie, S.: Higher order learning with graphs. In: Proceedings of the 23rd International Conference on Machine Learning, pp. 17–24. ACM, New York (2006)
3. Alashwal, H., El Halaby, M., Crouse, J., Abdalla, A., Moustafa, A.: The application of unsupervised clustering methods to Alzheimer's disease. Front. Comput. Neurosci. **13**, 31 (2019). https://doi.org/10.3389/fncom.2019.00031
4. Aldous, D., Fill, J.: Reversible Markov chains and random walks on graphs (1995)
5. Bach, F.R., Jordan, M.I.: Learning spectral clustering, with application to speech separation. J. Mach. Learn. Res. **7**, 1963–2001 (2006)
6. Bickel, P.J., Levina, E., et al.: Regularized estimation of large covariance matrices. Ann. Stat. **36**(1), 199–227 (2008)
7. Cano, C., Adarve, L., López, J., Blanco, A.: Possibilistic approach for biclustering microarray data. Comput. Biol. Med. **37**(10), 1426–1436 (2007)

8. Celeux, G., Soromenho, G.: An entropy criterion for assessing the number of clusters in a mixture model. J. Classif. **13**(2), 195–212 (1996)
9. Chakrabarti, D., Kumar, R., Tomkins, A.: Evolutionary clustering. In: Proceedings of the 12th ACM SIGKDD International Conference on Knowledge Discovery and Data Mining, pp. 554–560. ACM, New York (2006)
10. Chandrasekaran, V., Parrilo, P.A., Willsky, A.S.: Latent variable graphical model selection via convex optimization. In: 2010 48th Annual Allerton Conference on Communication, Control, and Computing (Allerton), pp. 1610–1613. IEEE, Piscataway (2010)
11. Charikar, M., Chekuri, C., Feder, T., Motwani, R.: Incremental clustering and dynamic information retrieval. SIAM J. Comput. **33**(6), 1417–1440 (2004)
12. Chaudhuri, K., Kakade, S.M., Livescu, K., Sridharan, K.: Multi-view clustering via canonical correlation analysis. In: Proceedings of the 26th Annual International Conference on Machine Learning, pp. 129–136. ACM, New York (2009)
13. Chen, H., Li, K., Zhu, D., Jiang, X., Yuan, Y., Lv, P., Zhang, T., Guo, L., Shen, D., Liu, T.: Inferring group-wise consistent multimodal brain networks via multi-view spectral clustering. IEEE Trans. Med. Imaging **32**(9), 1576–1586 (2013)
14. Chen, S., Ma, S., Xue, L., Zou, H.: An alternating manifold proximal gradient method for sparse principal component analysis and sparse canonical correlation analysis. INFORMS J. Optim. **2**(3), 192–208 (2020)
15. Chen, X., Cai, D.: Large scale spectral clustering with landmark-based representation. In: Twenty-Fifth AAAI Conference on Artificial Intelligence (2011)
16. Cheng, Y., Church, G.M.: Biclustering of expression data. Intell. Syst. Mol. Biol. **8**(**2000**), 93–103 (2000)
17. Chi, Y., Song, X., Zhou, D., Hino, K., Tseng, B.L.: Evolutionary spectral clustering by incorporating temporal smoothness. In: Proceedings of the 13th ACM SIGKDD International Conference on Knowledge Discovery and Data Mining, pp. 153–162. ACM, New York (2007)
18. Chi, Y., Song, X., Zhou, D., Hino, K., Tseng, B.L.: On evolutionary spectral clustering. ACM Trans. Knowl. Disc. Data **3**(4), 17 (2009)
19. Chung, F.R., Graham, F.C.: Spectral Graph Theory. American Mathematical Society, Providence (1997)
20. Craddock, R.C., James, G.A., Holtzheimer III, P.E., Hu, X.P., Mayberg, H.S.: A whole brain fMRI atlas generated via spatially constrained spectral clustering. Hum. Brain Mapp. **33**(8), 1914–1928 (2012)
21. Davis, C., Kahan, W.M.: The rotation of eigenvectors by a perturbation. III. SIAM J. Numer. Anal. **7**(1), 1–46 (1970)
22. Dhanjal, C., Gaudel, R., Clémençon, S.: Efficient eigen-updating for spectral graph clustering. Neurocomputing **131**, 440–452 (2014)
23. Dhillon, I.S.: Co-clustering documents and words using bipartite spectral graph partitioning. In: Proceedings of the Seventh ACM SIGKDD International Conference on Knowledge Discovery and Data Mining, pp. 269–274. ACM, New York (2001)
24. Dhillon, I.S., Guan, Y., Kulis, B.: Kernel k-means: spectral clustering and normalized cuts. In: Proceedings of the Tenth ACM SIGKDD International Conference on Knowledge Discovery and Data Mining, pp. 551–556. ACM, New York (2004)
25. Evanno, G., Regnaut, S., Goudet, J.: Detecting the number of clusters of individuals using the software structure: a simulation study. Mol. Ecol. **14**(8), 2611–2620 (2005)
26. Fowlkes, C., Belongie, S., Chung, F., Malik, J.: Spectral grouping using the Nystrom method. IEEE Trans. Pattern Anal. Mach. Intell. **26**(2), 214–225 (2004)
27. Fraley, C., Raftery, A.E.: Model-based clustering, discriminant analysis, and density estimation. J. Am. Stat. Assoc. **97**(458), 611–631 (2002)
28. Friedman, J., Hastie, T., Tibshirani, R.: The Elements of Statistical Learning. Springer Series in Statistics New York (2001)
29. Friedman, J., Hastie, T., Tibshirani, R.: Sparse inverse covariance estimation with the graphical lasso. Biostatistics **9**(3), 432–441 (2008)

30. Gepperth, A., Hammer, B.: Incremental learning algorithms and applications. In: European Symposium on Artificial Neural Networks (ESANN). Bruges, Belgium (2016). https://hal.archives-ouvertes.fr/hal-01418129
31. Hinton, G.E., Sejnowski, T.J., Poggio, T.A.: Unsupervised Learning: Foundations of Neural Computation. MIT Press, Cambridge (1999)
32. Kamthania, D., Pahwa, A., Madhavan, S.: Market segmentation analysis and visualization using k-mode clustering algorithm for e-commerce business. J. Comput. Inf. Technol. **26**, 57–68 (2018). https://doi.org/10.20532/cit.2018.1003863
33. Kamvar, K., Sepandar, S., Klein, K., Dan, D., Manning, M., Christopher, C.: Spectral learning. In: International Joint Conference of Artificial Intelligence. Stanford InfoLab (2003)
34. Kim, B., Lee, K.H., Xue, L., Niu, X.: A review of dynamic network models with latent variables. Stat. Surv. **12**, 105–135 (2018)
35. Kluger, Y., Basri, R., Chang, J.T., Gerstein, M.: Spectral biclustering of microarray data: coclustering genes and conditions. Genome Res. **13**(4), 703–716 (2003)
36. Kokate, U., Deshpande, A., Mahalle, P., Patil, P.: Data stream clustering techniques, applications, and models: comparative analysis and discussion. Big Data Cogn. Comput. **2**, 32 (2018). https://doi.org/10.3390/bdcc2040032
37. Kong, T., Tian, Y., Shen, H.: A fast incremental spectral clustering for large data sets. In: 2011 12th International Conference on Parallel and Distributed Computing, Applications and Technologies, pp. 1–5. IEEE, Piscataway (2011)
38. Kumar, A., Daumé, H.: A co-training approach for multi-view spectral clustering. In: Proceedings of the 28th International Conference on Machine Learning (ICML-11), pp. 393–400 (2011)
39. Kumar, A., Rai, P., Daume, H.: Co-regularized multi-view spectral clustering. In: Advances in Neural Information Processing Systems, pp. 1413–1421 (2011)
40. Lauritzen, S.L.: Graphical Models, vol. 17. Clarendon Press, Oxford (1996)
41. Ledoit, O., Wolf, M.: Improved estimation of the covariance matrix of stock returns with an application to portfolio selection. J. Empir. Financ. **10**(5), 603–621 (2003)
42. Lee, K.H., Chen, Q., DeSarbo, W., Xue, L.: Latent mixture Gaussian graphical models for ordinal response data. Technical Report, Penn State University (2020)
43. Lee, K.H., Xue, L.: Nonparametric finite mixture of Gaussian graphical models. Technometrics **60**(4), 511–521 (2018)
44. Lee, K.H., Xue, L., Hunter, D.R.: Model-based clustering of time-evolving networks through temporal exponential-family random graph models. J. Multivar. Anal. **175**, 104540 (2020)
45. Li, Y., Nie, F., Huang, H., Huang, J.: Large-scale multi-view spectral clustering via bipartite graph. In: Twenty-Ninth AAAI Conference on Artificial Intelligence (2015)
46. Li, Z., Liu, J., Tang, X.: Constrained clustering via spectral regularization. In: 2009 IEEE Conference on Computer Vision and Pattern Recognition, pp. 421–428. IEEE, Piscataway (2009)
47. Liu, F., Choi, D., Xie, L., Roeder, K.: Global spectral clustering in dynamic networks. Proc. Natl. Acad. Sci. **115**(5), 927–932 (2018)
48. Lovász, L.: Random walks on graphs: a survey. Comb. Paul Erdos Eighty **2**(1), 1–46 (1993)
49. Lu, C., Feng, J., Lin, Z., Yan, S.: Nonconvex sparse spectral clustering by alternating direction method of multipliers and its convergence analysis. In: Thirty-Second AAAI Conference on Artificial Intelligence (2018)
50. Lu, C., Yan, S., Lin, Z.: Convex sparse spectral clustering: single-view to multi-view. IEEE Trans. Image Process. **25**(6), 2833–2843 (2016)
51. Lu, Z., Carreira-Perpinan, M.A.: Constrained spectral clustering through affinity propagation. In: 2008 IEEE Conference on Computer Vision and Pattern Recognition, pp. 1–8. IEEE, Piscataway (2008)
52. Lugo-Martinez, J., Radivojac, P.: Classification in biological networks with hypergraphlet kernels. arXiv preprint arXiv:1703.04823 (2017)
53. Ma, S., Xue, L., Zou, H.: Alternating direction methods for latent variable Gaussian graphical model selection. Neural Comput. **25**(8), 2172–2198 (2013)

54. Michoel, T., Nachtergaele, B.: Alignment and integration of complex networks by hypergraph-based spectral clustering. Phys. Rev. E **86**(5), 056111 (2012)
55. Milligan, G.W., Cooper, M.C.: An examination of procedures for determining the number of clusters in a data set. Psychometrika **50**(2), 159–179 (1985)
56. Ng, A.Y., Jordan, M.I., Weiss, Y.: On spectral clustering: analysis and an algorithm. In: Advances in Neural Information Processing Systems, pp. 849–856 (2002)
57. Ning, H., Xu, W., Chi, Y., Gong, Y., Huang, T.: Incremental spectral clustering with application to monitoring of evolving blog communities. In: Proceedings of the 2007 SIAM International Conference on Data Mining, pp. 261–272. SIAM (2007)
58. Ning, H., Xu, W., Chi, Y., Gong, Y., Huang, T.S.: Incremental spectral clustering by efficiently updating the eigen-system. Pattern Recogn. **43**(1), 113–127 (2010)
59. Ochs, P., Brox, T.: Higher order motion models and spectral clustering. In: 2012 IEEE Conference on Computer Vision and Pattern Recognition, pp. 614–621. IEEE, Piscataway (2012)
60. Oyelade, J., Isewon, I., Oladipupo, F., Aromolaran, O., Uwoghiren, E., Ameh, F., Achas, M., Adebiyi, E.: Clustering algorithms: their application to gene expression data. Bioinf. Biol. Insights **10**, 237–253 (2016). https://doi.org/10.4137/BBI.S38316
61. Park, S., Zhao, H.: Spectral clustering based on learning similarity matrix. Bioinformatics **34**(12), 2069–2076 (2018)
62. Pearson, K.: Principal components analysis. Lond. Edinb. Dublin Philos. Mag. J. Sci. **6**(2), 559 (1901)
63. Pirim, H., Eksioglu, B., Perkins, A., Yceer, C.: Clustering of high throughput gene expression data. Comput. Oper. Res. **39**, 3046–3061 (2012)
64. Pontes, B., Giráldez, R., Aguilar-Ruiz, J.S.: Biclustering on expression data: a review. J. Biomed. Inf. **57**, 163–180 (2015)
65. Pritchard, J.K., Stephens, M., Donnelly, P.: Inference of population structure using multilocus genotype data. Genetics **155**(2), 945–959 (2000)
66. Rodriguez, J.A.: On the laplacian eigenvalues and metric parameters of hypergraphs. Linear Multilinear Algebra **50**(1), 1–14 (2002)
67. Rodriguez, J.A.: On the Laplacian spectrum and walk-regular hypergraphs. Linear and Multilinear Algebra **51**(3), 285–297 (2003)
68. Shi, J., Malik, J.: Normalized cuts and image segmentation. IEEE Trans. Pattern Anal. Mach. Intell. **22**(8), 888–905 (2000)
69. Smola, A.J., Schlkopf, B.: Sparse greedy matrix approximation for machine learning. In: Proceedings of the Seventeenth International Conference on Machine Learning, pp. 911–918. Morgan Kaufmann, Los Altos (2000)
70. Stewart, G.W.: Stochastic perturbation theory. SIAM Rev. **32**(4), 579–610 (1990)
71. Strehl, A., Ghosh, J.: Cluster ensembles—a knowledge reuse framework for combining multiple partitions. J. Mach. Learn. Res. **3**, 583–617 (2002)
72. Sugar, C.A., James, G.M.: Finding the number of clusters in a dataset: an information-theoretic approach. J. Am. Stat. Assoc. **98**(463), 750–763 (2003)
73. Templ, M., Filzmoser, P., Reimann, C.: Cluster analysis applied to regional geochemical data: Problems and possibilities. Appl. Geochem. **23**, 2198–2213 (2008). https://doi.org/10.1016/j.apgeochem.2008.03.004
74. Tibshirani, R., Walther, G., Hastie, T.: Estimating the number of clusters in a data set via the gap statistic. J. R. Stat. Soc. Ser. B Stat Methodol. **63**(2), 411–423 (2001)
75. Ting, D.T., Wittner, B.S., Ligorio, M., Jordan, N.V., Shah, A.M., Miyamoto, D.T., Aceto, N., Bersani, F., Brannigan, B.W., Xega, K.: Single-cell RNA sequencing identifies extracellular matrix gene expression by pancreatic circulating tumor cells. Cell Rep. **8**(6), 1905–1918 (2014)
76. Valgren, C., Duckett, T., Lilienthal, A.: Incremental spectral clustering and its application to topological mapping. In: Proceedings 2007 IEEE International Conference on Robotics and Automation, pp. 4283–4288. IEEE, Piscataway (2007)
77. Von Luxburg, U.: A tutorial on spectral clustering. Stat. Comput. **17**(4), 395–416 (2007)

78. Wang, B., Ma, S., Xue, L.: Riemannian stochastic proximal gradient methods for nonsmooth optimization over the Stiefel manifold (2020). arXiv preprint arXiv:2005.01209
79. Wang, X., Davidson, I.: Flexible constrained spectral clustering. In: Proceedings of the 16th ACM SIGKDD International Conference on Knowledge Discovery and Data Mining, pp. 563–572. ACM, New York (2010)
80. Wang, X., Qian, B., Davidson, I.: On constrained spectral clustering and its applications. Data Mining Knowl. Disc. **28**(1), 1–30 (2014)
81. Wang, Y., Wu, L., Lin, X., Gao, J.: Multiview spectral clustering via structured low-rank matrix factorization. IEEE Trans. Neural Netw. Learn. Syst. **29**(10), 4833–4843 (2018)
82. Wang, Z., Liu, B., Chen, S., Ma, S., Xue, L., Zhao, H.: A manifold proximal linear method for sparse spectral clustering with application to single-cell RNA sequencing data analysis (2020). arXiv preprint arXiv:2007.09524
83. Xia, R., Pan, Y., Du, L., Yin, J.: Robust multi-view spectral clustering via low-rank and sparse decomposition. In: Twenty-Eighth AAAI Conference on Artificial Intelligence (2014)
84. Xu, K.S., Kliger, M., Hero, A.O.: Evolutionary spectral clustering with adaptive forgetting factor. In: 2010 IEEE International Conference on Acoustics, Speech and Signal Processing, pp. 2174–2177. IEEE, Piscataway (2010)
85. Xu, Q., Desjardins, M., Wagstaff, K.: Constrained spectral clustering under a local proximity structure assumption. In: In Proceedings of the 18th International Conference of the Florida Artificial Intelligence Research Society (FLAIRS). Citeseer (2005)
86. Xue, L., Ma, S., Zou, H.: Positive-definite 1-penalized estimation of large covariance matrices. J. Am. Stat. Assoc. **107**(500), 1480–1491 (2012)
87. Xue, L., Zou, H.: Regularized rank-based estimation of high-dimensional nonparanormal graphical models. Ann. Stat. **40**(5), 2541–2571 (2012)
88. Xue, L., Zou, H.: Minimax optimal estimation of general bandable covariance matrices. J. Multivar. Anal. **116**, 45–51 (2013)
89. Xue, L., Zou, H.: Optimal estimation of sparse correlation matrices of semiparametric Gaussian copulas. Stat. Interface **7**(2), 201–209 (2014)
90. Xue, L., Zou, H.: Rank-based tapering estimation of bandable correlation matrices. Stat. Sin. **24**(1), 83–100 (2014)
91. Xue, L., Zou, H., Cai, T.: Nonconcave penalized composite conditional likelihood estimation of sparse Ising models. Ann. Stat. **40**(3), 1403–1429 (2012)
92. Yu, S.X., Shi, J.: Segmentation given partial grouping constraints. IEEE Trans. Pattern Anal. Mach. Intell. **26**(2), 173–183 (2004)
93. Yuan, M., Lin, Y.: Model selection and estimation in the Gaussian graphical model. Biometrika **94**(1), 19–35 (2007)
94. Zelnik-Manor, L., Perona, P.: Self-tuning spectral clustering. In: Advances in Neural Information Processing Systems, pp. 1601–1608 (2005)
95. Zhang, L., Yang, T., Yi, J., Jin, R., Zhou, Z.H.: Stochastic optimization for kernel PCA. In: Thirtieth AAAI Conference on Artificial Intelligence (2016)
96. Zhou, D., Burges, C.J.: Spectral clustering and transductive learning with multiple views. In: Proceedings of the 24th International Conference on Machine Learning, pp. 1159–1166. ACM, New York (2007)
97. Zhou, D., Huang, J., Schölkopf, B.: Beyond Pairwise Classification and Clustering Using Hypergraphs. Max Plank Institute for Biological Cybernetics, Tübingen (2005)
98. Zhou, D., Huang, J., Schölkopf, B.: Learning with hypergraphs: Clustering, classification, and embedding. In: Advances in Neural Information Processing Systems, pp. 1601–1608 (2007)
99. Zien, J.Y., Schlag, M.D., Chan, P.K.: Multilevel spectral hypergraph partitioning with arbitrary vertex sizes. IEEE Trans. Comput. Aided Des. Integr. Circuits Syst. **18**(9), 1389–1399 (1999)
100. Zou, H., Hastie, T., Tibshirani, R.: Sparse principal component analysis. J. Comput. Graph. Stat. **15**(2), 265–286 (2006)
101. Zou, H., Xue, L.: A selective overview of sparse principal component analysis. Proc. IEEE **106**(8), 1311–1320 (2018)

A Review on Modern Computational Optimal Transport Methods with Applications in Biomedical Research

Jingyi Zhang, Wenxuan Zhong, and Ping Ma

1 Introduction

There is a long and rich history of optimal transport (OT) problems initiated by Gaspard Monge (1746–1818), a French mathematician, in the eighteenth century. During recent decades, OT problems have found fruitful applications in our daily lives [90]. Consider the resource allocation problem, as illustrated in Fig. 1. Suppose that an operator runs n warehouses and m factories. Each warehouse contains a certain amount of valuable raw materials, i.e., the resources, that are needed by the factories to run properly. Furthermore, each factory has a certain demand for raw materials. Suppose the total amount of the resources in the warehouse equals the total demand for the raw materials in the factories. The operator aims to move all the resources from warehouses to factories, such that all the demands for the factories could be successfully met, and the total transport cost is as small as possible.

The resource allocation problem is a typical OT problem in practice. To put these problems in mathematical language, one can regard the resources as a whole and the demands as a whole as two probability distributions. For example, the resources from warehouses in Fig. 1 can be regarded as a non-uniform discrete distribution supported on three discrete points, and each of the points represents the geographical location of a particular warehouse. OT methods aim to find a transport map (or plan) between these two probability distributions with the minimum transport cost. Formal definitions for the transport map, the transport plan, and the transport cost are given in Sect. 2.

J. Zhang
Center for Statistical Science, Tsinghua University, Beijing, China

W. Zhong · P. Ma (✉)
Department of Statistics, University of Georgia, Athens, GA, USA
e-mail: wenxuan@uga.edu; pingma@uga.edu

Y. Zhao, (Din) D.-G. Chen (eds.), *Modern Statistical Methods for Health Research*, Emerging Topics in Statistics and Biostatistics,
https://doi.org/10.1007/978-3-030-72437-5_13

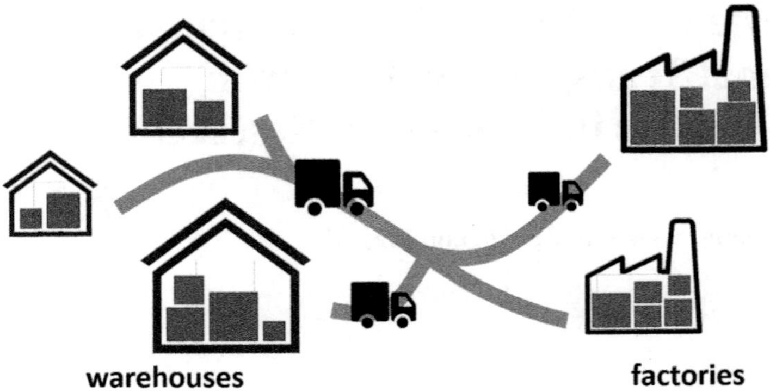

Fig. 1 Illustration for the resource allocation problem. The resources in warehouses are marked in blue, and the demand for each factory is marked in red

Nowadays, many modern statistical and machine learning problems can be recast as finding the optimal transport map (or plan) between two probability distributions. For example, domain adaptation [16, 29, 71] aims to learn a well-trained model from a source data distribution and transfer this model to adopt a target data distribution. Another example is deep generative models [4, 13, 39, 65] that target at mapping a fixed distribution, e.g., the standard Gaussian or uniform distribution, to the underlying population distribution of the genuine sample. During recent decades, OT methods have been reinvigorated in a remarkable proliferation of modern data science applications, including machine learning [3, 4, 11, 16, 28, 65, 75], statistics [12, 18, 73], and computer vision [25, 75, 78, 88].

Although OT finds a large number of applications in practice, the computation of OT meets challenges in the big data era. Traditional methods estimate the optimal transport map (OTM) by solving differential equations [5, 9] or by solving a problem of linear programming [74, 81]. Consider two p-dimensional samples with n observations within each sample. The calculation of the OTM between these two samples using these traditional methods requires $O(n^3 \log(n))$ computational time [75, 84]. Such a sizable computational cost hinders the broad applicability of optimal transport methods.

To alleviate the computational burden for OT, there have been a large number of works dedicated to develop efficient computational tools in the recent decade. One class of methods, starting from [17], considers solving a regularized OT problem instead of the original one. By utilizing the Sinkhorn algorithm (detailed in Sect. 3), the computational cost for solving such a regularized problem can be reduced to $O(n^2 \log(n))$, which is a significant reduction from $O(n^3 \log(n))$. Based on this idea, various computational tools are developed to solve the regularized OT problem as quickly as possible [2, 75]. By combining the Sinkhorn algorithm and the idea of low-rank matrix approximation, recently, [1] proposed an efficient algorithm with a computational cost that is approximately proportional to n. Although not covered in this chapter, regularization-based optimal transport methods even appear to have better theoretical properties than the unregularized counterparts; see [35, 68, 80] for details.

Another class of methods aims to estimate the OTM efficiently using random or deterministic projections. These so-called projection-based methods tackle the problem of estimating a p-dimensional OTM by breaking down the problem into a series of subproblems, each of which finds a one-dimensional OTM using projected samples [7, 76, 77, 79]. The subproblems can be easily solved since the one-dimensional OTM is equivalent to sorting, under some mild conditions. The projection-based methods reduce the computational cost for calculating OTMs from $O(n^3 \log(n))$ to $O(Kn \log(n))$, where K is the number of iterations until convergence.

With the help of these computational tools, OT methods have been widely applied to various biomedical researches. Taking single-cell RNA sequencing data as an example, OT methods can be used to study developmental time courses to infer ancestor–descendant fates for cells and help researchers to better understand the molecular programs that guide differentiation during development. For another example, OT methods can be used as data augmentation tools to increase the number of observations and thus to improve the accuracy and stability of various downstream analyses.

The rest of this chapter is organized as follows. We start in Sect. 2 by introducing the essential background of the OT problem. In Sect. 3, we present the details of regularization-based OT methods and their extensions. Section 4 is devoted to projection-based OT methods, including both random projection methods and deterministic projection methods. In Sect. 5, we show several applications of OT methods on real-world problems in biomedical research.

2 Background of the Optimal Transport Problem

In the aforementioned resource allocation problem, the goal is to transport the resources in the warehouse to the factories with the least cost, say the total fuel consumption of trucks. Here, the resources in the warehouse and the demand in the factories can be regarded as discrete distributions. We now introduce the following example that extends the discrete setting to the continuous setting. Suppose there is a worker who has to move a large pile of sand using a shovel in his hand. The goal of the worker is to use all that sand to construct a target pile with a prescribed shape, say a sandcastle. Naturally, the worker wishes to minimize the total "effort," which intuitively, in the sense of physical, can be regarded as the "work," the product of force and displacement. A French mathematician Gaspard Monge (1746–1818) once considered such a problem and formulated it into a general mathematical problem, i.e., the optimal transport problem [75, 90]: among all the possible transport maps ϕ between two probability measures μ and ν, how to find the one with the minimum transport cost? Mathematically, the optimal transport problem can be formulated as follows. Let $\mathscr{P}(\mathbb{R}^p)$ be the set of Borel probability measures in $\mathbb{R}^p$, and let

$$\mathscr{P}_2(\mathbb{R}^p) = \left\{ \mu \in \mathscr{P}(\mathbb{R}^p) \middle| \int ||x||^2 \mathrm{d}\mu(x) < \infty \right\}.$$

For $\mu, \nu \in \mathscr{P}_2(\mathbb{R}^p)$, let Φ be the set of all the so-called measure-preserving maps $\phi : \mathbb{R}^p \to \mathbb{R}^p$, such that $\phi_{\#}(\mu) = \nu$ and $\phi_{\#}^{-1}(\nu) = \mu$. Here, # represents the push-forward operator, such that for any measurable $\Omega \subset \mathbb{R}^d$, $\phi_{\#}(\mu)(\Omega) = \mu(\phi^{-1}(\Omega))$. Among all the maps in Φ, the optimal transport map defined under a cost function $c(\cdot, \cdot)$ is

$$\phi^{\dagger} := \arg\inf_{\phi \in \Phi} \int_{\mathbb{R}^p} c(x, \phi(x)) \mathrm{d}\mu(x). \tag{1}$$

One popular choice for the cost function is $c(x, y) = \|x - y\|^2$, with which Eq. (1) becomes

$$\phi^{\dagger} := \arg\inf_{\phi \in \Phi} \int_{\mathbb{R}^p} \|x - \phi(x)\|^2 \mathrm{d}\mu(x). \tag{2}$$

Equation (2) is called the Monge formulation, and its solution $\phi^{\dagger}$ is called the optimal transport map (OTM), or the Monge map. The well-known Brenier's Theorem [8] stated that when the cost function $c(x, y) = \|x - y\|^2$, if at least one of μ and ν has a density with respect to the Lebesgue measure, then the OTM $\phi^{\dagger}$ in Eq. (2) exists and is unique. In other words, the OTM $\phi^{\dagger}$ may not exist, i.e., the solution of Eq. (2) may not be a map, when the conditions of Brenier's Theorem are not met. To overcome such a limitation, Kantorovich [42] considered the following set of "couplings,"

$$\begin{aligned} \mathscr{M}(\mu, \nu) = \{\pi \in \mathscr{P}(\mathbb{R}^p \times \mathbb{R}^p) \; s.t. \; \forall \text{ Borel set } A, B \subset \mathbb{R}^p, \\ \pi(A \times \mathbb{R}^p) = \mu(A), \; \pi(\mathbb{R}^p \times B) = \nu(B)\}. \end{aligned} \tag{3}$$

Intuitively, a coupling $\pi \in \mathscr{M}(\mu, \nu)$ is a joint distribution of μ and ν, such that two particular marginal distributions of π are equal to μ and ν, respectively. Instead of finding the OTM, Kantorovich formulated the optimal transport problem as finding the optimal coupling,

$$\pi^* := \arg\inf_{\pi \in \mathscr{M}(\mu, \nu)} \int \|x - y\|^2 \mathrm{d}\pi(x, y). \tag{4}$$

Equation (4) is called the Kantorovich formulation (with L_2 cost), and its solution π^* is called the optimal transport plan (OTP). The key difference between the

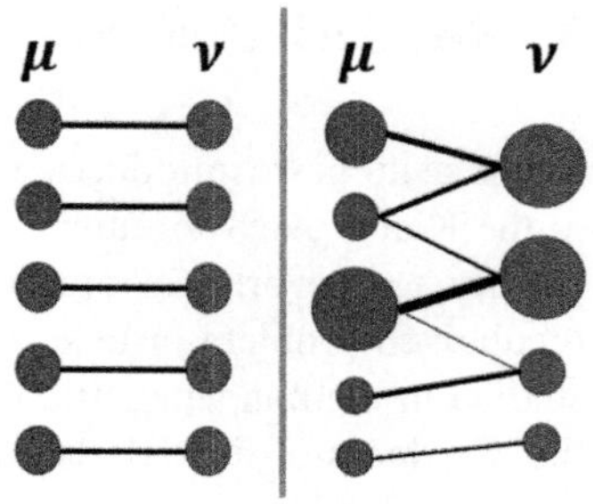

Fig. 2 Comparison between optimal transport map (OTM) and optimal transport plan (OTP). Left: An illustration of OTM, which is a one-to-one map. Right: An illustration of OPT, which may not necessarily be a map

Monge formulation and the Kantorovich formulation is that the latter does not require the solution to be a one-to-one map, as illustrated in Fig. 2.

The Kantorovich formulation is more realistic in practice, compared with the Monge formulation. Take the resource allocation problem as an example, as described in Sect. 1. It is unreasonable to assume that there always exists a one-to-one map between warehouses and factories, which can meet all the demands for the factories. The optimal solution of such resource allocation problems is thus usually an OTP instead of an OTM. Note that although the Kantorovich formulation is more flexible than the Monge formulation, it can be shown that when the OTM exists, the OTP is equivalent to the OTM.

Closely related to the optimal transport problem is the so-called Wasserstein distance. Intuitively, if we think the optimal transport problem (either in the Monge formulation or the Kantorovich formulation) as an optimization problem, then the Wasserstein distance is simply the optimal objective value of such an optimization problem, with certain power transform. Suppose the OTM $\phi^\dagger$ exists, the Wasserstein distance of order k is defined as

$$W_k(\mu, \nu) := \left(\int_{\mathbb{R}^p} \|X - \phi^\dagger(X)\|^k \mathrm{d}\mu \right)^{1/k}. \tag{5}$$

Let $\{x_i\}_{i=1}^n$ and $\{y_i\}_{i=1}^n$ be the two samples generated from μ and ν, respectively. One can thus estimate $\phi^\dagger$ using these two samples, and we let $\widehat{\phi}^\dagger$ to denote the corresponding estimator. The Wasserstein distance $W_k(\mu, \nu)$ can thus be estimated by

$$\widehat{W}_k(\mu, \nu) := \left(\frac{1}{n} \sum_{i=1}^{n} \|x_i - \widehat{\phi}^\dagger(x_i)\|^k \right)^{1/k}.$$

The Wasserstein distance respecting to the Kantorovich formulation can be defined analogously. We refer to [19, 73, 96] and the reference therein for theoretical properties of Wasserstein distances. Without further notification, we focus on the L_2 norm throughout this chapter, i.e., $k = 2$ in Eq. (5), and we abbreviate $W_2(\mu, \nu)$ by $W(\mu, \nu)$.

3 Regularization-Based Optimal Transport Methods

In this section, we introduce a family of numerical schemes to approximate solutions to the Kantorovich formulation (4). Such numerical schemes add a regularization penalty to the original optimal transport problem, and one can then solve the regularized problem instead. Such a regularization-based approach has long been studied in the nonparametric regression literature to balance the trade-off between the goodness-of-fit and the model and the roughness of a nonlinear function [40, 56, 67, 99].

Cuturi first introduced the regularization approach in OT problems [17] and showed that the regularized problem could be solved using a simple alternate minimization scheme, requiring $O(n^2 \log(n)\, p)$ computational time. Moreover, it can be shown that the solution to the regularized OT problem can well-approximate the solution to its unregularized counterpart. We call such numerical schemes the regularization-based optimal transport methods. We now present the details and some extensions of these methods as follows.

3.1 Computational Cost for OT Problems

We first introduce how to calculate the empirical Wasserstein distance by solving a linear system. Let $\boldsymbol{p}$ and $\boldsymbol{q}$ be the two probability distributions supported on a discrete set $\{\boldsymbol{x}_i\}_{i=1}^n$, where $\boldsymbol{x}_i \in \Omega$ for $i = 1, \ldots, n$, and $\Omega \subset \mathbb{R}^d$ is bounded. We identify $\boldsymbol{p}$ and $\boldsymbol{q}$ as the vectors located on the simplex

$$\Delta_n := \left\{ \boldsymbol{v} \in \mathbb{R}^n : \sum_{i=1}^{n} \boldsymbol{v}_i = 1, \text{ and } \boldsymbol{v}_i \geq 0, \ i = 1, \ldots, n. \right\},$$

whose entries denote the weight of each distribution assigned to the points of $\{\boldsymbol{x}_i\}_{i=1}^n$. Let $\mathbf{C} \in \mathbb{R}^{n\times n}$ be the pair-wise distance matrix, where $\mathbf{C}_{ij} = \|\boldsymbol{x}_i - \boldsymbol{x}_j\|^2$, and $\mathbf{1}_n$ be the all-ones vector with n elements. Recall the definition of coupling in Eq. (3), and analogously, we denote by $\mathscr{M}(\boldsymbol{p}, \boldsymbol{q})$ the set of coupling matrices between $\boldsymbol{p}$ and $\boldsymbol{q}$, i.e.,

$$\mathscr{M}(\boldsymbol{p}, \boldsymbol{q}) = \left\{ \mathbf{P} \in \mathbb{R}^{n\times n} : \mathbf{P}\mathbf{1}_n = \boldsymbol{p}, \ \mathbf{P}^\intercal \mathbf{1}_n = \boldsymbol{q} \right\}.$$

For brevity, this chapter focuses on square matrices $\mathbf{C}$ and $\mathbf{P}$, since extensions to rectangular cases are straightforward.

Let $\langle \cdot, \cdot \rangle$ denote the summation of the element-wise multiplication, such that, for any two matrix $\mathbf{A}, \mathbf{B} \in \mathbb{R}^{n\times n}$, $\langle \mathbf{A}, \mathbf{B} \rangle = \sum_{i=1}^n \sum_{j=1}^n \mathbf{A}_{ij}\mathbf{B}_{ij}$. According to the Kantorovich formulation in Eq. (4), calculating the Wasserstein distance between $\boldsymbol{p}$ and $\boldsymbol{q}$ is thus equivalent to solve the following optimization problem:

$$\min_{\mathbf{P} \in \mathcal{M}(\boldsymbol{p},\boldsymbol{q})} \langle \mathbf{P}, \mathbf{C} \rangle , \tag{6}$$

which is a linear program with $O(n)$ linear constraints. The coupling matrix $\mathbf{P}$ is called the optimal coupling matrix, when the optimization problem (6) achieves the minimum value, i.e., the optimal coupling matrix is the minimizer of the optimization problem (6). Note that when the OTM exists, the optimal coupling matrix $\mathbf{P}$ is a sparse matrix, such that there is exactly one non-zero element in each row and each column of $\mathbf{P}$, respectively.

Practical algorithms for solving the problem (6) through linear programming require a computational time of the order $O(n^3 \log(n))$ for fixed p [75]. Such a sizable computational cost hinders the broad applicability of OT methods in practice for the datasets with large sample size.

3.2 *Sinkhorn Distance*

To alleviate the computation burden for OT problems, [17] considered a variant of the minimization problem in Eq. (6), which can be solved within $O(n^2 \log(n)\, p)$ computational time using the Sinkhorn scaling algorithm, originally proposed in [86]. The solution of such a variant is called the Sinkhorn "distance",[1] defined as

$$W_\eta(\boldsymbol{p}, \boldsymbol{q}) = \min_{\mathbf{P} \in \mathcal{M}(\boldsymbol{p},\boldsymbol{q})} \langle \mathbf{P}, \mathbf{C} \rangle - \eta^{-1} H(\mathbf{P}), \tag{7}$$

where $\eta > 0$ is the regularization parameter, and $H(\mathbf{P}) = \sum_{i=1}^{n} \sum_{j=1}^{n} \mathbf{P}_{ij} \log\left(1/\mathbf{P}_{ij}\right)$ is the Shannon entropy of $\mathbf{P}$. We adopt the standard convention that $0 \log(1/0) = 0$ in the Shannon entropy. We present a fundamental definition as follows [86].

Definition 1 Given $\boldsymbol{p}, \boldsymbol{q} \in \Delta_n$ and $\mathbf{K} \in \mathbb{R}^{n \times n}$ with positive entries, the Sinkhorn projection $\Pi_{\mathcal{M}(\boldsymbol{p},\boldsymbol{q})}(\mathbf{K})$ of $\mathbf{K}$ onto $\mathcal{M}(\boldsymbol{p}, \boldsymbol{q})$ is the unique matrix in $\mathcal{M}(\boldsymbol{p}, \boldsymbol{q})$ of the form $\mathbf{D}_1 \mathbf{K} \mathbf{D}_2$ for positive diagonal matrices $\mathbf{D}_1, \mathbf{D}_2 \in \mathbb{R}^{n \times n}$.

Let $\mathbf{P}^\eta$ be the minimizer, i.e., the optimal coupling matrix, of the optimization problem (7). Throughout this chapter, all matrix exponentials and logarithms will be taken entry-wise, i.e., $(e^{\mathbf{A}})_{ij} := e^{\mathbf{A}_{ij}}$ and $(\log \mathbf{A})_{ij} := \log \mathbf{A}_{ij}$ for any matrix $\mathbf{A} \in \mathbb{R}^{n \times n}$. Cuturi [17] built a simple but key connection between the Sinkhorn distance and the Sinkhorn projection,

$$\mathbf{P}^\eta = \operatorname*{argmin}_{\mathbf{P} \in \mathcal{M}(\boldsymbol{p},\boldsymbol{q})} \langle \mathbf{P}, \mathbf{C} \rangle - \eta^{-1} H(\mathbf{P})$$

[1] We use quotations here since it is not technically a distance; see Section 3.2 of [17] for details. The quotes are dropped henceforth.

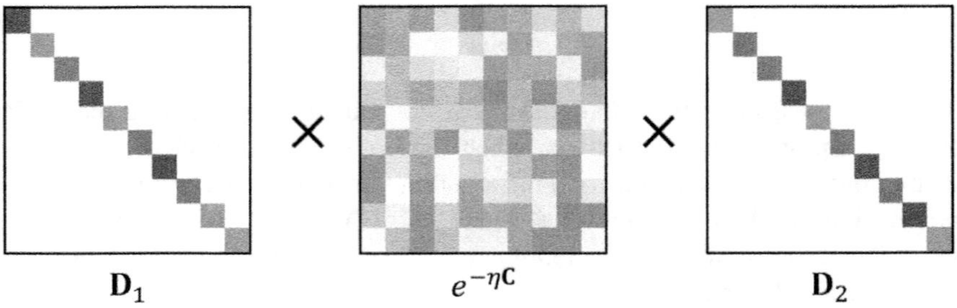

Fig. 3 The minimizer of the regularized optimal transport problem (7) takes the form $\mathbf{D}_1(e^{-\eta\mathbf{C}})\mathbf{D}_2$, for some unknown diagonal metrics $\mathbf{D}_1$ and $\mathbf{D}_2$

$$
\begin{aligned}
&= \underset{\mathbf{P}\in\mathcal{M}(\boldsymbol{p},\boldsymbol{q})}{\text{argmin}} \ \langle \eta\mathbf{C}, \mathbf{P}\rangle - \eta^{-1}H(\mathbf{P}) \\
&= \underset{\mathbf{P}\in\mathcal{M}(\boldsymbol{p},\boldsymbol{q})}{\text{argmin}} \ \left\langle -\log\left(e^{-\eta\mathbf{C}}\right), \mathbf{P}\right\rangle - \eta^{-1}H(\mathbf{P}) \\
&= \Pi_{\mathcal{M}(\boldsymbol{p},\boldsymbol{q})}\left(e^{-\eta\mathbf{C}}\right).
\end{aligned} \tag{8}
$$

Equation (8) suggests the minimizer of the optimization problem (7) takes the form $\mathbf{D}_1(e^{-\eta\mathbf{C}})\mathbf{D}_2$, for some positive diagonal matrices $\mathbf{D}_1, \mathbf{D}_2 \in \mathbb{R}^{n\times n}$, as illustrated in Fig. 3. Moreover, it can be shown that the minimizer in Eq. (8) exists and is unique due to the strict convexity of $-H(\mathbf{P})$ and the compactness of $\mathcal{M}(\boldsymbol{p},\boldsymbol{q})$.

Based on Eq. (8), [17] proposed a simple iterative algorithm, which is also known as the Sinkhorn–Knopp algorithm, to approximate $\mathbf{P}^{\eta}$. Let x_i, y_i, p_i, q_i be the i-th elements of the vectors $\boldsymbol{x}$, $\boldsymbol{y}$, $\boldsymbol{p}$, and $\boldsymbol{q}$, respectively, for $i = 1, \ldots, n$. For simplicity, we now use $\mathbf{A}$ to denote the matrix $e^{-\eta\mathbf{C}}$. Intuitively, the Sinkhorn–Knopp algorithm works as an alternating projection procedure that renormalizes the rows and columns of $\mathbf{A}$ in turn, so that they match the desired row and column marginals $\boldsymbol{p}$ and $\boldsymbol{q}$. In specific, at each step, it prescribes to either modify all the rows of $\mathbf{A}$ by multiplying the i-th row by $(p_i/\sum_{j=1}^{n}\mathbf{A}_{ij})$, for $i = 1, \ldots, n$, or do the analogous operation on the columns. Here, $\sum_{j=1}^{n}\mathbf{A}_{ij}$ is simply the i-th row sum of $\mathbf{A}$. Analogously, we also use $\sum_{i=1}^{n}\mathbf{A}_{ij}$ to denote the j-th column sum of $\mathbf{A}$. The standard convention that $0/0 = 1$ is adopted in the algorithm if it occurs. The algorithm terminates when the matrix $\mathbf{A}$, after k-th iteration, is sufficiently close to the polytope $\mathcal{M}(\boldsymbol{p},\boldsymbol{q})$. The pseudocode for the Sinkhorn–Knopp algorithm is shown in Algorithm 1.

One question remaining for Algorithm 1 is how to determine the size of η that balances the trade-off between the computation time and the estimation accuracy. In specific, a small η is associated with a more accurate estimation of the Wasserstein distance as well as longer computation time [33]. In practice, one can determine the size of η using cross-validation [17].

Algorithm 1 requires a computational cost of the order $O(n^2\log(n)pK)$, where K is the number of iterations. It is known that $K = O(\epsilon^{-2})$ in order to let

Algorithm 1 SINKHORN($\mathbf{A}$, $\mathcal{M}(\boldsymbol{p}, \boldsymbol{q})$, ϵ)

Initialize: $k \leftarrow 0$; $\mathbf{A}^{[0]} \leftarrow \mathbf{A}/\|\mathbf{A}\|_1$; $\boldsymbol{x}^{[0]} \leftarrow \mathbf{0}$; $\boldsymbol{y}^{[0]} \leftarrow \mathbf{0}$
repeat
  $k \leftarrow k+1$
  if k is odd **then**
    $x_i \leftarrow \log\left(p_i / \sum_{j=1}^{n} \mathbf{A}_{ij}^{[k-1]}\right)$, for $i = 1, \ldots, n$
    $\boldsymbol{x}^{[k]} \leftarrow \boldsymbol{x}^{[k-1]} + \boldsymbol{x}$; $\boldsymbol{y}^{[k]} \leftarrow \boldsymbol{y}^{[k-1]}$
  else
    $y_j \leftarrow \log\left(q_i / \sum_{i=1}^{n} \mathbf{A}_{ij}^{[k-1]}\right)$, for $j = 1, \ldots, n$
    $\boldsymbol{y}^{[k]} \leftarrow \boldsymbol{y}^{[k-1]} + \boldsymbol{y}$; $\boldsymbol{x}^{[k]} \leftarrow \boldsymbol{x}^{[k-1]}$
  $\mathbf{D}_1 \leftarrow \mathrm{diag}(\exp(\boldsymbol{x}^{[k]}))$; $\mathbf{D}_2 \leftarrow \mathrm{diag}(\exp(\boldsymbol{y}^{[k]}))$
  $\mathbf{A}^{[k]} = \mathbf{D}_1\mathbf{A}\mathbf{D}_2$
until $\mathrm{dist}(\mathbf{A}^{[k]}, \mathcal{M}(\boldsymbol{p}, \boldsymbol{q})) \le \epsilon$
Output: $\mathbf{P}^{\eta} = \mathbf{A}^{[k]}$

Algorithm 1 to achieve the desired accuracy. Recently, [2] proposed a new greedy coordinate descent variant of the Sinkhorn algorithm with the same theoretical guarantees and a significantly smaller number of iterations. With the help of Algorithm 1, the regularized optimal transport problem can be solved reliably and efficiently in the cases when $n \approx 10^4$ [17, 34].

3.3 *Sinkhorn Algorithms with the Nyström Method*

Although the Sinkhorn–Knopp algorithm has already yielded impressive algorithmic benefits, its computational complexity and memory usage are of the order of n^2, since such an algorithm involves the calculation of the $n \times n$ matrix $e^{-\eta C}$. Such a quadratic computational cost makes the calculation of Sinkhorn distances prohibitively expensive on the datasets with millions of observations.

To alleviate the computation burden, [1] proposed to replace the computation of the entire matrix $e^{-\eta C}$ with its low-rank approximation. Computing such approximations is a problem that has long been studied in machine learning under different names, including Nyström method [95, 97], sparse greedy approximations [87], incomplete Cholesky decomposition [26], and CUR matrix decomposition [63]. These methods draw great attention in the subsampling literature due to their close relationship to the *algorithmic leveraging* approach [58, 59, 66, 99], which has been widely applied in linear regression models [22, 57, 61], logistic regression [92], and streaming time series [98]. Among the aforementioned low-rank approximation methods, the Nyström method is arguably the most extensively used one in the literature [62, 93]. We now briefly introduce the Nyström method, followed by the fast Sinkhorn algorithm proposed in [1] that utilizes the Nyström method for low-rank matrix approximation.

Let $\mathbf{K} \in \mathbb{R}^{n \times n}$ be the matrix that we aim to approximate. Let $s < n$ be a positive integer, $\mathbf{S}$ be a $n \times s$ column selection matrix,[2] and $\mathbf{R} = \mathbf{KS} \in \mathbb{R}^{n \times s}$ be the so-called sketch matrix of $\mathbf{K}$. In other words, $\mathbf{R}$ is a matrix that contains certain columns of $\mathbf{K}$. Consider the optimization problem

$$\widetilde{\mathbf{X}} = \underset{\mathbf{X} \in \mathbb{R}^{s \times s}}{\operatorname{argmin}} \|\mathbf{S}^\intercal (\mathbf{K} - \mathbf{RXR}^\intercal)\mathbf{S}\|_F^2, \tag{9}$$

where $\|\cdot\|_F$ denotes the Frobenius norm. Equation (9) suggests the matrix $\mathbf{R}\widetilde{\mathbf{X}}\mathbf{R}^\intercal$ can be utilized as a low-rank approximation of $\mathbf{K}$ since such a matrix is the closest one to $\mathbf{K}$ among all the semi-positive definite metrics that have rank at most s. Let $(\cdot)^+$ denote the Moore–Penrose inverse of a matrix. It is known that the minimizer of the optimization problem (9) takes the form

$$\widetilde{\mathbf{X}} = (\mathbf{S}^\intercal\mathbf{R})^+(\mathbf{S}^\intercal\mathbf{KS})(\mathbf{R}^\intercal\mathbf{S})^+ = (\mathbf{S}^\intercal\mathbf{KS})^+;$$

see [93] for technical details. Consequently, we have the following low-rank approximation of $\mathbf{K}$,

$$\mathbf{K} \approx \mathbf{R}(\mathbf{S}^\intercal\mathbf{KS})^+\mathbf{R}^\intercal,$$

and such an approximation is called the Nyström method, as illustrated in Fig. 4. It is known that the Nyström method is highly efficient and could reliably be run on problems of size $n \approx 10^6$ [93].

Algorithm 2 introduces NYS-SINK [1], i.e., the Sinkhorn algorithm implemented with the Nyström method. The notations are analogous to the ones in Algorithm 1. Algorithm 2 requires a memory cost of the order $O(ns)$ and a computational cost of the order $O(ns^2p)$. When $s \ll n$, these costs are significant

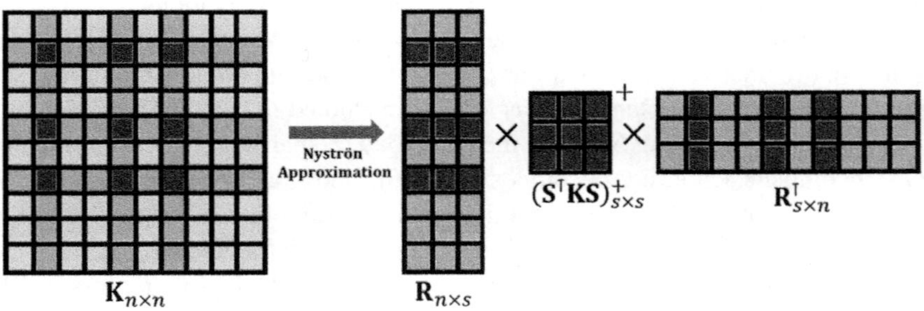

Fig. 4 Illustration for the Nyström method

[2] A column selection matrix is the one in which all the elements of which equal zero except that there exists one element in each column that equals one.

Algorithm 2 NYS-SINK($\mathbf{A}$, $\mathscr{M}(\boldsymbol{p}, \boldsymbol{q})$, ϵ,s)

Input: $\mathbf{A}$, $\boldsymbol{p}$, $\boldsymbol{q}$, s
Step 1: Calculate the Nyström approximation of $\mathbf{A}$ (with rank s), denoted by $\widetilde{\mathbf{A}}$.
Step 2: $\widetilde{\mathbf{P}}^{\eta}$ = SINKHORN($\widetilde{\mathbf{A}}$, $\mathscr{M}(\boldsymbol{p}, \boldsymbol{q})$, ϵ)
Output: $\widetilde{\mathbf{P}}^{\eta}$

reductions compared with $O(n^2)$ and $O(n^2 \log(n)\, p)$ for Algorithm 1, respectively. [1] reported that Algorithm 2 could reliably be run on problems of size $n \approx 10^6$ on a single laptop.

There are two fundamental questions when implementing the Nyström method in practice: (1) how to decide the size of s; and (2) given s, how to construct the column selection matrix $\mathbf{S}$. For the latter question, we refer to [36] for an extensive review of how to construct $\mathbf{S}$ through weighted random subsampling. There also exists a recursive strategy [70] for potentially more effective construction of $\mathbf{S}$. For the former question, various data-driven strategies have been proposed to determine the size of s that is adaptive to the low-dimensional structure of the data. These strategies are developed under different model setups, including kernel ridge regression [10, 36, 70], kernel K-means [41, 94], and so on. Considering the optimal transport problem that is of our interest, [1] assumed the data are lying on a low-dimensional manifold, and the authors developed a data-driven strategy to determine the effective dimension of such a manifold.

4 Projection-Based Optimal Transport Methods

In the cases when $n \gg p$, one can utilize projection-based optimal transport methods for potential faster calculation as well as smaller memory consumption, compared with regularization-based optimal transport methods. These projection-based methods build upon a key fact that the empirical one-dimensional OTM under the L_2 norm is equivalent to sorting. Utilizing such a fact, the projection-based OT methods tackle the problem of estimating a p-dimensional OTM by breaking down the problem into a series of subproblems, each of which finds a one-dimensional OTM using projected samples [7, 76, 77, 79]. The projection direction can be selected either at random or at deterministic, based on different criteria. Generally speaking, the computational cost for these projection-based methods are approximately proportional to n, and the memory cost of which is at the order of $O(np)$, which is a significant reduction from $O(n^2)$ when $p \ll n$. We will cover some representatives of the projection-based OT methods in this section.

4.1 Random Projection OT Method

The random projection method, also called the Radon probability density function (PDF) transformation method, is first proposed in [76] for transferring the color between different images. Intuitively, an image can be represented as a three-dimensional sample in the RGB color space, in which each pixel of the image is an observation. The goal of color transfer is to find a transport map ϕ such that the color of the transformed source image follows the same distribution of the color of the target image. Although the map ϕ does not have to be the OTM in this problem, the random projection method proposed in [76] can be regarded as an estimation method for OTM.

The random projection method is built upon the fact that two PDFs are identical if the marginal distributions, respecting all possible one-dimensional projection directions, of these two PDFs are identical. Since it is impossible to consider all possible projection directions in practice, the random projection method thus utilizes the Monte Carlo method and considers a sequence of randomly generated projection directions. The details of the random projection method are summarized in Algorithm 3. The computational cost for Algorithm 3 is at the order of $O(n \log(n) pK)$, where K is the number of iterations under convergence. We illustrate Algorithm 3 in Fig. 5.

Algorithm 3 Random projection method for OTM

Input: the source matrix $\mathbf{X} \in \mathbb{R}^{n\times p}$ and the target matrix $\mathbf{Y} \in \mathbb{R}^{n\times p}$
$k \leftarrow 0,\ \mathbf{X}^{[0]} \leftarrow \mathbf{X}$
repeat
(a) generate a random projection direction $\boldsymbol{\zeta}_k \in \mathbb{R}^p$
(b) find the one-dimensional OTM $\phi^{(k)}$ that matches $\mathbf{X}^{[k]}\boldsymbol{\zeta}_k$ to $\mathbf{Y}\boldsymbol{\zeta}_k$
(c) $\mathbf{X}^{[k+1]} \leftarrow \mathbf{X}^{[k]} + (\phi^{(k)}(\mathbf{X}^{[k]}\boldsymbol{\zeta}_k) - \mathbf{X}^{[k]}\boldsymbol{\zeta}_k)\boldsymbol{\zeta}_k^{\intercal}$
(d) $k \leftarrow k+1$
until converge
The final estimator is given by $\widehat{\phi} : \mathbf{X} \rightarrow \mathbf{X}^{[k]}$

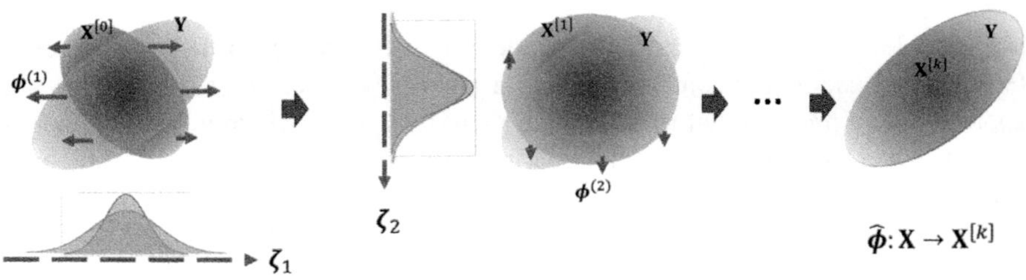

Fig. 5 Illustration of Algorithm 3. In the k-th iteration, a random projection direction $\boldsymbol{\zeta}_k$ is generated, and the one-dimensional OTM is calculated, which matches the projected sample $\mathbf{X}^{[k]}\boldsymbol{\zeta}_k$ to $\mathbf{Y}\boldsymbol{\zeta}_k$

Instead of randomly generating the projection directions using the Monte Carlo method, one can also generate a sequence of projection directions with "low-discrepancy," i.e., the directions that are distributed as disperse as possible on the unit sphere. The low-discrepancy sequence has been widely applied in the field of quasi-Monte Carlo and has been extensively employed for numerical integration [72] and subsampling in big data [67]. We refer to [20, 37, 48, 49] for more in-depth discussions on quasi-Monte Carlo methods. It is reported in [76] that using a low-discrepancy sequence of projection directions yields a potentially faster convergence rate.

Closely related to the random projection method is the sliced method. The sliced method modifies the random projection method by considering a large set of random directions from $\mathbb{S}^{d-1}$ in each iteration, where $\mathbb{S}^{d-1}$ is the d-dimensional unit sphere. The "mean map" of the one-dimensional OTMs over these random directions is considered as a component of the final estimate of the desired OTM. Let L be the number of projection directions considered in each iteration. Consequently, the computational cost of the sliced method is at the order of $O(n \log(n) pKL)$, where K is the number of iterations until convergence. Although the sliced method is L times slower than the random projection method, in practice, it is usually observed that the former yields a more robust estimation of the latter. We refer to [7, 79] for more implementation details of the sliced method.

4.2 Projection Pursuit OT Method

Despite the random projection method works reasonably well in practice, for moderate or large p, such a method suffers from slow or none convergence due to the nature of randomly selected projection directions. To address this issue, [65] introduced a novel statistical approach to estimate large-scale OTMs.[3] The proposed method, named projection pursuit Monge map (PPMM), combines the idea of projection pursuit [32] and sufficient dimension reduction [50]. The projection pursuit technique is similar to boosting that searches for the next optimal direction based on the residual of previous ones. In each iteration, PPMM aims to find the "optimal" projection direction, guided by sufficient dimension reduction techniques, instead of using a randomly selected one. Utilizing these informative projection directions, it is reported in [65] that the PPMM method yields a significantly faster convergence rate than the random projection method. We now introduce some essential background of sufficient dimension reduction techniques, followed by the details of the PPMM method.

Consider a regression problem with a univariate response T and a p-dimensional predictor Z. Sufficient dimension reduction techniques aim to reduce the dimension of Z while preserving its regression relation with T. In other words, such techniques

[3]The code is available at https://github.com/ChengzijunAixiaoli/PPMM.

seek a set of linear combinations of Z, say $\mathbf{B}^\intercal Z$ with some projection matrix $\mathbf{B} \in \mathbb{R}^{p \times q}$ $(q < p)$, such that T depends on Z only through $\mathbf{B}^\intercal Z$, i.e.,

$$T \perp\!\!\!\perp Z | \mathbf{B}^\intercal Z. \tag{10}$$

Let $\mathscr{S}(\mathbf{B})$ denote the column space of $\mathbf{B}$. We call $\mathscr{S}(\mathbf{B})$ a sufficient dimension reduction subspace (s.d.r. subspace) if $\mathbf{B}$ satisfies the formulation (10). Moreover, if the intersection of all possible s.d.r. subspaces is still an s.d.r. subspace, we call it the central subspace and denote it as $\mathscr{S}_{T|Z}$. Note that the central subspace is the s.d.r. subspace with the minimum number of dimensions. Some popular sufficient dimension reduction techniques include sliced inverse regression (SIR) [52], principal Hessian directions (PHD) [53], sliced average variance estimator (SAVE) [15], directional regression (DR) [51], among others. Under some regularity conditions, it can be shown that these methods can induce an s.d.r. subspace that equals the central subspace.

Consider estimating the OTM between a source sample and a target sample. One can form a regression problem using these two samples, i.e., add a binary response variable by labeling them as 0 and 1, respectively. The PPMM method utilizes sufficient dimension reduction techniques to select the most "informative" projection direction. Here, we call a projection direction $\boldsymbol{\xi}$ the most informative one, if the projected samples have the most substantial "discrepancy." The discrepancy can be measured by the difference of the kth order moments or central moments. For example, the SIR method measures the discrepancy using the difference of means, while the SAVE method measures the discrepancy using the difference of variances. The authors in [65] considered the SAVE method and showed that the most informative projection direction was equivalent to the eigenvector corresponding to the largest eigenvalue of the projection matrix $\mathbf{B}$, estimated by SAVE. The detailed algorithm for PPMM is summarized in Algorithm 4 as follows.

Algorithm 4 Projection pursuit Monge map (PPMM)

Input: two matrix $\mathbf{X} \in \mathbb{R}^{n \times p}$ and $\mathbf{Y} \in \mathbb{R}^{n \times p}$
$k \leftarrow 0$, $\mathbf{X}^{[0]} \leftarrow \mathbf{X}$
repeat
(a) calculate the most informative projection direction $\boldsymbol{\xi}_k \in \mathbb{R}^p$ between $\mathbf{X}^{[k]}$ and $\mathbf{Y}$ using SAVE
(b) find the one-dimensional OTM $\phi^{(k)}$ that matches $\mathbf{X}^{[k]}\boldsymbol{\xi}_k$ to $\mathbf{Y}\boldsymbol{\xi}_k$
(c) $\mathbf{X}^{[k+1]} \leftarrow \mathbf{X}^{[k]} + (\phi^{(k)}(\mathbf{X}^{[k]}\boldsymbol{\xi}_k) - \mathbf{X}^{[k]}\boldsymbol{\xi}_k)\boldsymbol{\xi}_k^\intercal$
(d) $k \leftarrow k + 1$
until converge
The final estimator is given by $\widehat{\phi} : \mathbf{X} \rightarrow \mathbf{X}^{[k]}$

The computational cost for Algorithm 4 mainly resides in steps (a) and (b). Within each iteration, steps (a) and (b) require the computational cost of the orders $O(np^2)$ and $O(n \log(n)$, respectively. Consequently, the overall computational cost for Algorithm 4 is at the order of $O(Knp^2 + Kn \log(n))$, where K is the number

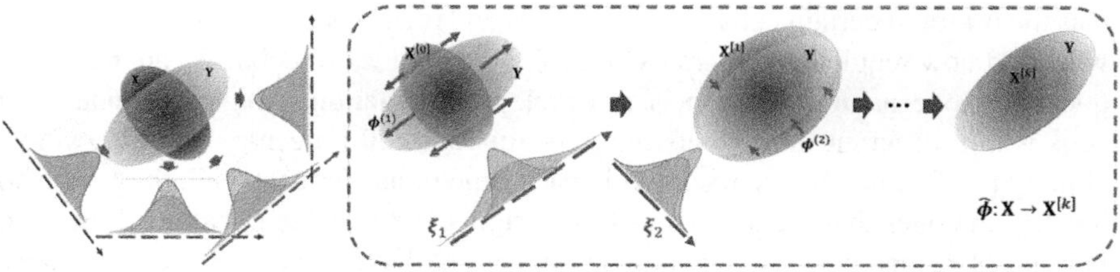

Fig. 6 Illustration of Algorithm 4. The left panel shows that in the k-th iteration, the most informative projection direction ξ_k is calculated by SAVE. The right panel shows that the one-dimensional OTM is calculated to match the projected sample $\mathbf{X}^{[k]}\xi_k$ to $\mathbf{Y}\xi_k$

of iterations. Although not theoretically guaranteed, it is reported in [65] that K is approximately proportional to p in practice, in which case the computational cost for PPMM becomes $O(np^3 + n\log(n)\,p)$. Compared with the computational cost for the Sinkhorn algorithm, i.e., $O(n^2\log(n)\,p)$, PPMM has a lower order of the computational cost when $p \ll n$. We illustrate Algorithm 4 in Fig. 6. Although not covered in this section, the PPMM method can be easily extended to calculate the OTP, with minor modifications [65].

5 Applications in Biomedical Research

In this section, we present some cutting-edge applications of optimal transport methods in biomedical research. We first present how optimal transport methods can be utilized to identify developmental trajectories of single cells [83]. We then review a novel method for augmenting the single-cell RNA-seq data [64]. The method utilizes the technique of generative adversarial networks (GANs), which is closely related to optimal transport methods, as we will discuss later.

5.1 Identify Development Trajectories in Reprogramming

The rapid development of single-cell RNA sequencing (scRNA-seq) technologies has enabled researchers to identify cell types in a population. These technologies help researchers to answer some fundamental questions in biology, including how individual cells differentiate to form tissues, how tissues function in a coordinated and flexible fashion, and which gene regulatory mechanisms support these processes [89].

However, scRNA-seq technologies are not the panacea. Since these technologies require to destroy cells in the course of sequencing their gene expression profiles, researchers cannot follow the expression of the same cell across time. Without further analysis, researchers are thus not able to answer the questions like what was the origin of certain cells at earlier stages and their possible fates at later stages; what and how regulatory programs control the dynamics of cells? To answer these questions, one natural solution is to develop computational tools to connect the cells within different time points into a continuous cell trajectory. In other words, although different cells are recorded in each time point, for each cell, the goal is to identify the ones that are analogous to its origins and its fates in earlier stages and late stages, respectively. A large number of methods have been developed to achieve this goal; see [24, 27, 43, 82] and the references therein.

A novel approach was proposed in [89] to reconstruct cell trajectories. They model the differentiating population of cells as a stochastic process on a high-dimensional expression space. Recall that different cells are recorded independently at different time points. Consequently, the unknown fact to the researchers is the joint distribution of expression of the unobserved cells between different pairs of time points. To infer how the differentiation process evolves over time, the authors assume the expression of each cell changes within a relatively small range over short periods. Based on such an assumption, one thus can infer the differentiation process though optimal transport methods that naturally give the transport map between two distributions, respecting to two time points, with the minimum transport cost.

Figure 7 illustrates an idea to search for the "cell trajectories." For gene expression $\mathbf{X}_t$ of any set of cells at time t, it can be transported to a later time point $t+1$ according to OTP from the distribution over $\mathbf{X}_t$ to the distribution over the cells at time $t + 1$. Analogously, $\mathbf{X}_t$ can be transported from a former time point $t - 1$ by back-winding the OPT from the distribution over $\mathbf{X}_t$ to the distribution over the cells at time $t - 1$ (the left and middle panels in Fig. 7). The trajectory combines the transportation between any two neighboring time points (the right panel in Fig. 7). Thus, OTP helps to infer the differentiation process of cells at any time along the trajectory.

The authors in [89] used optimal transport methods to calculate the differentiation process between consecutive time points and then compose all the transport maps together to obtain the cell trajectories over long time intervals. The authors also considered unbalanced transport [14] for modeling cellular proliferation, i.e.,

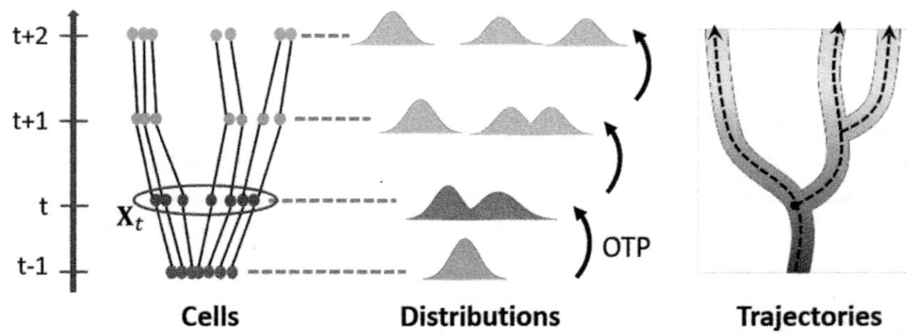

Fig. 7 Illustration for cell trajectories along time. Left: Cells at each time point. Middle: OPT between distributions over cells at each time point. Right: Cell trajectories based on OPT

cell growth and death. Analyzing around 315,000 cell profiles sampled densely across 18 days, the authors found reprogramming unleashes a much wider range of developmental programs and subprograms than previously characterized.

5.2 Data Augmentation for Biomedical Data

Recent advances in scRNA-seq technologies have enabled researchers to measure the expression of thousands of genes at the same time and to scrutinize the complex interactions in biological systems. Despite wide applications, such technologies may fail to quantify all the complexities in biological systems in the cases when the number of observations is relatively small, due to economic or ethical considerations or simply because the sample size of the available patients is low [69]. The problem of a small sample size results in biased results since a small sample may not be a decent representative of the population.

Not only arising from biomedical research, such a problem also arises from the research in various fields, including computer vision and deep learning, which require considerable quantity and diversity of data during the training process [38, 45]. In these fields, data augmentation is a widely applied strategy to alleviate the problem of small sample sizes, without actually collecting new data. In computer vision, some elementary algorithms for data augmentation include cropping, rotating, and flipping; see [85] for a survey. These algorithms, however, may not be suitable for augmenting data in biomedical research.

Compared with these elementary algorithms, a more sophisticated approach for data augmentation is to use generative models, including generative adversarial nets (GANs) [39], the "decoder" network in variational autoencoders [44], among others. Generative models aim to generate "fake" samples that are indistinguishable from the genuine ones. The fake samples can then be used, alongside the genuine ones, in downstream analysis to artificially increase sample sizes. Generative models have been widely used for generating realistic images [21, 55], songs [6, 23], and videos [54, 91]. Many variants of the GAN method have been proposed recently, and of particular interest is the Wasserstein GAN [4], which utilizes the Wasserstein distance instead of the Jensen–Shannon divergence in the standard GAN for measuring the discrepancy between two samples. The authors showed that the Wasserstein GAN yields a more stable training process compared with the standard GAN since Wasserstein distance appears to be a more powerful metric than the Jensen–Shannon divergence in GAN.

Nowadays, GAN has been widely used for data augmentation in various biomedical researches [30, 31, 60]. Recently, [64] proposed a novel data augmentation method for scRNA-seq data. The proposed method, called single-cell GAN, is developed based on Wasserstein GAN. The authors showed the proposed method improves downstream analyses such as the detection of marker genes, the robustness and reliability of classifiers, and the assessment of novel analysis algorithms, resulting in the potential reduction of the number of animal experiments and costs.

Note that generative models are closely related to optimal transport methods. Intuitively, a generative model is equivalent to finding a transport map from random noises with a simple distribution, e.g., Gaussian distribution or uniform distribution, to the underlying population distribution of the genuine sample. Recent studies suggest optimal transport methods outperform the Wasserstein GAN for approximating probability measures in some special cases [46, 47]. Consequently, researchers may consider using optimal transport methods instead of GAN models for data augmentation in biomedical research for potentially better performance.

Acknowledgments The authors would like to acknowledge the support from the U.S. National Science Foundation under grants DMS-1903226 and DMS-1925066 and the U.S. National Institute of Health under grant R01GM122080.

References

1. Altschuler, J., Bach, F., Rudi, A., Niles-Weed, J.: Massively scalable Sinkhorn distances via the Nyström method. In: Advances in Neural Information Processing Systems, pp. 4429–4439 (2019)
2. Altschuler, J., Weed, J., Rigollet, P.: Near-linear time approximation algorithms for optimal transport via Sinkhorn iteration. In: Advances in Neural Information Processing Systems, pp. 1964–1974 (2017)
3. Alvarez-Melis, D., Jaakkola, T., Jegelka, S.: Structured optimal transport. In: International Conference on Artificial Intelligence and Statistics, pp. 1771–1780 (2018)
4. Arjovsky, M., Chintala, S., Bottou, L.: Wasserstein generative adversarial networks. In: International Conference on Machine Learning, pp. 214–223 (2017)
5. Benamou, J.D., Brenier, Y., Guittet, K.: The monge–kantorovitch mass transfer and its computational fluid mechanics formulation. Int. J. Numer. Methods Fluids **40**(1–2), 21–30 (2002)
6. Blaauw, M., Bonada, J.: Modeling and transforming speech using variational autoencoders. In: Interspeech, pp. 1770–1774 (2016)
7. Bonneel, N., Rabin, J., Peyré, G., Pfister, H.: Sliced and radon Wasserstein barycenters of measures. J. Math. Imaging Vision **51**(1), 22–45 (2015)
8. Brenier, Y.: Polar factorization and monotone rearrangement of vector-valued functions. Commun. Pure Appl. Math. **44**(4), 375–417 (1991)
9. Brenier, Y.: A homogenized model for vortex sheets. Arch. Ration. Mech. Anal. **138**(4), 319–353 (1997)
10. Calandriello, D., Lazaric, A., Valko, M.: Analysis of Nyström method with sequential ridge leverage score sampling (2020)
11. Canas, G., Rosasco, L.: Learning probability measures with respect to optimal transport metrics. In: Advances in Neural Information Processing Systems, pp. 2492–2500 (2012)
12. Cazelles, E., Seguy, V., Bigot, J., Cuturi, M., Papadakis, N.: Geodesic PCA versus log-PCA of histograms in the Wasserstein space. SIAM J. Sci. Comput. **40**(2), B429–B456 (2018)
13. Chen, Y., Georgiou, T.T., Tannenbaum, A.: Optimal transport for Gaussian mixture models. IEEE Access **7**, 6269–6278 (2018)
14. Chizat, L., Peyré, G., Schmitzer, B., Vialard, F.X.: Scaling algorithms for unbalanced optimal transport problems. Math. Comput. **87**(314), 2563–2609 (2018)
15. Cook, R.D., Weisberg, S.: Sliced inverse regression for dimension reduction: comment. J. Am. Stat. Assoc. **86**(414), 328–332 (1991)

16. Courty, N., Flamary, R., Tuia, D., Rakotomamonjy, A.: Optimal transport for domain adaptation. IEEE Trans. Pattern Anal. Mach. Intell. **39**(9), 1853–1865 (2016)
17. Cuturi, M.: Sinkhorn distances: lightspeed computation of optimal transport. In: Advances in Neural Information Processing Systems, pp. 2292–2300 (2013)
18. Del Barrio, E., Gordaliza, P., Lescornel, H., Loubes, J.M.: Central limit theorem and bootstrap procedure for Wasserstein's variations with an application to structural relationships between distributions. J. Multivar. Anal. **169**, 341–362 (2019)
19. Del Barrio, E., Loubes, J.M.: Central limit theorems for empirical transportation cost in general dimension. Ann. Probab. **47**(2), 926–951 (2019). https://doi.org/10.1214/18-AOP1275
20. Dick, J., Kuo, F.Y., Sloan, I.H.: High-dimensional integration: the quasi-Monte Carlo way. Acta Numer. **22**, 133–288 (2013)
21. Dosovitskiy, A., Brox, T.: Generating images with perceptual similarity metrics based on deep networks. In: Advances in Neural Information Processing Systems, pp. 658–666 (2016)
22. Drineas, P., Magdon-Ismail, M., Mahoney, M.W., Woodruff, D.P.: Fast approximation of matrix coherence and statistical leverage. J. Mach. Learn. Res. **13**, 3475–3506 (2012)
23. Engel, J., Resnick, C., Roberts, A., Dieleman, S., Norouzi, M., Eck, D., Simonyan, K.: Neural audio synthesis of musical notes with wavenet autoencoders. In: Proceedings of the 34th International Conference on Machine Learning **70**, 1068–1077 (2017). JMLR.org
24. Farrell, J.A., Wang, Y., Riesenfeld, S.J., Shekhar, K., Regev, A., Schier, A.F.: Single-cell reconstruction of developmental trajectories during zebrafish embryogenesis. Science **360**(6392), eaar3131 (2018)
25. Ferradans, S., Papadakis, N., Peyré, G., Aujol, J.F.: Regularized discrete optimal transport. SIAM J. Imaging Sci. **7**(3), 1853–1882 (2014)
26. Fine, S., Scheinberg, K.: Efficient SVM training using low-rank kernel representations. J. Mach. Learn. Res. **2**, 243–264 (2001)
27. Fischer, D.S., Fiedler, A.K., Kernfeld, E.M., Genga, R.M., Bastidas-Ponce, A., Bakhti, M., Lickert, H., Hasenauer, J., Maehr, R., Theis, F.J.: Inferring population dynamics from single-cell RNA-sequencing time series data. Nat. Biotechnol. **37**(4), 461–468 (2019)
28. Flamary, R., Cuturi, M., Courty, N., Rakotomamonjy, A.: Wasserstein discriminant analysis. Mach. Learn. **107**(12), 1923–1945 (2018)
29. Flamary, R., Lounici, K., Ferrari, A.: Concentration bounds for linear Monge mapping estimation and optimal transport domain adaptation (2019). arXiv preprint arXiv:1905.10155
30. Frid-Adar, M., Diamant, I., Klang, E., Amitai, M., Goldberger, J., Greenspan, H.: GAN-based synthetic medical image augmentation for increased CNN performance in liver lesion classification. Neurocomputing **321**, 321–331 (2018)
31. Frid-Adar, M., Klang, E., Amitai, M., Goldberger, J., Greenspan, H.: Synthetic data augmentation using GAN for improved liver lesion classification. In: 2018 IEEE 15th international symposium on biomedical imaging (ISBI 2018), pp. 289–293. IEEE, Piscataway (2018)
32. Friedman, J.H., Stuetzle, W.: Projection pursuit regression. J. Am. Stat. Assoc. **76**(376), 817–823 (1981)
33. Genevay, A., Chizat, L., Bach, F., Cuturi, M., Peyré, G.: Sample complexity of Sinkhorn divergences. In: The 22nd International Conference on Artificial Intelligence and Statistics, pp. 1574–1583 (2019)
34. Genevay, A., Cuturi, M., Peyré, G., Bach, F.: Stochastic optimization for large-scale optimal transport. In: Advances in Neural Information Processing Systems, pp. 3440–3448 (2016)
35. Genevay, A., Peyré, G., Cuturi, M.: Learning generative models with Sinkhorn divergences (2017). arXiv preprint arXiv:1706.00292
36. Gittens, A., Mahoney, M.W.: Revisiting the Nyström method for improved large-scale machine learning. J. Mach. Learn. Res. **17**(1), 3977–4041 (2016)
37. Glasserman, P.: Monte Carlo Methods in Financial Engineering, vol. 53. Springer, Berlin (2013)
38. Goodfellow, I., Bengio, Y., Courville, A.: Deep Learning. MIT Press, Cambridge (2016)

39. Goodfellow, I., Pouget-Abadie, J., Mirza, M., Xu, B., Warde-Farley, D., Ozair, S., Courville, A., Bengio, Y.: Generative adversarial nets. In: Advances in Neural Information Processing Systems, pp. 2672–2680 (2014)
40. Gu, C.: Smoothing Spline ANOVA Models. Springer, Berlin (2013)
41. He, L., Zhang, H.: Kernel k-means sampling for Nyström approximation. IEEE Trans. Image Process. **27**(5), 2108–2120 (2018)
42. Kantorovich, L.: On translation of mass (in Russian), c r. In: Doklady. Acad. Sci. USSR, vol. 37, pp. 199–201 (1942)
43. Kester, L., van Oudenaarden, A.: Single-cell transcriptomics meets lineage tracing. Cell Stem Cell **23**(2), 166–179 (2018)
44. Kingma, D.P., Welling, M.: Auto-encoding variational Bayes (2013). arXiv preprint arXiv:1312.6114
45. LeCun, Y., Bengio, Y., Hinton, G.: Deep learning. Nature **521**(7553), 436–444 (2015)
46. Lei, N., An, D., Guo, Y., Su, K., Liu, S., Luo, Z., Yau, S.T., Gu, X.: A geometric understanding of deep learning. Engineering **6**(3), 361–374 (2020)
47. Lei, N., Su, K., Cui, L., Yau, S.T., Gu, X.D.: A geometric view of optimal transportation and generative model. Comput. Aided Geom. Des. **68**, 1–21 (2019)
48. Lemieux, C.: Monte Carlo and Quasi-Monte Carlo Sampling. Springer, New York (2009)
49. Leobacher, G., Pillichshammer, F.: Introduction to Quasi-Monte Carlo Integration and Applications. Springer, Berlin (2014)
50. Li, B.: Sufficient Dimension Reduction: Methods and Applications with R. Chapman and Hall/CRC, London (2018)
51. Li, B., Wang, S.: On directional regression for dimension reduction. J. Am. Stat. Assoc. **102**(479), 997–1008 (2007)
52. Li, K.C.: Sliced inverse regression for dimension reduction. J. Am. Stat. Assoc. **86**(414), 316–327 (1991)
53. Li, K.C.: On principal hessian directions for data visualization and dimension reduction: another application of Stein's lemma. J. Am. Stat. Assoc. **87**(420), 1025–1039 (1992)
54. Liang, X., Lee, L., Dai, W., Xing, E.P.: Dual motion GAN for future-flow embedded video prediction. In: Proceedings of the IEEE International Conference on Computer Vision, pp. 1744–1752 (2017)
55. Liu, Y., Qin, Z., Luo, Z., Wang, H.: Auto-painter: cartoon image generation from sketch by using conditional generative adversarial networks (2017). arXiv preprint arXiv:1705.01908
56. Ma, P., Huang, J.Z., Zhang, N.: Efficient computation of smoothing splines via adaptive basis sampling. Biometrika **102**(3), 631–645 (2015)
57. Ma, P., Mahoney, M.W., Yu, B.: A statistical perspective on algorithmic leveraging. J. Mach. Learn. Res. **16**(1), 861–911 (2015)
58. Ma, P., Sun, X.: Leveraging for big data regression. Wiley Interdiscip. Rev. Comput. Stat. **7**(1), 70–76 (2015)
59. Ma, P., Zhang, X., Xing, X., Ma, J., Mahoney, M.W.: Asymptotic analysis of sampling estimators for randomized numerical linear algebra algorithms. In: The 23nd International Conference on Artificial Intelligence and Statistics (2020)
60. Madani, A., Moradi, M., Karargyris, A., Syeda-Mahmood, T.: Chest x-ray generation and data augmentation for cardiovascular abnormality classification. In: Medical Imaging 2018: Image Processing, vol. 10574, p. 105741M. International Society for Optics and Photonics (2018)
61. Mahoney, M.W.: Randomized algorithms for matrices and data. Found. Trends® Mach. Learn. **3**(2), 123–224 (2011)
62. Mahoney, M.W.: Lecture notes on randomized linear algebra (2016). arXiv preprint arXiv:1608.04481
63. Mahoney, M.W., Drineas, P.: Cur matrix decompositions for improved data analysis. Proc. Natl. Acad. Sci. **106**(3), 697–702 (2009)
64. Marouf, M., Machart, P., Bansal, V., Kilian, C., Magruder, D.S., Krebs, C.F., Bonn, S.: Realistic in silico generation and augmentation of single-cell RNA-seq data using generative adversarial networks. Nat. Commun. **11**(1), 1–12 (2020)

65. Meng, C., Ke, Y., Zhang, J., Zhang, M., Zhong, W., Ma, P.: Large-scale optimal transport map estimation using projection pursuit. In: Advances in Neural Information Processing Systems, pp. 8116–8127 (2019)
66. Meng, C., Wang, Y., Zhang, X., Mandal, A., Ma, P., Zhong, W.: Effective statistical methods for big data analytics. In: Handbook of Research on Applied Cybernetics and Systems Science p. 280 (2017)
67. Meng, C., Zhang, X., Zhang, J., Zhong, W., Ma, P.: More efficient approximation of smoothing splines via space-filling basis selection. Biometrika **107**(3), 723–735 (2020)
68. Montavon, G., Müller, K.R., Cuturi, M.: Wasserstein training of restricted Boltzmann machines. In: Advances in Neural Information Processing Systems, pp. 3718–3726 (2016)
69. Munafò, M.R., Nosek, B.A., Bishop, D.V., Button, K.S., Chambers, C.D., Du Sert, N.P., Simonsohn, U., Wagenmakers, E.J., Ware, J.J., Ioannidis, J.P.: A manifesto for reproducible science. Nat. Hum. Behav. **1**(1), 1–9 (2017)
70. Musco, C., Musco, C.: Recursive sampling for the Nystrom method. In: Advances in Neural Information Processing Systems, pp. 3833–3845 (2017)
71. Muzellec, B., Cuturi, M.: Subspace detours: Building transport plans that are optimal on subspace projections. In: Advances in Neural Information Processing Systems, pp. 6914–6925 (2019)
72. Owen, A.B.: Quasi-Monte Carlo sampling. Monte Carlo Ray Tracing: Siggraph **1**, 69–88 (2003)
73. Panaretos, V.M., Zemel, Y.: Statistical aspects of Wasserstein distances. Ann. Rev. Stat. Appl. **6**, 405–431 (2019)
74. Pele, O., Werman, M.: Fast and robust Earth Mover's Distances. In: 2009 IEEE 12th International Conference on Computer Vision, pp. 460–467. IEEE, Piscataway (2009)
75. Peyré, G., Cuturi, M., et al.: Computational optimal transport. Found. Trends® Mach. Learn. **11**(5–6), 355–607 (2019)
76. Pitie, F., Kokaram, A.C., Dahyot, R.: N-dimensional probability density function transfer and its application to color transfer. In: Computer Vision, 2005. ICCV 2005. Tenth IEEE International Conference on, vol. 2, pp. 1434–1439. IEEE, Piscataway (2005)
77. Pitié, F., Kokaram, A.C., Dahyot, R.: Automated colour grading using colour distribution transfer. Comput. Vis. Image Underst. **107**(1–2), 123–137 (2007)
78. Rabin, J., Ferradans, S., Papadakis, N.: Adaptive color transfer with relaxed optimal transport. In: 2014 IEEE International Conference on Image Processing (ICIP), pp. 4852–4856. IEEE, Piscataway (2014)
79. Rabin, J., Peyré, G., Delon, J., Bernot, M.: Wasserstein barycenter and its application to texture mixing. In: International Conference on Scale Space and Variational Methods in Computer Vision, pp. 435–446. Springer, Berlin (2011)
80. Rigollet, P., Weed, J.: Entropic optimal transport is maximum-likelihood deconvolution. C.R. Math. **356**(11–12), 1228–1235 (2018)
81. Rubner, Y., Guibas, L.J., Tomasi, C.: The earth mover's distance, multi-dimensional scaling, and color-based image retrieval. In: Proceedings of the ARPA Image Understanding Workshop, vol. 661, p. 668 (1997)
82. Saelens, W., Cannoodt, R., Todorov, H., Saeys, Y.: A comparison of single-cell trajectory inference methods. Nat. Biotechnol. **37**(5), 547–554 (2019)
83. Schiebinger, G., Shu, J., Tabaka, M., Cleary, B., Subramanian, V., Solomon, A., Gould, J., Liu, S., Lin, S., Berube, P., et al.: Optimal-transport analysis of single-cell gene expression identifies developmental trajectories in reprogramming. Cell **176**(4), 928–943 (2019)
84. Seguy, V., Damodaran, B.B., Flamary, R., Courty, N., Rolet, A., Blondel, M.: Large-scale optimal transport and mapping estimation (2017). arXiv preprint arXiv:1711.02283
85. Shorten, C., Khoshgoftaar, T.M.: A survey on image data augmentation for deep learning. J. Big Data **6**(1), 60 (2019)
86. Sinkhorn, R.: Diagonal equivalence to matrices with prescribed row and column sums. Am. Math. Mon. **74**(4), 402–405 (1967)
87. Smola, A.J., Schölkopf, B.: Sparse greedy matrix approximation for machine learning (2000)

88. Su, Z., Wang, Y., Shi, R., Zeng, W., Sun, J., Luo, F., Gu, X.: Optimal mass transport for shape matching and comparison. IEEE Trans. Pattern Anal. Mach. Intell. **37**(11), 2246–2259 (2015)
89. Tanay, A., Regev, A.: Scaling single-cell genomics from phenomenology to mechanism. Nature **541**(7637), 331–338 (2017)
90. Villani, C.: Optimal Transport: Old and New. Springer, Berlin (2008)
91. Vondrick, C., Pirsiavash, H., Torralba, A.: Generating videos with scene dynamics. In: Advances in Neural Information Processing Systems, pp. 613–621 (2016)
92. Wang, H., Zhu, R., Ma, P.: Optimal subsampling for large sample logistic regression. J. Am. Stat. Assoc. **113**(522), 829–844 (2018)
93. Wang, S.: A practical guide to randomized matrix computations with MATLAB implementations (2015). arXiv preprint arXiv:1505.07570
94. Wang, S., Gittens, A., Mahoney, M.W.: Scalable kernel k-means clustering with Nyström approximation: relative-error bounds. J. Mach. Learn. Res. **20**(1), 431–479 (2019)
95. Wang, S., Zhang, Z.: Improving cur matrix decomposition and the Nyström approximation via adaptive sampling. J. Mach. Learn. Res. **14**(1), 2729–2769 (2013)
96. Weed, J., Bach, F.: Sharp asymptotic and finite-sample rates of convergence of empirical measures in Wasserstein distance. Bernoulli **25**(4A), 2620–2648 (2019)
97. Williams, C.K., Seeger, M.: Using the Nyström method to speed up kernel machines. In: Advances in Neural Information Processing Systems, pp. 682–688 (2001)
98. Xie, R., Wang, Z., Bai, S., Ma, P., Zhong, W.: Online decentralized leverage score sampling for streaming multidimensional time series. In: The 22nd International Conference on Artificial Intelligence and Statistics, pp. 2301–2311 (2019)
99. Zhang, X., Xie, R., Ma, P.: Statistical leveraging methods in big data. In: Handbook of Big Data Analytics, pp. 51–74. Springer, Berlin (2018)

Variable Selection Approaches in High-Dimensional Space

Bin Luo, Qian Yang, and Susan Halabi

1 Introduction

Advancements in molecular, imaging, and other laboratory tests have led to high-dimensional data, where a large number of variables (p) are observed on a relatively small sample (n), which is referred to as "large p, small n." For example, in biomedical studies, a huge number of magnetic resonance images (MRI) and functional MRI data are collected with only hundreds of patients involved. In cancer treatment, RNA expression, GWAS data, and microarray data are used to understand the biology of disease. There are plentiful of examples from diverse fields where massive high-throughput data are used to answer critical questions [10, 14].

The "curse of dimensionality" has posed several challenges in data analysis. One of them is the challenge to traditional statistical theory. For instance, in terms of asymptotic theory, the traditional approximation assumes that n goes to infinity, while p remains smaller order than n or usually fixed. However, in the high-dimensional scenario, the problem of statistical significance allows p to go to infinity faster than n [38]. Other challenges include the intensive computational costs that are inherent to high-dimensional problems and how to efficiently estimate model parameters and to obtain a model with a large number of meaningful variables that can be interpreted.

In order to enhance model interpretability and make statistical inference feasible in high-dimensional regression models, the sparsity condition has been proposed that among a large set of variables only a few of them are important [16]. In such

B. Luo · Q. Yang · S. Halabi (✉)
Department of Biostatistics and Bioinformatics, Duke University Medical Center, Durham, NC, USA
e-mail: bin.luo2@duke.edu; qian.yang658@duke.edu; susan.halabi@duke.edu

Y. Zhao, (Din) D.-G. Chen (eds.), *Modern Statistical Methods for Health Research*, Emerging Topics in Statistics and Biostatistics,
https://doi.org/10.1007/978-3-030-72437-5_14

cases, variable selection is a critical step to identify a parsimonious model and improve the estimation accuracy of predictive models.

In this chapter, we describe different variable selection approaches in high-dimensional space. We then apply these methods to a real example. We end the chapter with a brief review of high-dimensional inference. Throughout this chapter, we use the terms of variables, covariates, and features interchangeably.

2 Penalized Likelihood Approaches

Suppose the collected data $(\mathbf{x}_i, y_i)_{i=1}^n$ are independent samples, where $\mathbf{x}_i = (x_{i1}, x_{i2}, \cdots, x_{ip})^T$ is a p-dimensional covariate vector and y_i is a response variable. Note that in the high-dimensional setting, $p >> n$. It is frequently assumed that the conditional distribution of y_i given $\mathbf{x}_i$ depends on $\mathbf{x}^T\boldsymbol{\beta}$ with $\boldsymbol{\beta} = (\beta_1, \beta_2, \ldots, \beta_p)^T$. Under the sparse condition, $\boldsymbol{\beta} \in \mathbb{R}^p$ is usually assumed to be an s-sparse coefficient vector, i.e., only s elements are nonzero. The goal of variable selection approaches is to distinguish real signal from noise, namely, identifying important variables with nonzero coefficients and providing accurate estimates for those coefficients.

The penalized likelihood approach has been among the most popular methods to perform simultaneous variable selection and parameter estimation for the last decades [12, 56, 66, 68]. Suppose y_i has a density function $f(y_i; \mathbf{x}_i^T\boldsymbol{\beta})$ conditioning on $\mathbf{x}_i$. The penalized maximum log-likelihood estimator (PMLE) takes the following form:

$$\hat{\boldsymbol{\beta}} = \underset{\boldsymbol{\beta}\in\mathbb{R}^p}{\operatorname{argmax}} \frac{1}{n}\sum_{i=1}^{n} \ell\left(y_i; \mathbf{x}_i^T\boldsymbol{\beta}\right) - \sum_{j=1}^{p} \rho_\lambda(\beta_j), \tag{1}$$

where $\ell(y_i; \mathbf{x}_i^T\boldsymbol{\beta}) = \log f(y_i; \mathbf{x}^T\boldsymbol{\beta})$ is the conditional log-likelihood function of y_i given $\mathbf{x}_i$ and ρ_λ is the penalty function indexed by the regularized parameter $\lambda \geq 0$. Maximizing the penalized likelihood function with respect to $\boldsymbol{\beta}$ is equivalent to minimizing

$$-\frac{1}{n}\sum_{i=1}^{n} \ell\left(y_i; \mathbf{x}_i^T\boldsymbol{\beta}\right) + \sum_{j=1}^{p} \rho_\lambda(\beta_j). \tag{2}$$

While the penalty is designed to obtain exactly zeros for some coefficients, and nonzero for others, the PMLE can simultaneously estimate coefficients and select variables. From an optimization perspective, the PMLE minimizes the negative log-likelihood function with a constraint on the sum of penalty functions. Thus, the PMLE decreases the estimation variance and offers a model that can be interpreted.

2.1 Penalty Functions

We provide a brief review of selected penalty functions in this section. The Akaike Information Criterion (AIC) [1] and Bayesian Information Criterion (BIC) [52] choose a parameter $\boldsymbol{\beta}$ that minimizes the penalized log-likelihood function in (2) with the ℓ_0-norm penalty

$$\rho_\lambda(\beta_j) = \lambda \mathbf{I}(\beta_j \neq 0).$$

This method is referred to as the penalized ℓ_0-likelihood, which is essentially a model selection approach that penalizes the number of variables in the model. However, it is unstable with respect to small perturbations in the data, due to the non-continuity of the ℓ_0 penalty. In addition, it is equivalent to the best subset selection, and hence, it is not computationally feasible in the high-dimensional feature space.

Frank and Friedman [25] generalize the penalized ℓ_0-likelihood by using the bridge penalty as follows:

$$\rho_\lambda(\beta_j) = \lambda|\beta_j|^\gamma \text{ for } 0 < \gamma \leq 2.$$

It bridges the penalized ℓ_0 regression ($\gamma \to 0$) to the ridge regression [32] ($\gamma = 2$). When $\gamma \leq 1$, the components of $\hat{\boldsymbol{\beta}}$ in (2) shrink toward zero if λ is sufficiently large, thus achieving simultaneous coefficient estimation and variable selection. While the bridge penalty with $\gamma < 1$ is continuous, its infinite derivative at the origin may cause numerical problem.

The special case when $\gamma = 1$ is related to the least absolute shrinkage and selection operator (LASSO) [55], which is a very popular shrinkage method for variable selection. The ℓ_1 penalty can be viewed as a convex surrogate of the ℓ_0 penalty. However, it is more stable due to its continuity and also computationally feasible for high-dimensional data. From the Bayesian perspective, the LASSO estimator is essentially an estimate of Bayesian posterior mode, considering the unknown parameters follow independent Laplace priors [49].

Fan and Li [12] introduce the oracle property to characterize the model selection consistency of high-dimensional variable selection. An estimator $\hat{\boldsymbol{\beta}}$ has the oracle property if it correctly selects the true set, i.e., $\{j : \hat{\beta}_j \neq 0\} = \{j : \beta_j^* \neq 0\}$, with probability converging to 1 as $n \to \infty$, and $\hat{\boldsymbol{\beta}}_S$ obtains the same information bound as the oracle estimator. Here, $S := \{j : \beta_j^* \neq 0\}$ represents the true set with $\boldsymbol{\beta}^*$ denoting the true parameter vector, and $\hat{\boldsymbol{\beta}}_S$ is the subvector of $\hat{\boldsymbol{\beta}}$ formed by components in S. In other words, an estimator with the oracle property performs as good as the estimator under the true subset model. However, the LASSO penalty does not enjoy the oracle property in general. In fact, it tends to over shrink the large coefficients and includes many false positives in the selected model [12, 16, 68].

To address the bias of the LASSO, Zou [68] recommends the adaptive LASSO (ALASSO) that uses the weighted ℓ_1 penalty,

$$\rho_\lambda(\beta_j) = \lambda \tilde{w}_j |\beta_j|,$$

where $\tilde{w}_j = 1/|\tilde{\beta}_j|^\tau$ and $\tilde{\boldsymbol{\beta}}$ is a consistent estimator of $\boldsymbol{\beta}^*$ that serves as an initial estimator for the ALASSO procedure. Note that a consistent estimator $\tilde{\boldsymbol{\beta}}$ tends to produce larger initials for nonzero coefficients, which leads to smaller penalty for truly active parameters. Hence, the ALASSO is able to balance the penalization between zero and nonzero coefficients, yielding more accurate variable selection and nearly unbiased estimation of the coefficients. The ALASSO has the oracle property under certain conditions [33, 68].

The smoothly clipped absolute deviation (SCAD) [12] is another penalty that has the oracle property. It is defined as follows:

$$\rho_\lambda(t) = \begin{cases} \lambda|t| & \text{for } |t| \leq \lambda, \\ -\frac{t^2 - 2\gamma\lambda|t| + \lambda^2}{2(\gamma-1)} & \text{for } \lambda < |t| \leq \gamma\lambda, \\ \frac{(\gamma+1)\lambda^2}{2} & \text{for } |t| > \gamma\lambda, \end{cases} \tag{3}$$

where $\gamma > 2$ is a fixed parameter. The local minimizer $\hat{\boldsymbol{\beta}}$ of (2) with the SCAD penalty satisfies the oracle properties under some regular conditions [12, 17, 18].

The minimax concave penalty (MCP) [66] shares a similar penalty as the SCAD. The MCP takes the form

$$\rho_\lambda(t) = \lambda \int_0^{|t|} \left(1 - \frac{z}{\lambda\gamma}\right)_+ dz,$$

with a fixed parameter $\gamma > 0$. It minimizes the maximum concavity

$$\kappa(\rho) := \sup_{0<t_1<t_2} \left\{\rho'_\lambda(t_1) - \rho'_\lambda(t_2)\right\} / (t_2 - t_1)$$

subject to the unbiased and selection features

$$\rho'_\lambda(t) = 0 \quad \text{for } t \geq \gamma\lambda \quad \text{and} \quad \rho'_\lambda(0+) = \lambda.$$

The above-mentioned folded-concave penalties, i.e., the SCAD penalty and the MCP, can be viewed as interpolations between the ℓ_0 penalty and the ℓ_1 (LASSO) penalty. One the one hand, the folded-concave penalty possesses smoothness over the ℓ_0 penalty to gain flexibility and stability in computations. On the other hand, it can reduce the bias of the LASSO and thus improve model selection accuracy and obtain oracle properties. Fan and Lv [17] investigate the penalized likelihood approaches using a general class of folded-concave penalty functions in the context of generalized liner model. They demonstrate that such methods have oracle properties even in the ultra-high dimensional setting, where the dimensionality is allowed to grow in a non-polynomial order of the sample size, i.e. $\log p = \mathcal{O}(n^a)$ for some $a \in (0, 1)$. Table 1 summarizes the properties of different penalties in high-dimensional space.

Table 1 Summary of the properties of different penalties

Penalty	Continuity	Convexity	Unbiasedness	Oracle property
ℓ_0 norm				
Bridge	•			
LASSO	•	•		
ALASSO	•	•	•	•
SCAD	•		•	•
MCP	•		•	•

Although these methods enjoy many attractive statistical properties, they do not work well when the covariates are highly correlated or have certain grouping structures. For example, in gene expression analysis, genes from the same biological pathways may have strong correlations. Tibshirani [55] points out that when there are highly correlated predictors in high-dimensional settings, the prediction performance of the LASSO is dominated by the ridge regression. Zou and Hastie [69] demonstrate that the LASSO tends to select one variable among a group of highly correlated covariates.

To address these issues, Zou and Hastie [69] propose the elastic net (ENET) penalty, which is a linear combination of the ℓ_1 and ℓ_2 penalties

$$\rho_{\lambda,\alpha}(\boldsymbol{\beta}) = \alpha\lambda\|\boldsymbol{\beta}\|_1 + \frac{1}{2}(1-\alpha)\lambda\|\boldsymbol{\beta}\|_2^2, \tag{4}$$

where $\lambda > 0$ and $0 < \alpha < 1$ are the tuning parameters. The ENET penalty can encourage the sparsity and grouping effects simultaneously. Yuan and Lin [61] and Jia and Yu [37] investigate its selection consistency in the settings when p is fixed and $p \gg n$. They show that the variable selection with the ENET estimator is consistent under an irrepresentable condition and some other conditions [37, 61].

Zou and Zhang [71] propose the adaptive ENET estimator to reduce asymptotically the biasedness caused by the ℓ_1 component, following the same rationale behind the ALASSO estimator. However, their oracle results do not hold in the presence of highly correlated covariates and are only applicable to the case of $p < n$. To overcome these limitations, Huang et al. [34] replace the ℓ_1 component by the MCP and propose the Mnet approach. They show that the Mnet estimator has selection consistency and equals the oracle estimator under some regular conditions, which is applicable to the situation when $p \gg n$ [34]. Similarly, the SCAD-Ridge penalty is studied in [9, 62].

2.2 *Canonical Models in High Dimension*

We introduce the specific form of PMLE under several commonly used models in high-dimensional feature space in this section. In particular, we focus on the high-dimensional linear regression model, the logistic regression model, and the proportional hazards model, to deal with continuous, binary, and time-to-event outcomes, respectively. These three models share the same characteristics as the conditional distribution of y given $\mathbf{x}$ is assumed to depend on a certain linear form $\mathbf{x}^T\boldsymbol{\beta}$. As mentioned earlier, we suppose $\boldsymbol{\beta} \in \mathbb{R}^p$ is an s-sparse coefficient vector in a high-dimensional setting $p \gg n$, which indicates only s variables are importantly associated with the response based on a particular model. Note that if the underlying model requires a non-linear form of $f(\mathbf{x})$, we can either map the original feature space to a hyperspace to retain the linear form (e.g., the additive model) or use other non-linear approaches such as the random forest [5].

Linear Regression Model

We consider a high-dimensional linear regression model

$$y_i = \mathbf{x}_i^T\boldsymbol{\beta} + \epsilon_i, \quad 1 \le i \le n, \tag{5}$$

where y_i and $\mathbf{x}_i = (x_{i1}, \cdots, x_{ip})^T$ are the observed response variable and covariates vector and $\epsilon_1, \ldots, \epsilon_n$ are i.i.d. random variables with mean 0. If $\epsilon_i \sim N(0, \sigma^2)$, the PMLE $\hat{\boldsymbol{\beta}}$ in (2) is equivalent to the penalized least squares (PLS) estimator defined as follows:

$$\hat{\boldsymbol{\beta}} = \underset{\boldsymbol{\beta}\in\mathbb{R}^p}{\text{argmin}} \frac{1}{2n}\sum_{i=1}^{n}\left(y_i - \mathbf{x}_i^T\boldsymbol{\beta}\right)^2 + \sum_{j=1}^{p}\rho_\lambda(\beta_j). \tag{6}$$

The PLS method has become popular in high-dimensional linear regression analysis since the introduction of the LASSO [55]. It minimizes the sum of squared errors with a penalty on the coefficient vector. Using an appropriate penalty function introduced in Sect. 2.1, the PLS can simultaneously select important variables and estimate coefficient. By convention, the PLS with the LASSO, ALASSO, SCAD, and MCP are referred to as the LS-LASSO, LS-ALASSO, LS-SCAD, and LS-MCP, respectively. Note that the PLS method is still applicable even if the random errors do not follow the normal distribution.

Although the LS-LASSO does not have the oracle property, it has been widely used in many applications, due to its computational advantage of convexity. The statistical properties of the LASSO estimator have been extensively studied (e.g., [2, 42, 63, 67, 68]). Bickel et al. [2] present that the LASSO is asymptotically equivalent to the Dantzig selector [6], with the ℓ_2 error rate of prediction or estimation being $s \log(p)/n$, where the number of variables p can be much larger than the sample size n. To study the model selection consistency of the LASSO, Zhao and Yu [67] propose the property of sign consistency,

$$P\left(sgn(\boldsymbol{\beta}^*) = sgn(\hat{\boldsymbol{\beta}})\right) \to 1 \text{ as } n \to \infty,$$

where $sgn(\boldsymbol{\beta})$ is a vector of signs of β_js and $sgn(0)$ is defined as 0. They show that the LASSO is sign consistent if the following irrepresentable condition is satisfied [67],

$$\|\mathbf{X}_2^T\mathbf{X}_1\left(\mathbf{X}_1^T\mathbf{X}_1\right)^{-1} sgn(\boldsymbol{\beta}_1)\|_\infty < 1, \tag{7}$$

where $\boldsymbol{\beta}_1$ is the subvector formed by nonzero elements of $\boldsymbol{\beta}^*$, $\mathbf{X}_1$ and $\mathbf{X}_2$ are the sub-design matrices corresponding to the important and non-important variables, respectively. However, the irrepresentable condition is easily violated in the presence of highly correlated variables and is therefore very restrictive in high-dimension settings. This explains why the LASSO estimator tends to include many false positives in the selected model [16].

To address the inconsistent variable selection, Meinshausen and Bühlmann [46] propose stability selection based on sub-sampling. It provides finite-sample control of false discoveries and a transparent rule to determine the proper amount of penalizations. The randomized LASSO with stability selection is shown to select variables consistently even when the irrepresentable condition in (7) is violated [46].

Unlike the LS-LASSO, the LS-ALASSO is able to select the model consistently while preserving the convexity, when an appropriate estimation is used as an initial estimate. Despite the good statistical properties of the LS-SCAD and LS-MCP, their optimization programs are not convex and thus may suffer from multiple minima issues. For the LS-SCAD, Kim et al. [41] show that with high probability the oracle estimator $\hat{\boldsymbol{\beta}}^{\mathcal{O}}$ is actually a local minimum of the PLS procedure, allowing p to increase with n exponentially. They also provide sufficient conditions to check when a local minimum becomes a global minimum. For the LS-MCP, Zhang et al. [66] propose the penalized linear unbiased selection (PLUS) algorithm with MCP to obtain local minimizers that equal the oracle estimator $\hat{\boldsymbol{\beta}}^{\mathcal{O}}$, with the probability converging to 1. More details of the implementation of the PMLE are discussed in Sect. 2.3.

Logistic Regression Model

Suppose the response of the ith observation y_i is binary with a value either equal to 1 or 0. Such binary responses occur frequently in medicine and biostatistics applications, such as patients responded to a therapy or not. The logistic regression (LR) model aims to model the conditional probability of $y = 1$ given the covariate $\mathbf{x}$, which is defined as follows:

$$\mathbb{P}(y_i = 1|\mathbf{x}_i) = \frac{\exp\{\mathbf{x}_i^T\boldsymbol{\beta}\}}{1+\exp\{\mathbf{x}_i^T\boldsymbol{\beta}\}}, \quad i = 1, 2, \ldots, n. \tag{8}$$

To perform simultaneous variable selection and parameter estimation under the high-dimensional LR model, the corresponding PMLE takes the following form:

$$\hat{\boldsymbol{\beta}} = \underset{\boldsymbol{\beta}\in\mathbb{R}^p}{\operatorname{argmin}} -\frac{1}{n}\sum_{i=1}^{n}\{y_i \log p_i + (1-y_i)\log(1-p_i)\} + \sum_{j=1}^{p}\rho_\lambda(\beta_j), \tag{9}$$

where p_i denotes $\mathbb{P}(y_i = 1|\mathbf{x}_i)$. With different choices of penalty functions, we can obtain the LR-LASSO, LR-ALASSO, LR-SCAD, etc. Note that the statistical properties of PMLE introduced in Sect. 2.1 can be applied directly to the penalized logistic regression estimator, as the latter is a special case of the former.

Proportional Hazards Model

Consider $y_i = \min\{t_i, c_i\}$ as the observed time, where t_i and c_i are the survival time and the censoring time of the ith subject, respectively. Assume t_i and c_i are conditionally independent given $\mathbf{x}_i$ and the censoring mechanism is not informative. Let $\delta_i = I(t_i \le c_i)$ be the censoring indicator. Then, the collected data become $(y_i, \delta_i, \mathbf{x}_i)_{i=1}^n$.

To study the dependence of survival time t_i on covariate $\mathbf{x}_i$, the proportional hazards (PH) model includes a hazard function $h(t_i|\mathbf{x}_i)$ of a subject as follows:

$$h(t_i|\mathbf{x}_i) = h_0(t_i)\exp\left(\mathbf{x}_i^T\boldsymbol{\beta}\right), \tag{10}$$

with the baseline function $h_0(t)$ and coefficient vector $\boldsymbol{\beta}$. Under the sparsity condition in a high-dimensional setting with $p \gg n$, only a few variables are relevant to the survival time. The PMLE in (2) then becomes the penalized log partial likelihood estimator defined as follows:

$$\hat{\boldsymbol{\beta}} = \underset{\boldsymbol{\beta}\in\mathbb{R}^p}{\operatorname{argmin}} -\frac{1}{n}\sum_{i=1}^{n}\left\{\delta_i\mathbf{x}_i^T\boldsymbol{\beta} - \delta_i\log\left\{\sum_{j\in R_i}\exp\left(\mathbf{x}_j^T\boldsymbol{\beta}\right)\right\}\right\} + \sum_{j=1}^{p}\rho_\lambda(\beta_j),$$

where $R_i = \{j : y_j \ge y_i\}$ is the risk set right before the time y_i. Similarly, we refer to the PMLE under the PH model with different penalty functions such as PH-LASSO, PH-ALASSO, PH-SCAD, etc.

Tibshirani [57] proposes to use the LASSO for variable selection and shrinkage for the PH model. Gui and Li [29] apply the LARS algorithm to approximate the PH-LASSO and perform survival analysis with microarray gene expression data. Huang et al. [35] investigate the statistical properties of the PH-LASSO for $p \gg n$ data. In view of other penalized methods for survival, Zhang and Lu [64] establish the oracle property of the PH-ALASSO with a fixed number of covariates p when the maximum partial likelihood estimation is used as an initial estimate. Both Fan and Li [13] and Fan and Lv [17] study the SCAD type of penalty functions for the

PH model and show a local maximizer of the penalized log partial likelihood enjoys the oracle property, for fixed p and $p \gg n$ situations, respectively.

2.3 *Algorithm and Implementation*

When the penalty function is convex (e.g., the LASSO and ENET penalties), the objective function in (2) is convex and, hence, the optimization algorithm can be used. For the LASSO, Akaike [1] develops a fast and efficient angle regression (LARS) algorithm for computing the entire path of the LASSO solution. The LARS algorithm is based on the piecewise linearity of the LASSO solution path and can be extended to solve the ENET-penalized regression problem [69]. However, the nonconvex penalties, such as the SCAD and MCP, can introduce numerical challenges in fitting the penalized likelihood models. Zou and Li [70] propose a local linear approximation (LLA) to the penalty, thereby transforming the general PMLE to an iteratively reweighted LASSO-penalized regression that can be optimized using the LARS algorithm. Fan et al. [22] provide a general theory for obtaining the oracle solution via the LLA algorithm.

In this section, we introduce the coordinate descent algorithm for general penalized likelihood approaches. Such a coordinate-wise algorithm has been proved to be very competitive to the LARS procedure in the LASSO method, especially for the $p \gg n$ problem [27]. The application of coordinate descent algorithm to the PMLE approaches under the generalized linear model and the proportional hazards model has also been extensively studied [4, 28, 54].

The coordinate descent algorithm minimizes the objective function with respect to a single coordinate direction at a time, iteratively cycling through all coordinates until it converges. For optimizing the PMLE problem discussed in this chapter, each iteration over all parameters requires only $\mathcal{O}(np)$ operations. If we solve the problem along an entire path of values for the tuning parameter λ, the initial values using previous estimates will be close to the solution and thus only a few iterations are required. Since the computational cost is linear with respect to p, this algorithm is very efficient for the high-dimensional problems.

We first describe the coordinate descent algorithm for solving the penalized weighted least squares (PWLS) problem. Then, we illustrate how different types of PMLE can be solved by repeatedly solving a PWLS problem. Additional details for the convergence properties of the coordinate descent are provided in [4, 38].

Penalized Weighted Least Squares

We consider the collected data $(\mathbf{x}_i, y_i)_{i=1}^n$ under the linear regression model in (5). Suppose a weight w_i is associated with each observation. The PWLS estimator solves the following problem:

$$\hat{\boldsymbol{\beta}} = \underset{\boldsymbol{\beta}\in\mathbb{R}^p}{\operatorname{argmin}} \frac{1}{2n}\sum_{i=1}^{n} w_i \left(y_i - \mathbf{x}_i^T\boldsymbol{\beta}\right)^2 + \sum_{j=1}^{p} \rho_\lambda(\beta_j). \tag{11}$$

When $w_i = 1$ for each observation, the PWLS becomes the PLS in (6). Observations often receive different weights in iteratively reweighted PWLS algorithm for the general PMLE.

Let $Q(\boldsymbol{\beta})$ denote the objective function in (11). We describe the coordinate descent step for minimizing $Q(\boldsymbol{\beta})$. Suppose we would like to minimize $Q(\boldsymbol{\beta})$ with respect to β_k, while the estimates for β_j with $j \neq k$ are fixed. We compute the derivative

$$\begin{aligned}\frac{\partial Q}{\partial \beta_k} &= \tfrac{1}{n}\textstyle\sum_{i=1}^{n} w_i x_{ik}\left(y_i - \mathbf{x}_i^T\boldsymbol{\beta}\right) + \rho_\lambda'(\beta_k)\\ &= \tfrac{1}{n}\textstyle\sum_{i=1}^{n} w_i x_{ik}(y_i - \sum_{j\neq k} x_{ij}\beta_j) + \tfrac{1}{n}\sum_{i=1}^{n} w_i x_{ik}^2\beta_k + \rho_\lambda'(\beta_k)\\ &= z_k + t_k\beta_k + \rho_\lambda'(\beta_k),\end{aligned}$$

where $z_k = \frac{1}{n}\sum_{i=1}^{n} w_i x_{ik}(y_i - \sum_{j\neq k} x_{ij}\beta_j)$, $t_k = \frac{1}{n}\sum_{i=1}^{n} w_i x_{ik}^2$ and ρ_λ' is the derivative of ρ_λ. For a commonly used penalty function ρ_λ, the coordinate solution has a closed form

$$\beta_k = f(z_k, t_k, \lambda), \tag{12}$$

where f depends on the specific form of ρ_λ. We list some examples of function f for different types of penalty:

- The LASSO:

$$f_{LASSO}(z_k, t_k, \lambda) = \frac{S(z_k, \lambda)}{t_k}.$$

- The ALASSO:

$$f_{ALASSO}(z_k, t_k, \lambda) = \frac{S(z_k, \lambda\tilde{w}_k)}{t_k}.$$

- The ENET:

$$f_{ENET}(z_k, t_k, \lambda, \alpha) = \frac{S(z_k, \lambda)}{t_k + \lambda(1-\alpha)}.$$

- The SCAD:

$$f_{SCAD}(z_k, t_k, \lambda) = \begin{cases} \frac{S(z_k,\lambda)}{t_k} & \text{if } |z_k| \leq \lambda(t_k+1),\\ \frac{S(z_k,\gamma\lambda/(\gamma-1))}{t_k - 1/(\gamma-1)} & \text{if } \lambda(t_k+1) \leq |z_k| \leq t_k\gamma\lambda,\\ \frac{z_k}{t_k} & \text{if } |z_k| > t_k\gamma\lambda,\end{cases}$$

for $\gamma > 1 + 1/t_k$.

- The MCP:

$$f_{MCP}(z_k, t_k, \lambda) = \begin{cases} \frac{S(z_k,\lambda)}{t_k - 1/\gamma} & \text{if } |z_k| \le t\gamma\lambda, \\ \frac{z_k}{t_k} & \text{if } |z_k| > t\gamma\lambda, \end{cases}$$

for $\gamma > 1/t_k$.

Here, S is soft-thresholding operator defined for $\lambda \ge 0$ as

$$S(z, \lambda) = \begin{cases} z - \lambda & \text{if } z > \lambda, \\ 0 & \text{if } |z| \le \lambda, \\ z + \lambda & \text{if } z < -\lambda. \end{cases}$$

Note that t_k is calculated before any iteration. Let $r_i = y_i - \mathbf{x}_i^T \boldsymbol{\beta}$ be the residual of the ith observation based on the most recently updated value of $\boldsymbol{\beta}$. Hence, at step k of iteration (m+1), the following three calculations are made:

(1) Calculate

$$z_k = \frac{1}{n} \sum_{i=1}^{n} w_i x_{ik} r_i + t_k \beta_k^{(m)}.$$

(2) Update $\beta_k^{(m+1)} \leftarrow f(z_k, t_k, \lambda)$.
(3) Update $r_i = r_i + (\beta_k^{(m)} - \beta_k^{(m+1)}) x_{ik}$ for $i = 1, \ldots, n$.

Apparently, the computational cost of every single step is $\mathcal{O}(n)$, yielding $\mathcal{O}(np)$ for a full iteration.

Penalized Likelihoods

We now describe how to minimize the objective function in (2) by iteratively solving the PWLS problem. Suppose the log (partial)-likelihood $\ell(\boldsymbol{\beta}) = \sum_{i=1}^{n} \ell_i(\boldsymbol{\beta})$ is smooth with respect to $\boldsymbol{\beta}$ so that its first two partial derivatives are continuous. Let $\mathbf{X} = (\mathbf{x}_1, \ldots, \mathbf{x}_n)^T$ denote the design matrix and $\boldsymbol{\eta} = \mathbf{X}\boldsymbol{\beta}$. Let $\nabla\ell(\boldsymbol{\beta})$, $\nabla^2\ell(\boldsymbol{\beta})$, $\nabla\ell(\boldsymbol{\eta})$, $\nabla^2\ell(\boldsymbol{\eta})$ represent the gradient and Hessian of the log likelihood with respective to $\boldsymbol{\beta}$ and $\boldsymbol{\eta}$, respectively. We form a quadratic approximation to $\ell(\boldsymbol{\beta})$ by a two-term Taylor series expansion centered at current estimates $\tilde{\boldsymbol{\beta}}$, which is

$$\begin{aligned} \ell(\boldsymbol{\beta}) &\approx \ell(\tilde{\boldsymbol{\beta}}) + \nabla\ell(\tilde{\boldsymbol{\beta}})^T(\boldsymbol{\beta} - \tilde{\boldsymbol{\beta}}) + \tfrac{1}{2}(\boldsymbol{\beta} - \tilde{\boldsymbol{\beta}})^T \nabla^2\ell(\tilde{\boldsymbol{\beta}})(\boldsymbol{\beta} - \tilde{\boldsymbol{\beta}}) \\ &= \ell(\tilde{\boldsymbol{\beta}}) + \nabla\ell(\tilde{\boldsymbol{\eta}})(\mathbf{X}\boldsymbol{\beta} - \tilde{\boldsymbol{\eta}}) + \tfrac{1}{2}(\mathbf{X}\boldsymbol{\beta} - \tilde{\boldsymbol{\eta}})^T \nabla^2\ell(\tilde{\boldsymbol{\eta}})(\mathbf{X}\boldsymbol{\beta} - \tilde{\boldsymbol{\eta}}) \\ &= \tfrac{1}{2}(z(\tilde{\boldsymbol{\eta}}) - \mathbf{X}\boldsymbol{\beta})^T \nabla^2\ell(\tilde{\boldsymbol{\eta}})(z(\tilde{\boldsymbol{\eta}}) - \mathbf{X}\boldsymbol{\beta}) + C(\tilde{\boldsymbol{\eta}}, \tilde{\boldsymbol{\beta}}), \end{aligned} \tag{13}$$

where $\tilde{\boldsymbol{\eta}} = \mathbf{X}\tilde{\boldsymbol{\beta}}$ and $C(\tilde{\boldsymbol{\eta}}, \tilde{\boldsymbol{\beta}})$ does not depend on $\boldsymbol{\beta}$. Here, we define

$$z(\tilde{\boldsymbol{\eta}}) = \tilde{\boldsymbol{\eta}} - \nabla^2 \ell(\tilde{\boldsymbol{\eta}})^{-1} \nabla \ell(\tilde{\boldsymbol{\eta}}).$$

To simplify the calculation, we replace the Hessian $\nabla^2 \ell(\tilde{\boldsymbol{\eta}})$ by a diagonal matrix with the diagonal entries of $\nabla^2 \ell(\tilde{\boldsymbol{\eta}})$. In fact, $\nabla^2 \ell(\boldsymbol{\eta})$ is diagonal when $\ell_i(\boldsymbol{\beta})$ does not depend on $\boldsymbol{\eta}_k$ for $(k \neq i)$. This is true under the linear regression model and the logistic regression model. For other situations such as the proportional hazards model, Hastie and Tibshirani [31] also suggest this substitution since the off-diagonal entries are relatively small compared to the diagonal entries and the optimal $\boldsymbol{\beta}$ will remain a fixed point of the algorithm. Hence, the approximation in (13) becomes

$$\ell(\boldsymbol{\beta}) \approx -\frac{1}{2} \sum_{i=1}^{n} w(\tilde{\eta}_i) \left(z(\tilde{\eta}_i) - \mathbf{x}_i^T \boldsymbol{\beta} \right)^2 + C(\tilde{\boldsymbol{\eta}}, \tilde{\boldsymbol{\beta}}), \tag{14}$$

where

$$w(\tilde{\eta}_i) = -\ell''(\tilde{\eta}_i),$$

$$z(\tilde{\eta}_i) = \tilde{\eta}_i - \ell'(\tilde{\eta}_i)/\ell''(\tilde{\eta}_i),$$

with $\ell'(\tilde{\eta}_i)$ and $\ell''(\tilde{\eta}_i)$ being the ith entry of $\nabla \ell(\tilde{\boldsymbol{\eta}})$ and the diagonal of $\nabla^2 \ell(\tilde{\boldsymbol{\eta}})$ respectively. We list some examples of $w(\tilde{\eta}_i)$ and $z(\tilde{\eta}_i)$ under different models:

- Linear regression model:

$$w(\tilde{\eta}_i) = 1,$$

$$z(\tilde{\eta}_i) = y_i,$$

  with "$\approx$" in (14) being exactly "=".
- Logistic regression model:

$$w(\tilde{\eta}_i) = \tilde{p}_i(1 - \tilde{p}_i),$$

$$z(\tilde{\eta}_i) = \tilde{\eta}_i + \frac{y_i - \tilde{p}_i}{\tilde{p}_i(1 - \tilde{p}_i)},$$

  where $\tilde{p}_i = \exp(\tilde{\eta}_i)/(1 + \exp(\tilde{\eta}_i))$.

- Proportional hazards model:

$$w(\tilde{\eta}_i) = \delta_i \sum_{k \in C_i} \left\{ \frac{\exp(\tilde{\eta}_i) \sum_{j \in R_k} \exp(\tilde{\eta}_j) - (\exp(\tilde{\eta}_i))^2}{\left(\sum_{j \in R_k} \exp(\tilde{\eta}_j) \right)^2} \right\},$$

$$z(\tilde{\eta}_i) = \tilde{\eta}_i + \frac{1}{w(\tilde{\eta}_i)} \left\{ \delta_i - \delta_i \sum_{k \in C_i} \left(\frac{\exp(\tilde{\eta}_i)}{\sum_{j \in R_k} \exp(\tilde{\eta}_j)} \right) \right\},$$

where $C_i = \{k : y_k \leq y_i\}$ is the index set of observations that occur before or at y_i.

We summarize the algorithm below:

(1) Initialize $\tilde{\boldsymbol{\beta}}$ and set $\tilde{\eta} = \mathbf{X}^T \tilde{\boldsymbol{\beta}}$.
(2) Compute $w(\tilde{\eta}_i)$ and $z(\tilde{\eta}_i)$.
(3) Update $\hat{\boldsymbol{\beta}}$ by the minimizer of

$$\frac{1}{2n} \sum_{i=1}^{n} w(\tilde{\eta}_i) \left(z(\tilde{\eta}_i) - \mathbf{x}_i^T \boldsymbol{\beta} \right)^2 + \sum_{j=1}^{p} \rho_\lambda(\beta_j).$$

(4) Set $\tilde{\boldsymbol{\beta}} = \hat{\boldsymbol{\beta}}$ and set $\tilde{\eta} = \mathbf{X}^T \hat{\boldsymbol{\beta}}$.
(5) Repeat steps (2)–(4) until convergence of $\hat{\boldsymbol{\beta}}$.

The minimization of step (3) is a PWLS problem that can be solved by the coordinate descent, which was illustrated in Sect. 2.3.

Tuning Parameter Selection

The selection of tuning parameters plays a crucial role in the estimation of the penalized likelihood. When the penalty parameter $\lambda = 0$, the model includes all the variables and the approach reduces to the maximal likelihood method. When λ is sufficiently large, all the variables are excluded from the model. Hence, λ controls the complexity of the selected model: a smaller value of λ leads to a more complex model with smaller biases, whereas a larger value of λ yields a simpler model with smaller variances. We are interested in finding an optimal λ that balances the trade-off between bias and variance.

We usually compute a solution path for a sequence of λ and then choose the optimal one based on some criteria. In particular, we begin with λ sufficiently large to have $\hat{\boldsymbol{\beta}} = \mathbf{0}$ and decrease λ until we arrive near the unpenalized solution. When solving the problem for a new λ, we use current estimates as initial estimates so that the solution will not be far apart. This algorithm turns out to be efficient and stable. The strategy of warm starting together with the coordinate descent algorithm is frequently referred to as the pathwise coordinate descent.

Often the tuning parameter selection is done by using a multi-fold cross-validation. Other methods include the use of some information criteria such as the AIC or the BIC. However, the information criterion may not be suitable for penalized regression with $p > n$, since they are derived using asymptotic arguments for unpenalized regression models.

In addition to the penalized parameter λ, some penalties may also include other parameters, such as γ in SCAD or MCP. In this case, cross-validation can still be used but may suffer from intensive computation due to searching over a multi-dimensional grid of parameters. Breheny and Huang [4] suggest a hybrid method that combines the BIC and cross-validation to select the optimal λ and γ in SCAD or MCP. In some situations where the extra tuning parameter is not sensitive, it is reasonable to fix it to a certain value. For instance, Fan and Li [12] recommend to set $\gamma = 3.7$ for SCAD by a Bayesian argument.

3 Feature Screening for Ultra-High-Dimensional Data

In a high-dimensional setting, the dimensionality p may diverge to infinity at a certain order of sample size n. Specifically, we call a data set ultra-high-dimensional when p grows exponentially with n, i.e., $\log(p) = \mathcal{O}(n^a)$ for some $a > 0$ [11, 50]. Feature selection in ultra-high-dimensional data has become increasingly important in many scientific areas such as biomedical imaging, genomics, proteomics, and finance. For example, in a study of prostate cancer data, the number of probes can be on the order of millions, while the number of individuals can be on the order of hundreds. In such cases, it is challenging to identify significant features (e.g., genes) that contribute to the response and reliably predict the clinical prognosis (e.g., presence of metastasis) [40].

The variable selection methods introduced in Sect. 2 had been successfully applied to many high-dimensional data analyses and theoretically proved to retain good properties even under ultra-high-dimensional scenarios [3, 17]. However, the inherent computational complexity may prevent the direct use of those methods in ultra-high-dimensional settings. In particular, such ultra-high-dimensional data incurs several challenges, such as algorithm stability, computational expediency, and statistical accuracy [19].

A two-step approach has become popular in addressing the challenges incurred by a sparse ultra-high-dimensional model, since the introduction of the sure independence screening (SIS) [15]. The idea is to first reduce dimensionality p to a lower dimension using an efficient screening method and then apply well-established variable selection methods to the reduced feature space [40, 50]. We describe the SIS method and its extension for ultra-high-dimensional data.

3.1 Sure Independence Screening

The independence screening method aims to filter out features with weak marginal utility, which measures how useful a feature is for predicting the outcome independently. Fan and Lv [15] first introduce the concept of sure screening and propose the SIS in a sparse ultra-high-dimensional model. The sure screening refers to the property that all relevant variables will be covered in the subset derived from a screening procedure, with probability tending to 1, i.e.,

$$\mathbb{P}(M_* \subset M_s) \to 1 \text{ as } n \to 1,$$

where M_* and M_s are the true set of relevant features and the set of features selected from a screening procedure, respectively. The SIS is designed to reduce dimensionality p from a huge scale to a relatively large scale at the same order of sample size n while keeping all relevant features with high probability. After the SIS step, we can then apply a well-developed penalized regression approach illustrated in Sect. 2 to the reduced feature space, yielding a more stable algorithm and accurate estimates.

Correlation Ranking

Consider a high-dimensional linear model in (5). The SIS [15] measures the relevance of features using their marginal correlation to the response and keeps the variables with marginal correlations above a certain threshold. Specifically, let $\mathbf{Y} = (y_1, \ldots, y_n)^T$ and $\mathbf{X}_j = (x_{1j}, \ldots, x_{nj})^T$ be an n-dimensional vector of the response and the jth variable, respectively. Denote

$$\omega_j = \mathbf{X}_j^T \mathbf{Y}.$$

Suppose both $\mathbf{Y}$ and $\mathbf{X}_j$ are centered and standardized. Hence, ω_j is the sample correlation between the jth variable and the response. For any given size d_n, the SIS takes the submodel

$$\hat{M}_{d_n} = \left\{1 \le j \le p : |\omega_j| \text{ is among the } d_n \text{ largest}\right\}. \tag{15}$$

Thus, the original model is reduced from size $p \gg n$ to d_n, which can be at the same order of n. In practice, we can choose $d_n = n - 1$ or $d_n = [n/\log n]$. This screening procedure is very efficient with the computational cost as $\mathcal{O}(np)$. For classification problem with $y_i = \pm 1$, the correlation ranking in SIS becomes feature screening using two-sample t-statistics [11].

The SIS has been proved to have the sure screening property, under some regular conditions. It means that with high probability, the screened model $\hat{M}_d$ will contain all the important variables, even when p grows with n exponentially. However, this method may fail when some of the key conditions are not satisfied. Particularly, the sure screening property requires minimum strengths for both signals of predictors and marginal correlations, i.e.,

$$\min_{j \in M_*} |\beta_j| \geq cn^{-\kappa} \text{ and } \min_{j \in M_*} |\mathrm{Cov}(\beta_j^{-1}\mathbf{Y}, \mathbf{X}_j)| \geq c,$$

with $\kappa, c \geq 0$. In some applications, a relevant feature X_j can be marginally uncorrelated with the response $\mathbf{Y}$, i.e., $\mathrm{Cov}(\mathbf{Y}, \mathbf{X}_j) = 0$, due to certain joint correlations with some other relevant features. In such a case, the aforementioned condition does not hold and the SIS will miss this important feature. On the other hand, an unimportant feature can be selected with a higher chance via a "fake" high correlation with the outcome of interest due to the ultra-high-dimensionality. Such a "fake" correlation can be obtained when the unimportant features are strongly correlated with important ones. To overcome these issues, Fan and Lv [15] propose the iterative sure independence screening (ISIS), which is illustrated in Sect. 3.3.

Maximum Marginal Likelihoods

Consider an independent sample $\{\mathbf{x}_i, y_i\}_{i=1}^n$ with $\mathbf{x}_i = (x_{i1}, \ldots, x_{ip})^T$ as a p-dimensional covariate vector and y_i as a response. Recall that in ultra-high-dimensional setting, we have $p \gg n$ with $\log(p) = \mathcal{O}(n^a)$ for some $a > 0$. Suppose that the response y_i is associated with the covariate $\mathbf{x}_i$ through a p-dimensional parameter vector $\boldsymbol{\beta}$. In general, we aim to find the sparse parameter $\boldsymbol{\beta} = (\beta_1, \ldots, \beta_p)^T$ that minimizes the negative log likelihood of the form

$$Q(\boldsymbol{\beta}) = -\frac{1}{n}\sum_{i=1}^{n} \ell\left(y_i, \mathbf{x}_i^T \boldsymbol{\beta}\right).$$

Fan et al. [19] generalize the correlation-based SIS to a general likelihood framework, where the marginal utility of the jth feature is defined as the maximum marginal likelihood (MML) taking the form

$$L_j^M = \min_{\beta_j} \left\{ -\frac{1}{n}\sum_{i=1}^{n} \ell(y_i, x_{ij}\beta_j) \right\}, \tag{16}$$

for $j = 1, \ldots, p$, which can be regarded as the minimum loss of using the jth feature to predict the response. Hence, the feature with smaller L_j is more important. Note that we fit the model with one variable at a time, and thus solving [16] is quick and stable. By computing and ranking elements of the marginal utility vector $\mathbf{L} = (L_1, \ldots, L_p)^T$, the SIS selects the following submodel:

$$\hat{M}_{d_n} = \left\{ 1 \leq j \leq p : L_j^M \text{ is among the } d_n \text{ smallest} \right\}, \tag{17}$$

for any given size d_n. Fan et al. [19] suggest taking $d_n = \lfloor n/\log n \rfloor$. This method is reduced to the correlation ranking under the linear regression model with Gaussian errors.

Fan et al. [21] propose another version of SIS using the maximum marginal likelihood estimates (MMLE). By fitting the model with componentwise covariates, the MMLE for the jth feature $\hat{\beta}_j^M$ is defined as

$$\hat{\beta}_j^M = \underset{\beta_j}{\operatorname{argmin}} \left\{ -\frac{1}{n} \sum_{i=1}^{n} \ell(y_i, x_{ij}\beta_j) \right\},$$

for $j = 1, \ldots, p$. The SIS then selects a set of variables with the magnitude of $\hat{\beta}_j^M$ above a certain threshold, i.e.,

$$\hat{M}_{\gamma_n} = \left\{ 1 \leq j \leq p : |\hat{\beta}_j^M| \geq \gamma_n \right\},$$

where γ_n is a predefined threshold value. This method is shown to be equivalent to the MML ranking in (17) [21]. Fan et al. [21] also establish the sure screening property for the proposed SIS under certain conditions, with an appropriate choice of γ_n.

Fan et al. [20] extend the SIS to the PH model. Recall that in the PH model, we aim to find the sparse $\boldsymbol{\beta}$ to minimize the negative partial log likelihood defined as follows:

$$\ell(\boldsymbol{\beta}) = -\frac{1}{n} \sum_{i=1}^{n} \left\{ \delta_i \mathbf{x}_i^T \boldsymbol{\beta} - \delta_i \log \left\{ \sum_{j \in R_i} \exp(\mathbf{x}_j^T \boldsymbol{\beta}) \right\} \right\}.$$

Similar to the MML ranking, Fan et al. [20] define the marginal utility as the maximum marginal partial likelihood (MMPL) of the single variable:

$$U_k^M = \min_{\beta_k} -\frac{1}{n} \sum_{i=1}^{n} \left\{ \delta_i \mathbf{x}_{ik}^T \boldsymbol{\beta} - \delta_i \log \left\{ \sum_{j \in R_i} \exp(\mathbf{x}_{jk}^T \boldsymbol{\beta}) \right\} \right\},$$

for $k = 1, \ldots, p$. After computing all the marginal utilities U_k^M, the SIS selects a set of variables as follows:

$$\hat{M}_{d_n} = \left\{ 1 \leq k \leq p : U_k^M \text{ is among the } d_n \text{ smallest} \right\}.$$

3.2 Iterative Sure Independence Screening

In general, the SIS method will result in false negatives if a feature is jointly related but marginally unrelated to the response. It may also include false positives if a feature has a higher marginal utility than some important variables, but it is in fact unrelated to the response [16].

The aforementioned problems are essentially caused by the fact that the SIS only uses marginal information of features. To overcome these issues, Fan and Lv [15] propose the iterative SIS (ISIS) that uses joint information of variable under the linear regression model. Fan et al. [19, 20] improve the SIS by allowing iteratively variable deletion and extend the ISIS to a general likelihood framework. In particular, suppose we want to find the spare $\boldsymbol{\beta}$ to minimize

$$-\frac{1}{n}\ell_n(\mathbf{y}, \mathbf{X}\boldsymbol{\beta}) + \sum_{j=1}^{p} \rho_\lambda(\beta_j),$$

where ℓ_n is the log (partial)-likelihood function of $\mathbf{y}$ conditioning on $\mathbf{X}$ in an ultra-high-dimensional feature space. The ISIS algorithm works by the following steps:

(1) Apply the SIS to select a set I_1 of indices of size k_1. Then, perform a penalized maximum (partial) likelihood approach, such as the LASSO, ALASSO, SCAD, and MCP, to obtain a variable subset M_1 of I_1.

(2) Compute the marginal utility that measures the contribution of variable $\mathbf{X}_j$ in the presence of variable $\mathbf{X}_{M_1}$, which is defined as

$$U_{j|M_1} = \min_{\boldsymbol{\beta}_{M_1}, \beta_j} -\frac{1}{n}\ell_n(\mathbf{y}, \mathbf{X}_{M_1}\boldsymbol{\beta}_{M_1} + \mathbf{X}_j^T \beta_j),$$

for all $j \notin M_1$, where $\mathbf{X}_{M_1}$ is the sub-matrix of $\mathbf{X}$ of those features in M_1. Form the variable set I_2 consisting of the indices corresponding to the smallest k_2 elements in $\{U_{j|M_1}, j \notin M_1\}$.

(3) Use penalized variable selection methods to obtain

$$\hat{\boldsymbol{\beta}}_2 = \operatorname*{argmin}_{\boldsymbol{\beta}_{M_1}, \boldsymbol{\beta}_{I_2}} -\frac{1}{n}\ell_n(\mathbf{y}, \mathbf{X}_{M_1}\boldsymbol{\beta}_{M_1} + \mathbf{X}_{I_2}\boldsymbol{\beta}) + \sum_{j \in M_1 \cup I_2} \rho_\lambda(\beta_j).$$

The nonzero elements of $\hat{\boldsymbol{\beta}}_2$ give an active index M_2.

(4) Repeat steps (2)–(3) until d_n variables are selected or $M_l = M_{l-1}$, yielding the final estimates $\hat{\boldsymbol{\beta}}_{M_l}$.

Fan et al. [19] suggest to take $k_1 = \lfloor 2d_n/3 \rfloor$ and $k_r = d_n - |M_{r-1}|$ at the rth iteration.

3.3 Reduction of False Positive Rate

As a crude screening method, the SIS may include many false positive variables. Fan et al. [19] suggest to use sample splitting to reduce the false positive rate. Specifically, we randomly split the sample data into two halves and then apply the SIS or ISIS separately in each half, yielding two sets of active variables $\hat{I}_1$ and $\hat{I}_2$. We define a new set of indices by the intersection $\hat{I} = \hat{I}_1 \cup \hat{I}_2$. The indices set $\hat{I}$ should include all the important variables with probability tending to 1, due to the sure screening property of both $\hat{I}_1$ and $\hat{I}_2$. However, $\hat{I}$ should have fewer false positives as an unimportant variable is less likely to be selected by both $\hat{I}_1$ and $\hat{I}_2$ in the ultra-high-dimensional feature space. Under some exchangeable conditions on unimportant variable, Fan et al. [19] provide a non-asymptotic probability bound for the event that the intersection $\hat{I}$ selects at least r unimportant variables for any natural number r. Such probability is very small for ultra-high-dimensional data. Hence, the sample-splitting strategy is able to reduce the false positive rate.

4 Real Data Example

We provide an example of variable selection in ultra-high-dimensional space from a phase III clinical trial [39]. We demonstrate the performance of penalized (partial) likelihood and feature screening approaches introduced in Sects. 2 and 3, respectively. In particular, we consider the GWAS data from CALGB 90401. The GWAS has 498,081 single-nucleotide polymorphisms (SNPs) that were processed from blood samples from 623 Caucasian patients with metastatic castration-resistant prostate cancer. We are interested in identifying SNPs that would predict the overall survival in those patients [50].

We assume additive models for SNPs and consider the high-dimensional proportional hazards model in this example. We apply the PMLE estimators in (1) using the following penalties: LASSO, ALASSO, ENET, SCAD, and MCP. We also evaluate the performance of the sequential use of screening procedures (SIS, ISIS) with the PMLE. Thus, in combination, we have three classes of estimators (PMLE, SIS, and ISIS) with 21 different methods, as shown in Table 2. For the tuning parameter selection, we observe that the BIC tends to select a large number of variables in PMLE for this example, which may lead to model overfitting. Therefore, we use 10-fold cross-validation to choose the optimal tuning parameter λ.

We use the R library ncvreg [4] for PMLE methods, which implements the computational algorithm introduced in Sect. 2.3. In particular, the function cv.ncvsurv() can perform 10-fold cross-validation, with the argument "penalty" that specifies the type of penalizations for LASSO, MCP, and SCAD. For the ENET penalty, the argument "alpha" can be used to control the relative contribution between the ℓ_1 and ℓ_2 penalties, when setting the argument "penalty" to be "lasso." For the (I)SIS methods, we develop the R program based on the R library SIS [51]. Note that the

Table 2 Real data analysis results under high-dimensional proportional hazards model with SNP covariates

Selection approach	No. of variables selected	Original tAUC	Corrected tAUC
LASSO	2	0.585	0.462
ALASSO	2	0.589	0.464
ENET ($\alpha = 0.2$)	2	0.585	0.443
ENET ($\alpha = 0.5$)	2	0.585	0.455
ENET ($\alpha = 0.8$)	2	0.585	0.462
SCAD	2	0.585	0.462
MCP	2	0.585	0.487
SIS-LASSO	76	0.856	0.492
SIS-ALASSO	46	0.828	0.492
SIS-ENET ($\alpha = 0.2$)	87	0.861	0.491
SIS-ENET ($\alpha = 0.5$)	79	0.859	0.493
SIS-ENET ($\alpha = 0.8$)	77	0.857	0.491
SIS-SCAD	67	0.845	0.489
SIS-MCP	66	0.859	0.516
ISIS-LASSO	23	0.773	0.476
ISIS-ALASSO	23	0.790	0.484
ISIS-ENET ($\alpha = 0.2$)	24	0.758	0.473
ISIS-ENET ($\alpha = 0.5$)	24	0.767	0.476
ISIS-ENET ($\alpha = 0.8$)	23	0.773	0.479
ISIS-SCAD	23	0.778	0.479
ISIS-MCP	22	0.786	0.482

function SIS() allows only the LASSO penalty for the proportional hazards model. However, since it also utilizes the R package ncvreg for the penalized regression on variables selected by (I)SIS methods, we simply modify their source codes to support for other penalties.

To assess the performance of the estimators, we compute the time-dependence area under the curve(tAUC) using the function AUC.uno() in the R library survAUC. Table 2 shows the number of selected variables and the corresponding tAUC for each method. For the optimism correction, we find out that the bootstrapping method does not work well in this case. When applying a cross-validation procedure to a particular bootstrapping sample, we observe apparent overfitting in our numerical analysis. The reason could be that the cross-validation may fail to separate the training set and the validation set, due to duplicated observations in the bootstrapping sample. Such overfitting results in biased estimates of optimisms. To address this problem, we implement the Monte Carlo cross-validation to adjust for the optimism of the tAUCs: we randomly divide the data set into a training set ($n = 419$) and a testing set ($n = 204$) with a $2 : 1$ allocation ratio. We then apply each method to the training set and compute the tAUCs from both sets. We repeat this process 100 times and estimate the optimism using the average difference of tAUCs between the training set and the testing set. The corrected tAUCs are also reported in Table 2.

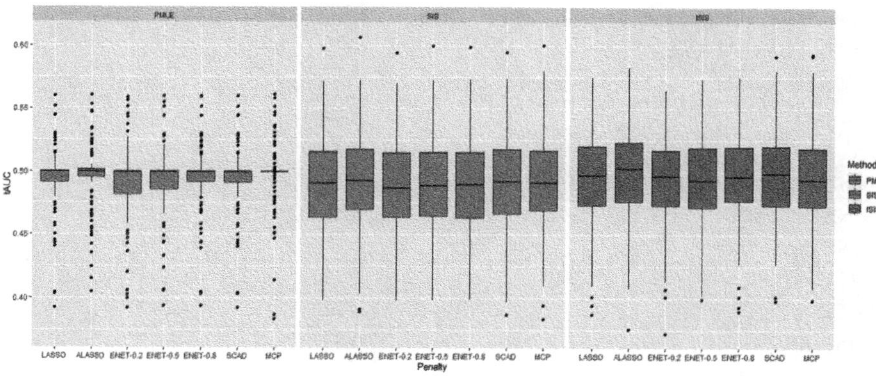

Fig. 1 The boxplots of tAUCs from the testing sets over 100 splits with SNP covariates

Across all the methods, the small values of tAUCs in Table 2 indicate that none of the selected SNPs are informative when predicting the overall survival of patients. It is also interesting to observe that the SIS and ISIS procedures tend to select a larger number of variables and thus have larger tAUCs on the original data set, regardless of the type of penalties used. In fact, the overfitting is not surprising since we screen variables based on all the samples, and thus the screened variables "have already seen" the validation set in the subsequent cross-validation [26]. The boxplots of tAUCs computed from the testing sets over 100 splits are displayed in Fig. 1.

We further adjust the model for the risk score based on the predicted survival model [30]. The results are displayed in Table 3 and Fig. 2. Table 3 shows that the risk score is highly predictive since it significantly increases the performance of all the variable selection approaches. Overall, the PMLE estimators have the best performance in terms of the corrected tAUCs, with only the risk score being selected. Similar to the result in Table 2, the SIS and ISIS methods select a relatively large number of variables, with large optimism between the original tAUCs and the corrected tAUCs.

5 High-Dimensional Inference

We focus on uncertainty assessment of high-dimensional estimates, e.g., hypothesis testing for individual variable ($H_{0,j} : \beta_j = 0$ versus $H_{a,j} : \beta_j \neq 0$) and confidence regions in this section. Compared to the well-explored consistency theory of variable selection approaches, the high-dimensional statistical inference is less developed until recently. The major challenge is that the limiting distribution of estimators is difficult to characterize in high-dimensional space. For example, Knight and Fu [42] show that the asymptotic distribution of the LASSO estimator is intractable with a point mass at zero. Hence, the standard sampling techniques such as bootstrapping fail to provide p-values or valid confidence intervals. Although some residual-type

Table 3 Real data analysis results under high-dimensional proportional hazards model with the risk score and SNP covariates

Selection approach	No. of variables selected	Original tAUC	Corrected tAUC
LASSO	1	0.740	0.724
ALASSO	1	0.740	0.680
ENET ($\alpha = 0.2$)	1	0.740	0.723
ENET ($\alpha = 0.5$)	1	0.740	0.724
ENET ($\alpha = 0.8$)	1	0.740	0.724
SCAD	1	0.740	0.724
MCP	1	0.740	0.727
SIS-LASSO	63	0.877	0.685
SIS-ALASSO	44	0.860	0.660
SIS-ENET ($\alpha = 0.2$)	75	0.875	0.680
SIS-ENET ($\alpha = 0.5$)	67	0.876	0.683
SIS-ENET ($\alpha = 0.8$)	63	0.877	0.685
SIS-SCAD	59	0.856	0.696
SIS-MCP	54	0.870	0.703
ISIS-LASSO	23	0.830	0.660
ISIS-ALASSO	22	0.841	0.651
ISIS-ENET ($\alpha = 0.2$)	24	0.821	0.671
ISIS-ENET ($\alpha = 0.5$)	24	0.823	0.664
ISIS-ENET ($\alpha = 0.8$)	23	0.824	0.658
ISIS-SCAD	23	0.836	0.633
ISIS-MCP	23	0.836	0.630

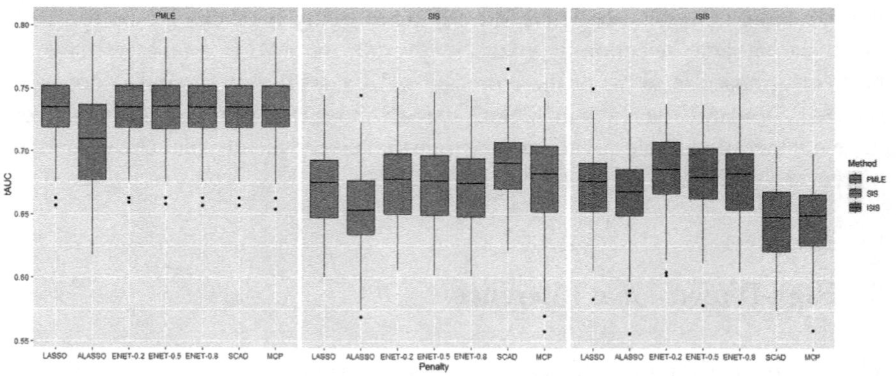

Fig. 2 The boxplots of tAUCs from the testing sets over 100 splits with the risk score and SNP covariates

bootstrapping methods [7, 44] are investigated in approximating the distribution of LASSO estimator, they may suffer from issues of nonuniform convergence to distributions and super-efficiency phenomenon [8].

A generic approach to assign significance in the high-dimensional model is based on sample splitting. Wasserman and Roeder [60] propose to split data into two halves, with high-dimensional variable selection methods applied to the first half and statistical inference of selected variables performed to the second half. For example, in high-dimensional linear regression, we can run the LASSO estimator in the first half to select "important" variables. Then, we confine the analysis to the reduced set of variables and apply ordinary least squares estimator to construct p-values and confidence intervals. The over-optimism is avoided by separating the selection and inference processes. However, the selection and the subsequent inference are sensitive to the choice of data splitting and thus may result in highly variant p-values. Additionally, such inferences based on single-sample splitting are only valid conditional on the selected model from the first half [24]. Meinshausen et al. [47] improve this procedure by using multiple-sample splitting, which performs the single-sample-splitting method multiple times and aggregates the dependent p-values for statistical inference. This method can control both the family-wise error rate (FWER) and false discover rates (FDR). The multiple-sample-splitting method is generic, which it is applicable to a wide variety of high-dimensional models, such as the generalized linear and proportional hazards models. One disadvantage of this approach is that it requires a minimum signal strength condition on unknown parameters, which may not hold in applications with small signals [8].

Taking a different perspective, the conditional inference approaches [43, 45, 58] focus on significance tests in the high-dimensional linear regression model, given a model is selected by the LASSO. Lockhart et al. [45] propose a covariance test that provides a sequence of p-values along the solution path of the LASSO estimator, conditional on all the relevant variables that are included in the current model. Although this method does not require perfect identification of important variables by the LASSO, it cannot test for the significance of individual variables. Extending the covariance test framework, Lee et al. [43] and Tibshirani et al. [58] construct confidence intervals or p-values for individual variables by characterizing the conditional distribution given a selected model. However, these approaches can only test the statistical significance for the set of variables selected by the LASSO that are sensitive to a specific sample data.

Another line of research considers debiased or desparsifying estimators [36, 59, 65] for uncertainty assessment of the LASSO in the high-dimensional linear or generalized linear model. These methods do not require the minimal signal strength condition and thus can make statistical inference for small nonzero coefficients. Specifically, Zhang and Zhang [65] propose a bias-corrected estimator based on a regularized projection. Following a similar idea, Javanmard and Montanari [36] study a version of debiased LASSO estimator and present an algorithm that constructs confidence intervals and p-values. Van de Geer et al. [59] extend the work of [65] to generalized linear model by inverting Karush–Kuhn–Tucker (KKT) conditions of the LASSO.

Most of the above-mentioned approaches focus on high-dimensional inference for the LASSO. Recently, Ning et al. [48] propose a decorrelated score test for individual coefficients in nonconvex penalized M-estimator for high-dimensional settings. Their framework is general and applicable to a wide range of regression models, such as linear regression, logistic regression, and Poisson regression. Their procedure can also provide valid inference for small signals since it does not require variable selection consistency. Fang et al. [23] extend their work and investigate the decorrelated score, the Wald test, and the partial likelihood ratio test for the proportional hazards model in high-dimensional space. Shi et al. [53] propose a score test, a Wald test, and a likelihood ratio test in a partial penalized regression framework for high-dimensional generalized linear models.

6 Conclusion

To summarize, we have provided a review on variable selection methods with a focus on penalized methods. We then applied these selection methods to a high-dimensional setting in patients with advanced prostate cancer. As costs of molecular tests become cheaper, we think that developing predictive models of outcomes based on high-dimensional data will become the standard research in every aspect of medicine and will impact patient diagnosis and treatment. It is important to note that many biological processes and mechanisms are not linearly associated with clinical outcomes and investigators may be interested in testing these variables and their effect on outcomes. Therefore, we expect to see more implementation of non-parametric approaches and high-dimensional inference to high-dimensional settings. We anticipate that advancement in laboratory technologies would lead to newer challenges in high-dimensional settings and would necessitate both novel statistical methods and efficient computational procedures to solve these critical problems.

Acknowledgments This research was partially supported by the United States Army Medical Research, Grant/Award Numbers: W81XWH-15-1-0467 and W81XWH-18-1-0278, National Institutes of Health R01 CA256157-01, and the Prostate Cancer Foundation.

References

1. Akaike, H.: Information theory and an extension of the maximum likelihood principle. In: Selected Papers of Hirotugu Akaike, pp. 199–213. Springer, Berlin (1998)
2. Bickel, P.J., Ritov, Y., Tsybakov, A.B.: Simultaneous analysis of Lasso and Dantzig selector. Ann. Stat. **37**(4), 1705–1732 (2009)
3. Bradic, J., Fan, J., Jiang, J.: Regularization for Cox's proportional hazards model with np-dimensionality. Ann. Stat. **39**(6), 3092 (2011)
4. Breheny, P., Huang, J.: Coordinate descent algorithms for nonconvex penalized regression, with applications to biological feature selection. Ann. Appl. Stat. **5**(1), 232 (2011)
5. Breiman, L.: Random forests. Mach. Learn. **45**(1), 5–32 (2001)
6. Candes, E., Tao, T.: The Dantzig selector: statistical estimation when p is much larger than n. Ann. Stat. **35**(6), 2313–2351 (2007)

7. Chatterjee, A., Lahiri, S.N.: Bootstrapping Lasso estimators. J. Am. Stat. Assoc. **106**(494), 608–625 (2011)
8. Dezeure, R., Bühlmann, P., Meier, L., Meinshausen, N.: High-dimensional inference: Confidence intervals, p-values and R-Software hdi. Stat. Sci. **30**(4), 533–558 (2015)
9. Dong, Y., Song, L., Amin, M.: SCAD-Ridge penalized likelihood estimators for ultra-high dimensional models. Hacettepe J. Math. Stat. **47**(2), 423–436 (2018)
10. Donoho, D.L., et al. High-dimensional data analysis: the curses and blessings of dimensionality. AMS Math Challenges Lecture, vol. 1, pp. 1–32 (2000)
11. Fan, J., Fan, Y.: High dimensional classification using features annealed independence rules. Ann. Stat. **36**(6), 2605 (2008)
12. Fan, J., Li, R.: Variable selection via nonconcave penalized likelihood and its oracle properties. J. Am. Stat. Assoc. **96**(456), 1348–1360 (2001)
13. Fan, J., Li, R.: Variable selection for Cox's proportional hazards model and frailty model. Ann. Stat., 74–99 (2002)
14. Fan, J., Li, R.: Statistical challenges with high dimensionality: Feature selection in knowledge discovery. arXiv preprint math/0602133 (2006)
15. Fan, J., Lv, J.: Sure independence screening for ultrahigh dimensional feature space. J. R. Stat. Soc. Ser. B (Stat. Methodol.) **70**(5), 849–911 (2008)
16. Fan, J., Lv, J.: A selective overview of variable selection in high dimensional feature space. Stat. Sin. **20**(1), 101 (2010)
17. Fan, J., Lv, J.: Nonconcave penalized likelihood with np-dimensionality. IEEE Trans. Inf. Theory **57**(8), 5467–5484 (2011)
18. Fan, J., Peng, H., et al.: Nonconcave penalized likelihood with a diverging number of parameters. Ann. Stat. **32**(3), 928–961 (2004)
19. Fan, J., Samworth, R., Wu, Y.: Ultrahigh dimensional feature selection: beyond the linear model. J. Mach. Learn. Res. **10**(Sep), 2013–2038 (2009)
20. Fan, J., Feng, Y., Wu, Y., et al.: High-dimensional variable selection for Cox's proportional hazards model. In: *Borrowing Strength: Theory Powering Applications–a Festschrift for Lawrence D. Brown*, pp. 70–86. Institute of Mathematical Statistics, New York (2010a)
21. Fan, J., Song, R. et al.: Sure independence screening in generalized linear models with np-dimensionality. Ann. Stat. **38**(6), 3567–3604 (2010b)
22. Fan, J., Xue, L., Zou, H.: Strong oracle optimality of folded concave penalized estimation. Ann. Stat. **42**(3), 819 (2014)
23. Fang, E.X., Ning, Y., Liu, H.: Testing and confidence intervals for high dimensional proportional hazards model. arXiv preprint arXiv:1412.5158 (2014)
24. Fithian, W., Sun, D., Taylor, J.: Optimal inference after model selection. arXiv preprint arXiv:1410.2597 (2014)
25. Frank, L.E., Friedman, J.H.: A statistical view of some chemometrics regression tools. Technometrics **35**(2), 109–135 (1993)
26. Friedman, J., Hastie, T., Tibshirani, R.: The Elements of Statistical Learning, vol. 1. Springer, New York (2001)
27. Friedman, J., Hastie, T., Höfling, H., Tibshirani, R. et al.: Pathwise coordinate optimization. Ann. Appl. Stat. **1**(2), 302–332 (2007)
28. Friedman, J., Hastie, T., Tibshirani, R.: Regularization paths for generalized linear models via coordinate descent. J. Stat. Softw. **33**(1), 1 (2010)
29. Gui, J., Li, H.: Penalized Cox regression analysis in the high-dimensional and low-sample size settings, with applications to microarray gene expression data. Bioinformatics **21**(13), 3001–3008 (2005)
30. Halabi, S., Lin, C.-Y., Kelly, W.K., Fizazi, K.S., Moul, J.W., Kaplan, E.B., Morris, M.J., Small, E.J.: Updated prognostic model for predicting overall survival in first-line chemotherapy for patients with metastatic castration-resistant prostate cancer. J. Clin. Oncol. **32**(7), 671 (2014)
31. Hastie, T.J., Tibshirani, R.J.: Generalized Additive Models, vol. 43. CRC press, New York (1990)

32. Hoerl, A.E., Kennard, R.W.: Ridge regression: Biased estimation for nonorthogonal problems. Technometrics **12**(1), 55–67 (1970)
33. Huang, J., Ma, S., Zhang, C.-H.: Adaptive Lasso for sparse high-dimensional regression models. Stat. Sinica, 1603–1618 (2008)
34. Huang, J., Breheny, P., Ma, S., Zhang, C.-H.: The Mnet method for variable selection. (Unpublished) Technical Report, vol. 402 (2010)
35. Huang, J., Sun, T., Ying, Z., Yu, Y., Zhang, C.-H.: Oracle inequalities for the Lasso in the Cox model. Ann. Stat. **41**(3), 1142 (2013)
36. Javanmard, A., Montanari, A.: Confidence intervals and hypothesis testing for high-dimensional regression. J. Mach. Learn. Res. **15**(1), 2869–2909 (2014)
37. Jia, J., Yu, B.: On model selection consistency of the elastic net when p n. Stat. Sinica. **20**(2), 595–611 (2010)
38. Johnstone, I.M., Titterington, D.M.: Statistical challenges of high-dimensional data. Philos. Trans. R. Soc. London A Math. Phys. Eng. Sci. **367**(1906), 4237–4253 (2009)
39. Kelly, W.K., Halabi, S., Carducci, M., George, D., Mahoney, J.F., Stadler, W.M., Morris, M., Kantoff, P., Monk, J.P., Kaplan, E. et al.: Randomized, double-blind, placebo-controlled phase iii trial comparing docetaxel and prednisone with or without bevacizumab in men with metastatic castration-resistant prostate cancer: Calgb 90401. J. Clin. Oncol. **30**(13), 1534 (2012)
40. Kim, S., Halabi, S.: High dimensional variable selection with error control. Biomed Res. Int. **2016** (2016)
41. Kim, Y., Choi, H., Oh, H.-S.: Smoothly clipped absolute deviation on high dimensions. J. Am. Stat. Assoc. **103**(484), 1665–1673 (2008)
42. Knight, K., Fu, W.: Asymptotics for Lasso-type estimators. Ann. Stat., 1356–1378 (2000)
43. Lee, J.D., Sun, D.L., Sun, Y., Taylor, J.E., et al.: Exact post-selection inference, with application to the Lasso. Ann. Stat. **44**(3), 907–927 (2016)
44. Liu, H., Yu, B. et al.: Asymptotic properties of Lasso+mLs and Lasso+Ridge in sparse high-dimensional linear regression. Electron. J. Stat. **7**, 3124–3169 (2013)
45. Lockhart, R., Taylor, J., Tibshirani, R.J., Tibshirani, R.: A significance test for the Lasso. Ann. Stat. **42**(2), 413 (2014)
46. Meinshausen, N., Bühlmann, P.: Stability selection. J. R. Stat. Soc. Series B (Stat. Methodol.) **72**(4), 417–473 (2010)
47. Meinshausen, N., Meier, L., Bühlmann, P.: P-values for high-dimensional regression. J. Am. Stat. Assoc. **104**(488), 1671–1681 (2009)
48. Ning, Y., Liu, H., et al.: A general theory of hypothesis tests and confidence regions for sparse high dimensional models. Ann. Stat. **45**(1), 158–195 (2017)
49. Park, T., Casella, G.: The Bayesian Lasso. J. Am. Stat. Assoc. **103**(482), 681–686 (2008)
50. Pi, L., Halabi, S.: Combined performance of screening and variable selection methods in ultra-high dimensional data in predicting time-to-event outcomes. Diagn. Progn. Res. **2**(1), 21 (2018)
51. Saldana, D.F., Feng, Y.: SIS: AnR package for sure independence screening in ultrahigh-dimensional statistical models. J. Stat. Softw. **83**(2), 1–25 (2018). https://doi.org/10.18637/jss.v083.i02
52. Schwarz, G., et al.: Estimating the dimension of a model. Ann. Stat. **6**(2), 461–464 (1978)
53. Shi, C., Song, R., Chen, Z., Li, R., et al.: Linear hypothesis testing for high dimensional generalized linear models. Ann. Stat. **47**(5), 2671–2703 (2019)
54. Simon, N., Friedman, J., Hastie, T., Tibshirani, R.: Regularization paths for Cox's proportional hazards model via coordinate descent. J. Stat. Softw. **39**(5), 1 (2011)
55. Tibshirani, R.: Regression shrinkage and selection via the Lasso. J. R. Stat. Soc. Ser. B (Methodol.), 267–288 (1996a)
56. Tibshirani, R.: Regression shrinkage and selection via the Lasso. J. R. Stat. Soc. Ser. B (Methodol.), 267–288 (1996b)
57. Tibshirani, R.: The Lasso method for variable selection in the Cox model. Stat. Med. **16**(4), 385–395 (1997)

58. Tibshirani, R.J., Taylor, J., Lockhart, R., Tibshirani, R.: Exact post-selection inference for sequential regression procedures. J. Am. Stat. Assoc. **111**(514), 600–620 (2016)
59. Van de Geer, S., Peter Bühlmann, Ritov, Y., Dezeure, R. et al.: On asymptotically optimal confidence regions and tests for high-dimensional models. Ann. Stat. **42**(3), 1166–1202 (2014)
60. Wasserman, L., Roeder, K.: High dimensional variable selection. Ann. Stat. **37**(5A), 2178 (2009)
61. Yuan, M., Lin, Y.: On the non-negative garrotte estimator. J. R. Stat. Soc. Ser. B (Stat. Methodol.) **69**(2), 143–161 (2007)
62. Zeng, L., Xie, J.: Group variable selection via SCAD-L2. Statistics **48**(1), 49–66 (2014)
63. Zhang, C.-H., Huang, J.: Model-selection consistency of the Lasso in high-dimensional linear regression. Ann. Statist **36**, 1567–1594 (2006)
64. Zhang, H.H., Lu, W.: Adaptive Lasso for Cox's proportional hazards model. Biometrika **94**(3), 691–703 (2007)
65. Zhang, C.-H., Zhang, S.S.: Confidence intervals for low dimensional parameters in high dimensional linear models. J. R. Stat. Soc. Ser. B Stat. Methodol., 217–242 (2014)
66. Zhang, C.-H. et al.: Nearly unbiased variable selection under minimax concave penalty. Ann. Stat. **38**(2), 894–942 (2010)
67. Zhao, P., Yu, B.: On model selection consistency of Lasso. J. Mach. Learn. Res. **7**, 2541–2563 (2006)
68. Zou, H.: The adaptive Lasso and its oracle properties. J. Am. Stat. Assoc. **101**(476), 1418–1429 (2006)
69. Zou, H., Hastie, T.: Regularization and variable selection via the elastic net. J. R. Stat. Soc. Ser. B (Stat. Methodol.) **67**(2), 301–320 (2005)
70. Zou, H., Li, R.: One-step sparse estimates in nonconcave penalized likelihood models. Ann. Stat. **36**(4), 1509 (2008)
71. Zou, H., Zhang, H.H.: On the adaptive elastic-net with a diverging number of parameters. Ann. Stat. **37**(4), 1733 (2009)

Estimation Methods for Item Factor Analysis: An Overview

Yunxiao Chen and Siliang Zhang

1 Introduction

Item-level response data are commonly encountered in social and behavioral sciences, including education, psychology, psychiatry, marketing, and political science. Such data are typically binary (e.g., disagree/agree) or ordinal (e.g., strongly disagree, disagree, neither, agree, and strongly agree), due to the way questionnaire items are designed. Due to the categorical nature of data, the traditional linear factor models are no longer suitable and item factor analysis models have been developed.

IFA models combine the idea of common factor analysis and the generalized linear modeling techniques for categorical data. The introduction of common factors allows IFA to characterize the joint distribution of a large set of observed variables by a smaller set of latent factors, leading to a reduction in data dimensionality. The latent factors are often interpreted substantively as common causal factors, such as personality factors, general intelligence, mental health factors, political standings, etc. The IFA models further provide a characterization of the relationship between the common factors and the observed variables, through the so-called item response functions which take a generalized linear model (GLM) regression form, where the response variables in the GLM regression are the observed variables (i.e., item responses) and the independent variables are the common factors. Thanks to its good interpretation, IFA models are widely used for generating and testing substantive theory.

The last decade has observed the need of solving large-scale IFA problems, where the sample size, the number of items, and the number of latent factors can all be large. For example, in psychiatry, there has been a need to better understand and

Y. Chen (✉) · S. Zhang
London School of Economics and Political Science, London, UK
e-mail: y.chen186@lse.ac.uk

Y. Zhao, (Din) D.-G. Chen (eds.), *Modern Statistical Methods for Health Research*,
Emerging Topics in Statistics and Biostatistics,
https://doi.org/10.1007/978-3-030-72437-5_15

classify mental disorders (e.g., [33]). This implies the need of applying IFA to many mental health symptoms from a large number of respondents, for which a large number of factors may be needed. In modern psychology, an important problem is to better characterize personality traits, for example by collecting large-scale data from the internet (e.g., [48, 54]). It means fitting IFA models to data with thousands of items and hundreds of thousands of respondents. In marketing, there are also needs to better analyze customers' preference choices by the IFA of large-scale e-commerce data. In this chapter, we will focus on reviewing estimation methods that are tailored to such large-scale IFA problems.

The rest of this chapter is organized as follows. In Sect. 2, we introduce the statistical frameworks of IFA. In Sect. 3, methods and algorithms for the estimation of IFA models are reviewed, followed by a survey of available computer software/packages in Sect. 4. We conclude this chapter with suggestions for the practical applications of IFA methods and discussions of future directions.

2 IFA Models

2.1 Modeling Framework

Consider N individuals answering J items, with Y_{ij} being the response from person i to item j and $Y = (Y_{ij})_{N\times J}$ being the data matrix. The data entry Y_{ij} is typically categorical, due to the nature of item-level response data. In particular, Y_{ij} takes values 0 or 1 for binary items, and Y_{ij} takes value $0, 1, \ldots, t_j$, for some $t_j \geq 2$ when the item is ordinal. An IFA model imposes a joint distribution on the data matrix $Y = (Y_{ij})_{N\times J}$. A typical IFA model makes the following three assumptions:

A1. Each individual is assumed to be represented by a latent trait vector $\boldsymbol{\theta}_i = (\theta_{i1}, \ldots, \theta_{iK})^\top$, for some $K \geq 1$. The distribution of person i's responses $\mathbf{Y}_i = (Y_{i1}, \ldots, Y_{iJ})^\top$ depends only on $\boldsymbol{\theta}_i$ but not other $\boldsymbol{\theta}_{i'}$s, for $i' \neq i$. The dimension K of the latent vector is typically chosen much smaller than the number of items J, so that a reduction in the data dimensionality is achieved. Depending on the types of applications, the value of K is either determined by substantive theory (typically in confirmatory analysis) or to be estimated from data (typically in exploratory analysis). IFA models with $K = 1$ are often known as unidimensional models and those with $K > 1$ are known as multidimensional models.

A2. Most IFA models assume local independence. That is, $Y_{i1}, \ldots, Y_{iJ}$ are assumed to be conditionally independent, given the latent vectors $\boldsymbol{\theta}_i$, for $i = 1, \ldots, N$.

A3. Making use of the previous two assumptions, an IFA model completes the specification of the joint distribution of Y by specifying the conditional distribution of each Y_{ij} given $\boldsymbol{\theta}_i$. A parametric model is typically assumed,

$$P(Y_{ij} = t|\boldsymbol{\theta}_i; \boldsymbol{\beta}_j) = f_j(t|\boldsymbol{\theta}_i; \boldsymbol{\beta}_j),$$

where $t \in \{0, 1\}$ for binary items and $t \in \{0, 1, \ldots, t_j\}$ for ordinal items, $\boldsymbol{\beta}_j$ is a generic notation for the item-specific parameters, and f_j is known as the item response function. Specific item response functions f_j will be discussed in Sect. 2.2.

These three assumptions lead to a joint distribution of the data matrix Y, given the person-specific latent factors $\boldsymbol{\theta}_i$ and the item-specific parameters $\boldsymbol{\beta}_j$. This leads to the joint likelihood function given observed data $y_{ij}, i = 1, \ldots, N, j = 1, \ldots, J$,

$$\begin{aligned} &L_{\mathrm{J}}(\boldsymbol{\theta}_i, \boldsymbol{\beta}_j, i = 1, \cdots, N, j = 1, \cdots, J) \\ &= \prod_{i=1}^{N} \prod_{j=1}^{J} f_j(y_{ij}|\boldsymbol{\theta}_i; \boldsymbol{\beta}_j). \end{aligned} \tag{1}$$

In this joint likelihood function, both the person-specific latent factors and the item-specific parameters are treated as unknown fixed parameters. Alternatively, the latent factors are often treated as random effects instead of fixed parameters, under the following assumption:

A4. The latent vectors $\boldsymbol{\theta}_i$ are independent and identically distributed, following a cumulative distribution function F. A parametric form is typically assumed for F, where we use $\boldsymbol{\gamma}$ to denote the parameters and use $F(\cdot|\boldsymbol{\gamma})$ to denote the parameterized cumulative distribution. In most IFA applications, F is assumed to be multivariate normal.

This additional assumption, together with the previous assumptions, implies the marginal likelihood function

$$\begin{aligned} &L_{\mathrm{M}}(\boldsymbol{\gamma}, \boldsymbol{\beta}_j, j = 1, \cdots, J) \\ &= \prod_{i=1}^{N} \int \left[\prod_{j=1}^{J} f_j(y_{ij}|\boldsymbol{\theta}; \boldsymbol{\beta}_j) \right] \phi(\boldsymbol{\theta}|\boldsymbol{\gamma}) d\boldsymbol{\theta}, \end{aligned} \tag{2}$$

where $\phi(\boldsymbol{\theta}|\boldsymbol{\gamma})$ denotes the density function of F. Fundamentally, the two different views of the latent factor come from different sampling foundations of the IFA models. In particular, the fixed effect view of the latent factors has a "stochastic subject" interpretation and the random effect view has a "random sampling" interpretation of the probability in IFA models. See [28] for detailed discussions. Technically, as will be discussed in Sect. 3, the estimations based on the two likelihood functions have different asymptotic behaviors.

Although our focus is on multivariate categorical data, the above modeling framework also includes the linear factor models as a special case. Specifically, a linear factor model takes the form of

$$Y_{ij} = d_j + \mathbf{a}_j^\top \boldsymbol{\theta}_i + \epsilon_{ij}, \tag{3}$$

where Y_{ij} is a continuous variable and ϵ_{ij} is a mean-zero independent error term with variance σ_j^2.

2.2 Examples of IFA Models

In what follows, we discuss some specific IFA models. We separate the discussion by the type of data.

Models for Binary Data When Y_{ij} is binary, one only needs to specify $P(Y_{ij} = 1|\boldsymbol{\theta}_i; \boldsymbol{\beta}_j) = f(1|\boldsymbol{\theta}_i; \boldsymbol{\beta}_j)$, which can be viewed as the specification of a generalized linear model for binary response, with Y_{ij} being the response and $\boldsymbol{\theta}_i$ being the independent variables. A commonly used parametrization is

$$f(1|\boldsymbol{\theta}_i; \boldsymbol{\beta}_j) = G(d_j + \mathbf{a}_j^\top \boldsymbol{\theta}_i), \tag{4}$$

where $G : \mathbb{R} \to (0, 1)$ is a pre-specified monotonically increasing function and item parameters $\boldsymbol{\beta}_j = (d_j, \mathbf{a}_j)$. Function G is often known as the inverse link function, using the terminology of generalized linear models. Commonly used choices of G include the logistic and probit forms, for which $G(x) = \exp(x)/(1 + \exp(x))$ and $G(x) = (\int_{-\infty}^x \exp(-z^2/2)dz)/\sqrt{2\pi}$, respectively. When viewing (4) as a generalized linear model that regresses Y_{ij} on $\boldsymbol{\theta}_i$, d_j can be viewed as the intercept parameter and $\mathbf{a}_j = (a_{j1}, \ldots, a_{jK})^\top$ are the slope parameters. The slope parameters are also known as the loading parameters in IFA.

When $K = 1$ and $G(x)$ takes the logistic form, then the model

$$f(1|\boldsymbol{\theta}_i; \boldsymbol{\beta}_j) = \frac{\exp(d_j + a_j\theta_i)}{1 + \exp(d_j + a_j\theta_i)}$$

is known as the two-parameter logistic model (2PL; [5]). When a_j is further restricted to be 1, then the model

$$f(1|\boldsymbol{\theta}_i; \boldsymbol{\beta}_j) = \frac{\exp(d_j + \theta_i)}{1 + \exp(d_j + \theta_i)}$$

becomes a reparametrization of the famous Rasch model [46]. Both models are widely used in the educational testing industry for the design, analysis, and scoring of tests. When $K > 1$, both the logistic and probit versions of model (4) are commonly used for multidimensional IFA analysis, with the logistic version typically known as the multidimensional two-parameter logistic model (M2PL; 47). As the two link functions can approximate each other well (see e.g., [5]), IFA result from the logistic model and that from the probit model are usually very similar.

Therefore, in practice, the choice of the link function is typically determined by computational consideration. Roughly speaking, the logistic form tends to be easier to handle computationally when treating the latent factors as fixed parameters, and the probit form has advantages under the random effect view. Further discussions will be provided in Sect. 3.

Equivalently, model (4) can be obtained through the introduction of a latent response. That is, we define a latent response

$$Y_{ij}^* = d_j + \mathbf{a}_j^\top \boldsymbol{\theta}_i + \epsilon_{ij}, \tag{5}$$

where ϵ_{ij} is an independent error term with zero mean. This equation takes the same form as (3) for linear factor model, except that the observed variables in (3) is replaced by the latent response in (5). The observed response is assumed to be a truncated version of the latent response, i.e.,

$$Y_{ij} = 1_{\{Y_{ij}^* \geq 0\}}. \tag{6}$$

When ϵ_{ij} follows the standard normal and logistic distributions, respectively, (5) and (6) together imply the probit and logistic versions of (4), respectively. The latent response formulation brings computational convenience for the probit model, when $\boldsymbol{\theta}_i$s are viewed as random effects and follow a multivariate normal distribution. This computational advantage is brought by a data argumentation trick for Monte Carlo sampling; see Sect. 3.2 for the details.

Models for Ordinal Data Ordinal responses are probably even more common than binary responses in practice due to the wide use of Likert-scale items in social and behavioral sciences. Models for ordinal data naturally generalize those for binary data by two different approaches. The first approach obtains $f_j(t|\boldsymbol{\theta}_i; \boldsymbol{\beta}_j)$ by specifying the cumulative probabilities of a response less than or equal to each threshold t. That is,

$$P(Y_{ij} \leq t|\boldsymbol{\theta}_i; \boldsymbol{\beta}_j) = G(d_{jt} + \mathbf{a}_j^\top \boldsymbol{\theta}_i),\ t = 0, \ldots, t_{j-1}, \tag{7}$$

where, the same as in (4), G is a pre-specified monotonically increasing function, and $\boldsymbol{\beta}_j = (d_{j0}, \ldots, d_{j,t_j-1}, \mathbf{a}_j)$ are the item-specific parameters. Recall that $Y_{ij} \in \{0, \ldots, t_j\}$, and thus $P(Y_{ij} \leq t_j|\boldsymbol{\theta}_i; \boldsymbol{\beta}_j) = 1$. It is worth noting that the intercept parameter in (7) depends on the response category while the slope parameter does not. Similar as the binary case, the inverse link function G is often chosen to take logistic or probit forms.

Due to the facts that $P(Y_{ij} \leq t + 1|\boldsymbol{\theta}_i; \boldsymbol{\beta}_j) \geq P(Y_{ij} \leq t|\boldsymbol{\theta}_i; \boldsymbol{\beta}_j)$ for each t and that G is monotonically increasing, we naturally have the constraints for the intercept parameters,

$$d_{j0} \leq d_{j1} \leq \cdots \leq d_{j,t_j-1}.$$

The cumulative probabilities (7) then imply the category-specific probabilities. That is,

$$f(t|\boldsymbol{\theta}_i;\boldsymbol{\beta}_j) = P(Y_{ij} \le t|\boldsymbol{\theta}_i;\boldsymbol{\beta}_j) - P(Y_{ij} \le t-1|\boldsymbol{\theta}_i;\boldsymbol{\beta}_j).$$

Depending on the dimension of the latent vector, the model (7) is referred to as the unidimensional and multidimensional graded response models [40, 53]. The model (7) has a similar latent response interpretation as the model for binary data. Therefore, it shares the same connection with linear factor models and has same computational advantage.

The second modeling approach is by specifying the conditional distributions based on the adjacent response categories. More precisely, the following conditional probabilities are specified:

$$P(Y_{ij} = t|\boldsymbol{\theta}_i, \boldsymbol{\beta}_j, Y_{ij} \in \{t-1, t\}) = G(d_{jt} + \mathbf{a}_j^\top \boldsymbol{\theta}_i),\ t = 1, \ldots, t_j. \tag{8}$$

Again, G is a pre-specified monotonically increasing function, and $\boldsymbol{\beta}_j = (d_{j1}, \ldots, d_{jt_j}, \mathbf{a}_j)$ are the item-specific parameters. In this model, the inverse link G is chosen to be the logistic form instead of the probit form. As a result, the conditional probability (8) implies that

$$\frac{f(t|\boldsymbol{\theta}_i;\boldsymbol{\beta}_j)}{f(t-1|\boldsymbol{\theta}_i;\boldsymbol{\beta}_j)} = \frac{G(d_{jt} + \mathbf{a}_j^\top \boldsymbol{\theta}_i)}{1 - G(d_{jt} + \mathbf{a}_j^\top \boldsymbol{\theta}_i)} = \exp(d_{jt} + \mathbf{a}_j^\top \boldsymbol{\theta}_i). \tag{9}$$

Note that the ratio of the probabilities in two adjacent categories does not have a simple form when using the probit link. The ratio (9) further leads to

$$f(t|\boldsymbol{\theta}_i;\boldsymbol{\beta}_j) = \begin{cases} 1/\left(1 + \sum_{s=1}^{t_j} \exp(s\mathbf{a}_j^\top \boldsymbol{\theta}_i + \sum_{v=1}^{s} d_{jv})\right), & \text{if } t = 0 \\ \exp(t\mathbf{a}_j^\top \boldsymbol{\theta}_i + \sum_{v=1}^{t} d_{jv})/\left(1 + \sum_{s=1}^{t_j} \exp(s\mathbf{a}_j^\top \boldsymbol{\theta}_i + \sum_{v=1}^{s} d_{jv})\right), & \text{if } t = 1, \ldots, t_j. \end{cases} \tag{10}$$

This model is known as the generalized partial credit model [38, 62].

The generalized partial credit model and the graded response models tend to have similar fit on empirical data. Computationally, the generalized partial credit model is easier to handle when the estimation is based on the joint likelihood function, thanks to the exponential family form of (10). When the latent factors are treated as random effect, the probit version of the graded response model with multivariate normal latent factors is computationally easier to handle; see Sect. 3.2 for more details.

2.3 Exploratory and Confirmatory Analyses

Like linear factor analysis, IFA is also used in two different settings, exploratory and confirmatory settings, respectively. Exploratory IFA assumes little or no prior knowledge about the data. It aims at learning the latent structure underlying the data through exploratory investigation procedures. Questions of interest include but not limited to: How many latent factors are needed to sufficiently describe the data? How do we interpret these factors? The first question is a model selection problem. Given a family of IFA models, the goal is to choose the dimension K of the latent factors so that the model best fits the data, in terms of model relative fit which may be measured by, for example, a suitable information criterion.

The second question is more complicated that is related to the identifiability of an exploratory IFA model. Therefore, we first discuss the model identifiability problem. An exploratory IFA model is not identifiable for several reasons. Take model (4) as an example, but the same reasons apply to the other models introduced above. First, the locations and the scales of the latent factors are not identifiable. A simultaneous linear transformation of the factors and the item parameters will lead to the same model. That is, we obtain exactly the same item response function with person parameters $\tilde{\boldsymbol{\theta}}_i$ and item parameters $\tilde{\boldsymbol{\beta}}_j = (\tilde{d}_j, \tilde{\boldsymbol{a}}_j)$, if we let $\tilde{\boldsymbol{\theta}}_i = \boldsymbol{\mu} + H\boldsymbol{\theta}_i$, $\tilde{\mathbf{a}}_j = H^{-1}\mathbf{a}_j$, and $\tilde{d}_j = d_j - \mathbf{a}_j^\top H^{-1}\boldsymbol{\mu}$, for any vector $\boldsymbol{\mu} \in \mathbb{R}^K$ and $K \times K$ invertible diagonal matrix H. This location and scale indeterminacy issue is solved by imposing identification constraints. Specifically, when the latent factors are treated as fixed effects, we can fix their locations and scales by requiring

$$\sum_{i=1}^{N} \theta_{ik} = 0, \text{ and } \frac{\sum_{i=1}^{N} \theta_{ik}^2}{N} = 1, k = 1, \ldots, K.$$

When $\boldsymbol{\theta}_i$s are treated as random effects, then these constraints are replaced by the corresponding population versions,

$$E(\theta_{ik}) = 0, \text{ and } Var(\theta_{ik}) = 1, k = 1, \ldots, K.$$

The second unidentifiability issue of exploratory IFA is due to rotational indeterminacy. That is, even with the locations and scales of the latent factors fixed using the above identification constraints, an exploratory IFA model is still not identifiable up to an oblique rotation of the factors.[1] More precisely, we obtain the same item response function if we simultaneously transform the latent factors and item parameters by letting $\tilde{\boldsymbol{\theta}}_i = H\boldsymbol{\theta}_i$, $\tilde{\mathbf{a}}_j = (H^{-1})^\top \mathbf{a}_j$, and $\tilde{d}_j = d_j$, where H is a $K \times K$ invertible matrix satisfying that the diagonal entries of $HH^\top$ are all one. Note that $\tilde{\boldsymbol{\theta}}_i$ given by this transformation still follows the identification constraints, regardless of whether the latent factors are treated as fixed or random effects.

Dealing with the rotational indeterminacy issue requires additional assumption on the loading matrix A. Roughly speaking, it is often assumed that the loading

[1]Orthogonal rotational methods (e.g., varimax rotation; 32) are available in factor analysis that requires the estimated factors to be orthogonal to each other. As the orthogonal requirement of the latent factors is somewhat artificial, we do not discuss them in this chapter.

matrix has a relatively simple structure, in the sense that many entries of the true loading matrix A^* are zero. Specifically, a^*_{jk} being zero implies that changing the value of the kth factor does not change the distribution of Y_{ij}. When many entries of the true loading matrix A^* are zero, then each latent factor is only measured by a small set of items. If this sparsity pattern can be learned from data, then each factor can be interpreted based on the items that are directly associated with it. Different methods have been developed for learning the sparsity pattern of the loading matrix. Traditionally, analytic rotation methods are used to find an approximate solution to this problem. An analytic rotation method starts from some estimate of the loading matrix $\hat{A}$, whose rotation may be fixed arbitrarily. It then finds a rotated loading matrix $\hat{A}H^{-1}$ by minimizing some complexity functions with respect to H, where the complexity function measures the sparsity of the loading matrix. Depending on different sparsity assumptions on the true loading matrix, different complexity functions have been proposed. We refer the readers to [8] for an overview of analytic rotation methods. It is worth noting that this type of estimators cannot produce loading matrix estimates with exactly zero entries. To avoid the ambiguity of analytic rotation methods for not producing exactly sparse loading estimates, recently, penalized estimators have been developed for the learning of a sparse loading matrix [57]. These estimators obtain a sparse $\hat{A}$ by maximizing a penalized likelihood, where LASSO-type penalty terms are used to enforce exact sparsity.

Confirmatory IFA aims at testing substantive theory or scaling individuals along multiple latent traits, by parameter estimation, model comparison, and assessment of model goodness-of-fit. In contrast to exploratory analysis, in conducting confirmatory IFA, the number of factors, the substantive meaning of each factor, and the factors each item is measuring are all specified a priori. More precisely, the factors each item measures are reflected by the sparsity pattern of the loading matrix. This sparsity pattern is typically known as the design matrix or the Q-matrix [17] in the context of confirmatory IFA. The Q-matrix is a $J \times K$ binary matrix, with each entry $q_{ij} = 0$ implying that $a_{ij} = 0$ and $q_{ij} = 1$ implying that a_{ij} is freely estimated. When the zero entries in the Q-matrix are well positioned, then the rotational indeterminacy issue that appears in exploratory IFA will disappear. As a result, with further identification constraints on the location and scale of the latent factors, the loading matrix and the latent factors can be identified and consistently estimated (see [2, 17] for rigorous treatment on this problem).

3 Estimation Methods

3.1 Estimation Based on Joint Likelihood

The joint maximum likelihood estimator was first proposed in [5]. Treating both the latent factors and the item parameters as fixed model parameters, the joint maximum likelihood estimator is defined as

$$(\hat{\boldsymbol{\theta}}_i, \hat{\boldsymbol{\beta}}_j : i = 1, \ldots, N, j = 1, \ldots, J)$$
$$= \underset{\boldsymbol{\theta}_i, \boldsymbol{\beta}_j, i=1,\cdots,N, j=1,\cdots,J}{\arg\max} \log L_J(\boldsymbol{\theta}_i, \boldsymbol{\beta}_j, i = 1, \cdots, N, j = 1, \cdots, J), \quad (11)$$

where the joint likelihood function is defined in (1) and the maximization in (11) may be required to satisfy certain identification constraints though they are not explicitly stated here.

This estimator is not favored for a long period of time in the history of IFA, which is largely due to the lack of good asymptotic properties. Under the conventional asymptotic regime that J is fixed and N grows to infinity, this joint estimator (11) has been shown to be inconsistent [1, 25, 27, 43]. This is not surprising, as the number of parameters grows linearly with the sample size N in this asymptotic setting, which makes the classical asymptotic theory for maximum likelihood estimation fail.

However, this traditional asymptotic regime may not be suitable for large-scale IFA applications where both N and J tend to be large. Instead, it may be more sensible to consider a double asymptotic setting with both N and J diverging. In fact, [27] showed under the Rasch model that a finite solution in (11) exists with probability tending to 1. This estimator is consistent under suitable identifiability conditions when both N and J diverge to infinity in suitable rates, and the estimator has asymptotic normality. Intuitively, under this asymptotic regime, the number of parameters grows in the rate of $O(N + J)$, while the number of data points is NJ. The consistency is due to that the growth of the data is much faster than the dimension of the parameter space, when both N and J grow to infinity.

The results of [27] rely heavily on the convex geometry of the Rasch parameter space and thus cannot be generalized to other IFA models. In analyzing joint likelihood-based estimation for a wider range of IFA models, [16, 17] considered a variant of (11) called the constrained joint maximum likelihood estimator (CJMLE). The CJMLE adds additional constraints on (11) that require $\|\boldsymbol{\theta}_i\| \leq C$ and $\|\boldsymbol{\beta}_j\| \leq C$, for some constant $C > 0$. These constraints restrict the estimated person parameters and item parameters to a compact ball, which not only provides technical convenience for the establishment of consistency results, but also brings numerical stability by avoiding the estimate of some person/item parameters being infinity due to the presence of extreme response patterns (e.g., $y_{ij} = 1$, for all $j = 1, \ldots, J$).

Due to the more complex geometry of the parameter space for general IFA models, the asymptotic results for the CJMLE are slightly weaker than that of the Rasch model. Specifically, [17] showed that for a general family of IFA models for binary data, the CJMLE leads to the convergence of the following average loss function:

$$\frac{\sum_{i=1}^{N}\sum_{j=1}^{J}\left(f_j(1|\boldsymbol{\theta}_i^*, \boldsymbol{\beta}_j^*) - f_j(1|\hat{\boldsymbol{\theta}}_i, \hat{\boldsymbol{\beta}}_j)\right)^2}{NJ} = O_p\left(\frac{1}{\min\{N, J\}}\right). \quad (12)$$

As shown in [17], when the dimension K is fixed, the rate in (12) is optimal in the minimax sense. That is, there does not exist other estimators that can beat the CJMLE in terms of the convergence rate of the loss function in (12). Moreover, by making use of (12) and matrix perturbation results [21, 60], one can show that under the exploratory IFA setting the loading matrix can be recovered up to a rotation, in the sense that

$$\frac{\min_{H \in \mathbb{R}^{K \times K}} \left\{ \sum_{j=1}^{J} \|\mathbf{a}_j^* - H\hat{\mathbf{a}}_j\|^2 \right\}}{JK} = O_p\left(\frac{1}{\min\{N, J\}} \right). \tag{13}$$

Under the confirmatory IFA setting, when the design matrix Q has a desirable structure, the convergence of the item parameters can be established as

$$\frac{\sum_{j=1}^{J} \|\mathbf{a}_j^* - \hat{\mathbf{a}}_j\|^2}{JK} = O_p\left(\frac{1}{\min\{N, J\}} \right), \tag{14}$$

which no longer involves a rotation matrix. We remark that these results can be easily generalized to IFA models for ordinal data.

We now discuss the computation of (11) and its constrained variants. A commonly used trick to solve such a problem is by alternating maximization. That is, one can decompose the parameters into two blocks, the person parameters and the item parameters. The optimization in (11) or that for the CJMLE can be realized by iteratively alternating between maximizing one block of parameters given the other block. Thanks to the factorization form of the joint likelihood, the maximization in each step can be performed in parallel for different people/items. Consequently, substantial computational advantage can be gained when parallel computing techniques are used. In addition, the maximization for each $\boldsymbol{\theta}_i$ or $\boldsymbol{\beta}_j$ can be viewed as finding the maximum likelihood estimate, either constrained or unconstrained, for a generalized linear regression problem. Certain IFA models have computational advantage in this step due to their exponential family forms when fixing one block of parameters. These models include the M2PL model for binary data and the generalized partial credit model for ordinal data. Finally, we remark that the optimization problem (11) is non-convex and thus there is no guarantee that the alternating maximization procedure converges to the global solution. Empirically, the performance of alternating maximization benefits from using a good initial value. See Sect. 3.4 for how a good initial value may be obtained.

3.2 Estimation Based on Marginal Likelihood

In the IFA literature, it is more common to estimate the item parameters based on the marginal likelihood, where the latent factors are treated as random effects. The marginal maximum likelihood estimator (MMLE) is defined as

$$(\hat{\boldsymbol{\gamma}}, \hat{\boldsymbol{\beta}}_j, j = 1, \cdots, J) = \underset{\boldsymbol{\gamma}, \boldsymbol{\beta}_j, j=1,\cdots,J}{\arg\max} \; \log L_{\mathrm{M}}(\boldsymbol{\gamma}, \boldsymbol{\beta}_j, j = 1, \cdots, J), \tag{15}$$

where the marginal likelihood function is defined in (2). In contrast to the joint likelihood-based estimators, as the latent factors are treated as nuisance parameters and integrated out in the likelihood function, this estimator can be analyzed using the classical theory for maximum likelihood estimation under the traditional asymptotic regime with J fixed and N diverging.

Similar to the joint likelihood, the marginal likelihood function is also non-convex and thus convergence to the global solution is not guaranteed in general. The computation for (15) tends to be much slower than (11), due to the more complex form of the marginal likelihood. Specifically, due to the integral in (2), its gradient is not easy to evaluate. As a result, (15) cannot be solved using standard numerical solvers like gradient ascent or coordinate ascent algorithms. The most classical method for solving (15) is the expectation-maximization (EM) algorithm [6, 22]. For ease of explanation, we simplify the notation by denoting $\Psi = (\boldsymbol{\gamma}, \boldsymbol{\beta}_j, j = 1, \cdots, J)$. Starting from an initial set of parameters $\Psi^{(0)}$, the EM algorithm iteratively performs two steps, the Expectation (E) step and the Maximization (M) step. In the $t + 1$th iteration, the E step constructs an objective function $Q(\Psi \mid \Psi^{(t)})$ given the parameter values from the previous step $\Psi^{(t)}$, where

$$Q(\Psi \mid \Psi^{(t)}) = \sum_{i=1}^{N} E_{\boldsymbol{\theta}_i|\Psi^{(t)},\mathbf{y}_i}\left[\log \phi(\boldsymbol{\theta}_i|\boldsymbol{\gamma}) + \sum_{j=1}^{J} \log f_j(y_{ij}|\boldsymbol{\theta}_i; \boldsymbol{\beta}_j)\right]. \tag{16}$$

The expectation in (16) is with respect to the latent factors $\boldsymbol{\theta}_i$ under its posterior distribution based on the current parameters $\Psi^{(t)}$. Then the M step produces the parameter values $\Psi^{(t+1)}$ by maximizing $Q(\Psi \mid \Psi^{(t)})$, i.e.,

$$\Psi^{(t+1)} = \underset{\Psi}{\arg\max}\, Q(\Psi \mid \Psi^{(t)}).$$

With a good starting point $\Psi^{(0)}$, the sequence $\Psi^{(t)}$ will converge to the marginal maximum likelihood estimate as defined in (15).

When the dimension K of the latent factors is large, the computational complexity of the E step is high, for the above vanilla version of the EM algorithm. This is because, the expectation with respect to $\boldsymbol{\theta}_i$ involves a K-dimensional integral that does not have a closed form. As a result, the expectation has to be evaluated by a numerical integral, whose complexity is exponential in the dimension K. Even for a moderate K (e.g., $K > 5$), the computation of the vanilla EM algorithm can hardly be affordable.

In dealing with the computation of large-scale IFA under the random effect view of the latent factors, several methods have been proposed. One way to improve the EM algorithm is by replacing the numerical integral in the E step using Monte Carlo integration, which leads to the Monte Carlo EM algorithm [37, 61] for IFA.

The Monte Carlo EM algorithm approximates the Q function by approximating the expectations in (16) by Monte Carlo integration, which means to sample from the posterior distribution of each $\boldsymbol{\theta}_i$ under the current model $\Psi^{(t)}$. As the posterior distribution of $\boldsymbol{\theta}_i$ typically does not have a simple closed form, Markov Chain Monte Carlo (MCMC) methods are often used. Even with the numerical integration avoided, the Monte Carlo EM still tends to be slow in practice. In a later stage of the Monte Carlo EM algorithm, the error in $\Psi^{(t)}$ will be dominated by the Monte Carlo error from the E step. To accurately approximate the MMLE, a very large number of Monte Carlo samples are needed in the last several iterations of the algorithm, which can cause a very high computational burden.

The computational inefficiency of the Monte Carlo EM algorithm is largely due to the inefficient use of the posterior samples of the latent factors. That is, the posterior samples of the latent factors are only used once and are immediately discarded in the next iteration. To avoid the inefficient use of the posterior samples, alternative methods have been proposed, including the stochastic EM algorithm [13, 29, 44, 66] and stochastic approximation with MCMC algorithms [9, 10, 26]. The stochastic EM algorithm differs from the EM algorithms by the following ways. Let $\Psi^{(t)}$ be the parameter estimate from the tth iteration. In the $(t+1)$th iteration, the stochastic EM algorithm replaces the E step of the EM algorithm by a stochastic E step. In this stochastic E step, we obtain one sample $\boldsymbol{\theta}_i^{(t+1)}$ for each $\boldsymbol{\theta}_i$ from its posterior distribution under the current model, then construct a Q-function in the form

$$Q(\Psi \mid \Psi^{(t)}) = \sum_{i=1}^{N} \left[\log \phi(\boldsymbol{\theta}_i^{(t+1)} | \boldsymbol{\gamma}) + \sum_{j=1}^{J} \log f_j(y_{ij} | \boldsymbol{\theta}_i^{(t+1)}; \boldsymbol{\beta}_j) \right].$$

Then in the M step of stochastic EM algorithm, we obtain

$$\Psi^{(t+1)} = \arg\max_{\Psi} Q(\Psi \mid \Psi^{(t)}).$$

Unlike the EM and Monte Carlo EM algorithms for which the final estimate is given by $\Psi^{(T)}$ from the last iteration, the final estimate of the stochastic EM algorithm is given by an average of $\Psi^{(t)}$s from the iterations after a sufficient burn-in period, i.e.,

$$\hat{\Psi} = \frac{\sum_{t=m+1}^{T} \Psi^{(t)}}{T - m}, \tag{17}$$

where iterations 1 to m are used as a burn-in period and the last $T - m$ iterations are used in the final estimate $\hat{\Psi}$. As shown in [44], the estimator (17) is almost asymptotically equivalent to the MMLE for a sufficiently large number of iterations T. Comparing with the Monte Carlo EM algorithm, the stochastic EM algorithm more efficiently makes use of the posterior samples of the latent factors, by including $\Psi^{(t)}$ from many iterations in the final estimate. The theoretical properties of the stochastic EM algorithm are studied comprehensively in [44]. Computational details and numerical examples of applying stochastic EM to large-scale IFA problems can be found in [66].

The stochastic approximation with MCMC algorithms [9, 10, 26] are developed based on the seminal work of [50] on stochastic approximation. It is worth pointing out that the work of [50] also lays the theoretical foundation for the gradient descent optimization method that is widely used in machine learning and artificial intelligence. Similar to the EM algorithm and its variants as introduced above, a stochastic approximation MCMC algorithm also iteratively alternates between two steps. Let the current iteration number be t and the current parameter estimate be $\Psi^{(t)}$. To proceed, the algorithm first does a stochastic E step. In this step, a small number of posterior samples for each $\boldsymbol{\theta}_i$ are obtained under the current model $\Psi^{(t)}$. These posterior samples are used to find a stochastic gradient of the marginal likelihood (2) at the current parameter $\Psi^{(t)}$. We denote this stochastic gradient as $H^{(t+1)}$. In some algorithms, an approximation to the Hessian matrix of (2) is also obtained in this step. We denote the Hessian matrix approximation by $\Gamma^{(t+1)}$. Then following the idea of stochastic approximation, in the second step of the iteration, the parameters are updated by a stochastic gradient ascent step

$$\Psi^{(t+1)} = \Psi^{(t)} + \gamma_{t+1} H^{(t+1)}, \tag{18}$$

or

$$\Psi^{(t+1)} = \Psi^{(t)} + \gamma_{t+1} \left[\Gamma^{(t+1)}\right]^{-1} H^{(t+1)}, \tag{19}$$

where γ_ts is a pre-specified constant that is typically chosen as $\gamma_t = 1/t$. This constant is known as the gaining constant in the stochastic approximation literature and it plays a very important role in the algorithm. Comparing the two updating methods (18) and (19), the second updating rule may lead to faster convergence when the Hessian matrix is accurately approximated [19, 24]. However, it can also lead to numerical instability and does not improve the convergence when the approximation is poor. This type of algorithms was first proposed by Gu and Kong [26] for handling general missing data problems. It is then tailored to large-scale IFA problems in [9, 10], with computational details and numerical examples provided.

A key step, which is also the most time-consuming part of all the above variants of the EM algorithm, is to sample from the posterior distribution of $\boldsymbol{\theta}_i$ under the current set of parameters. This problem can be non-trivial due to the lack of conjugacy, in particular, when the dimension K of the latent factors is high. Although the Gibbs sampler can always be used, it is likely to suffer from the slow-mixing issue, especially when K is large and the factors are highly correlated. However, there is one family of models, for which the posterior samples of $\boldsymbol{\theta}_i$ are easy to obtain. These models include model (4) and the graded response model (7), when the probit link is used and the marginal distribution F is multivariate normal. Under these models, $\boldsymbol{\theta}_i$ can be sampled using a blocked Gibbs sampler. This blocked

Gibbs sampler is designed using a data argumentation trick that is based on the latent response formulation. Take the model for binary data as an example. We consider the sampling of $\boldsymbol{\theta}_i$ given data $y_{i1}, \ldots, y_{iJ}$ and model parameters $\boldsymbol{\gamma}, \boldsymbol{\beta}_1, \ldots, \boldsymbol{\beta}_J$. The Gibbs sampler iterates between the following two steps, both of which can be easily implemented:

Step 1: Independently sample latent responses y_{ij}^*, $j = 1, \ldots, J$. Each y_{ij}^* is sampled from a unidimensional truncated normal distribution with density function

$$g(y) \propto \begin{cases} \exp\left(-(y - d_j - \mathbf{a}_j^\top \boldsymbol{\theta}_i)^2/2\right) 1_{\{y \geq 0\}}, & \text{if } y_{ij} = 1, \\ \exp\left(-(y - d_j - \mathbf{a}_j^\top \boldsymbol{\theta}_i)^2/2\right) 1_{\{y < 0\}}, & \text{if } y_{ij} = 0, \end{cases}$$

where the value of $\boldsymbol{\theta}_i$ is from the previous step.

Step 2: Update $\boldsymbol{\theta}_i$ by sampling from a multivariate normal distribution

$$h(\boldsymbol{\theta}) \propto \phi(\boldsymbol{\theta}|\boldsymbol{\gamma}) \prod_{j=1}^{J} \exp\left(-(y_{ij}^* - d_j - \mathbf{a}_j^\top \boldsymbol{\theta})^2/2\right),$$

where y_{ij}^*s are from Step 1.

We provide a brief comparison of the three stochastic variants of the EM algorithm. In terms of computational speed, the stochastic approximation with MCMC algorithm and the stochastic EM algorithm are similar in achieving the same accuracy, and the former may be slightly faster in some situations. Both methods tend to be substantially faster than the Monte Carlo EM algorithm. Further comparing the stochastic approximation method and the stochastic EM algorithm, the latter tends to be numerically more stable and thus easier to use for applied researchers. This is because, the stochastic EM algorithm is almost tuning free. In contrast, the performance of the stochastic approximation method is sensitive to the specification of the gaining constant and the accurate approximation of the Hessian matrix (when using updating rule (19)). As a result, good performance of the stochastic approximation method is sometimes subject to tuning, which can be labor-intensive.

Besides the variants of the EM algorithms described above, full Bayesian methods have also been developed to find approximate solutions to (15). A full Bayesian method imposes prior distributions on the parameters in (2), including $\boldsymbol{\gamma}$ and $\boldsymbol{\beta}_j$, $j = 1, \ldots, J$. Then posterior means/modes of these parameters are approximated using Markov Chain Monte Carlo Methods. See [4, 7], and [23] for applications of full Bayesian methods under various IFA settings. We point out that most applications of IFA take a frequentist setting. Even when full Bayesian methods are used for the computation, they tend to be used as a tool to approximate the marginal maximum likelihood estimator, making use of the asymptotic equivalence between posterior mean/mode and the maximum likelihood estimator in the frequentist sense (see e.g., [58, Chapter 10]).

3.3 Limited-Information Estimation

Methods introduced in Sects. 3.1 and 3.2 are typically known as the full-information estimation methods, as both the joint likelihood function and marginal likelihood function are based on the joint distribution of data. In contrast, limited-information estimation methods only make use of limited information such as univariate and bivariate proportions. In what follows, we review two commonly used limited-information methods.

The first method is called the composite likelihood-based estimator [31, 67]. This estimator is based on the marginal distributions of univariate and bivariate responses, in which the latent factors are still treated as random effects. This approach applies to all the models introduced above, as long as the latent factors follow a multivariate normal distribution. More precisely, the estimator is obtained by maximizing the following composite likelihood function:

$$(\hat{\boldsymbol{\gamma}}, \hat{\boldsymbol{\beta}}_j, j = 1, \cdots, J) = \underset{\boldsymbol{\gamma}, \boldsymbol{\beta}_j, j=1,\cdots,J}{\arg\max} \quad \log L_C(\boldsymbol{\gamma}, \boldsymbol{\beta}_j, j = 1, \cdots, J), \tag{20}$$

where

$$\begin{aligned} & L_C(\boldsymbol{\gamma}, \boldsymbol{\beta}_j, j = 1, \cdots, J) \\ & = \prod_{i=1}^{N} \left\{ \left[\prod_{j=1}^{J-1} \prod_{j'=j+1}^{J} \int f_j(y_{ij}|\boldsymbol{\theta}; \boldsymbol{\beta}_j) f_{j'}(y_{ij'}|\boldsymbol{\theta}; \boldsymbol{\beta}_{j'}) \phi(\boldsymbol{\theta}|\boldsymbol{\gamma}) d\boldsymbol{\theta} \right] \right. \\ & \quad \left. \times \left[\prod_{j=1}^{J} \int f_j(y_{ij}|\boldsymbol{\theta}; \boldsymbol{\beta}_j) \phi(\boldsymbol{\theta}|\boldsymbol{\gamma}) d\boldsymbol{\theta} \right] \right\}. \end{aligned} \tag{21}$$

This is a composite likelihood function as a product of all the univariate and bivariate likelihoods. When the latent factors follow a multivariate normal distribution, the computation of the estimator (20) tends to be much easier than that of (15) when the dimension K is large. This is because the integrals in (21) can be simplified to one- or two-dimensional integrals by a change of variables. For example, the integral

$$\int f_j(y_{ij}|\boldsymbol{\theta}; \boldsymbol{\beta}_j) f_{j'}(y_{ij'}|\boldsymbol{\theta}; \boldsymbol{\beta}_{j'}) \phi(\boldsymbol{\theta}|\boldsymbol{\gamma}) d\boldsymbol{\theta}$$

is two-dimensional, if we integrate with respect to $(\mathbf{a}_j^\top \boldsymbol{\theta}, \mathbf{a}_{j'}^\top \boldsymbol{\theta})^\top$, which follows a bivariate normal distribution.

When the number of items J is large, the computation of (20) tends to be slower than the CJMLE, stochastic EM, and stochastic approximation with MCMC algorithms. The gap in computational speed becomes even larger when parallel computing is allowed, as efficient parallel computing algorithms can be designed for the other methods but not the composite likelihood-based estimator. This is because the total number of parameters is in the order of J. All these parameters have to be optimized together in (20) due to the form of the objective function, while the optimizations and updates in the other algorithms can be decomposed into many small problems that can be performed in parallel. For example, in the alternating maximization of the joint likelihood, the maximization in each step can be performed independently for different people/items.

Under the classical asymptotic regime, the consistency and asymptotic normality of this estimator hold under standard assumptions, following the general theory for composite likelihood estimation (see [59] for an overview). Of course, comparing with the MMLE based on the full marginal likelihood, the composite likelihood-based estimator tends to be statistically less efficient, for only using univariate and bivariate information.

The second method is based on the concept of polychoric/tetrachoric correlation for binary/ordinal data [30, 34, 41]. This method makes use of the connection between the linear factor model and IFA models and only applies to model (4) and the graded response model (7) with a probit link and multivariate normal F. These models have a latent response interpretation and the latent responses $Y_{i1}^*, \ldots, Y_{iJ}^*$ are multivariate normal. The correlation between each pair $(Y_{ij}^*, Y_{ij'}^*)$ is known as the tetrachoric correlation when both variables are binary and the polychoric correlation when one or both of them are ordinal. This correlation can be consistently estimated based on observed data from the pair, $(y_{ij}, y_{ij'}), i = 1, \ldots, N$. By the definition of latent response (e.g., Eq. (5) for the binary case), the covariance matrix of the latent responses takes the form $A\Phi A^\top + I$, which further implies the polychoric/tetrachoric correlation matrix. Here, Φ is the covariance of $\boldsymbol{\theta}_i$ and I is a $K \times K$ identity matrix. With suitable identification constraints, the loading matrix A can be consistently estimated by minimizing a certain distance between the estimated polychoric/tetrachoric correlation matrix and the model implied one. Like the composite likelihood-based estimator above, under the classical asymptotic regime, this method also tends to be statistically less efficient than the MMLE.

3.4 Spectral Method

In linear factor analysis, principal component analysis (PCA) is commonly used as a spectral method for exploratory analysis. This approach is computationally much faster and does not suffer from convergence issue as in many other methods for involving non-convex optimization, as it only involves eigenvalue decomposition. Moreover, thanks to a close connection between PCA and linear factor models, the PCA solution to exploratory factor analysis is statistically consistent when data follow a linear factor model and both the sample size and the number of variables grow to infinity [56]. Thanks to both the computational advantage and theoretical guarantee, PCA is often the first estimation method to apply when conducting exploratory linear factor analysis. The PCA solution is also often used as the starting point in the computation of other estimators, which are often used after the PCA for providing more accurate estimation results and uncertainty quantification.

PCA cannot be used in IFA. Fortunately, a singular value decomposition (SVD) method has been proposed that can play a similar role as PCA in linear factor analysis [65]. Similar to PCA, the SVD method only involves singular value decomposition. Thus, it is computationally faster than other estimation methods and does not suffer from convergence issues. This method is built based on the SVD method for matrix estimation first proposed in [15]. In what follows, we discuss the main steps of this SVD method for analyzing binary data:

Step 1: Apply singular value decomposition to the binary data matrix $(y_{ij})_{N\times J}$.
Step 2: Denoise by truncating the small singular values to zero and obtain $\hat{P} = (\hat{p}_{ij})_{N\times J}$ as an estimate of the response probability matrix $(f_j(1|\boldsymbol{\theta}_i, \boldsymbol{\beta}_j))_{N\times J}$.
Step 3: Obtain an estimate $\bar{M}$ of the matrix $(\mathbf{a}_j^\top \boldsymbol{\theta}_i)_{N\times J}$ by truncating and transforming $\hat{P}$.
Step 4: Obtain estimates $\hat{\boldsymbol{\theta}}_i$, $\hat{\mathbf{a}}_j$, and d_j, $i = 1, \ldots, N$, $j = 1, \ldots, J$ by singular value decomposition of $\bar{M}$.

This method can also be used to analyze ordinal data, by dichotomizing the ordinal data to multiple binary data matrices.

As shown in [65], this method is also statistically consistent, in the sense that $\min_{H\in\mathbb{R}^{K\times K}} \left\{\sum_{j=1}^J \|\mathbf{a}_j^* - H\hat{\mathbf{a}}_j\|^2\right\}/(JK) = o_p(1)$, when both N and J grow to infinity, under similar conditions as those needed for the consistency of CJMLE [16, 17]. However, it is worth pointing out that the SVD method sacrifices statistical efficiency. Under suitable conditions, it can be shown that the loading matrix estimate $\hat{A}$ achieves the convergence rate

$$\frac{\min_{H\in\mathbb{R}^{K\times K}} \left\{\sum_{j=1}^J \|\mathbf{a}_j^* - H\hat{\mathbf{a}}_j\|^2\right\}}{JK} = O_p\left(\frac{1}{(\min\{N, J\})^{\frac{1}{K+2}}}\right), \tag{22}$$

while that same loss has the rate $O_p(1/\min\{N, J\})$ for the CJMLE. Thus, this SVD method is more suitable as an initial step for exploratory IFA to provide researchers a first impression on the data structure and to provide a starting point for the computation of other estimators.

4 Computer Implementations

In this section, we briefly introduce the commonly used statistical software and packages for IFA estimation. In the last decade, the large-scale IFA problem has received much attention in statistics and psychometrics and many computer implementations of IFA methods have emerged. In particular, several R packages have been developed and well-maintained that provide researchers computationally efficient tools for solving large-scale IFA problems. However, one has also to admit that the existing statistical software/packages have their own focus either on estimation methods or IFA models. There still lacks a statistical software/package that can implement all the state-of-the-art methods for all commonly used IFA models.

Commercial Software

- **Mplus** (Version 8.4; [42]) is a general latent variable modeling program available on major platforms including Windows, MacOS, and Linux. In particular, it is capable of doing exploratory and confirmatory factor analysis for binary or ordinal responses using weighted least square method, Gauss–Hermite EM algorithm, or full Bayesian approach via MCMC. A comparison of Mplus and IRTPRO for high-dimensional item factor analysis can be found in [3].
- **PARSCALE** (Version 4.10; [39]) is a Windows platform software for unidimensional item factor analysis. It is applicable for both binary and ordinal responses.
- **BILOG-MG** (Version 3.00; [52]) is a Windows platform software for binary response IRT analysis. It is an extension of BILOG with multiple-group respondents support.
- **IRTPRO** (Version 4.20; [12]) is a Windows-based software. It can be used for unidimensional and multidimensional item response theory models like 2PL, 3PL, generalized partial credit (GPC) model in both exploratory and confirmatory analysis. Multiple algorithms are implemented in IRTPRO such as Gauss–Hermite quadrature EM [6], MH-RM [10], MCMC [45], etc.
- **flexMIRT** (Version 3.5; [11]) is a Windows-based IRT analysis software. It works for unidimensional and multidimensional IRT models including 1–3PL models for dichotomous response, graded response model, generalized partial credit model for polytomous response through MML estimation. Gauss–Hermite EM, MH-RM algorithms are used in flexMIRT for the optimization procedure.

Free Software

- **WinBUGS** (Version 1.4; [55]) is a free software aiming at the Bayesian analysis on the Windows platform. It belongs to the BUGS (Bayesian inference Using Gibbs Sampling) project together with OpenBUGS. WinBUGS can be used for full Bayesian item factor analysis.

R Packages (Open Source)

- **ltm** (Version 1.1-1; [49]) is developed for the MML estimation of IRT models with Rasch, 2PL, 3PL, and Graded Response models, using Gauss–Hermite EM algorithm. It is written in pure R and it uses BFGS algorithm implemented "optim()" function in R's base **stats** package for the optimization.
- **eRm** (Version 1.0-0; [35]) is written in mixed C, Fortran, and R and focuses on the estimation of extended Rasch models using conditional maximum likelihood (CML) method.
- **TAM** (Version 3.3-10; [51]) is written in mixed C++, R. It could perform item response modeling under a variety of models, including Rasch model, 2PL/3PL model, generalized partial credit model, etc. It uses quasi Monte Carlo (QMC)

integration to prevent computational demanding in ordinary Gaussian quadrature integration.

- **MCMCpack** (Version 1.4-4; [36]) is written in C++ and R and aims for Bayesian inference by drawing MCMC samples from posterior under 18 statistical models including unidimensional and multidimensional IRT models. It is similar to BUGS and JAGS system but uses compiled and tailored code for the estimation of several pre-specified models, through which efficiency is gained.
- **mirt** (Version 1.31; [14]) is written in C++ and R. It contains functions for MML estimation of IRT models including Rasch, 2PL, and 3PL, ordinal response models, in an exploratory or confirmatory analysis. Gauss–Hermite quadrature EM, MH-RM, and stochastic EM algorithms are implemented in the package.
- **lvmcomp** (Version 1.2; [63]) is written in C++ and R. It implements the improved stochastic EM algorithm for full-information item factor analysis [66]. Boosted by parallel computing technique through the C++ OpenMP API [20], the **lvmcomp** package is especially suitable for medium-to-large scale estimation problems for multidimensional 2-parameter logistic (M2PL) and generalized partial credit (GPC) model under the confirmatory setting.
- **mirtjml** (Version 1.3.0; [64]) is written in C++ and R. Through the efficient constrainted joint maximum likelihood estimation (CJMLE, [16, 17]) algorithm and parallel computing technique, the **mirtjml** package is powerful in item factor analysis when the sample size, the number of items, and the number of factors are all large. For now, it provides functions for exploratory and confirmatory item factor analysis under the M2PL model.

5 Conclusions

In this chapter, we reviewed the modeling framework for IFA and the state-of-the-arts methods for its estimation. Our focus was on large-scale IFA applications, where the sample size, the number of items, and the number of factors are all large. In the recent decades, many works have been done on this topic and we believe that the problem of efficiently obtaining a point estimate has been solved well. Our tool box is now equipped with several powerful tools. For very large-scale problems, we tend to use the SVD method and the joint maximum likelihood estimation for a fast investigation of the data. For moderate-size problems, we would suggest to treat the person parameters as random effects and estimate the loading parameters by marginal likelihood-based methods, such as MCMC, stochastic EM, and stochastic approximation with MCMC. Among these marginal likelihood-based methods, the stochastic EM tends to achieve a better balance between computational efficiency and numerical stability. Several computer software/packages are available and well-maintained, though a comprehensive computation platform is needed to better support applied research that aggregates all these estimation methods under a wide range of models.

What has not been well-solved is the uncertain quantification for estimated IFA models (e.g., constructing confidence intervals/regions), especially for large-scale problems. The challenge lies in that when the sample size, the number of items, and the number of factors are all large, the classical asymptotic normality theory may no longer apply. New inference methods and asymptotic theory remain to be developed under a new regime that the sample size, the number of items, and possibly also the number of factors diverge. This is a challenging problem in general. Ideas from high-dimensional statistical inference (e.g., [18]) may be borrowed to solve the problem.

References

1. Andersen, E.B.: Conditional Inference and Models for Measuring. Mentalhygiejnisk Forlag, Copenhagen (1973)
2. Anderson, T.W., Rubin, H.: Statistical inference in factor analysis. In: Neyman J. (ed.) Proceedings of the Third Berkeley Symposium on Mathematical Statistics and Probability, Volume V: Contributions to Econometrics, Industrial Research, and Psychometry, pp. 111–150. University of California Press, Berkerley, CA (1956)
3. Asparouhov, T., Muthén, B.: Comparison of computational methods for high dimensional item factor analysis. Unpublished manuscript retrieved from www.statmodel.com (2012)
4. Béguin, A.A., Glas, C.A.: MCMC estimation and some model-fit analysis of multidimensional IRT models. Psychometrika **66**(4), 541–561 (2001)
5. Birnbaum, A.: Some latent trait models and their use in inferring an examinee's ability. In Lord F.M., Novick, M.R. (eds.) Statistical Theories of Mental Test Scores, pp. 397–479. Addison-Wesley, Reading, MA (1968)
6. Bock, R.D., Aitkin, M.: Marginal maximum likelihood estimation of item parameters: Application of an EM algorithm. Psychometrika **46**(4), 443–459 (1981)
7. Bolt, D.M., Lall, V.F.: Estimation of compensatory and noncompensatory multidimensional item response models using Markov chain Monte Carlo. Appl. Psychol. Meas. **27**(6), 395–414 (2003)
8. Browne, M.W.: An overview of analytic rotation in exploratory factor analysis. Multivar. Behav. Res. **36**(1), 111–150 (2001)
9. Cai, L.: High-dimensional exploratory item factor analysis by a Metropolis–Hastings Robbins–Monro algorithm. Psychometrika **75**(1), 33–57 (2010)
10. Cai, L.: Metropolis-Hastings Robbins-Monro algorithm for confirmatory item factor analysis. J. Educ. Behav. Stat. **35**(3), 307–335 (2010)
11. Cai, L., Wirth, R.: flexMIRT version 2: Flexible multilevel multidimensional item analysis and test scoring [Computer software]. Vector Psychometric Group, Chapel Hill, NC (2013)
12. Cai, L., Du Toit, S., Thissen, D.: IRTPRO: Flexible, Multidimensional, Multiple Categorical IRT Modeling [Computer software]. Scientific Software International, Chicago, IL (2011)
13. Celeux, G., Diebolt, J.: The SEM algorithm: A probabilistic teacher algorithm derived from the EM algorithm for the mixture problem. Comput. Stat. Q. **2**, 73–82 (1985)
14. Chalmers, R.P.: mirt: A multidimensional item response theory package for the *R* environment. J. Stat. Softw. **48**(6), 1–29 (2012)
15. Chatterjee, S.: Matrix estimation by universal singular value thresholding. Ann. Stat. **43**(1), 177–214 (2015)
16. Chen, Y., Li, X., Zhang, S.: Joint maximum likelihood estimation for high-dimensional exploratory item factor analysis. Psychometrika **84**(1), 124–146 (2019)
17. Chen, Y., Li, X., Zhang, S.: Structured latent factor analysis for large-scale data: Identifiability, estimability, and their implications. J. Am. Stat. Assoc **115**(532), 1756–1770 (2019)

18. Chernozhukov, V., Chetverikov, D., Demirer, M., Duflo, E., Hansen, C., Newey, W., Robins, J.: Double/debiased machine learning for treatment and structural parameters. Econom. J. **21**(1), C1–C68 (2018)
19. Chung, K.L.: On a stochastic approximation method. Ann. Math. Stat. **25**(3), 463–483 (1954)
20. Dagum, L., Menon, R.: OpenMP: An industry standard API for shared-memory programming. Comput. Sci. Eng. IEEE **5**(1), 46–55 (1998)
21. Davis, C., Kahan, W.M.: The rotation of eigenvectors by a perturbation. III. SIAM J. Numer. Anal. **7**(1), 1–46 (1970)
22. Dempster, A.P., Laird, N.M., Rubin, D.B.: Maximum likelihood from incomplete data via the EM algorithm. J. R. Stat. Soc. Ser. B (Methodol.) **39**(1), 1–22 (1977)
23. Edwards, M.C.: A Markov chain Monte Carlo approach to confirmatory item factor analysis. Psychometrika **75**(3), 474–497 (2010)
24. Fabian, V.: On asymptotic normality in stochastic approximation. Ann. Math. Stat. **39**(4), 1327–1332 (1968)
25. Ghosh, M.: Inconsistent maximum likelihood estimators for the Rasch model. Stat. Probab. Lett. **23**(2), 165–170 (1995)
26. Gu, M.G., Kong, F.H.: A stochastic approximation algorithm with Markov chain Monte-Carlo method for incomplete data estimation problems. Proc. Natl. Acad. Sci. **95**(13), 7270–7274 (1998)
27. Haberman, S.J.: Maximum likelihood estimates in exponential response models. Ann. Stat. **5**(5), 815–841 (1977)
28. Holland, P.W.: On the sampling theory roundations of item response theory models. Psychometrika **55**(4), 577–601 (1990)
29. Ip, E.H.: On single versus multiple imputation for a class of stochastic algorithms estimating max. Comput. Stat. **17**, 517–524 (2002)
30. Jöreskog, K.G.: On the estimation of polychoric correlations and their asymptotic covariance matrix. Psychometrika **59**(3), 381–389 (1994)
31. Jöreskog, K.G., Moustaki, I.: Factor analysis of ordinal variables: A comparison of three approaches. Multivar. Behav. Res. **36**(3), 347–387 (2001)
32. Kaiser, H.F.: The varimax criterion for analytic rotation in factor analysis. Psychometrika **23**(3), 187–200 (1958)
33. Kotov, R., Krueger, R.F., Watson, D., Achenbach, T.M., Althoff, R.R., Bagby, R.M., Brown, T.A., Carpenter, W.T., Caspi, A., Clark, L.A., et al.: The hierarchical taxonomy of psychopathology (HiTOP): A dimensional alternative to traditional nosologies. J. Abnorm. Psychol. **126**(4), 454–477 (2017)
34. Lee, S.-Y., Poon, W.-Y., Bentler, P.M.: A three-stage estimation procedure for structural equation models with polytomous variables. Psychometrika **55**(1), 45–51 (1990)
35. Mair, P., Hatzinger, R.: Extended Rasch modeling: The eRm package for the application of IRT models in *R*. J. Stat. Softw. **20**(9), 1–20 (2007)
36. Martin, A.D., Quinn, K.M., Park, J.H.: MCMCpack: Markov chain Monte Carlo in *R*. J. Stat. Softw. **42**(9), 1–21 (2011)
37. Meng, X.-L., Schilling, S.: Fitting full-information item factor models and an empirical investigation of bridge sampling. J. Am. Stat. Assoc. **91**(435), 1254–1267 (1996)
38. Muraki, E.: A generalized partial credit model: Application of an EM algorithm. Appl. Psychol. Meas. **16**(2), 159–176 (1992)
39. Muraki, E., Bock, D.: IRT Item Analysis and Test Scoring for Rating Scale Data [Computer software]. Scientific Software, Chicago, IL (1997)
40. Muraki, E., Carlson, J.E.: Full-information factor analysis for polytomous item responses. Appl. Psychol. Meas. **19**(1), 73–90 (1995)
41. Muthén, B.: A general structural equation model with dichotomous, ordered categorical, and continuous latent variable indicators. Psychometrika **49**(1), 115–132 (1984)
42. Muthén, L.K.: Mplus: The comprehensive modeling program for applied researchers: User's guide. Muthén & Muthén, Los Angeles, CA (1998)

43. Neyman, J., Scott, E.L.: Consistent estimates based on partially consistent observations. Econometrica 16(1), 1–32 (1948)
44. Nielsen, S.F.: The stochastic EM algorithm: Estimation and asymptotic results. Bernoulli **6**(3), 457–489 (2000)
45. Patz, R.J., Junker, B.W.: Applications and extensions of MCMC in IRT: Multiple item types, missing data, and rated responses. J. Educ. Behav. Stat. **24**(4), 342–366 (1999)
46. Rasch, G.: Probabilistic models for some intelligence and attainment tests. Danish Institute for Educational Research, Copenhagen (1960)
47. Reckase, M.: Multidimensional Item Response Theory. Springer, New York, NY (2009)
48. Revelle, W., Condon, D.M., Wilt, J., French, J.A., Brown, A., Elleman, L.G.: Web and phone based data collection using planned missing designs. In: Fielding, N.G., Lee, R.M., Blank, G. (eds.) Handbook of Online Research Methods, pp. 578–595. Sage Publications, Thousand Oaks, CA (2016)
49. Rizopoulos, D.: ltm: An *R* package for latent variable modeling and item response theory analyses. J. Stat. Softw. **17**(5), 1–25 (2006)
50. Robbins, H., Monro, S.: A stochastic approximation method. Ann. Math. Stat. **22**(3), 400–407 (1951)
51. Robitzsch, A., Kiefer, T., Wu, M.: TAM: Test analysis modules. R package version 3.3-10 (2019)
52. Rupp, A.A.: Item response modeling with BILOG-MG and MULTILOG for Windows. Int. J. Test. **3**(4), 365–384 (2003)
53. Samejima, F.: Estimation of latent ability using a response pattern of graded scores. ETS Res. Bull. Ser. **1968**(1), i–169 (1968)
54. Skitka, L.J., Sargis, E.G.: The internet as psychological laboratory. Annu. Rev. Psychol. **57**(1), 529–555 (2006)
55. Spiegelhalter, D., Thomas, A., Best, N., Lunn, D.: WinBUGS user manual: Version 1.4. MRC Biostatistics Unit, Cambridge (2003)
56. Stock, J.H., Watson, M.W.: Forecasting using principal components from a large number of predictors. J. Am. Stat. Assoc. **97**(460), 1167–1179 (2002)
57. Sun, J., Chen, Y., Liu, J., Ying, Z., Xin, T.: Latent variable selection for multidimensional item response theory models via L_1 regularization. Psychometrika **81**(4), 921–939 (2016)
58. van der Vaart, A.W.: Asymptotic Statistics. Cambridge University Press, Cambridge (1998)
59. Varin, C., Reid, N., Firth, D.: An overview of composite likelihood methods. Stat. Sin. **21**(1), 5–42 (2011)
60. Wedin, P.-Å.: Perturbation bounds in connection with singular value decomposition. BIT Numer. Math. **12**(1), 99–111 (1972)
61. Wei, G.C.G., Tanner, M.A.: A Monte Carlo implementation of the EM algorithm and the poor man's data augmentation algorithms. J. Am. Stat. Assoc. **85**(411), 699–704 (1990)
62. Yao, L., Schwarz, R.D.: A multidimensional partial credit model with associated item and test statistics: An application to mixed-format tests. Appl. Psychol. Meas. **30**(6), 469–492 (2006)
63. Zhang, S., Chen, Y.: lvmcomp: Stochastic EM algorithms for latent variable models with a high-dimensional latent space. R package version 1.3.0 (2019)
64. Zhang, S., Chen, Y., Li, X.: mirtjml: Joint maximum likelihood estimation for high-dimensional item factor analysis. R package version 1.3.0 (2019)
65. Zhang, H., Chen, Y., Li, X.: A note on exploratory item factor analysis by singular value decomposition. Psychometrika **85**, 358–372 (2020)
66. Zhang, S., Chen, Y., Liu, Y.: An improved stochastic EM algorithm for large-scale full-information item factor analysis. Br. J. Math. Stat. Psychol. **73**(1), 44–71 (2020)
67. Zhao, Y., Joe, H.: Composite likelihood estimation in multivariate data analysis. Can. J. Stat. **33**(3), 335–356 (2005)

Part IV
Survival Analysis and Functional Data Analysis

Functional Data Modeling and Hypothesis Testing for Longitudinal Alzheimer Genome-Wide Association Studies

Yehua Li, Ian Xu, and Catherine Liu

1 Introduction

Genome-Wide Association Studies (GWAS) have been successfully used to associate diseases or traits with genetic variants defined by Single Nucleotide Polymorphisms (SNPs) [28, 36]. One important goal in these studies is to identify the disease- or trait-related Single Nucleotide Polymorphisms (SNPs). A commonly used approach is to perform SNP level hypothesis tests and then make multiple comparison adjustments [5]. The current GWAS literature focuses on analyzing phenotype measured at a single time; however, in many aging studies the phenotypes are repeatedly measured over years where the measurement times are irregular and subject-specific. One example of such studies comes from the Alzheimer's Disease Neuroimaging Initiative (ADNI) (http://www.loni.ucla.edu/ADNI), where both longitudinal Alzheimer phenotypes and SNP level genotypes are available for all subjects. The longitudinal phenotype responses can be naturally modeled as

For the Alzheimer's Disease Neuroimaging Initiative
Data used in preparation of this article were obtained from the Alzheimer's Disease Neuroimaging Initiative (ADNI) database (http://adni.loni.usc.edu). As such, the investigators within the ADNI contributed to the design and implementation of ADNI and/or provided data but did not participate in analysis or writing of this book chapter. A complete listing of ADNI investigators can be found at: http://adni.loni.usc.edu/wp-content/uploads/how_to_apply/ADNI_Acknowledgement_List.pdf

Y. Li (✉)
University of California, Riverside, CA, USA
e-mail: yehuali@ucr.edu

I. Xu · C. Liu
Hong Kong Polytechnic University, Hong Kong, China
e-mail: sheng-ian.xu@connect.polyu.hk; macliu@polyu.edu.hk

Y. Zhao, (Din) D.-G. Chen (eds.), *Modern Statistical Methods for Health Research*, Emerging Topics in Statistics and Biostatistics,
https://doi.org/10.1007/978-3-030-72437-5_16

functional data [32, 42], and it is of scientific interest to test if the mean phenotype trajectories differ across different genotypes.

In this chapter, we introduce some state-of-the-art functional data modeling and inference methods to longitudinal GWAS. We model the longitudinal phenotype data by a class of generalized functional concurrent linear models, where the response is allowed to be either Gaussian or non-Gaussian. There is a large volume of recent literature on methods and applications of functional linear models and functional analysis of variance (fANOVA) under various designs [2, 26, 30, 40, 44, 46]. Most of these papers consider dense functional data, where repeated measurements on each subject are made on a dense grid. A comprehensive account of fANOVA methods for dense functional data is provided in the monograph of [43]. In contrast, data from many longitudinal studies are observed on irregular time points and contaminated with substantial measurement errors. These data are considered as sparse functional data, and many recent papers focus on estimating various functional parameters, such as the mean function, covariance function, and functional principal components [17, 23, 42, 45]. Recently, [35] also investigated nonparametric hypothesis testing problems for longitudinal data collected in a designed experiment. Their test is an extension of the generalized likelihood ratio test [6, 9, 24] to longitudinal setting. See [13] for a comprehensive review of nonparametric hypothesis test procedures.

We describe a profile local estimating equation approach to fit the generalized functional linear model for longitudinal GWAS phenotype data and compare two nonparametric hypothesis testing approaches, the generalized quasi-likelihood ratio (GQLR) test of [35] and the functional F-test of [43], to test the genotype effects. The GQLR enjoys a property called the Wilks phenomenon [9], meaning that the null distribution of the test statistic does not depend on the unknown model parameters. This important property makes it practical to perform GQLR tests to longitudinal GWAS data, saving us from repeating the bootstrap procedure on hundreds of thousands of SNPs. It is also known that the GQLR test attains the optimal minimax power rate under properly chosen bandwidth. In contrast, the functional F-test is not based on the likelihood principal, only applies to Gaussian type of data, and does not have the Wilks property. In addition, the asymptotic power for the functional F-test is largely unknown.

Neither the GQLR test nor the functional F-test has been applied to longitudinal GWAS data, where the responses are Alzheimer-related phenotypes modeled as sparse functional data. We provide both theoretical and numerical comparison to the performances of the two tests. We also provide practical strategies to address the implementation issues for the two tests, including bandwidth selection, estimating the within-subject covariance using nonparametric or semiparametric methods, and estimating the null distribution of the test statistics using bootstrap procedures.

The rest of the chapter is organized as follows. In Sect. 2, we describe the model and estimation procedure. In Sect. 3, we introduce the GQLR test and F-test for a hypothesis on genotype effects and discuss their asymptotic distributions under the null hypothesis. For the GQLR test, we also discuss its Wilks property and local power. We discuss some implementation issues in Sect. 4, including bandwidth selection, covariance estimation, and bootstrap procedure. We then illustrate the methodology by simulation studies in Sect. 5 and analyze the ADNI data in Sect. 6. Finally, some concluding remarks and discussions are provided in Sect. 7.

2 Functional Modeling of Longitudinal Phenotype Data and Estimation Procedure

2.1 Model Assumptions

Let $Y_i(t)$ be the phenotype of the ith subject observed at time $t \in \mathcal{T}, i = 1, \ldots, n$, where $\mathcal{T}$ is a closed time interval. Suppose $\boldsymbol{X}_i(t)$ is a p-dimensional subject-specific covariate vector which represents confounding environmental effects and can be time dependent. Let $\mathbf{Z}_i$ be a q-dim genetic predictor, which is time-invariant. We assume $E\{Y_i(t)|\mathbf{Z}_i, \boldsymbol{X}_i(s), s \in \mathcal{T}\} = E\{Y_i(t)|\mathbf{Z}_i, \boldsymbol{X}_i(t)\} = \mu_i(t)$ [31], and

$$g\{\mu_i(t)\} = \boldsymbol{X}_i^{\mathrm{T}}(t)\boldsymbol{\beta} + \mathbf{Z}_i^{\mathrm{T}}\boldsymbol{\theta}(t), \tag{1}$$

where $g(\cdot)$ is a known monotonic and differentiable link function, $\boldsymbol{\beta}$ is a p-vector of unknown coefficients representing environmental effects, and $\boldsymbol{\theta}(t) = (\theta_1, \ldots, \theta_q)^{\mathrm{T}}(t)$ is a vector of unknown smooth functions representing the genotype effect. In the ADNI data, some of the most important Alzheimer-related phenotypes include the hippocampal volume, the decay of which is known to be related to memory loss [34], and the Rey Auditory Verbal Learning Test (RAVLT) score; some environmental covariates include age, sex, education, marital status, etc.; and a genetic predictor can be the genotypes defined by a SNP, which are AA, AB, or BB defined by the two alleles of a SNP. To include the effects of one SNP in model (1), $\mathbf{Z}_i$ is a 3-dim vector of indicators for the three genotypes.

When $g(\cdot)$ is an identity link, model (1) is a functional concurrent linear model [32], since both the response Y and the covariate $\boldsymbol{X}$ are functions of time. When $\mathbf{Z}$ is a vector of group indicators, Model (1) is a functional analysis of covariance (fANCOVA) model [43] since the treatment effect for genotype k is represented by a nonparametric function $\theta_k(t)$. In semiparametric regression literature, Model (1) is also referred to as a generalized partially linear varying coefficient model. The parameter $\boldsymbol{\beta}$ is merely used to control the confounding effect of the environment covariates, and the primary interest is to make inference on the functional genotype effects $\boldsymbol{\theta}$. Specifically, we are interested in testing the following nonparametric hypotheses:

$$H_0 : \boldsymbol{C}\boldsymbol{\theta}(t) = \boldsymbol{c}(t) \quad \text{vs.} \quad H_1 : \boldsymbol{C}\boldsymbol{\theta}(t) \neq \boldsymbol{c}(t), \tag{2}$$

where $\boldsymbol{C}$ is an $r \times q$ matrix of linear contrasts, $\boldsymbol{c}(t)$ is an r-dim function, and $r = rank(\boldsymbol{C}) < q$. For the ADNI example, $\boldsymbol{\theta}(t) = (\theta_1, \theta_2, \theta_3)^{\mathrm{T}}(t)$ represents the genotype effects of a SNP, let

$$\boldsymbol{C} = \begin{pmatrix} 1 & 0 & -1 \\ 0 & 1 & -1 \end{pmatrix}, \quad \boldsymbol{c}(t) \equiv \begin{pmatrix} 0 \\ 0 \end{pmatrix}, \tag{3}$$

then hypothesis (2) an ANOVA test on $H_0 : \theta_1(t) = \theta_2(t) = \theta_3(t)$ and the SNP is disease/trait related if H_0 is rejected.

Although Model (1) is defined in continuum, observations on $Y_i(t)$ and $\boldsymbol{X}_i(t)$ are, in practice, made on discrete and subject-specific time points. Let $\boldsymbol{T}_i = (T_{i1}, \cdots, T_{im_i})^{\mathrm{T}}$ be the random observation time points for subject i in genotype k, where m_i is the number of repeated measurements. Denote $\boldsymbol{Y}_i = (Y_{i1}, \cdots, Y_{im_i})^{\mathrm{T}}$, $\boldsymbol{\mu}_i = (\mu_{i1}, \cdots, \mu_{im_i})^{\mathrm{T}}$, $\boldsymbol{X}_i = (\boldsymbol{X}_{i1}, \cdots, \boldsymbol{X}_{im_i})^{\mathrm{T}}$, where $Y_{ij} = Y_i(T_{ij})$, $\mu_{ij} = \mu_i(T_{ij})$, and $\boldsymbol{X}_{ij} = \boldsymbol{X}_i(T_{ij})$. We assume that the conditional covariance of $Y_i(t)$ is a bivariate positive semidefinite function

$$\mathscr{R}(t_1, t_2) = \operatorname{cov}\{Y_i(t_1), Y_i(t_2) | \boldsymbol{X}_i(s), s \in \mathscr{T}\}, \quad \text{for any } t_1, t_2 \in \mathscr{T}. \tag{4}$$

The covariance structure is assumed to be the same across subjects. Let $\boldsymbol{\Sigma}_i = \operatorname{cov}(\boldsymbol{Y}_i \mid \boldsymbol{X}_i, \boldsymbol{T}_i) = \{\mathscr{R}(T_{ij}, T_{ij'})\}_{j,j'=1}^{m_i}$ be the subject-specific covariance matrices. Since the true covariance function $\mathscr{R}$ is unknown, the covariance model $\mathscr{V}(t_1, t_2)$ adopted in data analysis is commonly referred to as a "working" covariance, which is subject to misspecification. Historically, a working covariance model is usually assumed to be member of a parametric family, such as the Matérn family. Let $\boldsymbol{V}_i = \{\mathscr{V}(T_{ij}, T_{ij'})\}_{j,j'=1}^{m_i}$ be the "working" covariance matrix for subject (k, i), which is the interpolation of the continuous covariance function $\mathscr{V}$ on the subject-specific time points. The simplest working covariance is the working independence (WI), i.e. $\boldsymbol{V}_i = \boldsymbol{I}_{m_i}$. It is known that misspecified working covariance can still lead to consistent estimators, although such estimators are not semiparametric efficient [37].

We refer to the model under the null hypothesis in (2) as the reduced model and that under the alternative hypothesis as the full model. Denote $\widehat{\boldsymbol{\beta}}_R$ and $\widehat{\boldsymbol{\theta}}_R(t)$ as the estimators under the reduced model and $\widehat{\boldsymbol{\beta}}_F$ and $\widehat{\boldsymbol{\theta}}_F(t)$ as the estimators under the full model. Our estimation procedures under both models are based on profile-kernel estimating equations.

2.2 Estimation Under the Full Model

We first consider estimation under the full model. By Taylor's expansion, for any T_{ij} in a neighborhood h of t, $\boldsymbol{\theta}(T_{ij})$ can be approximated locally by a linear polynomial

$$\boldsymbol{\theta}(T_{ij}) \approx \boldsymbol{\theta}(t) + \boldsymbol{\theta}'(t)(T_{ij} - t) = \boldsymbol{\alpha}_0 + \boldsymbol{\alpha}_1(T_{ij} - t)/h.$$

Let $K(\cdot)$ be a symmetric probability density function and denote $K_h(t) = h^{-1}K(t/h)$ where h is the bandwidth. Put $\mathbb{T}_i = (\boldsymbol{T}_i - t)/h$, $\boldsymbol{U}_{ij}(t) = \{\mathbf{Z}_i^{\mathrm{T}}, \mathbf{Z}_i^{\mathrm{T}}(T_{ij} -$

$t)/h\}^{\mathrm{T}}$ and $\boldsymbol{U}_i(t) = \{\boldsymbol{U}_{i1}(t), \ldots, \boldsymbol{U}_{im_i}(t)\}^{\mathrm{T}} = (\mathbf{1Z}_i^{\mathrm{T}}, \mathbb{T}_i\boldsymbol{Z}_i^{\mathrm{T}})$. For a given $\boldsymbol{\beta}$, $\boldsymbol{\theta}(t)$ is estimated by solving the following local linear estimating equation regarding $\boldsymbol{\alpha} = (\boldsymbol{\alpha}_0^{\mathrm{T}}, \boldsymbol{\alpha}_1^{\mathrm{T}})^{\mathrm{T}}$:

$$\sum_{i=1}^{n} \boldsymbol{U}_i(t)^{\mathrm{T}} \Delta_i(t) \mathscr{W}_i^{-1} \boldsymbol{K}_h(\boldsymbol{T}_i - t)\{\boldsymbol{Y}_i - \boldsymbol{\mu}_i(t)\} = 0, \tag{5}$$

where $\boldsymbol{K}_h(\boldsymbol{T}_i - t) = \mathrm{diag}\{K_h(T_{ij} - t)\}_{j=1}^{m_i}$, $\boldsymbol{\mu}_i(t) = (\mu_{i1}, \ldots, \mu_{im_i})^{\mathrm{T}}(t)$, $\mu_{ij}(t) = g^{-1}\{\boldsymbol{X}_{ij}^{\mathrm{T}}\boldsymbol{\beta} + \boldsymbol{U}_{ij}^{\mathrm{T}}(t)\boldsymbol{\alpha}\}$, $\Delta_i(t) = \mathrm{diag}\{\mu_{ij}^{(1)}(t)\}_{j=1}^{m_i}$, $\mu_{k,ij}^{(1)}(t)$ is the first derivative of $\mu(\cdot) = g^{-1}(\cdot)$ evaluated at $\boldsymbol{X}_{ij}^{\mathrm{T}}\boldsymbol{\beta} + \boldsymbol{U}_{ij}^{\mathrm{T}}(t)\boldsymbol{\alpha}$, and $\mathscr{W}_i$ is a weight matrix to be specified below. The local linear estimator is given by $\widehat{\boldsymbol{\theta}}_F(t; \boldsymbol{\beta}) = \widehat{\boldsymbol{\alpha}}_0$, where $(\widehat{\boldsymbol{\alpha}}_0^{\mathrm{T}}, \widehat{\boldsymbol{\alpha}}_1^{\mathrm{T}})^{\mathrm{T}}$ is the solution of (5). Then $\widehat{\boldsymbol{\beta}}_F$ is obtained by solving

$$\begin{aligned} \mathbf{0} = \sum_{i=1}^{n} \left\{ \boldsymbol{X}_i^{\mathrm{T}} + \sum_{k=1}^{q} Z_{ik} \frac{\partial \widehat{\theta}_{k,F}(\boldsymbol{T}_i; \boldsymbol{\beta})}{\partial \boldsymbol{\beta}} \right\} \Delta_i(\boldsymbol{T}_i) \mathscr{W}_i^{-1} \\ \times [\boldsymbol{Y}_i - g^{-1}\{\boldsymbol{X}_i\boldsymbol{\beta} + \widehat{\boldsymbol{\theta}}_F^{\mathrm{T}}(\boldsymbol{T}_i; \boldsymbol{\beta})\mathbf{Z}_i\}]. \end{aligned} \tag{6}$$

At convergence of the algorithm described above, the nonparametric estimator needs a final update as $\widehat{\boldsymbol{\theta}}_F(t) = \widehat{\boldsymbol{\theta}}_F(t, \widehat{\boldsymbol{\beta}}_F)$.

As shown by Lin and Carroll [27], the most efficient estimators within the class defined by (5) are obtained by setting $\mathscr{W}_i = \mathrm{diag}\{\omega(\mu_{ij})\}_{j=1}^{m_i}$ where $\omega(\cdot)$ is a working variance function. Similar kernel estimators are widely used in longitudinal and functional data analysis, see [7, 17, 23, 42]. The working variance function $\omega(\cdot)$ can be replaced by a nonparametric variance estimator described in Sect. 4.2.

Under the special case of identical link, $g(x) = x$, the solution of (5) is

$$\begin{aligned} \widehat{\boldsymbol{\alpha}} = \left\{ \sum_{i=1}^{n} \boldsymbol{U}_i(t)^{\mathrm{T}} \mathscr{W}_i^{-1} \boldsymbol{K}_h(\boldsymbol{T}_i - t) \boldsymbol{U}_i(t) \right\}^{-1} \\ \times \left\{ \sum_{i=1}^{n} \boldsymbol{U}_i(t)^{\mathrm{T}} \mathscr{W}_i^{-1} \boldsymbol{K}_h(\boldsymbol{T}_i - t)(\boldsymbol{Y}_i - \boldsymbol{X}_i\boldsymbol{\beta}) \right\}, \end{aligned}$$

then

$$\begin{aligned} \widehat{\boldsymbol{\theta}}(t, \boldsymbol{\beta}) = (\boldsymbol{I}, \mathbf{0}) \left\{ \sum_{i=1}^{n} \boldsymbol{U}_i(t)^{\mathrm{T}} \mathscr{W}_i^{-1} \boldsymbol{K}_h(\boldsymbol{T}_i - t) \boldsymbol{U}_i(t) \right\}^{-1} \\ \times \left\{ \sum_{i=1}^{n} \boldsymbol{U}_i(t)^{\mathrm{T}} \mathscr{W}_i^{-1} \boldsymbol{K}_h(\boldsymbol{T}_i - t)(\boldsymbol{Y}_i - \boldsymbol{X}_i\boldsymbol{\beta}) \right\}, \end{aligned}$$

$$\frac{\partial \widehat{\boldsymbol{\theta}}}{\partial \boldsymbol{\beta}^{\mathrm{T}}}(t, \boldsymbol{\beta}) = -(\boldsymbol{I}, \boldsymbol{0}) \left\{ \sum_{i=1}^{n} \boldsymbol{U}_i(t)^{\mathrm{T}} \mathscr{W}_i^{-1} \boldsymbol{K}_h(\boldsymbol{T}_i - t) \boldsymbol{U}_i(t) \right\}^{-1} \times \left\{ \sum_{i=1}^{n} \boldsymbol{U}_i(t)^{\mathrm{T}} \mathscr{W}_i^{-1} \boldsymbol{K}_h(\boldsymbol{T}_i - t) \boldsymbol{X}_i \right\}.$$

Define $\widetilde{\boldsymbol{X}}_i = (\widetilde{\boldsymbol{X}}_{i1}, \ldots, \widetilde{\boldsymbol{X}}_{im_i})^{\mathrm{T}}$ and $\widetilde{\boldsymbol{Y}}_i = (\widetilde{Y}_{i1}, \ldots, \widetilde{Y}_{im_i})^{\mathrm{T}}$, where

$$\begin{aligned} \widetilde{\boldsymbol{X}}_{ij}^{\mathrm{T}} &= \boldsymbol{X}_{ij}^{\mathrm{T}} + \mathbf{Z}_i^{\mathrm{T}} \frac{\partial \widehat{\boldsymbol{\theta}}}{\partial \boldsymbol{\beta}^{\mathrm{T}}}(T_{ij}, \boldsymbol{\beta}) \\ &= \boldsymbol{X}_{ij}^{\mathrm{T}} - (\mathbf{Z}_i^{\mathrm{T}}, \boldsymbol{0}) \left\{ \sum_{i'=1}^{n} \boldsymbol{U}_{i'}(T_{ij})^{\mathrm{T}} \mathscr{W}_{i'}^{-1} \boldsymbol{U}_{i'}(T_{ij}) \right\}^{-1} \left\{ \sum_{i'=1}^{n} \boldsymbol{U}_{i'}^{\mathrm{T}}(T_{ij}) \mathscr{W}_{i'}^{-1} \boldsymbol{X}_{i'} \right\}, \end{aligned}$$

$$\widetilde{Y}_{ij} = Y_{ij} - (\mathbf{Z}_i^{\mathrm{T}}, \boldsymbol{0}) \left\{ \sum_{i'=1}^{n} \boldsymbol{U}_{i'}(T_{ij})^{\mathrm{T}} \mathscr{W}_{i'}^{-1} \boldsymbol{U}_{i'}(T_{ij}) \right\}^{-1} \left\{ \sum_{i'=1}^{n} \boldsymbol{U}_{i'}^{\mathrm{T}}(T_{ij}) \mathscr{W}_{i'}^{-1} \mathbf{Y}_{i'} \right\}.$$

The solution of (6) is

$$\widehat{\boldsymbol{\beta}}_F = \left(\sum_{i=1}^{n} \widetilde{\boldsymbol{X}}_i^{\mathrm{T}} \mathscr{W}_i^{-1} \widetilde{\boldsymbol{X}}_i \right)^{-1} \left(\sum_{i=1}^{n} \widetilde{\boldsymbol{X}}_i^{\mathrm{T}} \mathscr{W}_i^{-1} \widetilde{\boldsymbol{Y}}_i \right).$$

2.3 Estimation Under the Reduced Model

We now consider estimation under the reduced model. We first partition the contrast matrix $\boldsymbol{C}$ in (2) into $\boldsymbol{C} = (\boldsymbol{C}_1, \boldsymbol{C}_2)$, where $\boldsymbol{C}_1$ is $r \times (q-r)$ and $\boldsymbol{C}_2$ is $r \times r$. Partition $\boldsymbol{\theta}$ accordingly into $(\boldsymbol{\theta}_1^{\mathrm{T}}, \boldsymbol{\theta}_2^{\mathrm{T}})^{\mathrm{T}}$, where $\dim(\boldsymbol{\theta}_2) = r$. Without loss of generality, suppose $\boldsymbol{C}_2$ is full rank, then under the null hypothesis $\boldsymbol{C}\boldsymbol{\theta}(t) = \boldsymbol{c}(t)$,

$$\boldsymbol{\theta}_1(t) = \boldsymbol{C}_1^{-1}\{\boldsymbol{c}(t) - \boldsymbol{C}_2\boldsymbol{\theta}_2(t)\}.$$

By a simple reparameterization, let $\boldsymbol{\vartheta}(t) = \boldsymbol{\theta}_2(t)$, then $\boldsymbol{\theta}(t) = \boldsymbol{c}^*(t) + \boldsymbol{D}\boldsymbol{\vartheta}(t)$, where

$$\boldsymbol{c}^*(t) = \begin{pmatrix} \boldsymbol{C}_1^{-1}\boldsymbol{c}(t) \\ \boldsymbol{0} \end{pmatrix}, \quad \boldsymbol{D} = \begin{pmatrix} -\boldsymbol{C}_1^{-1}\boldsymbol{C}_2 \\ \boldsymbol{I} \end{pmatrix}.$$

For a given $\boldsymbol{\beta}$, the profile local linear estimator for $\boldsymbol{\vartheta}(t)$ is given by $\widehat{\boldsymbol{\vartheta}}(t, \boldsymbol{\beta}) = \widehat{\boldsymbol{a}}_0$, where $\widehat{\boldsymbol{a}} = (\widehat{\boldsymbol{a}}_0, \widehat{\boldsymbol{a}}_1)^{\mathrm{T}}$ is the solution of

$$\sum_{i=1}^{n} \mathscr{U}_i(t)^T \Delta_i(t) \mathscr{W}_i^{-1} \boldsymbol{K}_h(\boldsymbol{T}_i - t)\{\boldsymbol{Y}_i - \boldsymbol{\mu}_i(t)\} = 0, \tag{7}$$

$\mathscr{U}_i(t) = \{\mathscr{U}_{i1}(t), \ldots, \mathscr{U}_{im_i}(t)\}$, $\boldsymbol{\mu}_i(t) = (\mu_{i1}, \ldots, \mu_{im_i})^{\mathrm{T}}(t)$, $\mathscr{U}_{ij}(t) = \{\mathbf{Z}_i^{\mathrm{T}}\boldsymbol{D}, \mathbf{Z}_i^{\mathrm{T}}\boldsymbol{D}(T_{ij} - t)/h\}^{\mathrm{T}}$, $\mu_{ij}(t) = g^{-1}\{\boldsymbol{X}_{ij}^{\mathrm{T}}\boldsymbol{\beta} + \mathbf{Z}_i\boldsymbol{c}^*(t) + \mathscr{U}_{ij}^{\mathrm{T}}(t)\boldsymbol{a}\}$, $\Delta_i(t) = \mathrm{diag}\{\mu_{ij}^{(1)}(t)\}_{j=1}^{m_i}$, and $\mu_{k,ij}^{(1)}(t)$ is the first derivative of $\mu(\cdot) = g^{-1}(\cdot)$ evaluated at $\boldsymbol{X}_{ij}^{\mathrm{T}}\boldsymbol{\beta} + \mathbf{Z}_i\boldsymbol{c}^*(t) + \mathscr{U}_{ij}^{\mathrm{T}}(t)\boldsymbol{a}$.

Denote $\mathscr{Z}_i = \boldsymbol{D}^{\mathrm{T}}\mathbf{Z}_i = (\mathscr{Z}_{i1}, \ldots \mathscr{Z}_{i,q-r})^{\mathrm{T}}$ and $\boldsymbol{\vartheta}(t) = (\vartheta_1, \ldots, \vartheta_{q-r})^{\mathrm{T}}(t)$. The reduced model estimator $\widehat{\boldsymbol{\beta}}_R$ is obtained by solving

$$\mathbf{0} = \sum_{i=1}^{n} \left\{ \boldsymbol{X}_i^{\mathrm{T}} + \sum_{j=1}^{q-r} \mathscr{Z}_{ij} \frac{\partial \widehat{\vartheta}_j(\boldsymbol{T}_i; \boldsymbol{\beta})}{\partial \boldsymbol{\beta}} \right\} \Delta_i(\boldsymbol{T}_i)\mathscr{W}_i^{-1}$$
$$\times [\boldsymbol{Y}_i - g^{-1}\{\boldsymbol{X}_i\boldsymbol{\beta} + \mathbf{Z}_i\boldsymbol{c}^*(t) + \mathscr{Z}_i^{\mathrm{T}}\widehat{\boldsymbol{\vartheta}}(\boldsymbol{T}_i; \boldsymbol{\beta})\}]. \tag{8}$$

At convergence, the nonparametric estimator is updated as $\widehat{\boldsymbol{\theta}}_R(t) = \boldsymbol{c}^*(t) + \boldsymbol{D}\widehat{\boldsymbol{\vartheta}}(t, \widehat{\boldsymbol{\beta}}_R)$.

3 Nonparametric Test on Genotype Effects

We now direct our focus back to testing the hypotheses in (2) and we will discuss two test procedures: the Generalized Quasi-Likelihood Ratio (GQLR) test and the functional F-test.

3.1 Generalized Quasi-Likelihood Ratio Test

The GQLR test is an extension of the generalized likelihood ratio test [6, 9]. For longitudinal data, especially when the response is non-Gaussian, the joint likelihood function is hard to correctly specify; we therefore build our test procedure based on a quasi-likelihood. A quasi-likelihood function [29] $\mathscr{Q}$ satisfies

$$\frac{\partial \mathscr{Q}(\boldsymbol{\mu}, \boldsymbol{Y})}{\partial \boldsymbol{\mu}} = \boldsymbol{V}(\boldsymbol{\mu})^{-1}(\boldsymbol{Y} - \boldsymbol{\mu}), \tag{9}$$

where $\boldsymbol{Y}$ is an m-vector of response within a subject, $\boldsymbol{\mu} = g^{-1}\{\boldsymbol{X}\boldsymbol{\beta} + \boldsymbol{\theta}^{\mathrm{T}}(\boldsymbol{T})\mathbf{Z}\}$ is the conditional mean vector, and $\boldsymbol{V}(\boldsymbol{\mu})$ is a working covariance matrix not necessarily the same as the true covariance $\boldsymbol{\Sigma}(\boldsymbol{\mu})$.

The quasi-likelihood of the data is

$$\ell(\boldsymbol{\theta}, \boldsymbol{\beta}) = \sum_{i=1}^{n} \mathscr{Q}[g^{-1}\{\boldsymbol{X}_i\boldsymbol{\beta} + \boldsymbol{\theta}^{\mathrm{T}}(\boldsymbol{T}_i)\mathbf{Z}_i\}, \boldsymbol{Y}_i]. \tag{10}$$

The GQLR test statistic is defined as the difference of the quasi-likelihoods under the full and reduced models

$$\lambda_n(H_0) = \ell(\widehat{\boldsymbol{\theta}}_F, \widehat{\boldsymbol{\beta}}_F) - \ell(\widehat{\boldsymbol{\theta}}_R, \widehat{\boldsymbol{\beta}}_R). \tag{11}$$

Asymptotic Distribution of GQLR Statistic Under the Null

Tang et al. [35] studied the asymptotic property of the GQLR test for the functional analysis of covariance (fANCOVA) model, which is a special case of (1) with $\mathbf{Z}_i$ being a vector of treatment group indicators, i.e. $Z_{ij} = 1$ if the ith subject is in the jth treatment group and 0 otherwise, $j = 1, \ldots, q$. And the hypothesis they tested is

$$H_0 : \theta_1(t) = \cdots = \theta_q(t), \quad \text{vs} \quad H_1 : \text{not all } \theta_k\text{'s are equal}. \tag{12}$$

For nonparametric hypothesis testing in independent data, Fan et al. [9] established a property called the Wilks phenomenon for the GLR test, i.e. the asymptotic distribution of the test statistic under the null hypothesis does not depend on the unknown true parameters. Indeed, when the likelihood function is used and correctly specified, this property holds for a wide range of problems. However, for generalized longitudinal data, working covariance matrices, generalized estimating equations and quasi-likelihoods are commonly used, and in many situations these models do not need to be correctly specified. When the variance (covariance) of ε depends on the mean, and if $\boldsymbol{V}$, $\mathscr{W}$, and $\boldsymbol{\Sigma}$ are different, the asymptotic distribution of $\lambda_n(H_0)$ depends on the true parameters $\boldsymbol{\beta}_0$ and $\theta_0(t)$. In this case, the Wilks phenomenon does not hold in general for the test statistic defined in (11).

The general asymptotic theory for the GQLR statistic is complicated, but under the important special case of working independence, the asymptotic null distribution is much simplified and provided in the following theorem. Let $\boldsymbol{\Sigma}_d$ be the variance matrix that contains only the diagonal of $\boldsymbol{\Sigma}$.

Theorem 1 *Under some regularity conditions, assuming $h \to 0$ and $nh^5 \to 0$ as $n \to \infty$, and if $\boldsymbol{V} = \mathscr{W} = \boldsymbol{\Sigma}_d$, the asymptotic distribution $\lambda_n(H_0)$ is*

$$\sigma_n^{-1}\{\lambda_n(H_0) - \mu_n - d_n\} \xrightarrow{d} Normal(0, 1),$$

where $d_n = o_p(h^{-1/2})$, $\mu_n = (q-1)h^{-1}|\mathscr{T}|\{K(0) - \nu_K/2\}$, $\sigma_n^2 = 2(q-1)h^{-1}|\mathscr{T}| \times \int\{K(t) - \frac{1}{2}K * K(t)\}^2 dt$, and $|\mathscr{T}|$ is the length of the time domain.

This result implies $r_K \lambda_n(H_0)$ follows an asymptotic χ^2 distribution with $r_K \mu_n$ degrees of freedom where

$$r_K = \frac{K(0) - \nu_K/2}{\int \{K(t) - \frac{1}{2}K * K(t)\}^2 dt}.$$

Remark 1 Theorem 1 implies that, if a working independence covariance is used in both estimation and hypothesis testing and if the true variance function is used, the asymptotic distribution of $\lambda_n(H_0)$ does not depend on $\boldsymbol{\beta}_0$, $\theta_0(t)$, or the true correlation structure $\mathscr{R}(\boldsymbol{\tau})$. This Wilks result makes it easy to assess the distribution of $\lambda_n(H_0)$ using bootstrap.

Remark 2 The Wilks property is particularly important in analyzing longitudinal GWAS data, where the longitudinal responses are repeated measures on disease related phenotypes, $\boldsymbol{X}$ contains the environmental covariates, and $\mathbf{Z}$ is the vector of genotype indicators defined by one SNP. The SNP level fANOVA tests are then repeated for hundreds of thousands of SNPs. The Wilks's property guarantees that the GQLR statistics have the same asymptotic distribution, so that we do not need to perform bootstrap hundreds of thousands of times.

Remark 3 By the central limit theorem, it is easy to see a χ^2 distribution with a diverging degree of freedom is approximately normal. The asymptotic χ^2 distribution in Theorem 1 has a degree of freedom $r_K \mu_n$, which is diverging to ∞ with the rate $O(h^{-1})$, and hence the connection with the asymptotic normal distribution. Similar χ^2 approximation was also used in Theorem 6 of [9].

Power of the GQLR Test

For the special case of fANCOVA models and the hypothesis (12), [35] also studies the local power of the GQLR test. They considered a contiguous alternative hypothesis

$$H_{1n} : \theta_k(t) = \theta_0(t) + G_{kn}(t), \quad k = 1, \ldots, q, \quad \text{with} \sum_{k=1}^{q} \pi_k G_{kn}(t) = 0, \quad (13)$$

where $\pi_k = n_k/n$, $n_k = \sum_{i=1}^{n} I(Z_{ik} = 1)$, $G_{kn}(t)$ are twice continuously differentiable smooth functions with $\sup_{t \in \mathscr{T}} G_{kn}(t) \to 0$ as $n \to \infty$, $k = 1, \ldots, q$.

Consider the test statistic in (11), and call it $\lambda_n(H_{1n})$ instead. The following theorem gives the asymptotic distribution of the test statistic under the local alternative (13) where the proof is given in the supplementary material.

Theorem 2 *Suppose the functions $G_{kn}(t)$'s are twice continuously differentiable. Denote $\mu_{1n} = \frac{1}{2}\sum_{k=1}^{q}\sum_{i=1}^{n_k} E\{G_{kn}^{\mathrm{T}}(\boldsymbol{T}_i)\Delta_i \boldsymbol{V}_{k,i}^{-1}\Delta_i G_{kn}(\boldsymbol{T}_i)\}$ and assume there exists a constant C_G such that*

$$h \times \mu_{1n} \to C_G < \infty. \tag{14}$$

Under the regularity conditions in Theorem 1 and the local alternative (13), the test statistic has the following limiting distribution:

$$\sigma_{1n}^{-1}\{\lambda_n(H_{1n}) - \mu_n - \mu_{1n}\} \xrightarrow{d} Normal(0, 1),$$

where $\sigma_{1n}^2 = \sigma_n^2 + \sum_{k=1}^{q}\sum_{i=1}^{n_k} E\{G_{kn}^{\mathrm{T}}(\boldsymbol{T}_i)\Delta_i \boldsymbol{V}_{k,i}^{-1}\boldsymbol{\Sigma}_{k,i}\boldsymbol{V}_{k,i}^{-1}\Delta_i G_{kn}(\boldsymbol{T}_i)\}$ *and* μ_n *and* σ_n^2 *are as defined in Theorem 1.*

An approximate level-α test based on the GQLR test statistic is $\varphi_n = I\{\lambda_n(H_{1n}) - \mu_n > z_\alpha \sigma_n\}$, where z_α is the upper $100 \times \alpha$ percentile of $N(0, 1)$, and we reject the null hypothesis if $\varphi_n = 1$. Let $\Phi(\cdot)$ be the cumulative distribution function of Normal$(0, 1)$. Then the type II error of the test is

$$\beta(\alpha, \boldsymbol{G}_n) = P(\lambda_n(H_{1n}) - \mu_n < z_\alpha \sigma_n) \approx \Phi(\sigma_{1n}^{-1}\sigma_n z_\alpha - \sigma_{1n}^{-1}\mu_{1n}), \tag{15}$$

where $\boldsymbol{G}_n = (G_{1n}, \ldots, G_{qn})^{\mathrm{T}}$. Define the class of functions

$$\mathcal{G}_n(\varrho) = \Big[\boldsymbol{G}_n = (G_{1n}, \ldots, G_{qn})^{\mathrm{T}} : \sum_{k=1}^{q} \pi_k E \times\{G_{kn}^{\mathrm{T}}(\boldsymbol{T}_k)\Delta_k \boldsymbol{V}_k^{-1}\Delta_k G_{kn}(\boldsymbol{T}_k)\} \geq \varrho^2\Big],$$

and the maximum probability of type II errors as

$$\beta(\alpha, \varrho) = \sup_{\boldsymbol{G}_n \in \mathcal{G}_n(\varrho)} \beta(\alpha, \boldsymbol{G}_n).$$

Following [21] and [9], define the minimax rate of a test φ with a type II error $\beta(\alpha, \varrho)$ as ϱ_n such that:

(a) For any $\varrho > \varrho_n$, $\alpha > 0$, and $\beta > 0$, there exists a constant c such that $\beta(\alpha, c\varrho) \leq \beta + o(1)$;
(b) For any sequence $\varrho_n^* = o(\varrho_n)$, there exist $\alpha > 0$ and $\beta > 0$ such that for any $c > 0$ $P(\varphi = 1|H_0) = \alpha + o(1)$ and $\liminf_{n\to\infty} \beta(\alpha, c\varrho_n^*) > \beta$.

The following theorem provides the minimax rate for our GQLR test procedure.

Theorem 3 *Under the regularity conditions in Theorem 1, the minimax rate of the GQLR test is* $\varrho_n(h) = n^{-4/9}$ *with* $h = c^* n^{-2/9}$ *for a constant* c^*.

Theorem 3 shows that the GQLR test achieves the minimax optimal rate of Ingster [21].

3.2 Functional F-Test

Zhang and Chen [44] and Zhang [43] (Chap. 6) proposed a functional F-test for hypothesis (2); however, their test was developed for Gaussian response under dense functional data setting and without covariates. We now extend their procedure into our setting with the link function $g(\cdot)$ restricted to be an identity link.

Define sum of squares

$$SSH_n(t) = \left\{\mathbf{C}\widehat{\boldsymbol{\theta}}(t) - \boldsymbol{c}(t)\right\}^{\mathrm{T}} \left\{\mathbf{C}(\mathbf{Z}^{\mathrm{T}}\mathbf{Z})^{-1}\mathbf{C}^{\mathrm{T}}\right\}^{-1} \left\{\mathbf{C}\widehat{\boldsymbol{\theta}}(t) - \boldsymbol{c}(t)\right\},$$

where $\mathbf{Z} = (\mathbf{Z}_1, \ldots, \mathbf{Z}_n)^{\mathrm{T}}$. The F-test statistic is defined as

$$F = \frac{\int SSH_n(t)dt/r}{\int \widehat{\mathscr{R}}(t,t)dt}, \tag{16}$$

where $\widehat{\mathscr{R}}(t,t)$ is an estimator of the variance function. For dense functional data, $\widehat{\mathscr{R}}(t,t)$ is expressed as mean square error in [43]. For sparse functional data, the covariance function needs to be estimated using methods described in Sect. 4.2.

According to [43] (p. 217),

$$F \sim F_{r\widehat{\kappa},(n-p-q)\widehat{\kappa}} \quad \text{approximately}, \tag{17}$$

where $\widehat{\kappa} = \frac{\mathrm{tr}^2(\widehat{\mathscr{R}})}{\mathrm{tr}(\widehat{\mathscr{R}}^{\otimes 2})}$ and $\widehat{\mathscr{R}}$ is an estimator of the covariance function (4). When the covariance function yields a spectral decomposition $\widehat{\mathscr{R}}(s,t) = \sum_{k=1}^{\infty} \widehat{\omega}_k \widehat{\psi}_k(s)\widehat{\psi}_k(t)$, where $\{\widehat{\psi}_k(t), k = 1, 2, \ldots\}$ are orthonormal eigenfunctions, then

$$\mathrm{tr}(\widehat{\mathscr{R}}) = \sum_k \widehat{\omega}_k, \quad \mathrm{tr}(\widehat{\mathscr{R}}^{\otimes 2}) = \sum_k \widehat{\omega}_k^2.$$

The approximate distribution (17) was developed under dense functional data and was never previously tested on longitudinal or sparse functional data. This approximation also suggests that the F-test does not enjoy the Wilks property that its null distribution does depend on nuisance parameters such as the eigenvalues of the covariance function.

4 Implementation Issues

4.1 Bandwidth Selection

For bandwidth selection, we adopt a leave-one-subject-out cross-validation [33] that is tailored to our data structure. Let $\widehat{h}_{cv}$ be the minimizer of

$$CV(h) = \sum_{i=1}^{n} \mathscr{Q}\left(g^{-1}\left[\boldsymbol{X}_i \widehat{\boldsymbol{\beta}}_h^{(-i)} + \{\widehat{\boldsymbol{\theta}}_h^{(-i)}(\boldsymbol{T}_i)\}^{\mathrm{T}} \mathbf{Z}_i, \boldsymbol{Y}_i\right]\right),$$

where $\mathscr{Q}(\cdot)$ is the quasi-likelihood function and $\widehat{\boldsymbol{\beta}}_h^{-(i)}$ and $\widehat{\boldsymbol{\theta}}_{k,h}^{-(i)}(\cdot)$ are the full model estimators with bandwidth h by removing the ith subject from the data set. It is well known that cross-validation estimates the optimal bandwidth for estimation, which is of order $n^{-1/5}$ [39]. To make the bandwidth follow the optimal order for hypothesis test suggested in Theorem 3, we propose to use $\widehat{h} = \widehat{h}_{cv} \times n^{-1/45}$. As shown in the empirical studies of Fan and Jiang [6], the hypothesis test results are quite robust against the choice of h as long as it is in the right order.

4.2 Covariance Estimation

There has been a vast volume of work on modeling covariance matrices in longitudinal data. Some recent work includes [19, 38]. However, most of these methods assume that the observations are made on a regular time grid, and therefore are not suitable for longitudinal data collected at irregular and subject-specific times. In this section, we will be mainly focused on two type of covariance models: (a) the semiparametric covariance models proposed by Fan and Wu [8]; (b) the nonparametric covariance models advocated by Yao et al. [42] and Li and Hsing [23]. For the rest of the subsection, we will focus on the case $g(\cdot)$ is an identity link, and let $\epsilon_i(t) = Y_i(t) - \{\boldsymbol{X}_i(t)^{\mathrm{T}}\beta + \mathbf{Z}_i^{\mathrm{T}}\boldsymbol{\theta}(t)\}$ be the error process.

Semiparametric Covariance Estimation

Fan et al. [10] modeled the variance function and correlation function separately. Specifically, in their setting the covariance function can be written as

$$\mathscr{R}(t_1, t_2) = \sigma(t_1)\sigma(t_2)\rho(t_1, t_2; \boldsymbol{\tau}),$$

where $\sigma^2(t)$ is the conditional variance of Y at time t modeled completely nonparametrically and $\rho(t_1, t_2; \boldsymbol{\tau})$ is a correlation function from a known family with only a few unspecified parameters. One example of the correlation model is the ARMA(1,1) correlation:

$$\rho(t_1, t_2; \gamma, \varphi) = \gamma \exp(-|t_1 - t_2|/\varphi), \tag{18}$$

for $0 \le \gamma \le 1$ and $\varphi > 0$.

The variance function is estimated applying a smoother to the squares of residuals. Let $\widehat{\boldsymbol{\beta}}$ and $\widehat{\boldsymbol{\theta}}(t)$ be the full model estimators described in Sect. 2, and define the residuals as $\widehat{\epsilon}_{ij} = Y_{ij} - \boldsymbol{X}_{ij}^{\mathrm{T}}\widehat{\beta} - \mathbf{Z}_i\widehat{\boldsymbol{\theta}}(T_{ij})$. Then $\sigma^2(t)$ can be estimated by a local linear estimator $\widehat{\sigma}^2(t) = \widehat{\alpha}_0$, where $(\widehat{\alpha}_0, \widehat{\alpha}_1)$ minimizes

$$\frac{1}{N}\sum_{i=1}^{n}\sum_{j=1}^{m_i}\{\widehat{\epsilon}_{ij}^2 - \alpha_0 - \alpha_1(T_{ij} - t)\}^2 K_h(T_{ij} - t), \tag{19}$$

and $K(\cdot)$ and h are the kernel function and bandwidth as described before.

Fan et al. [10] also proposed a quasi-maximum likelihood estimator (QMLE) for the correlation parameters. Letting $\widehat{\boldsymbol{\epsilon}}_i = (\widehat{\epsilon}_{i1}, \ldots, \widehat{\epsilon}_{im_i})^{\mathrm{T}}$, $\widehat{\boldsymbol{D}}_i = \mathrm{diag}\{\widehat{\sigma}(T_{i1}), \ldots, \widehat{\sigma}(T_{im_i})\}$, and $\boldsymbol{C}_i(\boldsymbol{\tau}) = \{\rho(T_{ij}, T_{ij'}; \boldsymbol{\tau})\}_{j,j'=1}^{m_i}$ be the correlation matrix for the ith cluster, then

$$\widehat{\boldsymbol{\tau}} = \mathrm{argmax}_{\boldsymbol{\tau}} \sum_{i=1}^{n}\left\{-\frac{1}{2}\log|\boldsymbol{C}_i(\boldsymbol{\tau})| - \frac{1}{2}\widehat{\boldsymbol{\epsilon}}_i^{\mathrm{T}}\widehat{\boldsymbol{D}}_i^{-1}\boldsymbol{C}_i^{-1}(\boldsymbol{\tau})\widehat{\boldsymbol{D}}_i^{-1}\widehat{\boldsymbol{\epsilon}}_i\right\}. \tag{20}$$

Fan and Wu [8] showed the consistency and asymptotic normality for the QMLE estimator in (20).

Nonparametric Covariance Estimation

The semiparametric covariance estimation in Sect. 4.2 provides valid yet flexible models for the covariance structure, but it depends on correctly specifying the correlation model. To extend this idea further, one can model the covariance function completely nonparametrically. Such models have become increasingly popular in functional data analysis [23, 32, 42].

We model $\mathscr{R}(t_1, t_2)$ as a bivariate nonparametric function, which is smooth except for the points on the diagonal line, $\{t_1 = t_2\}$, to allow possible nugget effects. To see this point, we assume that $\epsilon_i(t)$ can be decomposed into two independent components, $\epsilon_i(t) = \epsilon_{i0}(t) + \epsilon_{i1}(t)$, where $\epsilon_{i0}(\cdot)$ is a longitudinal process with smooth covariance function $\mathscr{R}_0(t_1, t_2)$ and $\epsilon_{i1}(\cdot)$ is a white noise process usually caused by measurement errors. Let $\sigma_1^2(t) = \mathrm{var}\{\epsilon_{i1}(t)\}$, then

$$\mathscr{R}(t_1, t_2) = \mathscr{R}_0(t_1, t_2) + \sigma_1^2(t_1) I(t_1 = t_2), \tag{21}$$

where $I(\cdot)$ is an indicator function. In Eq. (21), $\sigma_1^2(\cdot)$ is the nugget effect causing discontinuity in $\mathscr{R}(\cdot,\cdot)$. We assume that both $\mathscr{R}_0(\cdot,\cdot)$ and $\sigma_1^2(\cdot)$ are smooth functions. As a result, $\mathscr{R}(t_1, t_2)$ is a smooth surface except on the diagonal points where $t_1 = t_2$, and it is also smooth along the diagonal direction. For time series data, without additional assumptions, some confounding will occur if both the mean and covariance functions are modeled nonparametrically. However, this identifiability issue will not occur for longitudinal data, because of the independence structure between subjects.

Let $\widehat{\epsilon}_{ij} = Y_{ij} - \{\boldsymbol{X}_{ij}^{\mathrm{T}}\widehat{\boldsymbol{\beta}} + \mathbf{Z}_i^{\mathrm{T}}\widehat{\boldsymbol{\theta}}(T_{ij})\}$ be the residual of the full model in Sect. 2. Suppose $\mathscr{R}$ has a decomposition as in (21); we first estimate the smooth part $\mathscr{R}_0$ using a bivariate local linear smoother. Let $\widehat{\mathscr{R}}_0(t_1, t_2) = \widehat{\alpha}_0$, where $(\widehat{\alpha}_0, \widehat{\alpha}_1, \widehat{\alpha}_2)$ minimizes

$$\frac{1}{n}\sum_{i=1}^{n}\sum_{j=1}^{m_i}\sum_{j'\neq j}\left\{\widehat{\epsilon}_{ij}\widehat{\epsilon}_{ij'} - \alpha_0 - \alpha_1(T_{ij} - t_1) - a_2(T_{ij'} - t_2)\right\}^2 \times K_h(T_{ij} - t_1)K_h(T_{ij'} - t_2). \tag{22}$$

Define $N_R = \sum_{i=1}^{n} m_i(m_i - 1)$,

$$S_{pq} = \frac{1}{N_R}\sum_{i=1}^{n}\sum_{j=1}^{m_i}\sum_{j'\neq j}\left(\frac{T_{ij} - t_1}{h}\right)^p\left(\frac{T_{ij'} - t_2}{h}\right)^q K_h(T_{ij} - t_1)K_h(T_{ij'} - t_2),$$

$$R_{pq} = \frac{1}{N_R}\sum_{i=1}^{n}\sum_{j=1}^{m_i}\sum_{j'\neq j}\widehat{\epsilon}_{ij}\widehat{\epsilon}_{ik}\left(\frac{T_{ij} - t_1}{h}\right)^p\left(\frac{T_{ij'} - t_2}{h}\right)^q \times K_h(T_{ij} - t_1)K_h(T_{ij'} - t_2).$$

Then the following solution for (22) is given in [17]:

$$\widehat{\mathscr{R}}_0(s, t) = (\mathscr{A}_1 R_{00} - \mathscr{A}_2 R_{10} - \mathscr{A}_3 R_{01})\mathscr{B}^{-1}, \tag{23}$$

where $\mathscr{A}_1 = S_{20}S_{02} - S_{11}^2$, $\mathscr{A}_2 = S_{10}S_{02} - S_{01}S_{11}$, $\mathscr{A}_3 = S_{01}S_{20} - S_{10}S_{11}$, $\mathscr{B} = \mathscr{A}_1 S_{00} - \mathscr{A}_2 S_{10} - \mathscr{A}_3 S_{01}$.

As described above, the diagonal values on $\mathscr{R}(\cdot,\cdot)$ require a special treatment. The variance function can be written as $\sigma^2(t) = \mathscr{R}_0(t, t) + \sigma_1^2(t)$ and be estimated by the local linear smoother in (19). The covariance function is estimated by

$$\widehat{\mathscr{R}}(s, t) = \widehat{\mathscr{R}}_0(s, t)I(s \neq t) + \widehat{\sigma}^2(t)I(s = t). \tag{24}$$

Li [22] proved that the nonparametric covariance function estimator in (24) is uniformly consistent to the true covariance function

$$\sup_{s,t\in\mathscr{T}} |\widehat{\mathscr{R}}(s,t) - \mathscr{R}(s,t)| = O_p\left[h^2 + \{\log n/(nh^2)\}^{1/2}\right].$$

The detailed convergence rate for the nonparametric covariance estimator can be found in Li [22]. However, as noted in previous literature ([15, 25]), the kernel covariance estimator in (24) is not guaranteed to be positive semidefinite, and therefore some adjustment is needed to enforce the condition. One possible adjustment is though a spectral decomposition of the covariance estimator.

A commonly used spectral decomposition of the covariance functions for longitudinal data is [17, 42]

$$\mathscr{R}_0(s,t) = \sum_{k=1}^{\infty} \omega_k \psi_k(s)\psi_k(t),$$

where $\omega_1 \geq \omega_2 \geq \cdots \geq 0$ are the eigenvalues of the covariance function, and $\psi_k(t)$ are the corresponding eigenfunctions with $\int_{\mathscr{T}} \psi_k(t)\psi_{k'}(t)dt = I(k = k')$.

An adjustment procedure has been proposed and theoretically justified by Hall et al. [16] to transform $\widehat{\mathscr{R}}_0$ into a valid covariance function. We take a spectral decomposition of $\widehat{\mathscr{R}}_0$ and truncate the negative components. Letting $\widehat{\omega}_k$ and $\widehat{\psi}_k(\cdot)$, $k = 1, 2, \ldots$, be the eigenvalues and eigenfunctions of $\widehat{\mathscr{R}}_0$, and $K_n = \max\{k; \widehat{\omega}_k > 0\}$, then the adjusted estimator for $\mathscr{R}$ is

$$\widetilde{\mathscr{R}}_0(s,t) = \sum_{k=1}^{K_n} \widehat{\omega}_k \widehat{\psi}_k(s)\widehat{\psi}_k(t),$$

$$\widetilde{\mathscr{R}}(s,t) = \widetilde{\mathscr{R}}_0(s,t)I(s \neq t) + \widehat{\sigma}^2(t)I(s = t). \tag{25}$$

4.3 Wild Bootstrap

The numerical studies in [18] and [35] show that, under moderate sample size, the bootstrap can provide a better approximation to the distribution of $\lambda_n(H_0)$ than the asymptotic normal distribution in Theorem 1.

We now describe the wild bootstrap procedure of [35], which is an extension of the procedure of [18]. The idea is to generate data that satisfy the null hypothesis and closely resemble the true data, while preserving the within-subject correlation.

(i) Estimate both the full and reduced models from the original data and estimate the variance function by the nonparametric estimator $\widehat{\sigma}^2(t)$ described in Sect. 4.2 using residuals from the full model. Evaluate the GQLR test statistic $\lambda_n(H_0)$ under working independence.
(ii) For each subject, regenerate the response vector $Y_{ij}^* = g^{-1}(\mu_{ij}^*) + \varepsilon_{ij}^*$, where $\mu_{ij}^* = \boldsymbol{X}_{ij}^{\mathrm{T}}\widehat{\boldsymbol{\beta}}_R + \mathbf{Z}_i^{\mathrm{T}}\widehat{\boldsymbol{\theta}}_R(T_{ij})$, $\varepsilon_{k,ij}^* = \xi_i\widehat{\varepsilon}_{k,ij}$, $\widehat{\varepsilon}_{ij}$'s are the residuals from the full

model and ξ_i's are independent random perturbation factors with mean 0 and variance 1.

(iii) Calculate the GQLR test statistic $\lambda_n^*(H_0)$ from the bootstrap sample $\{\boldsymbol{Y}_i^*, \boldsymbol{X}_i, \boldsymbol{T}_i\}$ using the exact same procedure for the original data.

(iv) Repeat Steps (ii) and (iii) a large number of times to obtain the bootstrap replicates $\lambda_n^*(H_0)$. The estimated p-value is the percentage of $\lambda_n^*(H_0)$ that are greater than $\lambda_n(H_0)$.

Davidson and Flachaire [3] advocated to generate the perturbation factor ξ_i in Step (ii) from a simple Rademacher distribution, i.e. $P(\xi = 1) = P(\xi = -1) = 1/2$, which is also what we use in our numerical studies. Put $\mathscr{X} = \{(\boldsymbol{X}_i, \boldsymbol{T}_i),\ i = 1, \ldots, n\}$. For fANCOVA problem, Tang et al. [35] proved the following theorem on the consistency of the bootstrap procedure above.

Theorem 4 *Under the same assumptions as Theorem 1,*

$$P[\sigma_n^{-1}\{\lambda_n^*(H_0) - \mu_n - d_n\} < x \mid \mathscr{X}] \to \Phi(x) \quad \textit{in probability for any } x,$$

where σ_n, μ_n, and d_n are as defined in Theorem 1.

The theorem states that, conditioning on $\mathscr{X}$, $\lambda_n^*(H_0)$ from the working independent bootstrap procedure above has the same asymptotic normal distribution as $\lambda_n(H_0)$ in Theorem 1.

The approximate distribution (17) for the functional F-test was developed by Zhang [43] under dense functional data, which we found to be inaccurate for sparse functional data and under moderate sample size. In practice, the distribution of the functional F-test can also be estimated by the same bootstrap procedure.

5 Simulations

5.1 Gaussian Case

For Gaussian-type sparse functional data, both GQLR test and functional F-test can be used to test hypothesis (2); however, their powers have not been previously compared. We now provide such a comparison through simulation studies.

We generate data from model (1) with an identity link, $p = 2$ environmental predictors, and $q = 4$ genetic predictors. There are $m_i = 5$ repeated measures of Y on each subject, where the observation times are iid with $T_{ij} \sim Unif(0, 1)$. The first environmental predictor is time dependent with $X_{1,ij} = T_{ij} + U_{ij}$, where $U_{ij} \sim Unif(-1, 1)$; and the second environmental predictor $X_{2,i}$ is a binary, time-invariant covariate that equals 0 or 1 with probability 0.5. Suppose the subjects are classified into four groups according to genetic traits, and $\mathbf{Z}_i$ is a 4-dim vector of indicators for the groups. We simulate a total of $n = 200$ subjects with $n_k = 50$ subjects in each genetic group, $k = 1, \ldots, 4$. The goal is to test if there are any genetic effects, i.e.

$$H_0 : \theta_1(t) = \cdots = \theta_4(t) \equiv \theta_0(t). \tag{26}$$

We generate the errors ϵ_{ij} as discrete observations on a zero-mean Gaussian process $\epsilon_i(t)$ and consider two covariance settings: (i) ARMA(1,1) covariance as defined in (18) with $\gamma = 0.75$, $\varphi = 1$, and variance function $\sigma^2(t) = 0.5$; (ii) a nonparametric covariance induced by the mixed model $\epsilon_{ij} = \xi_{0,ij} + \sum_{l=1}^{3} \xi_{li}\phi_l(T_{ij})$, where $\xi_{0,ij}, \xi_{li} \sim \text{Normal}(0, 0.3)$ are independent random effects and $\phi_1(t) = t^2 + 0.5$, $\phi_2(t) = \sin(3\pi t)$, $\phi_3(t) = \cos(3\pi t)$.

We set $\boldsymbol{\beta} = (1, 1)^{\mathrm{T}}$, and $\theta_1(t) = \theta_0(t) - 2\delta S(t)$, $\theta_2(t) = \theta_0(t) - \delta S(t)$, $\theta_3(t) = \theta_0(t) + \delta S(t)$ and $\theta_4(t) = \theta_0(t) + 2\delta S(t)$, where $\theta_0 = \sin(2\pi t)$ and $S(t) = \sin(6\pi t)$. We set $\delta = \{0, 0.05, 0.1, 0.15, 0.2, 0.25\}$, where $\delta = 0$ correspond to the null hypothesis (26) and the true model deviates further from H_0 as δ increases. For each value of δ, we simulate 200 data sets and apply both the GQLR test and the F-test to test the null hypothesis (26).

Note that the hypothesis (26) is an ANOVA hypothesis, under which case the F-test statistic can be written as

$$F = \frac{\int_{\mathcal{T}} \sum_{k=1}^{q} n_k \{\widehat{\theta}_{F,k}(t) - \widehat{\theta}_R(t)\}^2 dt/(q-1)}{\int_{\mathcal{T}} \widehat{\mathscr{R}}(t, t) dt}.$$

There are two ways to estimate null distribution of the F statistic: the asymptotic F distribution given in Sect. 3.2 (F**-asymp**) with the covariance function estimated using the nonparametric method described in Sect. 4.2 and the bootstrap method (F**-boot**) described in Sect. 4.3. For the GQLR test statistic, we use a Gaussian quasi-likelihood $\mathscr{Q}(\boldsymbol{\mu}, \boldsymbol{Y}) = -(\boldsymbol{Y} - \boldsymbol{\mu})^{\mathrm{T}} \boldsymbol{V}^{-1} (\boldsymbol{Y} - \boldsymbol{\mu})/2$, where $\boldsymbol{V}$ is a diagonal variance matrix using the estimated variance function (19) interpolated at subject-specific time points. The null distribution of the GQLR test is estimated by bootstrap.

The empirical powers of the three tests as functions of δ are shown in Fig. 1, where the two panels correspond to the two covariance settings. The F-test based on asymptotic theory does not hold the nominal size in our second covariance setting, which is understandable since the asymptotic distribution in Sect. 3.2 was developed under dense functional data. This result shows that the asymptotic F approximation for the F-test may not be legitimate under our sparse functional data setting. Both the GQLR and F-test hold the nominal size when the null hypothesis is estimated by bootstrap; however, the GQLR test is more powerful under both simulation settings.

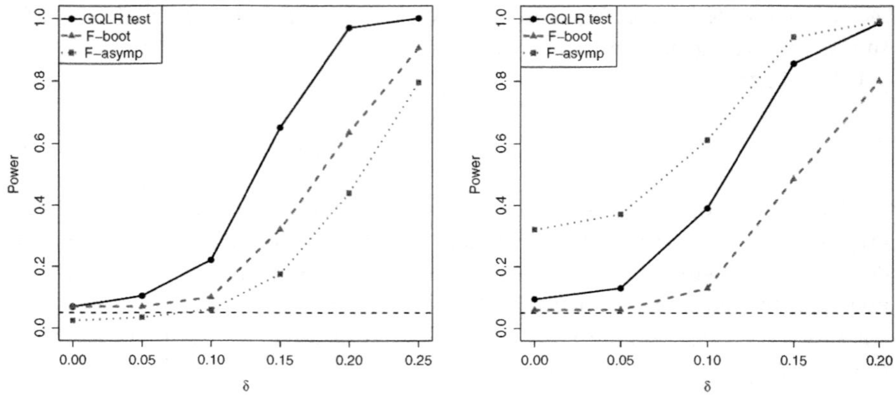

Fig. 1 Empirical power of three tests. The horizontal dotted line is set at 0.05. The left panel is the result under covariance setting (1) where the true covariance is ARMA(1,1); the right panel is the result under covariance setting (2) where the errors are generated from a mixed model with nonparametric factors

5.2 Non-Gaussian Response

To demonstrate the use of the methods described, we also simulate data from model (1) under a logarithm link. The covariates $\boldsymbol{X}$ and $\mathbf{Z}$ are simulated in the same way as in Sect. 5.1. Suppose there are $m_i = 4$ repeated measures on each subject with observation times uniformly distributed in $[0, 1]$. Conditional on $\boldsymbol{X}_{ij}$ and $\mathbf{Z}_i$, Y_{ij} are generated from a multivariate Poisson distribution with mean values $\mu_{ij} = \exp\{\boldsymbol{X}_{ij}^{\mathrm{T}}\boldsymbol{\beta} + \mathbf{Z}_i^{\mathrm{T}}\boldsymbol{\theta}(T_{ij})\}$ and exchangeable correlation within the same subject.

The correlated multivariate Poisson random variables are simulated by the method of [41], using auxiliary normal distributions. To be more specific, we generate standard normal distribution Y'_{ij} with exchangeable within-cluster correlation such that $corr(Y'_{ij}, Y'_{ij'}) = \rho_{jj'} = 0.3$ for $j \neq j'$ and generate $Y_{ij} = F_{ij}^{-1}\{\Phi(Y'_{ij})\}$ where $\Phi(\cdot)$ is the distribution function of standard normal and $F_{ij}(\cdot)$ is the distribution function of a Poisson distribution with mean μ_{ij}.

We test the same ANOVA hypothesis in (26). Note that the F-test was not developed for non-Gaussian response; we therefore only consider the GQLR test using a Poisson quasi-likelihood $\mathscr{Q}(\boldsymbol{\mu}_i, \boldsymbol{Y}_i) = \boldsymbol{Y}_i^{\mathrm{T}} \log\left(\boldsymbol{\mu}_i\right) - \boldsymbol{\mu}_i^{\mathrm{T}}\mathbf{1}$.

To demonstrate the Wilks phenomenon of the GQLR test, we consider the following three scenarios with different setting of $\boldsymbol{\beta}$ and θ_0:

$$\text{Scenario I}: \beta_1 = 1,\ \beta_2 = 1,\ \theta_0(t) = \sin(2\pi t);$$

$$\text{Scenario II}: \beta_1 = 0.5,\ \beta_2 = 1.5,\ \theta_0(t) = \sin(2\pi t);$$

$$\text{Scenario III}: \beta_1 = 1,\ \beta_2 = 1.5,\ \theta_0(t) = \cos(2\pi t).$$

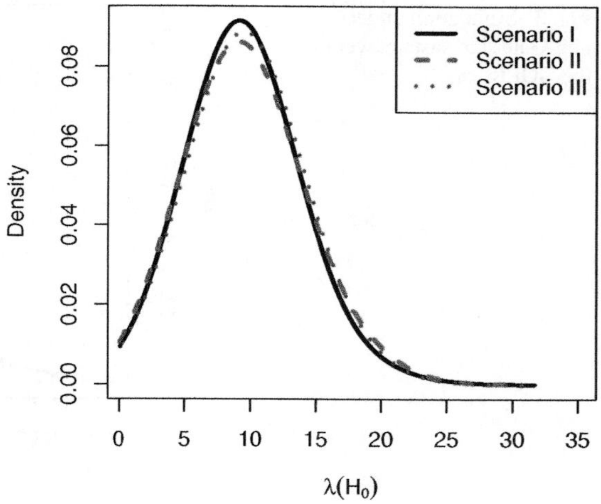

Fig. 2 Simulation under non-Gaussian case: demonstration of the Wilks phenomenon. The three curves are the estimated distribution of $\lambda_n(H_0)$ under the three simulation scenarios

We simulate 200 data sets for each scenario and apply the GQLR test to each simulated data set. Figure 2 shows the estimated densities for $\lambda_n(H_0)$ under the three scenarios using kernel smoothing. We perform a k-sample Anderson–Darling test and find no significant difference among the three distributions (p-value: 0.53). These results show Wilks phenomenon holds for the GQLR test under non-Gaussian case that the distribution of $\lambda_n(H_0)$ does not depend on the true value of the parameters.

Next, we study the power of the GQLR test. We focus on the simulation setting described in Scenario I and consider local alternatives with $\theta_1(t) = \theta_0(t) - 2\delta G(t)$, $\theta_2(t) = \theta_0(t) - \delta G(t)$, $\theta_3(t) = \theta_0(t) + \delta G(t)$, and $\theta_4(t) = \theta_0(t) + 2\delta G(t)$. We set $G(t) = \sin(4\pi t)$ and consider different δ values. The null hypothesis is true when $\delta = 0$ and as δ increases the model deviates further away from H_0. Specifically, we set the significance level at $\alpha = 0.05$ and use the wild bootstrap procedure in Sect. 4.3 to estimate the null distribution. Figure 3 shows the power of the GQLR test as a function of δ. As we can see, the test holds the nominal size and the power increases to 1 as δ increases.

6 Analysis of Longitudinal GWAS Data from ADNI

The Alzheimer's Disease Neuroimaging Initiative (ADNI) is an NIH-funded longitudinal observational study, the goal of which is to develop biomarkers to detect and track Alzheimer's Disease (AD). The original ADNI cohort included a total of 800 subjects, many of whom have repeated measurements on AD related biomarkers, such as the hippocampal volume (HV) and Rey Auditory Verbal Learning Tests (RAVLT), over 10 years of follow-ups. The HV is a Gaussian-type continuous

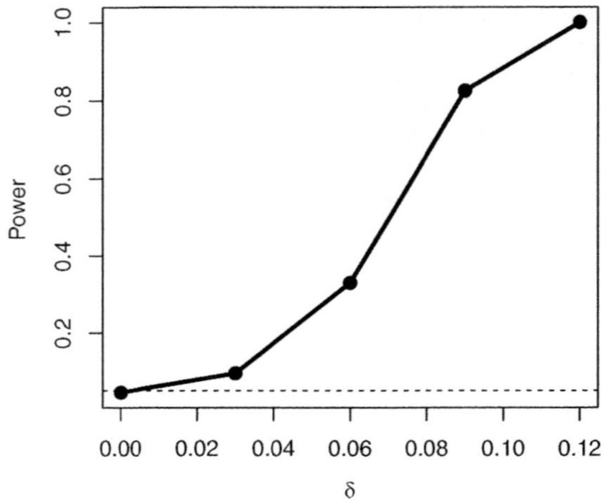

Fig. 3 Simulation under non-Gaussian case: power of the GQLR test

variable, which can be modeled by Model (1) with an identity link; in contrast, the RAVLT data are non-Gaussian count data.

Genotype of 620,901 SNPs was measured for the ADNI subjects, and our goal is to identify the SNPs related to AD biomarkers such as HV and RAVLT. As mentioned before, the genotypes for each SNP are AA, AB, and BB, determined by the two alleles of the SNP. After excluding SNPs with large portions of missing values and unevenly distributions, our analysis focuses on 311,417 SNPs with at least 5% subjects in each of the three genotypes. Demographical variables, such as baseline age, sex, years of education, race, and marital status, are collected as covariates.

6.1 Analysis of the Hippocampal Volume Data

The hippocampus is a functional region in a human brain that is related to memory and interpreting environmental contexts. There has been some documented evidence that loss of hippocampal volume (HV) may be associated with memory loss and AD [4, 34]. In the ADNI cohort, 629 subjects have repeatedly measured HV using neuroimaging methods during the 10-year follow-up, where the number of repeated measures ranges between 2 and 11 with a median of 4. The observation times are random and subject-specific, the distribution of which is highly skewed. We therefore take a log-transformation to time and let $t = \log(1 + \text{actual visit time})$, which brings the time domain to $\mathcal{T} = [0, 2.4]$.

Repeated for each of the 311,417 SNPs, we fit Model (1) with an identity link to the HV data where $\boldsymbol{X}$ contains the demographical variables (baseline age, sex, years of education, race, and marital status) and $\mathbf{Z}$ is a vector of genotype indicators defined by the SNP. We then test the hypothesis (2) with the specification (3). We repeat the test for each SNP, taking into account of the multiple hypothesis testing issue by a Bonferroni procedure.

To perform SNP level tests for hundreds of thousands of times, we encounter two technical difficulties. First, it is computationally infeasible to run bootstrap for hundreds of thousands of SNPs. Second, the commonly used genome-wide significant levels are 10^{-5} or 10^{-7} [5, 20]; hence, it requires a gigantic bootstrap sample for the bootstrap p-value to reach such accuracy.

Between the two tests discussed in Sect. 3, the GQLR test is more feasible to address these statistical challenges. First, the Wilks phenomenon described in Theorem 1 implies that the null distribution the GQLR test is the same for all SNPs so that there is no need to repeat bootstrap for hundreds of thousands of SNPs. In contrast, no Wilks property is established for the F-test. Second, our simulation study also suggest that the GQLR test is more power than the F-test. We therefore perform the GQLR test to all SNPs but only apply the proposed wild bootstrap procedure on 20 randomly selected SNPs, with 1000 bootstrap samples for each SNP. We then combine these bootstrap test statistics from the 20 SNPs and fit a χ^2 distribution to the combined sample using maximum likelihood estimation, and we use the fitted χ^2 distribution to evaluate the p-values for all SNPs.

The GQLR test detects 3 SNPs associated with HV at 10^{-7} significance level and 52 SNPs at 10^{-5} significance level. The 50 most significant SNPs are reported in Table 1, where we report the name of the SNP, the corresponding gene and chromosome, and the position of the SNP on chromosome. The most significant SNP is in gene TOMM40, which has been identified by multiple independent studies to be related to HV and AD [11, 14]. The second most significant SNP is located at gene ABLIM2, the association of which with AD was found by Gasparoni et al. [12]. The third SNP "rs2800235" on the list is not found in any existing literature and thus merits further investigation. We also show in Fig. 4 the functional genotype effects for the top three most significant SNPs. The solid curve in each plot is the overall mean function, while the dashed, dotted, and dash-dot curves are the estimated genotype effects for AA, AB, and BB, respectively.

6.2 *Analysis of the RAVLT Data*

The RAVLT is a neuropsychological assessment designed to evaluate verbal memory in patients and it can also be used to evaluate the nature and severity of memory dysfunction. During the test, the patient hears a list of 15 nouns (List A) and is asked to recall as many words from the list as possible. After five repetitions of free-recall, a second interference list (List B) is presented, and the participant is asked to recall as many words from List B as possible. The participant is asked to recall the words from List A immediately after the interference trial and after a 30 min delay. The delayed RAVLT score is the number of words that the participant correctly recalls from List A after the delay interval, which has been used for identifying patients at high risks of cognitive decline and subsequent dementia [1].

Table 1 Top 50 SNPs associated with HV, with the names of SNP and corresponding gene, the chromosome, and the position of the SNP on chromosome

Order	SNP	Gene	Chr	Position	Order	SNP	Gene	Chr	Position
1	rs2075650	TOMM40	19	44892363	26	rs13420500	C2orf88	2	190070149
2	rs11936149	ABLIM2	4	8120770	27	rs7068990	LOC105378515	10	120329401
3	rs2800235	–	1	224861046	28	rs1673887	–	3	103882935
4	rs1673874	–	3	103868142	29	rs11247613	SLC9A1	1	27149295
5	rs2061345	–	3	103869583	30	rs2516104	–	6	117770467
6	rs17300532	LOC105379028	5	72084529	31	rs1474359	C2orf88	2	190068281
7	rs6044895	DSTN	20	17586934	32	rs4518082	–	3	139685328
8	rs1885082	RRBP1	20	17613340	33	rs4980200	–	10	123698107
9	rs2655997	TMEM63C	14	77204147	34	rs10936959	LINC02015	3	177873287
10	rs10495753	DTNB	2	25452827	35	rs1361417	–	6	102290539
11	rs10439990	ZBTB20	3	114396188	36	rs4920338	PAX7	1	18664300
12	rs4972625	–	2	173988067	37	rs433627	LOC105376126	9	87212499
13	rs10895739	–	11	97410246	38	rs2257468	ABR	17	1083503
14	rs7889761	FRMPD4	X	12520193	39	rs405509	APOE	19	44905580
15	rs4740801	–	9	4790166	40	rs3909086	–	20	6270993
16	rs10931440	C2orf88	2	190018635	41	rs12713521	AFTPH	2	64590123
17	rs10995440	–	10	63108822	42	rs29327	ANK2	4	113286511
18	rs1345516	–	2	64476153	43	rs1890202	MCF2L	13	112900737
19	rs228815	–	6	39139170	44	rs10518258	–	19	29185868
20	rs6136143	DSTN	20	17592113	45	rs4947936	–	7	50839056
21	rs9874829	–	3	139681798	46	rs7233189	EPB41L3	18	5480543
22	rs11633192	THSD4	15	71555974	47	rs6054058	–	20	6281541
23	rs733217	–	3	69671518	48	rs5030938	LOC101928994	10	69216161
24	rs2395891	LOC107985278	19	2032150	49	rs10992211	–	9	90129734
25	rs972795	FHIT	3	59774393	50	rs1062980	IREB2	15	78500186

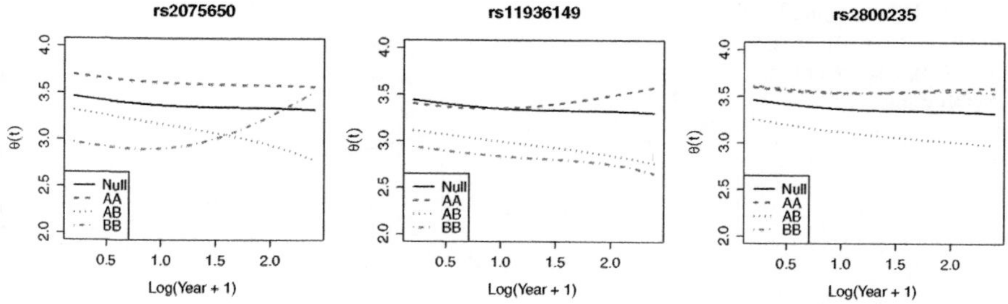

Fig. 4 Estimated genotype effects for the top three SNPs related to HV in the ADNI data

Fig. 5 The histogram of all observed RAVLT delay scores

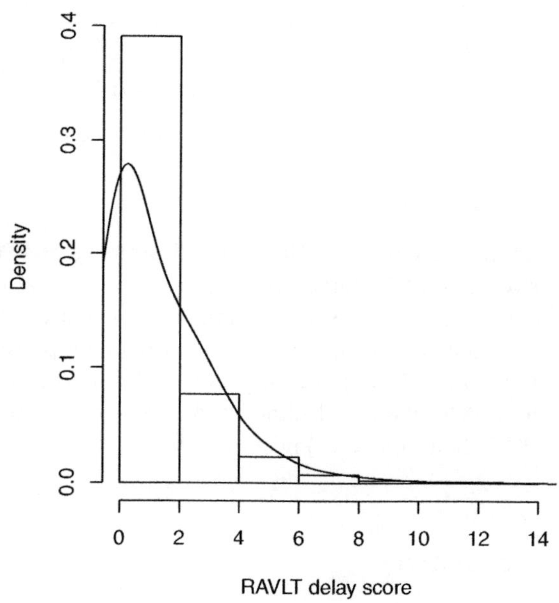

In the ADNI cohort, 358 subjects with mild cognitive impairment (MCI) were administered the RAVLT test at months 0, 6, 12, 18, 24, and 36, but actual measurement times varied randomly around the scheduled dates. A histogram of delay RAVLT scores is provided in Fig. 5. These scores are count data, skew to the right, and obviously non-Gaussian. Our goal is to establish the association between RAVLT test score and the gene APOE.

We fit Model (1) with log link to RAVLT data, where $\boldsymbol{X}$ includes the baseline age and sex (0 for man and 1 for woman) and $\mathbf{Z}$ is a vector of indicators for APOE alleles numbers (0, 1 or 2). The estimated coefficients for age and sex are $\hat{\beta}_{\mathtt{age}} = -0.0024$ and $\hat{\beta}_{\mathtt{sex}} = -0.1992$ with standard errors 0.006382 and 0.09997, respectively, indicating a significant effect of sex. To test the significance of the effect of APOE on RAVLT scores, the proposed GQLR test is applied. The obtained p-value for the null hypothesis: $\theta_1(t) = \theta_2(t) = \theta_3(t)$ is 0.039 by the wild bootstrap procedure

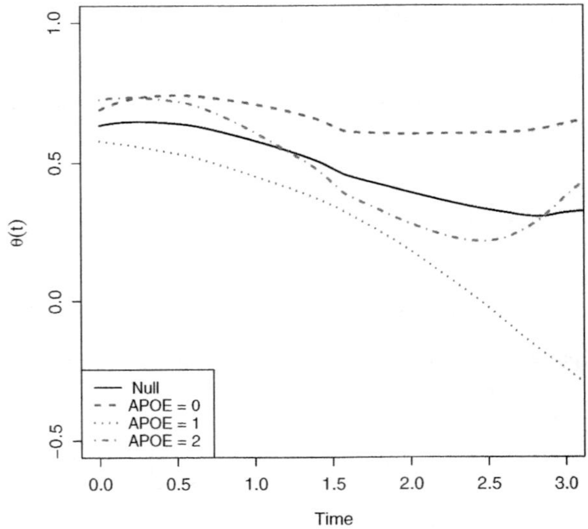

Fig. 6 The estimated functional effects of APOE on RAVLT scores in the ADNI data

with sample size 1000. This result illustrated that APOE is significant with the mean curve of RAVLT curve. The estimated functional effects of APOE are shown in Fig. 6, where the dark solid curve is $\widehat{\theta}(t)$ under the null hypothesis representing the overall mean curve and the other three curves represent the group mean functions for APOE alleles 0, 1, and 2, respectively. It shows that RAVLT scores of MCI patients with APOE allele(s) decline dramatically over time, while scores of those without APOE alleles remain almost the same level.

7 Summary

In this chapter, we demonstrate the use of functional data modeling and inference methods to analyze longitudinal GWAS data, where aging disease related phenotypes are repeatedly measured over time. The method can be used to analyze both Gaussian-type (such as the HV data in ADNI) and non-Gaussian (such as the RAVLT scores) response, taking into account the parametric effects of environmental covariates and functional effects of genotypes. In testing the functional genotype effects, we compare the effectiveness of two widely used nonparametric tests and show the advantages of the GQLR test over the functional F-test when analyzing sparse functional data from longitudinal GWAS. First, the GQLR test can be used for both Gaussian and non-Gaussian responses, but the F-test was only developed for Gaussian response. Second, the GQLR test enjoys the Wilks property making it feasible for large scale multiple SNP level hypotheses testing, but the F-test does not enjoy such property. Third, the GQLR test is shown to enjoy the minimax optimal power, while the local power of the F-test is largely unknown.

Our simulation studies suggest the GQLR test has higher power than the F-test, where there is inhomogeneity and correlation in the data.

Acknowledgments Li's research was supported partially by National Institute of Aging grant 5R21AG058198. Xu's research was supported by The Hong Kong Polytechnic University Ph.D. Studentship. Liu's research was partially supported by the General Research Fund (15301519), Research Grants of Council (RGC), Hong Kong.

Data collection and sharing for this project was funded by the Alzheimer's Disease Neuroimaging Initiative (ADNI) (National Institutes of Health Grant U01 AG024904) and DOD ADNI (Department of Defense award number W81XWH-12-2-0012). ADNI is funded by the National Institute on Aging, the National Institute of Biomedical Imaging and Bioengineering, and through generous contributions from the following: AbbVie, Alzheimer's Association; Alzheimer's Drug Discovery Foundation; Araclon Biotech; BioClinica, Inc.; Biogen; Bristol-Myers Squibb Company; CereSpir, Inc.; Cogstate; Eisai Inc.; Elan Pharmaceuticals, Inc.; Eli Lilly and Company; EuroImmun; F. Hoffmann-La Roche Ltd and its affiliated company Genentech, Inc.; Fujirebio; GE Healthcare; IXICO Ltd.; Janssen Alzheimer Immunotherapy Research & Development, LLC.; Johnson & Johnson Pharmaceutical Research & Development LLC.; Lumosity; Lundbeck; Merck & Co., Inc.; Meso Scale Diagnostics, LLC.; NeuroRx Research; Neurotrack Technologies; Novartis Pharmaceuticals Corporation; Pfizer Inc.; Piramal Imaging; Servier; Takeda Pharmaceutical Company; and Transition Therapeutics. The Canadian Institutes of Health Research is providing funds to support ADNI clinical sites in Canada. Private sector contributions are facilitated by the Foundation for the National Institutes of Health (www.fnih.org). The grantee organization is the Northern California Institute for Research and Education, and the study is coordinated by the Alzheimer's Therapeutic Research Institute at the University of Southern California. ADNI data are disseminated by the Laboratory for Neuro Imaging at the University of Southern California.

References

1. Andersson, C., Lindau, M., Almkvist, O., Engfeldt, P., Johansson, S.-E., Jönhagen, M E.: Identifying patients at high and low risk of cognitive decline using Rey Auditory Verbal Learning Test among middle-aged memory clinic outpatients. Dement. Geriatr. Cogn. Disord. **21**(4), 251–259 (2006)
2. Brumback, B., Rice, J.A.: Smoothing spline models for the analysis of nested and crossed samples of curves (with discussion). J. Am. Stat. Assoc. **93**, 961–994 (1998)
3. Davidson, R., Flachaire, E.: The wild bootstrap, tamed at last. J. Econometrics, 146, 162–169 (2008)
4. den Heijer, T., van der Lijn, F., Koudstaal, P.J., Hofman, A., van der Lugt, A., Krestin, G.P., Niessen, W.J., Breteler, M.M.: A 10-year follow-up of hippocampal volume on magnetic resonance imaging in early dementia and cognitive decline. Brain **133**(4), 1163–1172 (2010)
5. Fadista, J., Manning, A.K., Florez, J.C., Groop, L.: The (in) famous GWAS P-value threshold revisited and updated for low-frequency variants. Eur. J. Hum. Genet. **24**, 1202 (2016)
6. Fan, J., Jiang, J.: Nonparametric inferences for additive models. J. Am. Stat. Assoc. **100**, 890–907 (2005)
7. Fan, J., Li, R.: New estimation and model selection procedures for semiparametric modeling in longitudinal data analysis. J. Am. Stat. Assoc. **99**, 710–723 (2004)
8. Fan, J., Wu, Y.: Semiparametric estimation of covariance matrixes for longitudinal data. J. Am. Stat. Assoc. **103**, 1520–1533 (2008)
9. Fan, J., Zhang, C., Zhang, J.: Generalized likelihood ratio statistics and Wilks phenomenon. Ann. Stat. **29**, 153–193 (2001)

10. Fan, J., Huang, T., Li, R.: Analysis of longitudinal data with semiparametric estimation of covariance function. J. Am. Stat. Assoc. **102**(478), 632–641 (2007)
11. Ferencz, B., Laukka, E.J., Lövdén, M., Kalpouzos, G., Keller, L., Graff, C., Wahlund, L.-O., Fratiglioni, L., Bäckman, L.: The influence of APOE and TOMM40 polymorphisms on hippocampal volume and episodic memory in old age. Front. Hum. Neurosci. **7**, 198 (2013)
12. Gasparoni, G., Bultmann, S., Lutsik, P., Kraus, T.F., Sordon, S., Vlcek, J., Dietinger, V., Steinmaurer, M., Haider, M., Mulholland, C.B., et al.: DNA methylation analysis on purified neurons and glia dissects age and Alzheimer's disease-specific changes in the human cortex. Epigenetics Chromatin **11**(1), 41 (2018)
13. González-Manteiga, W., Crujeiras, R.M.: An updated review of goodness-of-fit tests for regression models. Test **22**, 361–411 (2013)
14. Grupe, A., Abraham, R., Li, Y., Rowland, C., Hollingworth, P., Morgan, A., Jehu, L., Segurado, R., Stone, D., Schadt, E.: Evidence for novel susceptibility genes for late-onset Alzheimer's disease from a genome-wide association study of putative functional variants. Hum. Mol. Genet. **16**(8), 865–873 (2007)
15. Hall, P., Fisher, N.I., Hoffmann, B.: On the nonparametric estimation of covariance functions. The Annals of Statistics. JSTOR. **22**(4), 2115–2134 (1994)
16. Hall, P., Müller, H.G., Yao, F.: Modeling sparse generalized longitudinal observations with latent Gaussian processes. JRSSB. **70**, 703–723 (2008)
17. Hall, P., Müller, H. G., Wang, J. L.: Properties of principal component methods for functional and longitudinal data analysis. Ann. Stat. **34**, 1493–1517 (2006)
18. Härdle, W., Mammen, E.: Comparing nonparametric versus parametric regression fits. Ann. Stat. **21**, 1926–1947 (1993)
19. Huang, J.Z., Liu, L., Liu, N.: Estimation of large covariance matrices of longitudinal data with basis function approximations. J. Comput. Graph. Stat. **16**, 189–209 (2007)
20. Huang, C., Thompson, P., Wang, Y., Yu, Y., Zhang, J., Kong, D., Colen, R.R., Knickmeyer, R.C., Zhu, H., Initiative, T. A. D. N.: FGWAS: Functional genome wide association analysis. Neuroimage **159**, 107–121 (2017)
21. Ingster, Y.I.: Asymptotic minimax hypothesis testing for nonparametric alternatives. Math. Methods Stat. **2**, 85–114 (1993)
22. Li, Y.: Efficient semiparametric regression for longitudinal data with nonparametric covariance estimation. Biometrika 98, 355–370 (2011)
23. Li, Y., Hsing, T.: Uniform convergence rates for nonparametric regression and principal component analysis in functional/longitudinal data. Ann. Stat. **38**, 3321–3351 (2010)
24. Li, R., Liang, H.: Variable selection in semiparametric regression modeling. Ann. Stat. **36**, 261–286 (2008)
25. Li, Y., Wang, N., Hong, M., Turner, N.D., Lupton, J.R., Carroll, R.J.: Nonparametric estimation of correlation functions in longitudinal and spatial data, with application to colon carcinogenesis experiments. Ann. Stat. **35**(4), 1608–1643 (2007)
26. Li, H., Keadle, S.K., Staudenmayer, J., Assaad, H., Huang, J.Z., Carroll, R.J.: Methods to assess an exercise intervention trial based on 3-level functional data. Biostatistics **16**, 754–771 (2015)
27. Lin, X., Carroll, R.J.: Semiparametric regression for clustered data using generalized estimating equations. J. Am. Stat. Assoc. **96**, 1045–1056 (2001)
28. Liu, Z., Lin, X.: Multiple phenotype association tests using summary statistics in genome-wide association studies. Biometrics **74**, 165–175 (2017)
29. McCullagh, P., Nelder, J.: Generalized linear models. Chapman & Hall, London. 2nd, (1989)
30. Morris, J.S., Carroll, R.J.: Wavelet-based functional mixed models. J. R. Stat. Soc. Ser. B **68**, 179–199 (2006)
31. Pepe, M.S., Couper, D.: Modeling partly conditional means with longitudinal data. J. Am. Stat. Assoc. **92**, 991–998 (1997)
32. Ramsay, J.O., Silverman, B.W.: Functional data analysis, 2nd edn. Springer, New York (2005)
33. Rice, J., Silverman, B.: Estimating the mean and covariance structure nonparametrically when the data are curves. J. R. Stat. Soc. Ser. B. **53**, 233–243 (1991)

34. Schuff, N., Woerner, N., Boreta, L., Kornfield, T., Shaw, L., Trojanowski, J., Thompson, P., Jack Jr, C., Weiner, M., Initiative, A.D.N.: MRI of hippocampal volume loss in early Alzheimer's disease in relation to ApoE genotype and biomarkers. Brain **132**, 1067–1077 (2009)
35. Tang, J., Li, Y., Guan, Y.: Generalized quasi-likelihood ratio tests for semiparametric analysis of covariance models in longitudinal data. J. Am. Stat. Assoc. **111**, 736–747 (2016)
36. Visscher, P.M., Wray, N.R., Zhang, Q., Sklar, P., McCarthy, M.I., Brown, M.A., Yang, J.: 10 years of GWAS discovery: biology, function, and translation. Am. J. Hum. Genet. **101**, 5–22 (2017)
37. Wang, N., Carroll, R.J., Lin, X.: Efficient semiparametric marginal estimation for longitudinal/clustered data. J. Am. Stat. Assoc. **100**, 147–157 (2005)
38. Wu, W.B., Pourahmadi, M.: Nonparametric estimation of large covariance matrices of longitudinal data. Biometrika **90**, 831–844 (2003)
39. Xia, Y., Li, W.K.: Asymptotic behavior of bandwidth selected by cross-validation method under dependence. Journal Multivariate Analysis. **83**, 265–287 (2002)
40. Xu, Y., Li, Y., Nettleton, D.: Nested hierarchical functional data modeling and inference for the analysis of functional plant phenotypes. J. Am. Stat. Assoc. **113**, 593–606 (2018)
41. Yahav, I., Shmueli, G.: On generating multivariate Poisson data in management science applications. Appl. Stoch. Model. Bus. Ind. **28**(1), 91–102 (2012)
42. Yao, F., Müller, H.-G., Wang, J.-L.: Functional data analysis for sparse longitudinal data. J. Am. Stat. Assoc. **100**(470), 577–590 (2005)
43. Zhang, J.T.: Analysis of Variance for Functional Data. CRC Press, New York (2013)
44. Zhang, J.T., Chen, J.W.: Statistical inferences for functional data. Ann. Stat. **35**, 1052–1079 (2007)
45. Zhang, X., Wang, J.L.: From sparse to dense functional data and beyond. Ann. Stat. **44**(5), 2281–2321 (2016)
46. Zhou, L., Huang, J., Martinez, J.G., Maity, A., Baladandayuthapani, V., Carroll, R.J.: Reduced rank mixed effects models for spatially correlated hierarchical functional data. J. Am. Stat. Assoc. **105**, 390–400 (2010)

Mixed-Effects Negative Binomial Regression with Interval Censoring: A Simulation Study and Application to Aridity and All-Cause Mortality Among Black South Africans Over 1997–2013

Christian M. Landon, Robert H. Lyles, Noah C. Scovronick, Azar M. Abadi, Rocky Bilotta, Mathew E. Hauer, Jesse E. Bell, and Matthew O. Gribble

1 Background

In public health research, models with count response variables are often used to describe patterns such as the number of deaths in a defined population, the number of days absent from school or work, the number of alcoholic drinks consumed per day, or the number of bacteria in dilution assays [1]. Poisson regression is a generalized linear model form commonly used to address research questions about counts, with the key assumption that the variance equals the mean and that observations are independent. However, in many areas of research, real-world count data is over-dispersed and may be more adequately described by negative binomial models that assume variance is proportionate, but not necessarily equal, to the mean [2]. Other extensions to the basic Poisson model are often necessitated by quirks of the data-generating processes being studied.

C. M. Landon (✉) · N. C. Scovronick
Department of Environmental Health, Rollins School of Public Health, Emory University, Atlanta, GA, USA
e-mail: cmlando@alumni.emory.edu; scovronick@emory.edu

R. H. Lyles
Department of Biostatistics and Bioinformatics, Rollins School of Public Health, Emory University, Atlanta, GA, USA
e-mail: rlyles@sph.emory.edu

A. M. Abadi · J. E. Bell
Department of Environmental, Agricultural, and Occupational Health, University of Nebraska Medical Center, Omaha, NE, USA
e-mail: azar.abadi@unmc.edu; jesse.bell@unmc.edu

Y. Zhao, (Din) D.-G. Chen (eds.), *Modern Statistical Methods for Health Research*, Emerging Topics in Statistics and Biostatistics,
https://doi.org/10.1007/978-3-030-72437-5_17

Observations in real-world studies are seldom independent; for example, in many surveillance studies, data on event counts are collected repeatedly from the same places over time (e.g., county-years of surveillance). Mixed-effect models account for this hierarchical clustering of observations by estimating an underlying distribution of cluster-specific parameters (e.g., random intercepts representing cluster-specific differences from the grand mean) and fitting the rest of the model (i.e., fixed effects) conditional on these cluster-specific parameters [3].

Censoring of the outcome variable is a frequent complication of applied research [4, 5]. Censoring can arise in applied analyses of count data when events are rare, such as the number of deaths that occur in rural or very small populations. Data administrators (e.g., government agencies) often censor the precise number of events in order to protect the privacy of persons who experienced those events [6], providing data analysts only with an interval within which the correct number of counts is contained. When the probability of censoring is related to the underlying exposure-outcome dose-response, this is an example of informative missingness and can introduce bias if unaddressed [7]. Statistical methods exist to account for this censoring process directly [8, 9].

Mixed-effects Poisson and negative binomial regression models accounting for censoring of counts were used previously in a few applications [6, 10], but assessment of the performance of interval censored mixed-effects negative binomial regression models, vis-à-vis simplified alternatives, and versus mixed-effects negative binomial regression models fitted to uncensored complete data, remains to be explored.

The objective of this simulation study is to assess the performance of these methods, regarding the bias in parameter estimates and standard errors, the 95% confidence interval coverage, the statistical power, and the type I error rates. The contrasts between these approaches are then further illustrated using real-world data on aridity and monthly mortality rates among black South Africans over 1997–2013.

R. Bilotta
National Oceanic and Atmospheric Administration's National Centers for Environmental Information and ISciences, L.L.C., Asheville, NC, USA
e-mail: rocky.bilotta@noaa.gov

M. E. Hauer
Department of Sociology, College of Social Sciences and Public Policy, Florida State University, Tallahassee, FL, USA
e-mail: mehauer@fsu.edu

M. O. Gribble
Department of Environmental Health, Rollins School of Public Health, Emory University, Atlanta, GA, USA

Department of Epidemiology, Rollins School of Public Health, Emory University, Atlanta, GA, USA
e-mail: matt.gribble@emory.edu

2 Methods

2.1 Simulation

We developed a macro for SAS 9.4 software (SAS, Cary, NC) to conduct the simulations. The SAS IML ("interactive matrix language") procedure is utilized within the macro to create the matrices and variables and to set the parameter values for the simulations. In this study, we ran 1000 simulations for each set of explored parameter values, including the baseline log-count (β_0), the variance of the random intercept reflecting differences in baseline log-counts (σ^2), the effect of the exposure on the outcome (β_1), the effect of the covariate on the outcome (β_2), the negative binomial dispersion factor (α), the number of counties (K), and the number of study-years (N), resulting in 140,000 total simulations.

In order to examine how the models' performance was influenced by sample size, five possible combinations of cluster-years were considered. We will refer to the cluster-years as county-years throughout this paper as an aesthetic simplification because longitudinal count data are collected with county as the study unit in relevant motivating studies. The number of counties in our simulations ranged from 10 to 500, and the number of years of observation per county ranged from 10 to 20 years. This resulted in a range of simulations with a minimum of 100 county-years and a maximum of 10,000 county-years. The combinations of county-years considered in this simulation study are described in Table 1.

A uniformly distributed variable (X_{ij}) ranging from 0 to 10 was generated as the primary independent variable ("exposure") for the simulations. A uniformly distributed covariate (Z_j) ranging from 1 to 20 was also generated. The outcome variable in the simulations was a negative binomial count variable. Collectively, these results are expressed in the following linear predictive form:

$$\ln\left(\mu_{ij}\right) = (\beta_0 + b_{0i}) + \beta_1 X_{ij} + \beta_2 Z_j$$

which varies slightly across models and is further detailed in the subsequent section.

Data were simulated under seven true values of β_1 (the fixed effect of continuous exposure on the outcome): −0.30, −0.20, −0.10, 0.01, 0.10 0.20, and 0.30. The remaining parameters were held constant with β_0 (the log-scale mean of the outcome when the exposure and covariate values are at zero) = 2.25, $\sigma^2 = 0.05$, $\beta_2 = 0$, and $\alpha = 0.25$. This resulted in the following combinations of true parameter values for simulation across the different county-year levels:

$$\beta_0 = 2.25, \beta_1 = -0.30, \beta_2 = 0.00, \alpha = 0.25, \sigma^2 = 0.05.$$

$$\beta_0 = 2.25, \beta_1 = -0.20, \beta_2 = 0.00, \alpha = 0.25, \sigma^2 = 0.05.$$

Table 1 Simulation design and sample size

True β_1: 0.01				True β_1: 0.10			
K	N	K*N	Simulations	K	N	K*N	Simulations
10	10	100	4000	10	10	100	4000
50	10	500	4000	50	10	500	4000
50	20	1000	4000	50	20	1000	4000
250	20	5000	4000	250	20	5000	4000
500	20	10,000	4000	500	20	10,000	4000
True β_1: 0.20				True β_1: 0.30			
K	N	K*N	Simulations	K	N	K*N	Simulations
10	10	100	4000	10	10	100	4000
50	10	500	4000	50	10	500	4000
50	20	1000	4000	50	20	1000	4000
250	20	5000	4000	250	20	5000	4000
500	20	10,000	4000	500	20	10,000	4000
True β_1: −0.10				True β_1: −0.20			
K	N	K*N	Simulations	K	N	K*N	Simulations
10	10	100	4000	10	10	100	4000
50	10	500	4000	50	10	500	4000
50	20	1000	4000	50	20	1000	4000
250	20	5000	4000	250	20	5000	4000
500	20	10,000	4000	500	20	10,000	4000
True β_1: −0.30							
K	N	K*N	Simulations				
10	10	100	4000	Where K represents the number of counties, N represents the number of years that counties were observed, and K*N represents the number of county-years (sample size)			
50	10	500	4000				
50	20	1000	4000				
250	20	5000	4000				
500	20	10,000	4000				

$$\beta_0 = 2.25, \beta_1 = -0.10, \beta_2 = 0.00, \alpha = 0.25, \sigma^2 = 0.05.$$

$$\beta_0 = 2.25, \beta_1 = 0.01, \beta_2 = 0.00, \alpha = 0.25, \sigma^2 = 0.05.$$

$$\beta_0 = 2.25, \beta_1 = 0.10, \beta_2 = 0.00, \alpha = 0.25, \sigma^2 = 0.05.$$

$$\beta_0 = 2.25, \beta_1 = 0.20, \beta_2 = 0.00, \alpha = 0.25, \sigma^2 = 0.05.$$

$$\beta_0 = 2.25, \beta_1 = 0.30, \beta_2 = 0.00, \alpha = 0.25, \sigma^2 = 0.05.$$

Statistical Analysis of Simulated Data

Model 1 was a mixed-effects negative binomial regression of the following form fit to the complete simulated dataset

$$\ln\left(\mu_{ij}\right) = (\beta_0 + b_{0i}) + \beta_1 X_{ij} + \beta_2 Z_j$$

where X_{ij} was the exposure for county (or district) i in year j, Z_j was the covariate, and (b_{0i}) was a normally distributed random intercept. Model 1 used the following likelihood contribution for county i in year j:

$$\Pr\left(Y_{ij} = y_{ij} | X_{ij} = x_{ij}, Z_j = z_j\right) = \frac{\Gamma\left(\alpha^{-1} + y_{ij}\right)}{\Gamma\left(\alpha^{-1}\right) y_{ij}!}\left(\frac{\alpha\mu_{ij}}{1+\alpha\mu_{ij}}\right)^{y_{ij}}\left(\frac{1}{1+\alpha\mu_{ij}}\right)^{\frac{1}{\alpha}}$$

In our simulations and data analysis, we set the covariate Z_j equal to j, that is, the time-varying covariate was identically equal to the year.

Model 2 had a similar linear predictive form, and when the outcome (Y_{ij}) was not censored (counts of 0 or $\geq$ 10), the same likelihood contribution was used. However, $\Pr\left(Y_{ij} = y_{ij} | X_{ij} = x_{ij}, Z = z\right) = \frac{\Gamma(\alpha^{-1}+y_{ij})}{\Gamma(\alpha^{-1})y_{ij}!}\left(\frac{\alpha\mu_{ij}}{1+\alpha\mu_{ij}}\right)^{y_{ij}}\left(\frac{1}{1+\alpha\mu_{ij}}\right)^{\frac{1}{\alpha}}$ when the number of outcomes was in the censoring window [1–9], the conditional likelihood contribution became

$$\Pr\left(1 \leq Y_{ij} \leq 9 | b_{0i}, X_{ij}, Z_j\right)$$

based on the negative binomial model.

We used the SAS NLMIXED procedure to specify this log-likelihood conditional on the random effects. Taking advantage of the recursive properties of the gamma function, contributions for the censored outcomes were specified, and the indicator for outcomes existing within the censoring window was defined within the procedure.

Model 3 had the same likelihood contribution as Models 1 and 2 when outcome counts were 0 or $\geq$ 10, but when the number of events was in the censoring window [1,9], Y_{ij} was set to 5. This analytic approach is equivalent to deterministic imputation of censored counts by a count in the middle of the censoring window.

Model 4 accounted for censoring but not for the hierarchical structure of the data, and therefore its linear predictive form and conditional likelihood contribution were slightly different from the other models. The linear predictive form failed to account for the random intercept, dropping b_{0i} from the equation

$$\ln\left(\mu_{ij}\right) = \beta_0 + \beta_1 X_{ij} + \beta_2 Z_j$$

and when the number of outcomes was in the censoring window [1–9], the likelihood contribution was

Table 2 Model descriptions and forms

Model	Form	Description
1	$\ln(\mu_{ij}){=}(\beta_0 + b_{0i}) + \beta_1 X_{ij} + \beta_2 Z_j$ $\Pr\left(Y_{ij} = y_{ij} \vert b_{0i}, X_{ij}, Z_j\right) =$ $\frac{\Gamma(\alpha^{-1}+y_{ij})}{\Gamma(\alpha^{-1})y_{ij}!}\left(\frac{\alpha\mu_{ij}}{1+\alpha\mu_{ij}}\right)^{y_{ij}}\left(\frac{1}{1+\alpha\mu_{ij}}\right)^{\frac{1}{\alpha}}$	Mixed negative binomial model and likelihood contribution for county i in year j
2	$\ln(\mu_{ij}) = (\beta_0 + b_{0i}) + \beta_1 X_{ij} + \beta_2 Z_j$ If Y_{ij}observed : Same as model 1 If Y_{ij} censored : $\Pr\left(1 \leq Y_{ij} \leq 9 \vert\, b_{0i}, X_{ij}, Z_j\right)$	Interval censored (on deaths 1–9) mixed-effects negative binomial model and conditional likelihood contribution
3	$\ln(\mu_{ij}){=}(\beta_0 + b_{0i}) + \beta_1 X_{ij} + \beta_2 Z_j$ If $\mathrm{Y_{ij}}$observed : Same as model 1 If Y_{ij} censored : Same as model 1 with Y_{ij} set to 5	Midpoint imputed mixed-effects negative binomial model and conditional likelihood contribution
4	$\ln(\mu_{ij}) = \beta_0 + \beta_1 X_{ij} + \beta_2 Z_j$ If Y_{ij} observed : Same as model 1 with $b_{0i} = 0$ If Y_{ij} censored : $\Pr\left(1 \leq Y_{ij} \leq 9 \vert\, X_{ij}, Z_j\right)$	Interval censored (on deaths 1–9) fixed-effects negative binomial model and conditional likelihood contribution

$$\Pr\left(1 \leq Y_{ij} \leq 9 \vert\, X_{ij}, Z_j\right)$$

A summary of all the model forms and likelihood contributions can be found in Table 2.

Simulation Summaries

Applying these four models to the simulated datasets for each set of parameter values generated a set of 1000 β_1 estimates and 1000 β_1 standard errors of those estimates per approach for each data-generating process. The SAS MEANS procedure was applied to this distribution of β_1 estimates and distribution of β_1 standard errors to obtain the averages of those estimates for each modeling approach, applied to data from each data-generating process.

Confidence intervals (CIs) with intended 95% coverage for β_1 estimates were calculated under normality assumptions. Confidence interval coverage was calculated as the percentage of the 1000 simulations wherein the confidence intervals generated within each dataset contained the true data-generating parameter value β_1. Statistical power was calculated as the percentage of the 1000 simulations wherein the confidence intervals excluded zero. Both these conditions were tabulated using the SAS FREQ procedure.

The percentage bias of each β_1 parameter estimate was obtained by calculating the absolute value of the difference between the true value of β_1 and the estimated β_1, dividing by the true β_1, and then multiplying by 100 to express as a percentage. The SAS Compare procedure was used to perform this calculation.

Type I error rates were calculated as the percentage of the simulations, under a given set of parameter values where the true β_1 was 0, wherein the confidence intervals generated within each dataset excluded 0. The SAS FREQ procedure was used to tally the number of times per set of 1000 simulations that this condition was met.

2.2 *South African Data Analysis*

Mortality Data

District-level monthly mortality data for black South Africans was provided by Statistics South Africa, the country's national statistical service. The mortality dataset is from the civil registration system and is estimated to be ~89% to ~ 94% complete during the study period of January 1, 1997, to December 31, 2013 [11, 12]. This resulted in a total sample size of 10,608 district-months. Population estimates of black South Africans at risk of contributing to mortality outcomes were based on linear interpolation for census years 1996, 2001, and 2011 and linear extrapolation for 2011–2013 based on the period 1996–2011.

Standardized Precipitation Index

The primary exposure variable in the South African dataset was the Standardized Precipitation Index (SPI). The SPI characterizes local relative aridity over a defined timescale. Different timescales of the SPI distinguish different types of drought conditions, such as short-term changes in precipitation (~1-month SPI), changes in soil water content (3–6-month SPI), and longer-term variations in groundwater storage (>12-month SPI). For this study, a 6-month timescale was used as an indicator of climatological drought conditions [13]. SPI quantifies observed precipitation as a departure from the expected precipitation given the historical record for a given region. Historical precipitation data are typically fitted to a gamma or a Pearson Type III distribution, and then transformed to a normal distribution [14]. SPI values can be interpreted as the number of standard deviations by which the observed anomaly deviates from the long-term mean. The dataset used for our analysis included 6-month SPI values for every district in South Africa as a monthly time-series. SPI values were generated using gridded monthly precipitation data from the Global Precipitation Climatology Centre. Gridded SPI values were assigned to each district using an area-weighted average approach [15]. The 6-month SPI values ranged from -3 to 3, with values above 0 representing increasingly wet conditions and values below 0 representing increasingly dry conditions compared to the local historical average. The 6-month SPI was treated as a continuous variable for the main analysis but also coded as increasingly dry quartiles for a sensitivity analysis.

Model Specification and Statistical Analysis

Models analogous to Models 1–4 in the simulation study were fitted to the South African aridity and mortality dataset. These models had the following general linear predictive form:

$$\ln\left(\mu_{ij}\right) = (\beta_0 + b_{0i}) + \beta_1 X_{ij} + \beta_2 Z_j + f_{ij}$$

where SPI was the exposure variable (X_{ij}), the covariate ($Z_j = j$) was the 17-year time period variable, and the offset f_{ij} reflected the ln(population) of each district at risk of developing mortality events for each month during the study period. The linear predictive forms and likelihood contributions of the four models were akin to those in the simulation study described in Table 2, but with an offset term added.

In contrast to the simulation study, the true value for the effect of the exposure (SPI) on mortality is not known. As a result, the β_1 estimate from Model 1, based on complete data, is used as the basis for comparison for the β_1 estimates obtained from Models 2–4, which treat some of the outcomes as censored or imputed. The SAS procedure GLIMMIX was used to obtain plausible initial values for the negative binomial parameters used in the PARMS statement of the SAS NLMIXED procedure.

In addition to the main analysis modeling SPI as a continuous linear predictor, a sensitivity analysis was conducted to confirm that a linear dose-response was adequate. For this, the SPI variable was transformed into quartiles to allow for a possibly nonlinear dose-response. The SAS procedure GLIMMIX was used to obtain the β_1 regression parameter estimates corresponding to the SPI quartiles in this sensitivity analysis. Model results were visualized using ggplot2 package [16] in the R programming language [17]. Only Model 1 was used to conduct the sensitivity analysis since it was the only model that analyzes the complete uncensored dataset.

3 Results

3.1 Simulation Study

All simulation results were displayed in Figs. 1 and 2 and Appendix 1. When $\beta_1 = -0.30$, all the models had similar performances with the exception of Model 3. Average percent bias of the β_1 parameter estimate for Models 1, 2, and 4 ranged from 0.22% to 0.36%. However, Model 3 presented an average percent bias of 52.56% while having the smallest average standard error (0.010). Models 1, 2, and 4 had empirical confidence interval coverage that was similar to the desired coverage level. Model 3 had negligible confidence interval coverage (0.04%), compared to 93.90%, 94.40%, and 94.30% for Models 1, 2, and 4, respectively. Statistical power was ~100% for all models at all sample sizes.

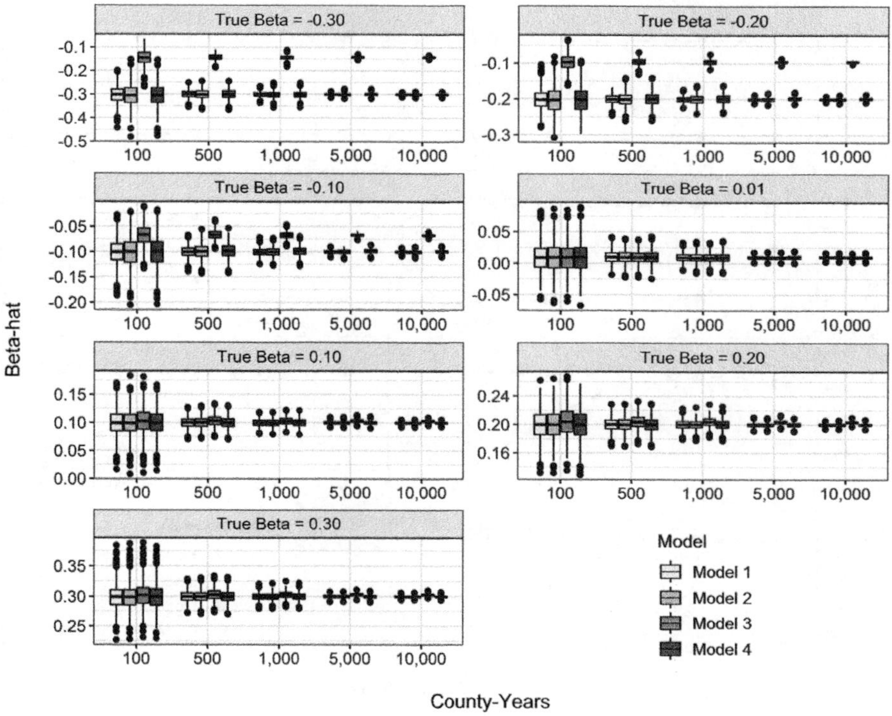

Fig. 1 Simulated boxplots estimating the effect of the exposure (β_1) on the outcome. Models 1–4 are displayed numerically from left to right at each level of county-year and true beta value

When $\beta_1 = -0.20$ similar results were obtained. The mean percent bias was small for Model 1 (0.17%), Model 2 (0.32%), and Model 4 (0.81%), whereas Model 3 had an average percent bias of 52.32% and the smallest standard error (0.008). Model 3 failed to achieve acceptable confidence interval coverage, with an average coverage of 0.10% across county-year sample sizes, compared to 94.2% for Model 1, 94.7% for Model 2, and 93.8% for Model 4. Statistical power was greater than 99% for all models at all sample sizes.

When $\beta_1 = -0.10$, Model 3 had a lower percent bias (33.32%) than at β_1 values of -0.30 and -0.20 yet was still far more biased at $\beta_1 = -0.10$ than Model 1 (0.25%), Model 2 (0.40%), or Model 4 (1.53%). Model 3 had the smallest average standard error size across county-year sample sizes (0.007) compared to Model 1 (0.009), Model 2 (0.012), and Model 4 (0.012). Model 3 continued to yield poor confidence interval coverage, averaging 11% coverage across all county-year sample sizes. Models 1, 2, and 4 achieved more reasonable confidence interval coverage across all county year sample sizes, with mean coverage ranging from 93% to 95%. At 100 county-years, statistical power ranged from 93% to 99%; however, 100% power was reached for all models once the sample size was increased.

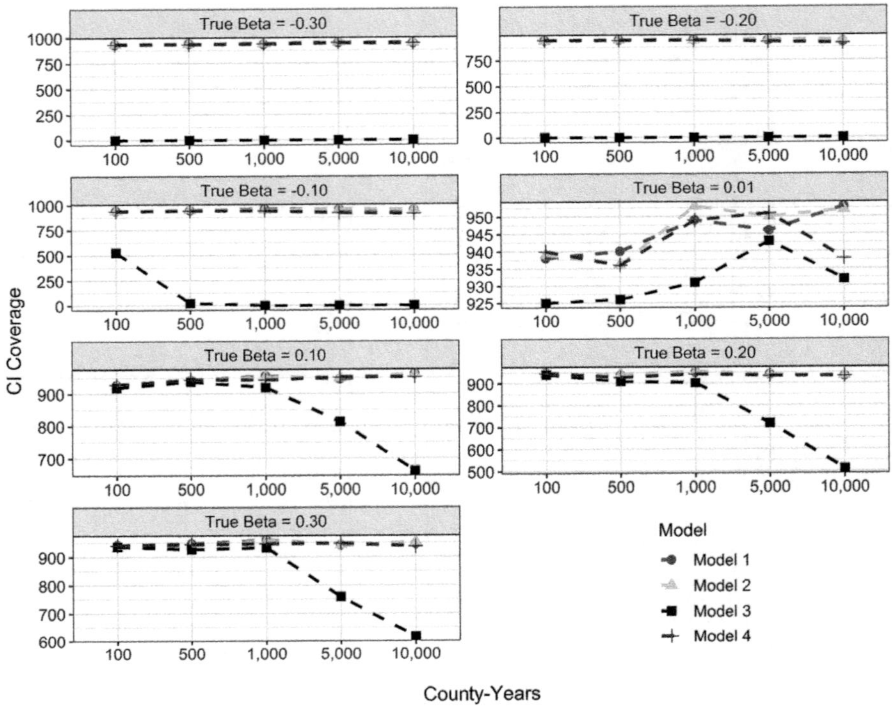

Fig. 2 Line plots displaying β_1 confidence interval coverage per 1000 simulations. Confidence intervals (CIs) with intended 95% coverage for β_1 estimates were calculated under normality assumptions. CI coverage is displayed as the frequency of the 1000 simulations wherein the confidence intervals generated within each dataset contained the true data-generating parameter value β_1

When $\beta_1 = 0.01$, differences between the models became less apparent. Model 3 had an average percent bias of 2.31% across all county-year sample sizes, which was similar to Model 1 (2.19%), Model 2 (1.34%), and Model 4 (0.83%). Model 3 presented the smallest average standard error size across county-year sample sizes (0.008) but was similar to a mean standard error of 0.009 for each of Models, 1, 2, and 4. The confidence interval coverage ranged from 93% to 95% across all county-year sample sizes, across the four models. Power varied from ~8% to ~99% depending on sample size.

When β_1 was set to 0.10, this resulted in mean percent biases of 0.06% (Model 1), 0.07% (Model 2), 3.22% (Model 3), and 0.15% (Model 4). Models 1–3 had an average standard error size of 0.008 across county-year sample sizes, whereas Model 4 had an average standard error size of 0.009. Mean confidence interval coverage ranged from 94% to 95% for Models 1, 2, and 4. Model 3 achieved 91–94% coverage until the larger county-year sample sizes of 5000 and 10,000, where coverage proceeded to decline to 81.3% and 66.1%, respectively. Statistical power was greater than or equal to 99% across all models and county-year sample sizes.

Increasing β_1 to 0.20 resulted in Model 3 having the largest percent bias (2.13%), observed at 1000 county-years. All four models presented an average standard error size of 0.008 across county-year sample sizes. Confidence interval coverage for Models 1, 2, and 4 ranged from 92% to 95% for every county-year sample size with Model 2 having the highest mean confidence interval coverage across all of the county-years out of the models. Model 3 reached coverage levels of approximately 90–94% until the simulations at 5000 and 10,000 county-years, where coverage dropped to 71.80% and 51.20%, respectively. Power was ~100% for all models at all sample sizes.

When $\beta_1 = 0.30$, Models 1, 2, and 4 had percent biases below 0.25% at every county-year sample size, and Model 3 had slightly more bias (0.82% being the minimum and 1.10% being the maximum). Models 1, 2, and 4 had confidence interval coverages ranging from 94% to 95%. Model 3 achieved peak coverage at 100 county-years (93.7%) but then declined to 75.9% and 61.7% at the county-year sample sizes of 5000 and 10,000, respectively. Power was ~100% for all models at all sample sizes.

All models had similar type I error rates (4–5%). Model 3 had the highest type I error rate of 6.10% at 100 county-years, and Model 1 had the lowest with 3.90% at 1000 county-years.

In order to explore the effect of increased between-county variance (σ^2) on model performance, additional simulations were conducted post hoc. In these simulations, all the parameter values were the same as the primary simulation study when $\beta_1 = -0.30$, except σ^2 was increased from 0.05 to 1.00 and only a county-year sample size of 1000 was explored. Under these conditions, Models 1 and 2 had percent biases below 0.13%, Model 3 had a bias of 38.63%, and Model 4 exhibited an increased bias of 3.04%. Models 1 and 2 achieved confidence interval coverage ranging from 94% to 95%, Model 3 had negligible confidence interval coverage (0.0%), and Model 4 displayed decreased confidence interval coverage (84.2%). Complete results and model parameters are described in Appendix 1, Table 7.

3.2 *Aridity and Mortality Among Black South Africans*

The approximate population size of the districts in the South African dataset ranged from 3370 to 3,594,087 persons, with a mean of 720,993 over the study period. In models relating the numbers of deaths per district-month to aridity (Fig. 3), Model 1 estimated a rate ratio of 0.96 (95% CI 0.95, 0.97), Model 2 estimated a rate ratio of 0.96 (95% CI 0.95, 0.97), Model 3 estimated a rate ratio of 0.96 (95% CI 0.95, 0.97), and Model 4 produced an estimated rate ratio of 0.97 (95% CI 0.96, 0.98) after adjusting for possible linear temporal trends. The estimated rate ratios presented correspond to a one-unit increase of 6-month SPI.

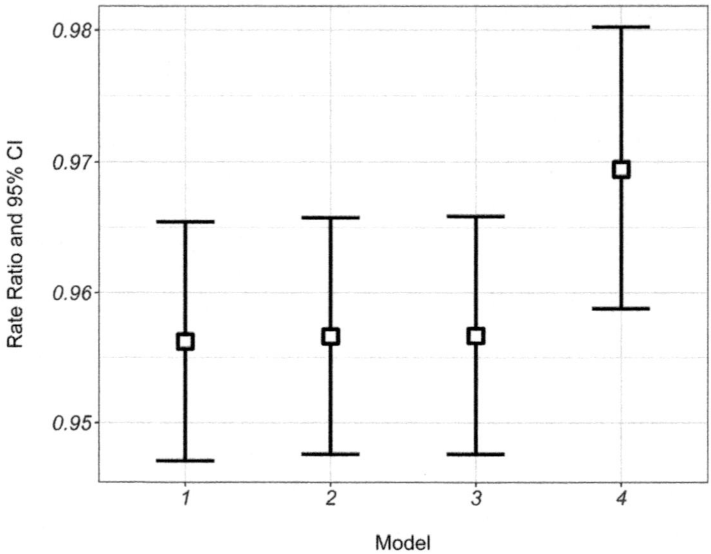

Fig. 3 Overall model results from the association between aridity (SPI) and mortality among black South Africans from 1997 to 2013, adjusting for possible linear temporal trends

In a sensitivity analysis for possible nonlinearity of the dose-response using mixed-effects negative binomial regression fitted to the complete dataset (Fig. 4), there was a monotonic dose-response of increasing mortality with increasingly drought-like conditions. After adjusting for possible linear temporal trends, comparing the second-wettest quartile of district-months to the wettest quartile of district-months resulted in a mortality rate ratio of 1.02, (95% CI 1.00, 1.04). Comparing the second-driest quartile of district-months to the wettest quartile of district-months resulted in a mortality rate ratio of 1.05 (95% CI 1.03, 1.07). Contrasting the driest quartile of district-months against the wettest quartile of district months resulted in a mortality rate ratio of 1.11 (95% CI 1.09, 1.13). Thus, a linear model for the dose-response appears to be a reasonable, if reductionist, summary of the dose-response association of mortality with 6-month SPI.

4 Discussion

The simulation study indicates that these models perform similarly at a true β_1 value of 0.01. However, when the true β_1 value was increased or decreased across the different sets of simulations, differences in the models' performances became more apparent. Here, Model 3 begins to be increasingly influenced by differential

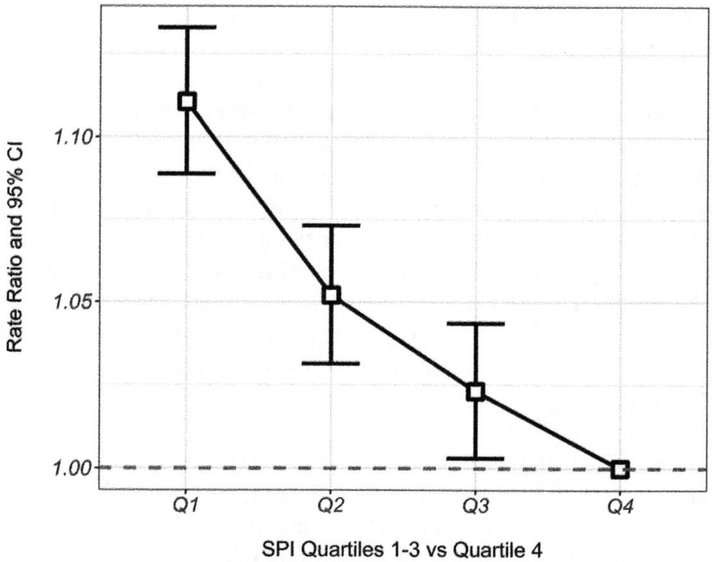

Fig. 4 Sensitivity analysis results for the association between aridity (SPI) and mortality among black South Africans from 1997 to 2013, adjusting for possible linear temporal trends. The wettest period (Q4) was used as the reference against increasingly drier periods (Q1 being the driest). Because Model 1 was the only model that analyzes the complete, uncensored dataset, only it was explored for the sensitivity analysis

measurement error of outcome by exposure, resulting in the large percent bias observed. When there is a true positive association between the exposure and outcome, as the exposure increases, the number of events in a county should increase. As a result, counties at higher levels of exposure will have fewer events in the censoring interval, and Model 3 may require relatively little imputation. When the true dose-response is negative, then there are more censored counts among the more exposed than among the less exposed. If after censoring the outcomes are imputed with error, as in Model 3, then the differential measurement error in outcomes by exposure will contribute to information bias in dose-response estimates [18], as was observed when Model 3 was applied to data simulated under the β_1 true values of −0.30, −0.20, and −0.10. Model 3 also had negligible confidence interval coverage, and falsely small standard error sizes, under a variety of simulated conditions, likely due to the decreased variation in the imputed outcomes compared to the true variability in the uncensored count data. In the simulations exploring the effects of increased random-effects variance between counties (σ^2), Model 4s confidence interval coverage decreased as the σ^2 parameter values increased; in contrast, Models 1 and 2, which accounted for the structure of the data hierarchy, performed well.

The application of these models to the real-world dataset suggests a significant association between 6-month SPI and all-cause mortality rates among black South Africans. The positive association of aridity with mortality rates is a potentially important finding for public health and should be investigated further in follow-up substantive research. Aridity could affect health outcomes in South Africa through several pathways. Alteration in the rainfall pattern and the change in the temperature may have a significant impact on the agricultural sector and crop and livestock production, potentially causing food insecurity and malnutrition [19–21]. A study on the 1973 drought in the Sahelian region showed that there were more than 100,000 human deaths, and up to 40% of the livestock died, as a result of the prolonged drought [22]. Droughts may also contribute to water-borne diseases such as cholera and dysentery as a consequence of diminished water availability and quality [23, 24]. Drought and warmer conditions may also change disease vector populations and intensify the spread of vector-borne diseases such as malaria, tick-borne diseases, Rift Valley fever, and dengue [25–28]. In addition to these potential mechanisms for elevated mortality, droughts could potentially also contribute to population displacement and respiratory issues driven by desert dust [29, 30]. Additional research is needed to investigate possible mechanisms underlying the observed positive associations in this preliminary study and to exclude other possible confounding explanations distinct from drought.

Understanding the salience of climatic conditions for health in South Africa is especially important in the context of climate change. Mean temperature has increased much faster in South Africa compared to the global average, and this trend is expected to continue [31]. Much of the African continent, including in Southern Africa, is expected to shift to a drier climate as the century progresses due to accelerated evaporation from drier soils in hotter weather [31]. Although a few studies have linked daily temperature to adverse health outcomes [32, 33], the relationship of drought to health outcomes in South Africa is largely unknown. Our findings from this preliminary analysis are consistent with droughts contributing to excess mortality in black South Africans; further research is needed.

The South African data analysis highlighted conditions when different modeling approaches perform well or poorly. Model 3, which accounted for the data hierarchy while imputing censored values, had a similar performance to the Model 1 analysis of complete data, but Model 4, which ignored the hierarchical structure of the data, had greater β_1 estimation bias. This likely occurred due to the limited number of censored observations in the South African dataset, reducing the impact of censored-value imputation error, and large between-district variance of the outcome observed in the South African data.

Few studies have examined the performance of mixed-effect negative binomial models with interval censoring. Similar models have been employed in research conducted by Bartell and Lewandowski [6] and Quiroz et al. [10], but to our knowledge, this is the first study to compare interval censored mixed-effect negative binomial models' performance versus mixed-effects models with deterministic imputation of censored values and versus censored regression models without random effects. Our simulation study provides insights beyond the guidance of Bartell and Lewandowski [6] regarding when deterministic imputation of censored outcomes is problematic. Their study suggested that the information bias from deterministic imputation is negligible when two conditions were met: (1) few observations were below the censoring cutoff, and (2) the censoring cutoff was relatively small compared to most of the measurements. We found out that these two conditions are not necessary for low bias, because in our simulations where $\beta_1 = 0.01$, the imputation resulted in negligible bias, even with 50% of the data falling within the censoring interval. Our findings indicate that additional considerations beyond the censoring process influence the information bias introduced by deterministic imputation of censored outcomes. Despite the largest percentage of outcomes in our simulations being censored when β_0 was 2.25 and β_1 was -0.10 (77 to 82 percent depending upon sample size), there was greater bias under Model 3 for true β_1 values of -0.20 and -0.30. Under more extreme dose-response functions, study units with extreme exposure values will on average have greater divergence between their imputed outcome and their true outcome, resulting in a differential measurement error that scales with the strength of the true dose-response. In summary, the true data-generating process and the investigator's decision about which value to use for deterministic imputation, rather than only the particulars of the censoring process, may impact the information bias resulting from deterministic imputation-based analysis.

Even though this study included 140,000 simulated datasets, and illustrated the issues through analysis of a real-world dataset, this project was still somewhat limited in its scope. We considered two methods commonly used in applied research (i.e., censored negative binomial regression and multilevel negative binomial regression with deterministic imputation of censored outcomes) and a comparison method (i.e., interval-censored mixed-effects negative binomial regression) but did not consider the performance of other potentially appropriate comparison techniques such as mixed-effects negative binomial models with multiple imputation of censored values. We also considered a limited range of censoring window sizes, as our current implementation of the simulation code makes it cumbersome to expand the censoring interval to a much larger size (see Appendix 2). For future research, taking advantage of recursive properties or arrays within the SAS procedure NLMIXED or its analogues in other software could simplify this issue and allow for examination of larger censoring intervals.

When working with real data, as with the South Africa dataset, the true effect of exposure on outcome is not known. In our study we used analysis of the complete dataset as an approximation for the true association; however, this association could be affected by issues such as unmeasured confounding, and there may not be a true underlying relationship between aridity and mortality rates for black South Africans. Future epidemiological research is needed on the topic of aridity and mortality in South Africa. Additionally, we used a linear extrapolation model for estimating the black South African population at risk of dying. Errors in the estimates for the population at risk of mortality in each district would influence the district-month-specific offsets, which could affect estimation of district-level random intercepts, and thereby possibly the jointly estimated fixed effect for mean slope conditional on district-level baseline rates. Future research focused on unbiased estimation of the effects of aridity on mortality rates in South Africa might consider sensitivity analyses with alternative approaches for estimation of the populations at risk.

5 Conclusion

Interval-censored mixed-effects negative binomial regression performs well when there is both censoring and strong hierarchical structure in the count outcome data. This approach may be useful in epidemiological research with longitudinal datasets that involve interval-censored exposures.

Acknowledgments We thank Statistics South Africa for supplying the mortality data. Statistics South Africa had no role in the design, data analysis, or interpretation of this study.

Appendix 1: Simulation Results

Table 3 Maximum likelihood estimates and standard errors

Mean β_1 maximum likelihood estimates and standard errors: negative beta values									
County-years	True β_1	Model 1		Model 2		Model 3		Model 4	
		MLE	S.E.	MLE	S.E.	MLE	S.E.	MLE	S.E.
100	−0.30	−0.303	0.033	−0.304	0.044	−0.144	0.025	−0.304	0.043
500	−0.30	−0.300	0.015	−0.300	0.019	−0.142	0.011	−0.300	0.019
1000	−0.30	−0.300	0.010	−0.301	0.013	−0.142	0.008	−0.300	0.013
5000	−0.30	−0.300	0.005	−0.300	0.006	−0.142	0.003	−0.299	0.006
10,000	−0.30	−0.300	0.003	−0.300	0.004	−0.142	0.002	−0.300	0.004
Mean	−0.30	**−0.301**	**0.013**	**−0.301**	**0.017**	**−0.142**	**0.010**	**−0.301**	**0.017**
100	−0.20	−0.201	0.027	−0.202	0.038	−0.096	0.021	−0.201	0.038
500	−0.20	−0.200	0.012	−0.201	0.017	−0.095	0.009	−0.199	0.017
1000	−0.20	−0.200	0.009	−0.200	0.012	−0.095	0.006	−0.198	0.012
5000	−0.20	−0.200	0.004	−0.200	0.005	−0.095	0.003	−0.198	0.005
10,000	−0.20	−0.200	0.003	−0.200	0.004	−0.095	0.002	−0.198	0.004
Mean	−0.20	**−0.200**	**0.011**	**−0.201**	**0.015**	**−0.095**	**0.008**	**−0.199**	**0.015**
100	−0.10	−0.101	0.023	−0.101	0.029	−0.067	0.018	−0.101	0.029
500	−0.10	−0.100	0.011	−0.100	0.013	−0.066	0.008	−0.098	0.013
1000	−0.10	−0.100	0.007	−0.100	0.009	−0.067	0.006	−0.098	0.009
5000	−0.10	−0.100	0.003	−0.100	0.004	−0.067	0.003	−0.098	0.004
10,000	−0.10	−0.100	0.002	−0.100	0.003	−0.067	0.002	−0.098	0.003
Mean	−0.10	**−0.100**	**0.009**	**−0.100**	**0.012**	**−0.067**	**0.007**	**−0.099**	**0.012**

Model 1 (Mixed-effects negative binomial model). Model 2 (Interval censored (on outcomes 1–9) mixed-effects negative binomial model). Model 3 (Midpoint imputed mixed-effects negative binomial model). Model 4 (Interval censored (on outcomes 1–9) fixed-effects negative binomial model)

(continued)

Table 3 (continued)

Mean β_1 maximum likelihood estimates and standard errors: positive beta values

County-years	True β_1	Model 1		Model 2		Model 3		Model 4	
		MLE	S.E.	MLE	S.E.	MLE	S.E.	MLE	S.E.
100	0.01	0.010	0.021	0.010	0.022	0.010	0.021	0.010	0.023
500	0.01	0.010	0.010	0.010	0.010	0.010	0.009	0.010	0.010
1000	0.01	0.010	0.007	0.010	0.007	0.010	0.007	0.010	0.007
5000	0.01	0.010	0.003	0.010	0.003	0.010	0.003	0.010	0.003
10,000	0.01	0.010	0.002	0.010	0.002	0.010	0.002	0.010	0.002
Mean	0.01	**0.010**	**0.009**	**0.010**	**0.009**	**0.010**	**0.008**	**0.010**	**0.009**
100	0.10	0.100	0.020	0.099	0.021	0.103	0.021	0.099	0.021
500	0.10	0.100	0.009	0.100	0.009	0.103	0.009	0.100	0.010
1000	0.10	0.100	0.006	0.100	0.006	0.103	0.007	0.100	0.007
5000	0.10	0.100	0.003	0.100	0.003	0.103	0.003	0.100	0.003
10,000	0.10	0.100	0.002	0.100	0.002	0.103	0.002	0.100	0.002
Mean	0.10	**0.100**	**0.008**	**0.100**	**0.008**	**0.103**	**0.008**	**0.100**	**0.009**
100	0.20	0.200	0.020	0.200	0.020	0.204	0.020	0.200	0.021
500	0.20	0.200	0.009	0.200	0.009	0.204	0.009	0.200	0.009
1000	0.20	0.200	0.006	0.200	0.006	0.204	0.006	0.200	0.007
5000	0.20	0.200	0.003	0.200	0.003	0.204	0.003	0.200	0.003
10,000	0.20	0.200	0.002	0.200	0.002	0.204	0.002	0.200	0.002
Mean	0.20	**0.200**	**0.008**	**0.200**	**0.008**	**0.204**	**0.008**	**0.200**	**0.008**
100	0.30	0.299	0.019	0.299	0.020	0.302	0.020	0.300	0.020
500	0.30	0.300	0.009	0.300	0.009	0.303	0.009	0.300	0.009
1000	0.30	0.300	0.006	0.300	0.006	0.303	0.006	0.300	0.006
5000	0.30	0.300	0.003	0.300	0.003	0.303	0.003	0.300	0.003
10,000	0.30	0.300	0.002	0.300	0.002	0.303	0.002	0.300	0.002
Mean	0.30	**0.300**	**0.008**	**0.300**	**0.008**	**0.303**	**0.008**	**0.300**	**0.008**

Model 1 (Mixed-effects negative binomial model). Model 2 (Interval censored (on outcomes 1–9) mixed-effects negative binomial model). Model 3 (Midpoint imputed mixed-effects negative binomial model). Model 4 (Interval censored (on outcomes 1–9) fixed-effects negative binomial model)

Table 4 Confidence interval performance and statistical power

Results for β_1 mean confidence interval performance and statistical power: true values of −0.30 and −0.20

County-years	True β_1	CI coverage	Power	CI coverage	Power
		Model 1		Model 2	
100	−0.30	93.3	100.0	93.7	99.9
500	−0.30	94.0	100.0	93.9	100.0
1000	−0.30	93.5	100.0	94.1	100.0
5000	−0.30	94.6	100.0	95.4	100.0
10,000	−0.30	94.2	100.0	94.7	100.0
Mean	−0.30	**93.9**	**100.0**	**94.4**	**100.0**
		Model 3		Model 4	
100	−0.30	0.2	100.0	93.6	100.0
500	−0.30	0.0	100.0	93.6	100.0
1000	−0.30	0.0	100.0	94.3	100.0
5000	−0.30	0.0	100.0	95.2	100.0
10,000	−0.30	0.0	100.0	94.6	100.0
Mean	−0.30	**0.0**	**100.0**	**94.3**	**100.0**
		Model 1		Model 2	
100	−0.20	94.4	100.0	94.2	100.0
500	−0.20	94.8	100.0	94.8	100.0
1000	−0.20	94.9	100.0	94.6	100.0
5000	−0.20	94.3	100.0	95.1	100.0
10,000	−0.20	92.8	100.0	94.7	100.0
Mean	−0.20	**94.2**	**100.0**	**94.7**	**100.0**
		Model 3		Model 4	
100	−0.20	0.3	99.8	94.8	100.0
500	−0.20	0.0	100.0	94.5	100.0
1000	−0.20	0.0	100.0	94.6	100.0
5000	−0.20	0.0	100.0	93.3	100.0
10,000	−0.20	0.0	100.0	91.7	100.0
Mean	−0.20	**0.1**	**100.0**	**93.8**	**100.0**

Model 1 (Mixed-effects negative binomial model). Model 2 (Interval censored (on outcomes 1–9) mixed-effects negative binomial model). Model 3 (Midpoint imputed mixed-effects negative binomial model). Model 4 (Interval censored (on outcomes 1–9) fixed-effects negative binomial model)

(continued)

Table 4 (continued)

Results for β_1 mean confidence interval performance and statistical power: true values of −0.10 and 0.01

County-years	True β_1	CI coverage	Power	CI coverage	Power
		Model 1		Model 2	
100	−0.10	94.1	98.8	94.0	93.7
500	−0.10	94.6	100.0	95.1	100.0
1000	−0.10	96.0	100.0	95.3	100.0
5000	−0.10	95.5	100.0	96.0	100.0
10,000	−0.10	94.7	100.0	95.3	100.0
Mean	−0.10	**95.0**	**99.8**	**95.1**	**98.7**
		Model 3		Model 4	
100	−0.10	52.9	94.2	93.9	94.0
500	−0.10	2.3	100.0	94.3	100.0
1000	−0.10	0.0	100.0	94.3	100.0
5000	−0.10	0.0	100.0	92.2	100.0
10,000	−0.10	0.0	100.0	91.4	100.0
Mean	−0.10	**11.0**	**98.8**	**93.2**	**98.8**
		Model 1		Model 2	
100	0.01	93.8	8.9	93.9	8.5
500	0.01	94.0	20.1	93.6	18.2
1000	0.01	94.9	32.6	95.3	29.6
5000	0.01	94.6	93.6	95.0	90.0
10,000	0.01	95.3	99.8	95.2	99.4
Mean	0.01	**94.5**	**51.0**	**94.6**	**49.1**
		Model 3		Model 4	
100	0.01	92.5	10.1	94.0	8.3
500	0.01	92.6	20.8	93.6	18.3
1000	0.01	93.1	32.7	94.9	28.5
5000	0.01	94.3	91.5	95.1	86.6
10,000	0.01	93.2	99.5	93.8	99.1
Mean	0.01	**93.1**	**50.9**	**94.3**	**48.2**

Model 1 (Mixed-effects negative binomial model). Model 2 (Interval censored (on outcomes 1–9) mixed-effects negative binomial model). Model 3 (Midpoint imputed mixed-effects negative binomial model). Model 4 (Interval censored (on outcomes 1–9) fixed-effects negative binomial model)

(continued)

Table 4 (continued)

Results for β_1 mean confidence interval performance and statistical power: true values of 0.10 and 0.20

County-years	True β_1	CI coverage	Power	CI coverage	Power
		Model 1		Model 2	
100	0.10	92.8	99.5	92.6	99.4
500	0.10	94.2	100.0	94.1	100.0
1000	0.10	95.6	100.0	95.4	100.0
5000	0.10	94.6	100.0	95.0	100.0
10,000	0.10	96.2	100.0	96.2	100.0
Mean	0.10	**94.7**	**99.9**	**94.7**	**99.9**
		Model 3		Model 4	
100	0.10	91.9	99.4	92.9	99.0
500	0.10	93.8	100.0	94.5	100.0
1000	0.10	92.0	100.0	94.4	100.0
5000	0.10	81.3	100.0	95.3	100.0
10,000	0.10	66.1	100.0	95.3	100.0
Mean	0.10	**85.0**	**99.9**	**94.5**	**99.8**
		Model 1		Model 2	
100	0.20	94.8	100.0	94.5	100.0
500	0.20	93.7	100.0	94.1	100.0
1000	0.20	95.1	100.0	95.4	100.0
5000	0.20	94.1	100.0	94.1	100.0
10,000	0.20	93.3	100.0	93.6	100.0
Mean	0.20	**94.2**	**100.0**	**94.3**	**100.0**
		Model 3		Model 4	
100	0.20	94.1	100.0	94.7	100.0
500	0.20	90.9	100.0	92.8	100.0
1000	0.20	90.3	100.0	94.3	100.0
5000	0.20	71.8	100.0	93.6	100.0
10,000	0.20	51.2	100.0	93.4	100.0
Mean	0.20	**79.7**	**100.0**	**93.8**	**100.0**

Model 1 (Mixed-effects negative binomial model). Model 2 (Interval censored (on outcomes 1–9) mixed-effects negative binomial model). Model 3 (Midpoint imputed mixed-effects negative binomial model). Model 4 (Interval censored (on outcomes 1–9) fixed-effects negative binomial model)

(continued)

Table 4 (continued)

Results for β_1 mean confidence interval performance and statistical power: true value of 0.30					
County-years	True β_1	CI coverage	Power	CI coverage	Power
		Model 1		Model 2	
100	0.30	94.2	100.0	93.4	100.0
500	0.30	94.7	100.0	94.1	100.0
1000	0.30	95.9	100.0	95.8	100.0
5000	0.30	94.2	100.0	94.2	100.0
10,000	0.30	94.5	100.0	95.2	100.0
Mean	0.30	**94.7**	**100.0**	**94.5**	**100.0**
		Model 3		Model 4	
100	0.30	93.7	100.0	94.1	100.0
500	0.30	92.7	100.0	94.5	100.0
1000	0.30	93.3	100.0	94.7	100.0
5000	0.30	75.9	100.0	94.9	100.0
10,000	0.30	61.7	100.0	93.8	100.0
Mean	0.30	**83.5**	**100.0**	**94.4**	**100.0**

Model 1 (Mixed-effects negative binomial model). Model 2 (Interval censored (on outcomes 1–9) mixed-effects negative binomial model). Model 3 (Midpoint imputed mixed-effects negative binomial model). Model 4 (Interval censored (on outcomes 1–9) fixed-effects negative binomial model)

Table 5 Mean bias

β_1 mean bias: negative beta values					
County-years	True β_1	Model 1	Model 2	Model 3	Model 4
		Percent different	Percent different	Percent different	Percent different
100	−0.30	0.90	1.20	51.99	1.25
500	−0.30	0.11	0.02	52.79	0.15
1000	−0.30	0.04	0.27	52.58	0.09
5000	−0.30	0.04	0.00	52.75	0.18
10,000	−0.30	0.03	0.05	52.71	0.14
Mean	−0.30	**0.22**	**0.31**	**52.56**	**0.36**
100	−0.20	0.62	1.19	51.82	0.64
500	−0.20	0.15	0.29	52.47	0.50
1000	−0.20	0.05	0.10	52.46	0.97
5000	−0.20	0.03	0.01	52.44	0.94
10,000	−0.20	0.00	0.03	52.42	0.98
Mean	−0.20	**0.17**	**0.32**	**52.32**	**0.81**
100	−0.10	0.67	1.18	33.33	0.53
500	−0.10	0.05	0.44	33.78	2.06
1000	−0.10	0.25	0.08	33.20	1.56
5000	−0.10	0.25	0.28	33.24	1.94
10,000	−0.10	0.01	0.04	33.05	1.57
Mean	−0.10	**0.25**	**0.40**	**33.32**	**1.53**

Model 1 (Mixed-effects negative binomial model). Model 2 (Interval censored (on outcomes 1–9) mixed-effects negative binomial model). Model 3 (Midpoint imputed mixed-effects negative binomial model). Model 4 (Interval censored (on outcomes 1–9) fixed-effects negative binomial model)

(continued)

Table 5 (continued)

β_1 mean bias: positive beta values					
County-years	True β_1	Model 1	Model 2	Model 3	Model 4
		Percent different	Percent different	Percent different	Percent different
100	0.01	4.84	0.20	2.97	0.67
500	0.01	4.18	4.31	2.13	2.52
1000	0.01	0.71	1.60	3.45	0.28
5000	0.01	0.42	0.03	1.81	0.02
10,000	0.01	0.79	0.57	1.21	0.65
Mean	0.01	**2.19**	**1.34**	**2.31**	**0.83**
100	0.10	0.04	0.13	3.08	0.03
500	0.10	0.17	0.16	3.40	0.13
1000	0.10	0.01	0.00	3.22	0.15
5000	0.10	0.00	0.01	3.24	0.27
10,000	0.10	0.06	0.06	3.16	0.17
Mean	0.10	**0.06**	**0.07**	**3.22**	**0.15**
100	0.20	0.03	0.11	2.10	0.07
500	0.20	0.03	0.06	2.04	0.13
1000	0.20	0.16	0.17	2.13	0.24
5000	0.20	0.02	0.01	1.95	0.08
10,000	0.20	0.02	0.02	1.93	0.10
Mean	0.20	**0.05**	**0.07**	**2.03**	**0.12**
100	0.30	0.23	0.25	0.82	0.15
500	0.30	0.01	0.01	1.10	0.04
1000	0.30	0.06	0.06	1.01	0.04
5000	0.30	0.00	0.01	1.08	0.06
10,000	0.30	0.01	0.01	1.06	0.05
Mean	0.30	**0.06**	**0.07**	**1.01**	**0.07**

Model 1 (Mixed-effects negative binomial model). Model 2 (Interval censored (on outcomes 1–9) mixed-effects negative binomial model). Model 3 (Midpoint imputed mixed-effects negative binomial model). Model 4 (Interval censored (on outcomes 1–9) fixed-effects negative binomial model)

Table 6 Type I error rate

County-years	Model 1	Model 2	Model 3	Model 4
	Type I error	Type I error	Type I error	Type I error
100	5.00	5.10	6.10	5.20
500	5.40	4.90	5.40	4.80
1000	4.80	5.10	5.70	4.90
5000	3.90	3.60	4.00	3.10
10,000	4.30	4.10	4.70	4.00
Mean	**4.68**	**4.56**	**5.18**	**4.40**

Model 1 (Mixed-effects negative binomial model). Model 2 (Interval censored (on outcomes 1–9) mixed-effects negative binomial model). Model 3 (Midpoint imputed mixed-effects negative binomial model). Model 4 (Interval censored (on outcomes 1–9) fixed-effects negative binomial model)

Table 7 Increased between-cluster variance simulations

Results for mean β_1 maximum likelihood estimates, standard errors, and confidence interval coverage: true β_1 value of −0.30							
County- years	Trueβ_1	MLE	SE	CI coverage	MLE	SE	CI coverage
		Model 1			Model 2		
1000	−0.30	−0.300	0.010	95.200	−0.300	0.012	94.600
		Model 3			Model 4		
1000	−0.30	−0.184	0.009	0.000	−0.291	0.017	84.200

Supplemental simulations were conducted to examine model performance when the data was both highly structured and had extensive censoring. Model 1 (Mixed-effects negative binomial model). Model 2 (Interval censored (on outcomes 1–9) mixed-effects negative binomial model). Model 3 (Midpoint imputed mixed-effects negative binomial model). Model 4 (Interval censored (on outcomes 1–9) fixed-effects negative binomial model)

True parameter values: $\beta_0 = 2.25$, $\beta_1 = -0.30$, $\beta_2 = 0.00$, $\alpha = 0.25$, $\sigma^2 = 1.00$

Appendix 2: SAS Code Examples

Simulation Data Generation and Sample Models

```
libname Drought 'h:\bob\Gribble';
options ps=66 ls=90 nodate nonumber nonotes;
title1 'PROGRAM: Sim Pgm Template 09_13_18.sas';
title2 'Simulating data from Negative Binomial model';
ods listing;
%let nsim=1000;
%macro  iternb;
   %do q=1 %to & nsim;
proc iml worksize=70 symsize=250;
k=50;       ** Number of counties **;
n=20;          ** # observations (years)per county **;
ntot=n*k;
sig1sq=.05;
**Set parameters for NB regression simulation**;
**NOTE: 1/alpha has to be an integer to generate data, but not in
analysis of data **;
  bet0=2.25;  bet1= 0.2;  bet2=0;
  alpha=.25;  r=1/alpha;
t={1 2 3 4 5 6 7 8 9 10 11 12 13 14 15 16 17 18 19 20};    ** Let
years go from 1 to 20 **;
tmat=j(n,k,0);
w=j(n,k,0);
  do j1=1 to n;
    w[j1,]=1:k; *** matrix with ID #s for exporting to proc
nlmixed **;
  end;
  do i=1 to k;
  tmat[,i]=t'; *** matrix with obs. times for exporting to proc
nlmixed **;
  end;
```

```
 wvec=shape(w',ntot,1);        ***STRING OUT W and T INTO
VECTORS***;
 tvec=shape(tmat',ntot,1);
START DATAGEN;
gamm0is=j(k,1,0);
ymat=j(n,k,0);
indexmat=j(n,k,0);
linpred=j(n,k,0);
mumat=j(n,k,0);
pmat=j(n,k,0);
RVx=j(r,1,0);
t={1 2 3 4 5 6 7 8 9 10 11 12 13 14 15 16 17 18 19 20};   ** Let
years go from 1 to 20 **;
tprime=t';
   do i=1 to k;
      gamm0is[i,]=0 + sqrt(sig1sq)*RANNOR(0);
   do j=1 to n;
      indexmat[j,i]=10*RANUNI(0); **Generate drought index for
each county/year as uniform(0,10);
         linpred[j,i]=(bet0 + gamm0is[i,])
+ bet1*indexmat[j,i] + bet2*tprime[j,];
         mumat[j,i]=exp(linpred[j,i]);
         pmat[j,i]=1/(1+mumat[j,i]/r);
**Generating each NB outcome**;
do randindx=1 to r;
     u=RANUNI(0);
     RVx[randindx,]=floor(log(u)/log(1-pmat[j,i]));
    end;
  **print RVx;
  ymat[j,i]=sum(RVx);
   end;
   end;
yvec=shape(ymat',ntot,1);    ***STRING OUT Y INTO A VECTOR***;
indexvec=shape(indexmat',ntot,1); ***STRING OUT Drought Indices
INTO A VECTOR***;
FINISH DATAGEN;
run datagen;
datmat=wvec||tvec||yvec||indexvec;
create dat from datmat;
append from datmat;
truevals=bet0||bet1||bet2||alpha||sig1sq;
create truevals from truevals;
append from truevals;
QUIT;
data dat; set dat;
  rename COL1=id;
  rename COL2=year;
  rename COL3=Ydeaths;
  rename COL4=DroughtIndx;
run;
data dat; set dat;
  Ylt10=0;
  if Ydeaths < 10 then Ylt10=1;
  Yobserved=0;
```

```
  if Ydeaths=0 | Ydeaths ge 10 then Yobserved=1;
run;

****** Model 1 ******;
proc nlmixed data=dat;
        parms bet0=2.25, bet1=.2, bet2=0, alpha=.2, sigsq1=.05;
        bounds sigsq1 >= 0;
        alphainv=1/alpha;
        linp=(bet0+g0i) + bet1*DroughtIndx + bet2*year;
        mu=exp(linp);
        p=1/(1+mu*alpha);
        loglike=lgamma(alphainv+Ydeaths) - lgamma(alphainv) -
lgamma(1+Ydeaths)
               + Ydeaths*log(1-p) + alphainv*log(p);
        model Ydeaths ~ general(loglike);
        random g0i ~ normal(0, sigsq1) subject=id;
  run;

****** Model 2 ******;
proc nlmixed data=dat;
        parms bet0=2.25, bet1=.2, bet2=0, alpha=.2, sigsq1=.05;
        bounds sigsq1 >= 0;
        alphainv=1/alpha;
        linp=(bet0+g0i) + bet1*DroughtIndx + bet2*year;
        mu=exp(linp);
        p=1/(1+mu*alpha);
        prYeq0=p**alphainv;
        prYeq1=alphainv*(p**alphainv)*(1-p);
        prYeq2=((alphainv+1)*alphainv/fact(2))*(p**alphainv)
*(1-p)**2;
       prYeq3=((alphainv+2)*(alphainv+1)*alphainv/fact(3))
*(p**alphainv)*(1-  p)**3;
        prYeq4=((alphainv+3)*(alphainv+2)*(alphainv+1)
*alphainv/fact(4))*(p**alphainv)*(1-p)**4;
        prYeq5=((alphainv+4)*(alphainv+3)*(alphainv+2)
*(alphainv+1)*alphainv/fact(5))*(p**alphainv)*(1-p)**5;
        prYeq6=((alphainv+5)*(alphainv+4)*(alphainv+3)
*(alphainv+2)*(alphainv+1)*alphainv/fact(6))*(p**alphainv)
*(1-p)**6;
        prYeq7=((alphainv+6)*(alphainv+5)*(alphainv+4)
*(alphainv+3)*(alphainv+2)*(alphainv+1)*alphainv/fact(7))
*(p**alphainv)*(1-p)**7;
        prYeq8=((alphainv+7)*(alphainv+6)*(alphainv+5)
*(alphainv+4)*(alphainv+3)*(alphainv+2)*(alphainv+1)
*alphainv/fact(8))*(p**alphainv)*(1-p)**8;
        prYeq9=((alphainv+8)*(alphainv+7)*(alphainv+6)
*(alphainv+5)*(alphainv+4)*(alphainv+3)*(alphainv+2)*(alphainv+1)
*alphainv/fact(9))*(p**alphainv)*(1-p)**9;
       CDFterm=prYeq0 + prYeq1 + prYeq2 + prYeq3 + prYeq4
+ prYeq5 + prYeq6 + prYeq7 + prYeq8 + prYeq9;
   ** log-likelihood function when Y values are detectable ***;
       if Yobserved=1 then do;
       loglike=lgamma(alphainv+Ydeaths) - lgamma(alphainv)
- lgamma(1+Ydeaths)
          + Ydeaths*log(1-p) + alphainv*log(p);
```

```
  end;
 ** log-likelihood function when Y values are interval censored
on [1,9] ***;
       else if Yobserved=0 then do;
       loglike=log(CDFterm - prYeq0);
  end;
       model Ydeaths ~ general(loglike);
       random g0i ~ normal(0, sigsq1) subject=id;
  run;

****** Model 3 ******;
proc nlmixed data=dat;
       parms bet0=2.25, bet1=.2, bet2=0, alpha=.2, sigsq1=.05;
       bounds sigsq1 >= 0;
       alphainv=1/alpha;
       linp=(bet0+g0i) + bet1*DroughtIndx + bet2*year;
       mu=exp(linp);
       p=1/(1+mu*alpha);
       if Ydeaths lt 10 and Ydeaths gt 0 then Ydeaths = 5;
       loglike=lgamma(alphainv+Ydeaths) - lgamma(alphainv)
- lgamma(1+Ydeaths)
          + Ydeaths*log(1-p) + alphainv*log(p);
       model Ydeaths ~ general(loglike);
       random g0i ~ normal(0, sigsq1) subject=id;
  run;

****** Model 4 ******;
proc nlmixed data=dat;
        parms bet0=2.25, bet1=.2, bet2=0, alpha=.2, sigsq1=.05;
        bounds sigsq1 >= 0;
        alphainv=1/alpha;
        linp=(bet0) + bet1*DroughtIndx + bet2*year;
        mu=exp(linp);
        p=1/(1+mu*alpha);
        prYeq0=p**alphainv;
        prYeq1=alphainv*(p**alphainv)*(1-p);
        prYeq2=((alphainv+1)*alphainv/fact(2))*(p**alphainv)
*(1-p)**2;
        prYeq3=((alphainv+2)*(alphainv+1)*alphainv/fact(3))
*(p**alphainv)*(1-p)**3;
         prYeq4=((alphainv+3)*(alphainv+2)*(alphainv+1)
*alphainv/fact(4))*(p**alphainv)*(1-p)**4;
         prYeq5=((alphainv+4)*(alphainv+3)*(alphainv+2)
*(alphainv+1)*alphainv/fact(5))*(p**alphainv)*(1-p)**5;
         prYeq6=((alphainv+5)*(alphainv+4)*(alphainv+3)
*(alphainv+2)*(alphainv+1)*alphainv/fact(6))*(p**alphainv)*(1-p)
**6;
         prYeq7=((alphainv+6)*(alphainv+5)*(alphainv+4)
*(alphainv+3)*(alphainv+2)*(alphainv+1)*alphainv/fact(7))
*(p**alphainv)*(1-p)**7;
         prYeq8=((alphainv+7)*(alphainv+6)*(alphainv+5)
*(alphainv+4)*(alphainv+3)*(alphainv+2)*(alphainv+1)
*alphainv/fact(8))*(p**alphainv)*(1-p)**8;
```

```
        prYeq9=((alphainv+8)*(alphainv+7)*(alphainv+6)
*(alphainv+5)*(alphainv+4)*(alphainv+3)*(alphainv+2)*(alphainv+1)
*alphainv/fact(9))*(p**alphainv)*(1-p)**9;
      CDFterm=prYeq0 + prYeq1 + prYeq2 + prYeq3 + prYeq4
+ prYeq5 +   prYeq6 + prYeq7 + prYeq8 + prYeq9;
  ** log-likelihood function when Y values are detectable ***;
      if Yobserved=1 then do;
      loglike=lgamma(alphainv+Ydeaths) - lgamma(alphainv)
- lgamma(1+Ydeaths)
        + Ydeaths*log(1-p) + alphainv*log(p);
  end;
 ** log-likelihood function when Y values are interval censored
on [1,9] ***;
      else if Yobserved=0 then do;
      loglike=log(CDFterm - prYeq0);
  end;
      model Ydeaths ~ general(loglike);run;
```

South African Data SAS Code

```
****** Model 1 ******;
proc nlmixed data=format;
      parms bet0=3.2076, bet1= -0.04197, bet2=.000151,
alpha=.1950, sigsq1= 1.3586;
      bounds sigsq1 >= 0;
      alphainv=1/alpha;
      linp=(bet0+g0i) + bet1*exposure + bet2*date + lnpop;
      mu=exp(linp);
      p=1/(1+mu*alpha);
      loglike=lgamma(alphainv+deaths) - lgamma(alphainv)
- lgamma(1+deaths)+ deaths*log(1-p) + alphainv*log(p);
      model deaths ~ general(loglike);
      random g0i ~ normal(0, sigsq1) subject=district;
      ods output parameterestimates=ests1;
      title1 'NB regression with random effects, using general
LL facility';
run;
data ests1;
      set ests1;
      model = '1';
run;
proc print data = ests1;
run;

****** Model 2 ******;
  proc nlmixed data=format;
      parms bet0=3.2076, bet1= -0.04197, bet2=.000151,
alpha=.1950, sigsq1= 1.3586;
      bounds sigsq1 >= 0;
      alphainv=1/alpha;
      linp=(bet0+g0i) + bet1*exposure + bet2*date + lnpop;
```

```
        mu=exp(linp);
        p=1/(1+mu*alpha);
        prYeq0=p**alphainv;
         prYeq1=alphainv*(p**alphainv)*(1-p);
         prYeq2=((alphainv+1)*alphainv/fact(2))*(p**alphainv)
*(1-p)**2;
          prYeq3=((alphainv+2)*(alphainv+1)*alphainv/fact(3))
*(p**alphainv)*(1-p)**3;
          prYeq4=((alphainv+3)*(alphainv+2)*(alphainv+1)
*alphainv/fact(4))*(p**alphainv)*(1-p)**4;
          prYeq5=((alphainv+4)*(alphainv+3)*(alphainv+2)
*(alphainv+1)*alphainv/fact(5))*(p**alphainv)*(1-p)**5;
          prYeq6=((alphainv+5)*(alphainv+4)*(alphainv+3)
*(alphainv+2)*(alphainv+1)*alphainv/fact(6))*(p**alphainv)
*(1-p)**6;
          prYeq7=((alphainv+6)*(alphainv+5)*(alphainv+4)
*(alphainv+3)*(alphainv+2)*(alphainv+1)*alphainv/fact(7))
*(p**alphainv)*(1-p)**7;
          prYeq8=((alphainv+7)*(alphainv+6)*(alphainv+5)
*(alphainv+4)*(alphainv+3)*(alphainv+2)*(alphainv+1)
*alphainv/fact(8))*(p**alphainv)*(1-p)**8;
          prYeq9=((alphainv+8)*(alphainv+7)*(alphainv+6)
*(alphainv+5)*(alphainv+4)*(alphainv+3)*(alphainv+2)
*(alphainv+1)*alphainv/fact(9))*(p**alphainv)*(1-p)**9;
CDFterm=prYeq0
+ prYeq1 + prYeq2 + prYeq3 + prYeq4 + prYeq5 + prYeq6 + prYeq7
+ prYeq8 + prYeq9;
   ** log-likelihood function when Y values are detectable ***;
        if Yobserved=1 then do;
        loglike=lgamma(alphainv+deaths) - lgamma(alphainv)
-     lgamma(1+deaths)
           + deaths*log(1-p) + alphainv*log(p);
  end;
   ** log-likelihood function when Y values are interval censored
on [1,9] ***;
        else if Yobserved=0 then do;
        loglike=log(CDFterm - prYeq0);
  end;
  model deaths ~ general(loglike);
  random g0i ~ normal(0, sigsq1) subject=district;
  ods output parameterestimates=ests2;
title1 'NB regression with random effects, Interval censored
[1-9]';
run;
data ests2;
set ests2;
model = '2';
run;
proc print data = ests2;
run;

****** Model 3 ******;
proc nlmixed data=format;
```

```
       parms bet0=3.2076, bet1= -0.04197, bet2=.000151,
alpha=.1950,sigsq1= 1.3586;
       bounds sigsq1 >= 0;
       alphainv=1/alpha;
       linp=(bet0+g0i) + bet1*exposure + bet2*date + lnpop;
       mu=exp(linp);
        p=1/(1+mu*alpha);
       if deaths lt  10 and deaths gt 0 then deaths = 5;
       loglike=lgamma(alphainv+deaths) - lgamma(alphainv)
- lgamma(1+deaths) + deaths*log(1-p) + alphainv*log(p);
       model deaths ~ general(loglike);
       random g0i ~ normal(0, sigsq1) subject=district;
       ods output parameterestimates=ests3;
       title1 'NB regression W/ Midpoint Imputation';
run;
data ests3;
set ests3;
model = '3';
run;
proc print data = ests3;
run;

****** Model 4 ******;
  proc nlmixed data=format;
       parms bet0=3.2076, bet1= -0.04197, bet2=.000151,
alpha=.1950, sigsq1= 1.3586;
       bounds sigsq1 >= 0;
       alphainv=1/alpha;
       linp=(bet0) + bet1*exposure + bet2*date + lnpop;
       mu=exp(linp);
       p=1/(1+mu*alpha);
       prYeq0=p**alphainv;
       prYeq1=alphainv*(p**alphainv)*(1-p);
       prYeq2=((alphainv+1)*alphainv/fact(2))*(p**alphainv)
*(1-p)**2;
         prYeq3=((alphainv+2)*(alphainv+1)*alphainv/fact(3))
*(p**alphainv)*(1-p)**3;
         prYeq4=((alphainv+3)*(alphainv+2)*(alphainv+1)
*alphainv/fact(4))*(p**alphainv)*(1-p)**4;
         prYeq5=((alphainv+4)*(alphainv+3)*(alphainv+2)
*(alphainv+1)*alphainv/fact(5))*(p**alphainv)*(1-p)**5;
         prYeq6=((alphainv+5)*(alphainv+4)*(alphainv+3)
*(alphainv+2)*(alphainv+1)*alphainv/fact(6))*(p**alphainv)
*(1-p)**6;
         prYeq7=((alphainv+6)*(alphainv+5)*(alphainv+4)
*(alphainv+3)*(alphainv+2)*(alphainv+1)*alphainv/fact(7))
*(p**alphainv)*(1-p)**7;
         prYeq8=((alphainv+7)*(alphainv+6)*(alphainv+5)
*(alphainv+4)*(alphainv+3)*(alphainv+2)*(alphainv+1)
*alphainv/fact(8))*(p**alphainv)*(1-p)**8;
         prYeq9=((alphainv+8)*(alphainv+7)*(alphainv+6)
*(alphainv+5)*(alphainv+4)*(alphainv+3)*(alphainv+2)
*(alphainv+1)*alphainv/fact(9))*(p**alphainv)*(1-p)**9;
        CDFterm=prYeq0 + prYeq1 + prYeq2 + prYeq3 + prYeq4
+ prYeq5 + prYeq6 + prYeq7 + prYeq8 + prYeq9;
```

```
   ** log-likelihood function when Y values are detectable ***;
        if Yobserved=1 then do;
        loglike=lgamma(alphainv+deaths) - lgamma(alphainv)
- lgamma(1+deaths)   + deaths*log(1-p) + alphainv*log(p);
  end;
   ** log-likelihood function when Y values are interval censored
on [1,9] ***;
       else if Yobserved=0 then do;
       loglike=log(CDFterm - prYeq0);
  end;
       model deaths ~ general(loglike);
       ods output parameterestimates=ests4;
       title1 'NB regression with fixed effects';
run;
data ests4;
set ests4;
model = '4';
run;
proc print data = ests4;
run;

****** Examine the Exposure in Quartiles ******;
proc glimmix data = Quartiles;
      class district Quarter (ref = '4');
      model deaths = Quarter date / dist=negbin link=log
solution offset=lnpop;
      random intercept / sub= district;
      estimate 'Rate ratio of Q1 vs Q4' Quarter 1 0 0 / exp cl;
      estimate 'Rate ratio of Q2 vs Q4' Quarter 0 1 0 / exp cl;
      estimate 'Rate ratio of Q3 vs Q4' Quarter 0 0 1 / exp cl;
run;
```

References

1. Coxe, S., West, S.G., Aiken, L.S.: The analysis of count data: A gentle introduction to Poisson regression and its alternatives. J. Pers. Assess. **91**(2), 121–136 (2009). https://doi.org/10.1080/00223890802634175
2. Smithson, M., Merkle, E.: Generalized linear models for categorical and continuous limited dependent variables. CRC Press, Taylor & Francis Group, Boca Raton, FL (2014)
3. Laird, N., Ware, J.: Random-effects models for longitudinal data. Biometrics. **38**(4), 963–974 (1982). https://doi.org/10.2307/2529876
4. Touloumi, G., Pocock, S.J., Babiker, A.G., Darbyshire, J.H.: Estimation and comparison of rates of change in longitudinal studies with informative drop-outs. Stat. Med. **18**(10), 1215–1233 (1999). https://doi.org/10.1002/(SICI)1097-0258(19990530)18:10<1215::AID-SIM118>3.0.CO;2-6
5. Wu, M.C.: Sample size for comparison of changes in the presence of right censoring caused by death, withdrawal, and staggered entry. Control. Clin. Trials. **9**(1), 32–46 (1988). https://doi.org/10.1016/0197-2456(88)90007-4
6. Bartell, S.M., Lewandowski, T.A.: Administrative censoring in ecological analyses of autism and a Bayesian solution. J. Environ. Public Health. **2011**, 1–5 (2011). https://doi.org/10.1155/2011/202783

7. Schluter, M.D.: Methods for the analysis of informatively censored longitudinal data. Stat. Med. **11**, 1861–1870 (1992)
8. Hilbe, J.M., Judson, D.H.: sg94: Right, left, and uncensored Poisson regression. Stata Tech. Bull. **46**, 18–20 (1998). College Station, TX: Stata Press
9. Terza, J.V.: A Tobit-type estimator for the censored Poisson regression model. Econ. Lett. **18**(4), 361–365 (1985). https://doi.org/10.1016/0165-1765(85)90053-9
10. Quiroz, J., Wilson, J.R., Roychoudhury, S.: Statistical analysis of data from dilution assays with censored correlated counts. Pharm. Stat. **11**, 63–73 (2012). https://doi.org/10.1002/pst.499
11. Statistics South Africa: Mortality and causes of death in South Africa, 2011: Findings from death notification. Stats SA, Pretoria, South Africa (2014a)
12. Statistics South Africa: Mortality and causes of death in South Africa, 2013: Findings from death notification. Stats SA, Pretoria, South Africa (2014b)
13. Keyantash, J., & National Center for Atmospheric Research Staff (Eds). The Climate Data Guide: Standardized Precipitation Index (SPI) (2018). https://climatedataguide.ucar.edu/climate-data/standardized-precipitation-index-spi.
14. McKee, T.B., Doesken, N.J., Kliest, J.: The relationship of drought frequency and duration to time scales. In: Proceedings of the 8th conference of applied climatology, 17–22 January, Anaheim, CA, pp. 179–118. American Meteorological Society, Boston, MA (1993)
15. Ziese, M., Becker, A., Finger, P., Meyer-Christoffer, A., Rudolf, B., Schneider, U.: GPCC First Guess product at 1.0°: Near real-time First Guess monthly land-surface precipitation from rain-gauges based on SYNOP data. [Data File]. Global Precipitation Climatology Centre, Deutscher Wetterdienst, Germany (2011). https://doi.org/10.5676/DWD_GPCC/FG_M_100
16. Wickham, H.: ggplot2: Elegant graphics for data analysis. Springer-Verlag, New York, NY (2016)
17. R Core Team. R: A language and environment for statistical computing. Vienna, Austria: R Foundation for Statistical Computing (2018). https://www.R-project.org/.
18. Copeland, K.T., Checkoway, H., McMichael, A.J., Holbrook, R.H.: Bias due to misclassification in the estimation of relative risk. Am. J. Epidemiol. **105**(5), 488–495 (1977). https://doi.org/10.1093/oxfordjournals.aje.a112408
19. Mason, J.B., Bailes, A., Mason, K.E., Yambi, O., Jonsson, U., Hudspeth, C. . . . .M.: AIDS, drought, and child malnutrition in southern Africa. Public Health Nutr. **8**(6), 551–563 (2005)
20. O'Keefe, S.J.: Malnutrition among adult hospitalized patients in Zululand during the drought of 1983. S. Afr. Med. J. **64**(16), 628–629 (1983)
21. Vogel, C.H., Moser, S., Kasperson, R., Daebelko, G.: Linking vulnerability, adaptation and resilience science to practice: pathways, players and partnerships. Glob. Environ. Chang. **17**, 349–364 (2007). https://doi.org/10.1016/j.gloenvcha.2007.05.002
22. Glantz, M.H.: The value of long-range weather forecast for the Western Sahel. Bull. Am. Meteorol. Soc. **58**, 150–158 (1977)
23. Bandyopadhyay, S., Kanji, S., Wang, L.M.: The impact of rainfall and temperature variation on diarrheal prevalence in Sub-Saharan Africa. Appl. Geogr. **33**(1), 63–72 (2012)
24. Effler, P., Isaacson, M., Arntzen, L., Heenan, R., Canter, P., Barrett, T., et al.: Factors contributing to the emergence of Escherichia coli O157 in Africa. Emerg. Infect. Dis. **7**(5), 812–819 (2001)
25. Byass, P.: Climate change and population health in Africa: where are the scientists? Glob. Health Action. **2**(1), 2065 (2009). https://doi.org/10.3402/gha.v2i0.2065
26. Gage, K.L., Burkot, T.R., Eisen, R.J., Hayes, E.B.: Climate and vector-borne diseases. Am. J. Prev. Med. **35**(5), 436–450 (2008)
27. Myers, J., Young, T., Galloway, M., Manyike, P., Tucker, T.: A public health approach to the impact of climate change on health in southern Africa—Identifying priority modifiable risks. S. Afr. Med. J. **101**(11), 817–820 (2011)
28. Stanke, C., Kerac, M., Prudhomme, C., Medlock, J., Murray, V.: Health effects of drought: a systematic review of the evidence. PLoS Curr. **2013**, 5 (2013). https://doi.org/10.1371/currents.dis.7a2cee9e980f91ad7697b570bcc4b004

29. Barios, S., Bertinelli, L., Strobl, E.: Climactic change and rural-urban migration: the case of sub-Saharan Africa. J. Urban Econ. **60**, 357–371 (2006)
30. de Longueville, F., Ozer, P., Doumbia, S., Henry, S.: Desert dust impacts on human health: an alarming worldwide reality and a need for studies in West Africa. Int. J. Biometeorol. **57**(1), 1–19 (2012). https://doi.org/10.1007/s00484-012-0541-y
31. Engelbrecht, F., Adegoke, J., Bopape, M.J., Naidoo, M., Garland, R., Thatcher, M., et al.: Projections of rapidly rising surface temperatures over Africa under low mitigation. Environ. Res. Lett. **10**, 8 (2015). https://doi.org/10.1088/1748-9326/10/8/085004
32. Scovronick, N., Sera, F., Acquaotta, F., Garzena, D., Fratianni, S., Wright, C.Y., Gasparrini, A.: The association between ambient temperature and mortality in South Africa: a time-series analysis. Environ. Res. **161**, 229–235 (2018). https://doi.org/10.1016/j.envres.2017.11.001
33. Wichmann, J.: Heat effects of ambient apparent temperature on all-cause mortality in Cape Town, Durban and Johannesburg, South Africa: 2006–2010. Sci. Total Environ. **587–588**, 266–272 (2017). https://doi.org/10.1016/j.scitotenv.2017.02.135

Online Updating of Nonparametric Survival Estimator and Nonparametric Survival Test

Yishu Xue, Elizabeth D. Schifano, and Guanyu Hu

1 Introduction

Survival analysis is widely used in many different fields such as biostatistics [4], finance [8], and reliability analysis [7]. With the development of advanced technology generating massive amounts of data, even simple analyses of such data have become a challenge. For survival data [5, 6] focused on massive sample size, high-dimensional scenarios and used cyclic coordinate descent to enable fast estimation for parametric and Cox models. Wang et al. [11] proposed using divide-and-conquer for Cox regression in conjunction with LASSO for variable selection. To ensure appropriateness of the Cox model, Xue et al. [12] proposed an online updating approach to test the validity of proportional hazards assumption. However, there are several important nonparametric survival estimators and statistics, whose calculation has not been fully studied in the massive-data setting.

The Nelson–Aalen estimator [1] is a universally used nonparametric estimator of the cumulative hazard function in survival analysis. It has been shown by Zhou [13] that the maximum empirical likelihood estimator of cumulative hazard function has the same form as the Nelson–Aalen estimator. Zhou [13] also provided statistical properties of the maximum empirical likelihood estimator of the cumulative hazard function. In general, the empirical likelihood estimator is also a nonparametric estimator. These traditional estimation methods are often not feasible for analyzing big survival data, however, as huge datasets cannot always be loaded into a

Y. Xue · E. D. Schifano
Department of Statistics, University of Connecticut, Storrs, CT, USA
e-mail: yishu.xue@uconn.edu; elizabeth.schifano@uconn.edu

G. Hu (✉)
Department of Statistics, University of Missouri-Columbia, Columbia, MO, USA
e-mail: Guanyu.hu@missouri.edu

Y. Zhao, (Din) D.-G. Chen (eds.), *Modern Statistical Methods for Health Research*, Emerging Topics in Statistics and Biostatistics,
https://doi.org/10.1007/978-3-030-72437-5_18

computer's memory and analyzed as a whole. As estimation of the hazard function is fundamental to analysis of survival data, it is desirable that the big data problem be tackled from this starting point for nonparametric estimators and test statistics.

In this chapter, we propose online updating nonparametric estimators and a testing procedure of the cumulative hazard function when the data arrives sequentially in large chunks, i.e., in streams [9]. Our proposed methods are computationally efficient and require storage of only a few summaries of historical data rather than the full dataset. The rest of this chapter is organized as follows. In Sect. 2, we briefly review the nonparametric survival estimators for the cumulative hazard function, the empirical likelihood approach for cumulative hazard functions, and a two-group nonparametric test for cumulative hazard. Estimation of the cumulative hazard function and calculation of the two-group nonparametric test statistic in the online updating setting are detailed in Sect. 3. Simulation study results are presented in Sect. 4, followed by analysis of survival for lymphoma patients in the Surveillance, Epidemiology, and End Results (SEER) program in Sect. 5. A brief discussion concludes in Sect. 6.

2 Notation and Preliminaries

2.1 Nonparametric Survival Estimator

Let (T_i, δ_i), $i = 1, \ldots, n$, denote an independent sample of survival data, where T_i is the observed time, and δ_i is an indicator variable that equals 0 if observation i is censored, and 1 otherwise. Also, let $Y_i(t) = 1$ when subject i is still at risk at time t, and 0 otherwise, and further denote $Y(t) = \sum_{i=1}^{n} Y_i(t)$ as the number of observations at risk at time t. We can formulate the empirical log likelihood in terms of the hazard function using the Binomial extension of empirical log likelihood from [13] as

$$\log EL = \sum_{i=1}^{n}(\delta_i \log(\Delta\Lambda(T_i)) + \sum_{i=1}^{n}\sum_{j=1}^{n} I(T_j \leq T_i)\log\left(1 - \Delta\Lambda(T_j)\right), \tag{1}$$

where Λ denotes the cumulative hazard function, and $\Delta\Lambda(T_i)$ denotes its jump at T_i. The maximizer for the hazard corresponding to this empirical likelihood is

$$\Delta\widehat{\Lambda}(t) = \frac{N(t)}{Y(t)}, \tag{2}$$

where $N(t)$ is the number of events occurring at time t and equals $\sum_{i=1}^{n} N_i(t)$ with $N_i(t)$ being the number of events for subject i at time t. It is worth noting that this is exactly the same form as in the Nelson–Aalen estimator, where the cumulative hazard function at time t is given by

$$\widehat{\Lambda}(t) = \sum_{s \le t} \frac{N(s)}{Y(s)}, \tag{3}$$

with estimated variance

$$\widehat{\mathrm{Var}}(\widehat{\Lambda}(t)) = \sum_{s \le t} \frac{(Y(s) - N(s))N(s)}{(Y(s) - 1)Y^2(s)} = \sum_{s \le t} \frac{(1 - \Delta\widehat{\Lambda}(s))\Delta\widehat{\Lambda}(s)}{Y(s) - 1}. \tag{4}$$

2.2 *Two-Group Nonparametric Test*

Using Λ_g to denote the cumulative hazard for group g, $g = 1, 2$, the relevant null hypothesis for a two-group comparison can be written as

$$H_0 : \Lambda_1(t) = \Lambda_2(t), \quad \forall t > 0. \tag{5}$$

It is natural to construct such a test by utilizing the Nelson–Aalen estimators of the cumulative hazards for the two groups. Our proposed test resembles the well-known procedures in survival analysis in Fleming and Harrington [3]. The continuous version of log rank test is defined via the following general form:

$$W = \int_0^\infty K(s)(\Delta\widehat{\Lambda}_1(s) - \Delta\widehat{\Lambda}_2(s))ds, \tag{6}$$

where K is a bounded, nonnegative predictable process adapted to $\{\mathscr{F}_{t-} : t \ge 0\}$ with $\mathscr{F}_{t-}$ being the smallest σ-algebra containing all sets in $\cup_{h>0}\mathscr{F}_{t-h}$.

The formulation (6) can be alternatively discretized as

$$W = \sum_{t=0}^{\infty} K(t)(\Delta\widehat{\Lambda}_1(t) - \Delta\widehat{\Lambda}_2(t)), \tag{7}$$

with estimated variance:

$$\widehat{\mathrm{Var}}(W) = \sum_{t=0}^{\infty} K^2(t) \left(\frac{Y_1(t) + Y_2(t)}{Y_1(t)Y_2(t)}\right) \left(1 - \frac{N_1(t) + N_2(t) - 1}{Y_1(t) + Y_2(t) - 1}\right) \frac{N_1(t) + N_2(t)}{Y_1(t) + Y_2(t)}, \tag{8}$$

where $Y_g(t)$ is the number of observations at risk at time t in group g, and $N_g(t)$ is the number of events at time t from group g, $g = 1, 2$.

Standard theory from [3] suggests that W, computed from either (6) or (7), is asymptotically normal as the total sample size $n \to \infty$, and therefore under H_0,

$$Z_0 = \frac{W}{\sqrt{\widehat{\text{Var}}(W)}} \tag{9}$$

will be asymptotically $N(0, 1)$. For large n, an approximate level α test is obtained by rejecting H_0 when $|Z_0| > z_{\alpha/2}$, where $z_{\alpha/2}$ is the usual $1 - \alpha/2$ quantile from the standard normal distribution.

3 Online Updating

3.1 Online Updating for Nonparametric Estimator

In the online updating setting, data become available in chunks and are processed sequentially. We index the chunks using $\ell = 1, 2, \ldots$ and denote the number of observations in the chunks as $n_1, n_2, \ldots$. Many public health study datasets, including those from the SEER program, report rounded integer-valued survival times, where the estimated cumulative hazard functions for such datasets would only have possible jumps at these integer values. For the rest of this chapter, we focus on a sequence of such pre-specified jump locations, denoted as $a_0, \ldots, a_J$. Denote the unknown true jumps at $a_0, \ldots, a_J$ as $\boldsymbol{\theta}^* = (\Delta\Lambda(a_0), \ldots, \Delta\Lambda(a_J))$, and the cumulative hazard values as $\boldsymbol{\theta}$. The score function for $\boldsymbol{\theta}^*$ based on block ℓ can be obtained using the log empirical likelihood approach as

$$\boldsymbol{U}_{n_\ell,\ell}(\boldsymbol{\theta}^*) = \sum_{i=1}^{n_\ell} \frac{\delta_{i\ell}}{\Delta\Lambda(T_{i\ell})} + \sum_{i=1}^{n_\ell} \frac{\sum_{j=1}^{J} I(T_{i\ell} < a_j)}{\Delta\Lambda(T_{i\ell}) - 1}, \tag{10}$$

where $T_{i\ell}$ is the observed time for observation i in block ℓ, and $\delta_{i\ell}$ is the corresponding event indicator. Let the maximizer of (10) be $\widehat{\boldsymbol{\theta}}^*_{n_\ell,\ell}$. Similar to the approach in [9], we take the Taylor expansion of $-\boldsymbol{U}_{n_\ell,\ell}(\boldsymbol{\theta}^*)$ and have

$$-\boldsymbol{U}_{n_\ell,\ell}(\boldsymbol{\theta}^*) = \boldsymbol{A}_{n_\ell,\ell}(\boldsymbol{\theta}^* - \widehat{\boldsymbol{\theta}}^*_{n_\ell,\ell}) + \boldsymbol{R}_{n_\ell,\ell},$$

where

$$\boldsymbol{A}_{n_\ell,\ell} = -\sum_{i=1}^{n_\ell} \frac{\partial \boldsymbol{U}_{n_\ell,\ell}(\widehat{\boldsymbol{\theta}}^*_{n_\ell,\ell})}{\partial \boldsymbol{\theta}^*},$$

and $\boldsymbol{R}_{n_\ell,\ell}$ is a remainder. The cumulative estimating equation (CEE) estimator for $\boldsymbol{\theta}^*$ similar to in [9] can be obtained at block k as

$$\widehat{\boldsymbol{\theta}}^*_k = \left(\sum_{\ell=1}^{k} \boldsymbol{A}_{n_\ell,\ell}\right)^{-1} \left(\sum_{\ell=1}^{k} \boldsymbol{A}_{n_\ell,\ell}\widehat{\boldsymbol{\theta}}^*_{n_\ell,\ell}\right), \tag{11}$$

i.e., the estimator is online-updated as

$$\widehat{\boldsymbol{\theta}}_k^* = \left(\boldsymbol{A}_{k-1} + \boldsymbol{A}_{n_k,k}\right)^{-1}\left(\boldsymbol{A}_{k-1}\widehat{\boldsymbol{\theta}}_{k-1}^* + \boldsymbol{A}_{n_k,k}\widehat{\boldsymbol{\theta}}_{n_k,k}^*\right),$$

with $\boldsymbol{A}_{k-1} = \sum_{\ell=1}^{k-1} \boldsymbol{A}_{n_\ell,\ell}$, $\boldsymbol{A}_0 = \boldsymbol{0}_{(J+1)\times(J+1)}$ and $\widehat{\boldsymbol{\theta}}_0^* = \boldsymbol{0}_{(J+1)\times 1}$.

Note that in the case where there is no event at a_j in blocks $\ell = 1, \ldots, k$, the jth diagonal element of $\sum_{\ell=1}^{k} \boldsymbol{A}_{n_\ell,\ell}$ would be 0, causing it to be singular. This is, however, unlikely when the data size is huge, the censoring rate is not very high, and the block sample sizes n_ℓ remain large, particularly for the first block. Therefore, for the rest of this chapter, we will assume $\sum_{\ell=1}^{k} \boldsymbol{A}_{n_\ell,\ell}$ to be full rank and invertible for all k. An (cumulative) estimate of the cumulative hazard function over blocks $\ell = 1, \ldots, k$, denoted by $\widehat{\boldsymbol{\theta}}_k$, can be obtained by taking the cumulative sum of $\widehat{\boldsymbol{\theta}}_k^*$, i.e.,

$$\widehat{\boldsymbol{\theta}}_k = \begin{pmatrix} \widehat{\Lambda}_k(a_0) \\ \widehat{\Lambda}_k(a_1) \\ \vdots \\ \widehat{\Lambda}_k(a_J) \end{pmatrix} \equiv \boldsymbol{T}\widehat{\boldsymbol{\theta}}_k^* = \begin{pmatrix} 1 & 0 & 0 & \ldots & 0 \\ 1 & 1 & 0 & \ldots & 0 \\ \vdots & \vdots & \vdots & \ddots & \vdots \\ 1 & 1 & 1 & \ldots & 1 \end{pmatrix} \widehat{\boldsymbol{\theta}}_k^*, \tag{12}$$

and an estimator for the variance of $\widehat{\boldsymbol{\theta}}_k$ can be obtained as

$$\mathrm{Var}(\widehat{\boldsymbol{\theta}}_k) = \boldsymbol{T}\boldsymbol{A}_k^{-1}\boldsymbol{T}^\top.$$

3.2 *Bias-Corrected Online Updating Estimators*

The CEE-type estimator has been shown to be biased in finite samples, and debiasing techniques with the help of an intermediary estimator have been proposed under the generalized linear models framework [9]. Under the empirical likelihood formulation for survival times, we apply a similar technique. For ease of calculation in the next step, with block ℓ, for $\Delta\Lambda(a_j)$, the jth element of $\boldsymbol{\theta}^*$, we write its score function, i.e., the jth element of (10), as

$$U_{n_\ell,\ell}(\Delta\Lambda(a_j)) = \frac{\sum_{i=1}^{n_\ell} \delta_{i\ell} I(T_{i\ell} = a_j)}{\Delta\Lambda(a_j)} - \sum_{i=1}^{n_\ell} I(T_{i\ell} \geq a_j), \quad j = 1\ldots, J. \tag{13}$$

We consider a similar bias-correction technique by using a sequence of intermediary estimators $\breve{\boldsymbol{\theta}}_{n_\ell,\ell}^*$ to account for the omission of higher-order remainder terms. Note that without performing bias correction, we will ultimately obtain estimator (11). At accumulation point k, we choose $\breve{\boldsymbol{\theta}}_{n_k,k}^*$ to be

$$\widetilde{\boldsymbol{\theta}}^*_{n_k,k} = \left(\widetilde{\boldsymbol{A}}_{k-1} + \boldsymbol{A}_{n_k,k}\right)^{-1} \left(\sum_{\ell=1}^{k-1} \widetilde{\boldsymbol{A}}_{n_\ell,\ell}\widetilde{\boldsymbol{\theta}}^*_{n_\ell,\ell} + \boldsymbol{A}_{n_k,k}\widehat{\boldsymbol{\theta}}^*_{n_k,k}\right),$$

where $\widehat{\boldsymbol{\theta}}^*_{n_\ell,\ell}$ was defined above, $\widetilde{\boldsymbol{A}}_{n_\ell,\ell}$ is obtained by evaluating $\boldsymbol{A}_{n_k,k}$ at $\widetilde{\boldsymbol{\theta}}^*_{n_\ell,\ell}$, $\widetilde{\boldsymbol{A}}_0 = \mathbf{0}_{(J+1)\times(J+1)}$, $\widetilde{\boldsymbol{\theta}}^*_{n_0,0} = \mathbf{0}_{(J+1)\times 1}$, and $\widetilde{\boldsymbol{A}}_k = \sum_{\ell=1}^{k} \widetilde{\boldsymbol{A}}_{n_\ell,\ell}$. This intermediary estimator is the solution to the estimating equation

$$\sum_{\ell=1}^{k-1} \widetilde{\boldsymbol{A}}_{n_\ell,\ell}\left(\boldsymbol{\theta}^* - \widetilde{\boldsymbol{\theta}}^*_{n_\ell,\ell}\right) + \boldsymbol{A}_{n_k,k}\left(\boldsymbol{\theta}^* - \widehat{\boldsymbol{\theta}}^*_{n_k,k}\right) = \mathbf{0}_{(J+1)\times 1},$$

where the second term serves the bias-correction purpose. For more details, we refer the reader to Section 3.1 of [9]. The cumulatively updated estimating equation (CUEE)-like estimator of $\boldsymbol{\theta}^*$ at accumulation point k is given by

$$\widetilde{\boldsymbol{\theta}}^*_k = \left(\sum_{\ell=1}^{k} \widetilde{\boldsymbol{A}}_{n_\ell,\ell}\right)^{-1} \left(\sum_{\ell=1}^{k} \widetilde{\boldsymbol{A}}_{n_\ell,\ell}\widetilde{\boldsymbol{\theta}}^*_{n_\ell,\ell} + \sum_{\ell=1}^{k} \boldsymbol{U}_{n_\ell,\ell}(\widetilde{\boldsymbol{\theta}}^*_{n_\ell,\ell})\right), \tag{14}$$

where $\boldsymbol{U}_{n_\ell,\ell}(\widetilde{\boldsymbol{\theta}}^*_{n_\ell,\ell})$ is the score vector (13) evaluated at $\widetilde{\boldsymbol{\theta}}^*_{n_\ell,\ell}$, and its variance can be estimated as

$$\mathrm{Var}(\widetilde{\boldsymbol{\theta}}^*_k) = \left(\sum_{\ell=1}^{k} \widetilde{\boldsymbol{A}}_{n_\ell,\ell}\right)^{-1} \left(\sum_{\ell=1}^{k} \widetilde{\boldsymbol{A}}_{n_\ell,\ell}\boldsymbol{A}^{-1}_{n_\ell,\ell}\widetilde{\boldsymbol{A}}_{n_\ell,\ell}\right)\left(\sum_{\ell=1}^{k} \widetilde{\boldsymbol{A}}_{n_\ell,\ell}\right)^{-1}.$$

Similar to (12), the corresponding CUEE-like estimator for cumulative hazard, $\widetilde{\boldsymbol{\theta}}_k$, can be subsequently obtained as

$$\widetilde{\boldsymbol{\theta}}_k = \boldsymbol{T}\widetilde{\boldsymbol{\theta}}^*_k,$$

with variance estimator

$$\mathrm{Var}(\widetilde{\boldsymbol{\theta}}_k) = \boldsymbol{T}\left(\widetilde{\mathrm{Var}}(\widetilde{\boldsymbol{\theta}}^*_k)\right)\boldsymbol{T}^\top.$$

3.3 Online Updating for Nonparametric Test

In this section, we will introduce an online updating test for equality of cumulative hazard across two groups based on the blockwise estimators. Our null hypothesis is that there is no difference in the survival distributions of the two groups for the entire data stream, i.e.,

$$H_0 : \Lambda_1(t) = \Lambda_2(t), \quad \forall t > 0, \tag{15}$$

where $\Lambda_g(t)$ is the cumulative hazard for group g. In the online updating setting, we can calculate the Z_0^ℓ for ℓth block by the following form:

$$Z_0^\ell = \frac{W^\ell}{\sqrt{\widehat{\text{Var}}(W^\ell)}}, \tag{16}$$

where W^ℓ and $\widehat{\text{Var}}(W^\ell)$ are estimated by (7) and (8) within the ℓth block. In order to test the null hypothesis in (15), we construct the following test statistic:

$$T_k(Z_0) = \frac{1}{\sqrt{k}} \sum_{\ell=1}^{k} Z_0^\ell. \tag{17}$$

Under the Central Limit Theorem e.g., [10], the asymptotic distribution of $T_K(Z_0)$ under the null hypothesis is $N(0, 1)$. At the end of a data stream, i.e., when block ℓ, $\ell = 1, \ldots, K$, have arrived and been analyzed, we use the value of $T_K(Z_0)$ to decide if the two groups in the entire data stream follow the same survival distribution. The null hypothesis is rejected when $|T_K(Z_0)| > z_{\alpha/2}$, where $z_{\alpha/2}$ is the $1-\alpha/2$ quantile from the standard normal distribution.

4 Simulation Study

4.1 Simulation for Nonparametric Estimators

To evaluate the performance of the proposed online updating nonparametric estimators, an exponential survival model with $\lambda = 0.018$ is used to generate the survival times. Next, the censoring times are generated independently from a mixture distribution $0.9\text{Uniform}(0, 60) + 0.1\langle 60\rangle$, where $\langle 60\rangle$ denotes a point mass at 60, and the observed time for each subject is taken as the smaller of its survival time and censoring time. The resulting data has an average censoring rate of around 58%. Initially in each stream, observations are aggregated to ensure that $\boldsymbol{A}_{n_1,1}$ is invertible. Subsequent block sizes are set to 5000, 10000, or 15000 under three designs. For each design, a total of 1000 replicates with each stream of data containing 50 total blocks are performed.

For each data stream, the CEE estimator (11) and the CUEE estimator (14) are calculated, and their cumulative sums over the time grid $\{1, 2, \ldots, 60\}$ are obtained. Also, we utilize a Linux workstation with 128 GB memory to obtain the estimating equation (EE) estimator, which is calculated using (1) based on the dataset that pools the entire stream together. As each estimator contains 60 values, we choose to look at their values at $t \in \{10, 20, 30, 40, 50, 60\}$. The estimates at these time points were compared against their true underlying values, which equal $0.018t$ for each t. Performance is evaluated using average bias (AB), standard deviation (SD),

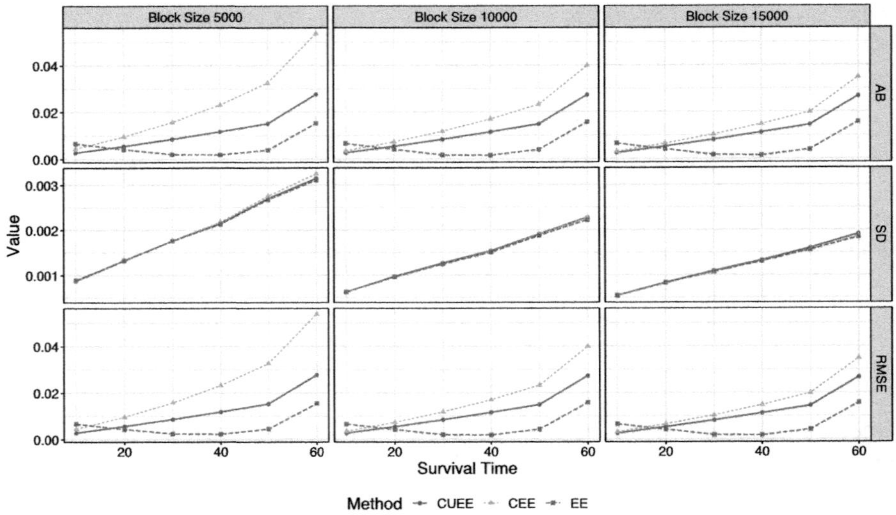

Fig. 1 Performance plots for the CUEE, CEE, and EE estimators at $t \in \{10, 20, 30, 40, 50, 60\}$

and root mean-squared error (RMSE). The three measurements for our considered scenarios are presented in Fig. 1.

A few observations can be made from Fig. 1. For all time points, the EE estimator has the smallest absolute bias except at $t = 10$, followed by the CUEE estimator, and finally the CEE estimator. The scales of biases decrease as a natural consequence of increasing block size. Also, for a fixed block size, the scale of bias for CUEE and CEE increases with respect to survival time, which is mainly caused by relative shortage of observed events near the end of follow-up time. The RMSE also displays an overall decreasing trend with increases in block size. Within each fixed block size, the CEE estimator has the largest RMSE (except for small time points) due to its large bias, followed by CUEE and EE estimators. The difference in SDs for the three estimators is minor. A closer look at the biases for the three estimators is given in Fig. 2. From the boxplots, the increase in bias of the CEE estimator is rather clear, and so is the bias correction of the CUEE estimator. The increasing pattern of bias for CEE and CUEE estimators is again verified. The difference between CEE and CUEE, however, becomes smaller with the increase in sample size.

4.2 Simulation for Nonparametric Test

We focus on the scenario of having streams of survival data with two different groups. An exponential survival model was used. After the survival times are generated, the censoring times are generated using the same mixture distribution in Sect. 4.1.

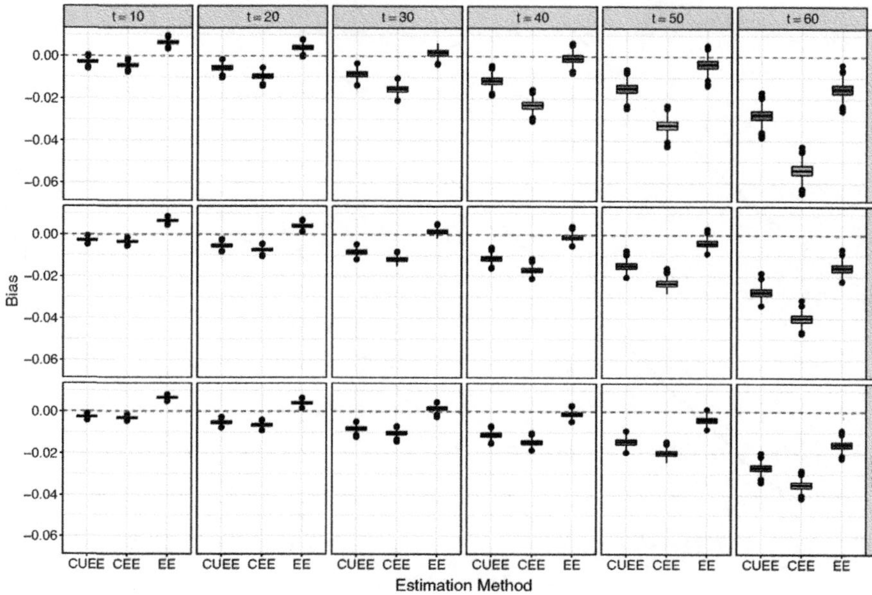

Fig. 2 Boxplot for biases of the CUEE, CEE, and EE estimators at selected time points for block sizes 5000, 10000, and 15000 scenarios

4.2.1 Under the Null Hypothesis

As before, for each block size $n_\ell \in \{5000, 10000, 15000\}$, we simulate 1000 streams of data each containing 50 blocks, with the observations aggregated in the first block to ensure that $A_{n_1,1}$ is invertible, and subsequent blocks have sizes 5000, 10000, or 15000. Every block consists of two equally sized groups coming from the same survival and censoring distribution. The online updating cumulative test statistic (17) is calculated at each update. At the end of each stream, we also calculate a cumulative log rank test statistic (9) based on all data in this stream. The results are summarized in Fig. 3. It can be seen that our proposed test statistic $T_k(Z_0)$ is approximately $N(0, 1)$ as desired under the null hypothesis.

4.2.2 Under the Alternative Hypothesis

Using the same setting, we vary the rate of the exponential distribution for one of the groups in each stream to study the power of our test statistic. Again, for each block size in $\{5000, 10000, 15000\}$, 1000 streams of survival data are simulated, each consisting of 50 blocks. Half of the observations in each block are generated using $\lambda_{01}(t) = 0.018$, and the other half are generated using $\lambda_{02}(t) \in \{0.0185, 0.01875, 0.019\}$. At each accumulation point, we calculate the log rank test statistic using cumulative data (i.e., with all datasets up to the current accumulation

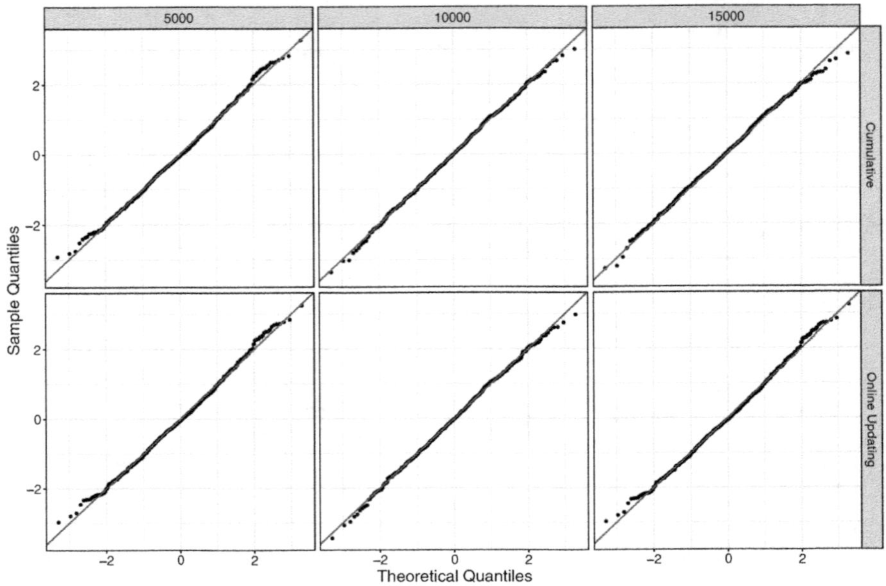

Fig. 3 Normal quantile–quantile plots of cumulative log rank test statistics (top) and online updating log rank test statistics (bottom) obtained for 1000 data streams with block sizes being 5000, 10000, and 15000

point combined), and the online updating log rank test statistic. The results are summarized in Fig. 4.

It can be seen that the empirical power for both versions keeps increasing with accumulation of data and hence discrepancies. For decision-making at the final block ($K = 50$), it is worth noticing that, for $\lambda_{02}(t) = 0.0185$, the power for block size 10000 is 0.867 for the cumulative data test statistic, while that for online updating statistic is 1 even when the block size is 5000. In fact, comparing between panels, it is easy to see that the empirical powers for the online updating statistic always increase to 1 faster than the cumulative statistic. This could be due to the existence of averaging effect when the data is considered as a whole, while breaking the data into pieces and examining the pieces allow discrepancies to be exposed more quickly. Similar findings have been made in [2, 12].

5 Real Data Application

We consider the 131960 patients diagnosed with lymphoma between 1973 and 2007 from the SEER program. We focus on the 5-year survival; therefore, deaths due to lymphoma or all other causes within 60 months of diagnosis count as events. The

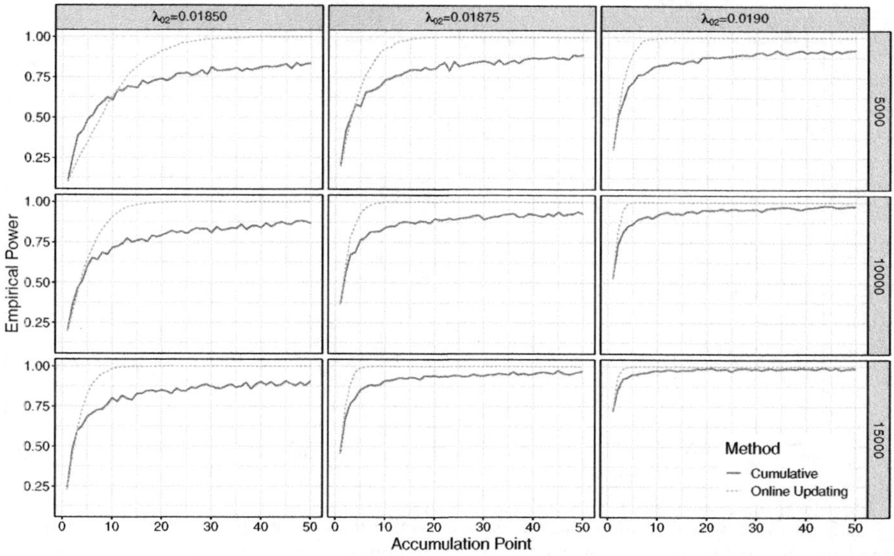

Fig. 4 Plot of proportion of absolute statistic values that exceed 1.96 against block index for cumulative log rank test and online updating log rank test obtained using 1000 data streams for each combination of alternative baseline hazard rate and block size. The empirical powers are the values of the curves at accumulation point 50

average censoring rate is 54.42%. There are 60432 females and 71528 males in the dataset.

5.1 Survival Estimator

The dataset is partitioned temporally into 2-year intervals, resulting in $K = 18$ blocks. Both the block size and the censoring rate increase with respect to time. We applied our proposed bias-corrected online updating cumulative hazard function estimator separately to the male and female subgroups from the dataset. The resulting estimates are plotted in Fig. 5. It can be seen from panel (a) that the blockwise cumulative hazard estimates are quite different across blocks, with the lower curves corresponding to more recent blocks due to higher censoring rate brought by the overall medical advancements. Such inconsistency is a violation of the underlying assumption for online updating—all blocks are assumed to have the same hazard or cumulative hazard functions. A consequence of such violation is seen from panel (b), where there are apparent discrepancies between the online-updated estimates and the full-data estimates.

To evaluate the performance of the proposed online updating estimator when the underlying assumptions are satisfied, we randomly permuted and re-partitioned the

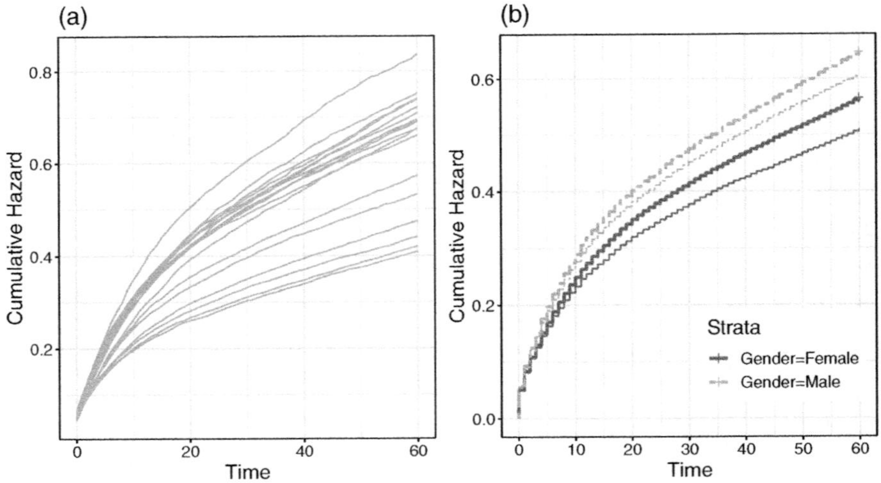

Fig. 5 (**a**) Blockwise cumulative hazard estimates under the temporal partition scheme; (**b**) online updating cumulative hazard estimates (thin lines) and full-data cumulative hazard estimates (thick lines) for female (solid lines) and male (dashed lines) subgroups

dataset while keeping block sizes consistent with the temporal partition scheme. The results are presented in Fig. 6. It can be seen that when the blockwise cumulative hazards all lie within a relatively tight band, satisfying the assumption of the online updating methodology, the discrepancies between the online-updated estimates and the full-data estimates become very minor. To verify this observation is not a special case but holds in general, different random seeds are used in the permutation, and the observations are consistent (individual scenarios not shown here).

5.2 *Nonparametric Test*

To test if males and females have the same survival distribution with 5 years after diagnosis, we apply our online updating nonparametric test to the two groups in each block. We also calculate the standard nonparametric test using the entire dataset. The online updating version statistic has a final value of -12.79, and the full-data statistic is calculated to be -12.84. While we only focus on the final block and make decision based on the final value from the online updating scheme, we also calculate, at each accumulation point $k = 1, \ldots, 18$, the full-data statistic using all blocks $1, \ldots, k$ as a whole for further comparison. Trajectories of the two statistics are plotted in Fig. 7. It can be seen that the two statistics align well, and both arrived at the conclusion of rejecting the equal survival distribution null hypothesis.

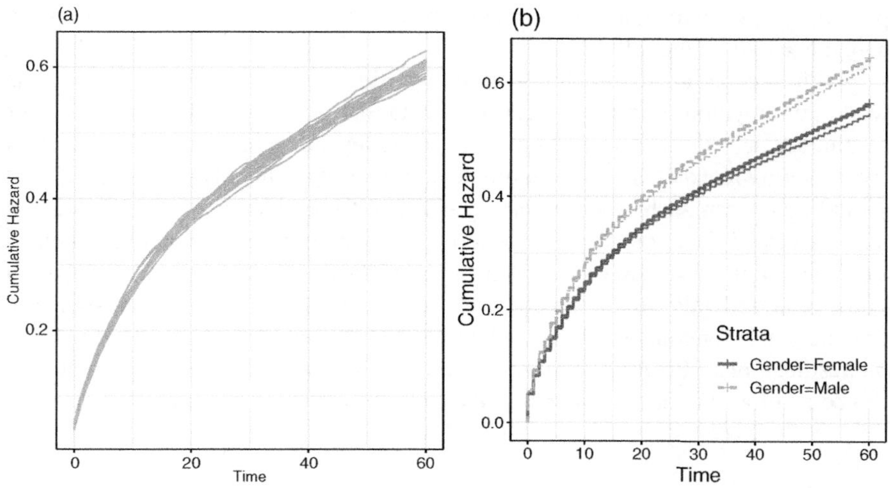

Fig. 6 (**a**) Blockwise cumulative hazard estimates under the randomized partition scheme; (**b**) online updating cumulative hazard estimates (thin lines) and full-data cumulative hazard estimates (thick lines) for female (solid lines) and male (dashed lines) subgroups

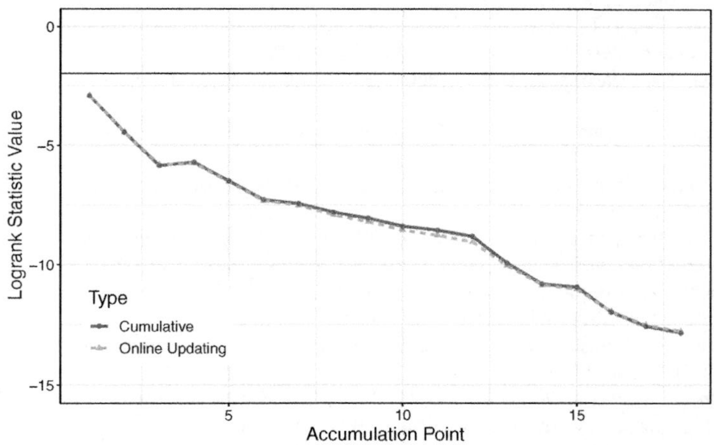

Fig. 7 Plot of trajectories for the cumulative data test statistic and the online updating test statistic versus accumulation point. The horizontal line with y-intercept -1.96 is illustrated

6 Conclusion

We developed an online updating algorithm for estimating and testing of cumulative hazard functions in the big data setting. Survival times in the data are discretized and treated in an interval-censored fashion under the empirical likelihood framework. In the simulation study and real data results, our estimation algorithm and testing procedure have comparable performance to the traditional estimating and testing methods based on the full dataset.

For future research, the choice of pre-specified time grid $(a_0, a_1, \ldots, a_J)$ is worth investigation. For interval-censored data, the grid is naturally available. For continuous data, the selection of time grid could depend on multiple factors, such as the censoring rate and the research problem of interest. Generally speaking, the grid should be chosen such that the curve yielded is representative of the information that a block of data contains. Furthermore, the testing procedure can be extended to address multiple-group comparisons. Closer study of the asymptotic distribution of the proposed online updating estimator, as well as construction of nonparametric statistic to test for equality of survival distribution based on this estimator, are other interesting topics. Finally, diagnostic procedures utilizing methods of scan statistics can be employed to detect changes in the cumulative hazard over time.

References

1. Aalen, O.: Nonparametric estimation of partial transition probabilities in multiple decrement models. Ann. Stat. **6**, 534–545 (1978)
2. Battey, H., Fan, J., Liu, H., Lu, J., Zhu, Z.: Distributed testing and estimation under sparse high dimensional models. Ann. Stat. **46**(3), 1352–1382 (2018)
3. Fleming, T.R., Harrington, D.P.: Counting Processes and Survival Analysis, vol. 169. Wiley, New York (2011)
4. Hosmer, D.W., Lemeshow, S., May, S.: Applied Survival Analysis. Wiley Blackwell, New York (2011)
5. Mittal, S., Madigan, D., Cheng, J.Q., Burd, R.S.: Large-scale parametric survival analysis. Stat. Med. **32**(23), 3955–3971 (2013)
6. Mittal, S., Madigan, D., Burd, R.S., Suchard, M.A.: High-dimensional, massive sample-size Cox proportional hazards regression for survival analysis. Biostatistics **15**(2), 207–221 (2014)
7. Rausand, M., Arnljot, H.: System Reliability Theory: Models, Statistical Methods, and Applications, vol. 396. Wiley, New York (2004)
8. Richards, S.: A handbook of parametric survival models for actuarial use. Scand. Actuar. J. **2012**(4), 233–257 (2012)
9. Schifano, E.D., Wu, J., Wang, C., Yan, J., Chen, M.-H.: Online updating of statistical inference in the big data setting. Technometrics **58**(3), 393–403 (2016)
10. Van der Vaart, A.W.: Asymptotic Statistics, vol. 3. Cambridge University, Cambridge (1998)
11. Wang, Y., Hong, C., Palmer, N., Di, Q., Schwartz, J., Kohane, I., Cai, T.: A fast divide-and-conquer sparse Cox regression. Biostatistics **22**(2), 381–401 (2019)
12. Xue, Y., Wang, H., Yan, J., Schifano, E.D.: An online updating approach for testing the proportional hazards assumption with streams of survival data. Biometrics **76**(1), 171–182 (2020)
13. Zhou, M.: Empirical Likelihood Method in Survival Analysis, vol. 79. CRC Press, New York (2015)

Part V
Statistical Modeling in Genomic Studies

Graphical Modeling of Multiple Biological Pathways in Genomic Studies

Yujing Cao, Yu Zhang, Xinlei Wang, and Min Chen

1 Introduction

Many complex diseases, like various types of cancer, type 2 diabetes, and psychiatric disorders, are known to be associated with a number of genetic factors and gene expression profiles. However, the current treatments of complex diseases often fail to work well for all patients. Some patients may respond differently to the same treatment, and may suffer from adverse side effects differently. The genome and transcriptome of an individual may affect the susceptibility to develop a disease and the variation in the responses to treatments. Identifying genomic and transcriptomic risk factors thus can help us to better understand the pathogenesis of a disease. It is also the very first step toward the development of successful prevention and intervention strategies. In addition, it may shed light on genomic and transcriptomic markers that may aid the decisions of precision medicine to improve the treatment efficiency and reduce the side effects. Here, we focus on developing a

---

Yujing Cao and Yu Zhang authors contributed equally.

Y. Cao · Y. Zhang
Department of Mathematical Sciences, University of Texas at Dallas, Dallas, TX, USA

X. Wang
Department of Statistical Science, Southern Methodist University, Richardson, TX, USA

M. Chen (✉)
Department of Mathematical Sciences, University of Texas at Dallas, Dallas, TX, USA

Department of Population and Data Sciences, UT Southwestern Medical Center, Richardson, TX, USA
e-mail: mchen@utdallas.edu

Y. Zhao, (Din) D.-G. Chen (eds.), *Modern Statistical Methods for Health Research*, Emerging Topics in Statistics and Biostatistics,
https://doi.org/10.1007/978-3-030-72437-5_19

novel statistical model to identify the genetic factors and genes that are associated with complex diseases.

Genome-wide association study (GWAS) is a popular approach to identifying genetic variants related to a complex disease [8, 18, 40]. Single nucleotide polymorphism (SNP) is among the most common types of genetic variations and is the basic unit of investigation in many GWASs. There are millions of SNPs in the human genome, accounting for a large portion of the genomic elements that affect many phenotypes. According to the NHGRI GWAS Catalog [7], GWASs have identified over 171,000 associations as candidate risk factors in complex diseases by the year 2020. Although the traditional GWAS methods based on single-marker analysis have been successful, they fail to account for much of the heritability of phenotypes. One limitation is related to multiple testing correction, which is required to control the overall type I error when testing a large number of hypotheses. To improve the power of detection, researchers have developed pathway-based approaches in GWAS, which allow one to take into account multiple genetic variants in different loci that interact with one another. The pathway-based analysis offers an opportunity to collectively evaluate genetic variants so that the dependence among themselves can be considered in the model. Also, pathway-based studies can include markers whose effects are small and thus are hard to detect through traditional single-marker tests.

A number of pathway-based approaches have been proposed in the literature. For example, Luo et al. [30] proposed a two-stage (gene and pathway) GWAS. Chen et al. [12] proposed a supervised principal component analysis [2] to test the association between a group of SNPs and variation in disease outcome. For association tests with pathways in the presence of both common and rare variants, Pan et al. [37] extended the sum of powered score tests [36], originally developed for analysis of rare variants, to a pathway-based test that is data-adaptive at both the gene and the SNP levels. Note that the widely used kernel machine tests [48, 49] can be regarded as special cases of the sum of powered score tests. ICSNPathway [45] was developed to identify candidate causal SNPs and their corresponding candidate causal pathways. This approach integrates linkage disequilibrium analysis, functional SNP annotation, and pathway-based analysis.

Other than GWAS, gene expression analysis has been widely employed to identify genes associated with disease. Gene expression measures the expression level of mRNA that is related to the protein abundance. The regulation variation of gene expression plays a key role in shaping phenotypic differences among individuals, and as a result, it is very likely to influence disease susceptibility [13, 34]. For example, gene expression profiles from cancer and normal cells are used for comparison and reveal new disease entities [39]. Also, the involvements of gene expression are found in risk loci of the inflammatory bowel disease [32]. Single-gene based analysis has the limitation similar to that of the GWAS, namely, the lack of statistical power when a large number of hypotheses are being tested simultaneously. Many studies have proposed to incorporate the topological structures of biological pathways with gene expression data to identify differentially expressed genes. Similar to disease association status of genes, the genes that interact with others tend to have similar expression status (differentially expressed and equally expressed) as well. Zhi et al. [51] used a discrete MRF to model the dependency of the differential expression patterns of genes in the network. Some researchers have extended the transitional enrichment analysis to topology-based enrichment approaches to identify pathways or gene sets that are significantly enriched with differentially expressed genes. Signaling pathway impact analysis (SPIA) [46] integrates the evidence of differentially expressed genes and topology structure of a signaling pathway. PathNet [15] is another enrichment method considering topology information of biological pathways.

There are many types of pathways, and most well-known ones include metabolic, gene regulatory, and signal transduction pathways. An example of a biological pathway is shown in Fig. 1. Metabolic pathways [50] are mainly concerned with a series of biochemical reactions, especially the chemical modification of the small molecule substrates of enzymes. For example, glucose is broken apart during cellular respiration to produce adenosine triphosphate (ATP), which is an energy source for the cell's functions. Gene-regulatory pathways control what genes are expressed and the expression levels of mRNA and proteins. Signal transduction pathways [25] transmit signals from cell's exterior to its interior. For instance, a chemical signal from outside the cell might direct the cell to produce protein inside the cell. Different pathways work together properly so that human body can function well and stay healthy. Much knowledge about biological pathways has been accumulated over the past decades. Consequently, a number of online resources for biological pathways are available. These knowledge bases are extensive, including

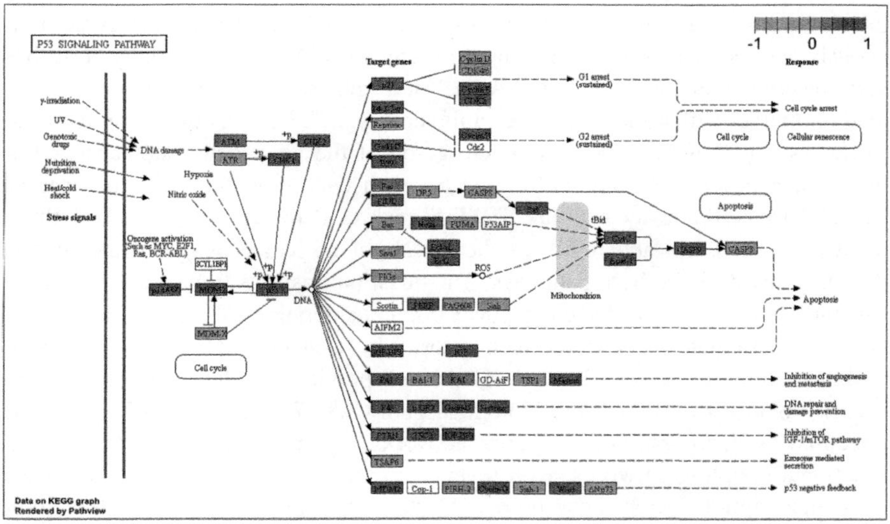

Fig. 1 p53 signaling pathway obtained from KEGG. The pathway shows the various genes, gene products, the interactions between genes, the directions of the signal propagation, and many other things

Kyoto Encyclopedia of Genes and Genomes (KEGG) [23, 24], WikiPathways [44], Reactome [21], and Pathway Commons [41].

The success of pathway-based approaches has been demonstrated in different studies. However, most pathway-based approaches utilize only partial information, that is, a pathway is treated as a list of genes and its topology structure is not considered. Indeed, a biological pathway describes a collection of interactions of molecules in cells, like mRNA, proteins, and metabolites, which coordinate with one another to perform cell functions or to direct cell responses to environmental changes. The topological structure of a biological pathway can be very informative. It reveals the interactions between genes, and it can help to improve the power of detection and to better understand risk factors of the disease. Different studies have demonstrated that incorporating the topological structure of a single biological pathway can improve the power to detect disease-related genes [10, 19, 22, 51]. Chen et al. [10] showed that the neighboring genes tend to have similar disease association statues. The proposed method introduced a Markov random field to model the topology structures of biological pathways. Hou et al. [20] proposed a novel guilt-by-rewiring principle, utilizing network information to prioritize disease genes. Freytag et al. [17] extended a logistic kernel machine into a network-based kernel machine test so that the topology structure of a biological pathway can be included in the model. Liu et al. [28] proposed the partial neighborhood selection (PNS) algorithm to estimate the gene dependence network, and a hidden Markov random field (HMRF) was adopted to combine the estimated network with genetic association scores.

The aforementioned studies only consider a single biological pathway. However, a single biological pathway only contains partial information about genes and interactions among genes. Genes participate in various biological processes simultaneously and they can interact in many different ways. A pathway usually describes very specific biological functions. As a result, genes, especially important ones, tend to interact with each other in several pathways. Therefore, combining multiple pathways can provide a more complete graph of the gene–gene interactions. For instance, genes IL23A and IL23R interact with each other in the Inflammatory Bowel Disease Pathway and Jak-STAT Signaling Pathway. Integration of these pathways can reveal and reinforce the effects of critical gene–gene interactions that play key roles in these pathways. The question arises as to whether or not we can further improve the detection power via consideration of multiple biological pathways simultaneously. Not much effort has been devoted to this important problem, although a very limited number of previous studies have shown the success of integrating multiple biological pathways. Wei and Pan [47] proposed a method to incorporate multiple gene networks, e.g., co-expression networks and functional coupling networks, with diverse genomic data to identify target genes of a transcription factor. They used a Markov random field-based mixture joint model (MRF-MJM) to merge gene networks. They assumed that the contribution of each gene network is additive and that a weight is assigned to each individual network. A larger weight indicates that there are more neighboring genes with similar status. In this method, the way to utilize multiple biological pathways is to sum over the contribution of each gene network. Their method focuses on identifying the regulatory target genes of a transcription factor. Bokanizad et al. [6] considered another approach to combining different biological pathways. Multiple biological pathways are linked together through a single gene, called interface gene, that connects two biological pathways through biological interactions and signal transduction.

Here, we propose to combine multiple biological pathways based on the common genes shared among different biological pathways. When we merge two or more biological pathways, the topological structures of the pathways will be preserved. Also, combining different biological pathways based on the common genes they share can account for the interactions among pathways. To model the topological structures of pathways, a probabilistic graphical model called Markov random field [10, 33] is employed. An MRF is a probabilistic measure assigned to an undirected graph. In the graph, genes are nodes and interactions are denoted by edges. One advantage of MRF is that it has the ability to capture the conditional independence among variables based on the graph topology. Thus, it can provide a compact and natural representation of the joint probability distribution of the set of variables in the graph. Another advantage of the MRF is that it can be used to control the false discovery rate in the presence of dependent relationships between genes [27]. Since MRF is capable of modeling the dependent structure in data, it has been applied to a wide range of fields. For example, Lin et al. [26] estimated the differentially expressed genes in the mouse transcriptome data, using a Markov random field to model the layer similarity, temporal dependency, and the similarity between sexes.

The rest of this chapter is organized as follows. Section 2 introduces our proposed methods. It includes the basic concepts that are relevant to the graph theory, a Gibbs measure assigned to the graph serving as a prior probability, different ways of setting weights to nodes and edges, the likelihood function, and the computational method. Simulation studies are presented in Sect. 3. A small-size graph and a relatively large graph are employed to show that combining multiple biological pathways can further improve the power of detection and control the false positive rate. Section 4 shows a case study that uses lung cancer data to demonstrate the performances of the proposed methods. Finally, Sect. 5 summarizes our methods with a discussion and possible future work.

2 Method

2.1 MRF Modeling of Biological Pathways

2.1.1 Undirected Graphs and Biological Pathways

A biological pathway consists of a collection of interacting molecules, which can be modeled as a graph through the use of graph theory [3, 38]. We will start with introducing some basic concepts in graph theory. A graph, defined as $G = (\mathcal{V}, \mathcal{E})$, is a collection of nodes that are connected by edges, where

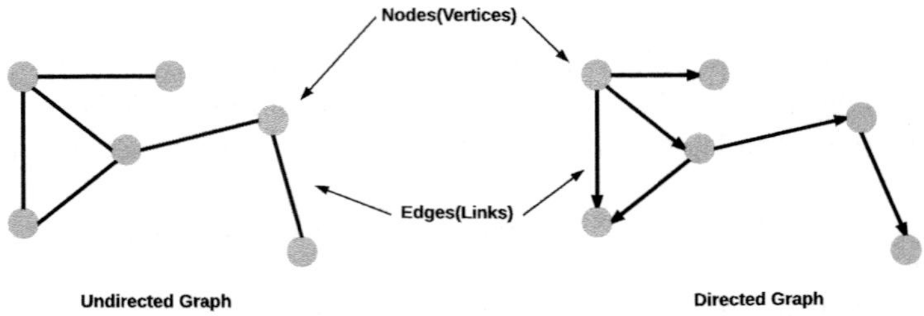

Fig. 2 Undirected graph and directed graph

$$\mathcal{V} = \{1, 2, \ldots, n\}$$
$$\mathcal{E} = \{< i, j >: i \text{ and } j \text{ are directly connected}\}.$$

If the edges do not have directions, the graph is called an undirected graph; otherwise, it is a directed graph (see Fig. 2). There are three key concepts in graph theory that will be useful to describe the structure of a graph. The first is the neighborhood of a node v, which, by definition, is a subset of all nodes that are directly connected to v by an edge. For the ith node in $\mathcal{V}$, we define the following terms:

$$\begin{aligned} N_i &= \{j :< i, j >\in \mathcal{E}\}, \\ d_i &= |N_i|, \\ E_{ij} &= \text{the number of edges connecting node } i \text{ and node } j, \\ E_i &= \sum_{j \in N_i} E_{ij}, \end{aligned}$$

where N_i is a set of neighbors of node i, d_i is the number of neighbors that node i has, E_{ij} is the number of edges linking node i and node j, and E_i is the number of total edges of node i. Note that $d_i = E_i$ if only one edge is present between any pair of nodes. In general, $d_i \leq E_i$ because multiple edges are allowed between node i and any of its neighbors, like in a combined graph to be discussed in Sect. 2.2. A complete graph is a simple undirected graph in which every pair of distinct nodes is connected by a unique edge. A clique is a complete subgraph of G. A clique of size k is called a k-clique (kth order clique). Each individual node is corresponding to a 1-clique. A pair of nodes can form a 2-clique and all triangles are 3-cliques. Examples are given in Fig. 3. In Fig. 3, there are six 1-cliques $\{1, 2, 3, 4, 5, 6\}$, six 2-cliques $\{(1, 2), (1, 3), (3, 6), (4, 5), (4, 6)\}$, and one 3-clique $\{(4, 6, 5)\}$. Note that since $\mathcal{V}$ is a set of nodes and $\mathcal{E}$ is a set of edges, from the perspective of cliques, $\mathcal{V}$ and $\mathcal{E}$ can also be treated as a set of 1-cliques and a set of 2-cliques, respectively.

Biological pathways represent the biological reaction and interaction network in a cell. Genes, proteins, and other molecules are involved and interact with each

Fig. 3 Cliques

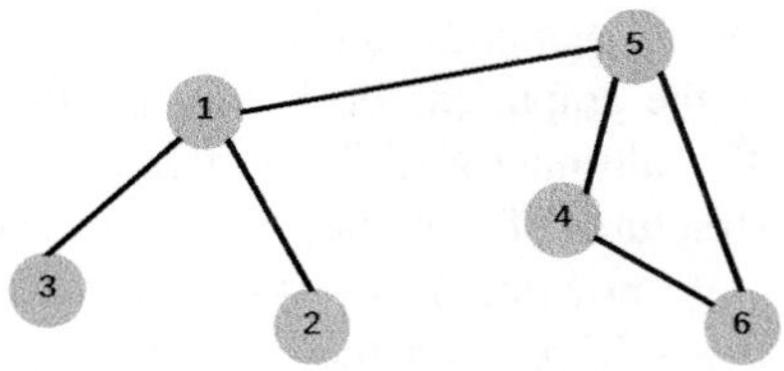

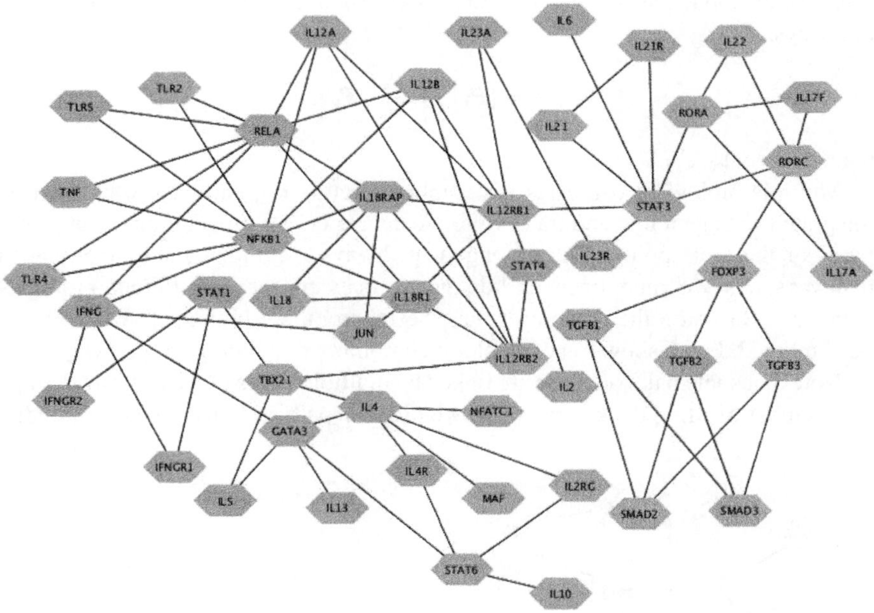

Fig. 4 Inflammatory Bowel Disease Pathway is represented as an UG (image is generated by Cytoscape [42])

other in a biological pathway. In our study, only gene–gene interactions are taken into consideration and we use an undirected graph (UG) to represent a biological pathway. An example of such a graph is shown in Fig. 4.

In the graph, genes are treated as nodes and gene–gene interactions are edges. Define S_i as the true status of gene i:

$$S_i = +1 \text{ if gene } i \text{ is associated with disease or is differentially expressed,}$$

$$S_i = -1 \text{ if gene } i \text{ is not associated with disease or is not differentially expressed.}$$

Hereafter, ± 1 are referred to as labels of nodes. Let $\mathbf{S} = (S_1, \ldots, S_n)$ be the labeling of $\mathcal{V}$. Thus, $\mathbf{S}$ is a spatial random vector whose element may be correlated to each other. Each node can be labeled as either $+1$ or -1. So, there are 2^n unique labelings of the graph, and each unique labeling of the graph is also called a configuration. The ultimate goal is to infer the value of $\mathbf{S}$ based on the underlying topological structures of biological pathways and observed data from biological experiments.

In practice, genes do not function in isolation. For complex diseases, multiple genes have been identified to collectively account for clinical phenotypes [29]. Moreover, the same pair of genes can interact in different biological pathways, which motivates us to combine multiple biological pathways to gather more information about gene–gene interactions. Let $\mathcal{P}$ denote a set of g distinct biological pathways:

$$\mathcal{P} = \{P_1, P_2, \ldots, P_g\},$$

where $P_l = (\mathcal{V}_l, \mathcal{E}_l), l = 1, \cdots, g$.

Multiple biological pathways are combined into a big pathway, which will be integrated with genomic and transcriptomic data later. We use an intuitive approach based on the overlapping genes among the pathways to combine multiple biological pathways. As we mentioned earlier, genes may appear in different biological pathways. Based on the common genes they share, these biological pathways can be combined. Fig. 5 shows an example of combining two biological pathways.

Note that some pairs of genes are linked by multiple edges in the combined graph. The number of edges denotes how many biological pathways that the corresponding

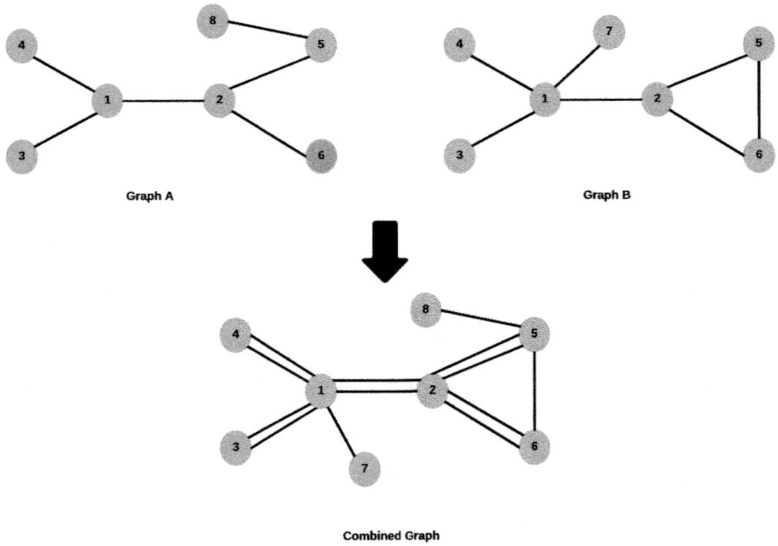

Fig. 5 An example of combining two biological pathways. Overlapping nodes in Graph A and Graph B are nodes (1, 2, 3, 4, 5, 6). Based on the shared nodes, Graphs A and B are integrated to a combined graph

genes interact with each other. In our study, we treat the multiple edges between neighboring genes as weighted single edge. The specific ways to assign weights to the weighted single edges will be discussed in section "A Nearest Gibbs Measure".

Genes interact with each other in the biological pathway. In the other words, there exist dependencies among the genes. In order to describe the topological structure and the dependencies, a Markov random field is employed [10], as will be introduced in the following section. An MRF not only describes the structures of biological pathways but also allows us to define a joint distribution for interdependent genes.

2.1.2 A Nearest Gibbs Measure

Speaking about the joint distribution of genes, we need to assign a probability measure to the combined biological pathway. The probability measure should reflect that the neighboring genes tend to have similar labels, and it should also quantify the effects of edges that connect the neighboring genes. Following [10], we can achieve both goals with one probability measure, a nearest Gibbs measure, as follows:

$$\mathbb{P}(\mathbf{S}|\theta_0) = \frac{1}{z(\theta_0)} \exp\left\{ h \sum_{i \in \mathcal{V}} I_1(S_i) + \tau_0 \sum_{<i,j> \in \mathcal{E}} (\omega_i + \omega_j) I_{-1}(S_i) I_{-1}(S_j) \right.$$
$$\left. + \tau_1 \sum_{<i,j> \in \mathcal{E}} (\omega_i + \omega_j) I_1(S_i) I_1(S_j) \right\}, \quad (1)$$

where $\theta_0 = (h, \tau_1, \tau_0)$, $I_1(\cdot)$ and $I_{-1}(\cdot)$ are indicator functions, and $z(\theta_0)$ is a normalizing function that is the sum over all 2^n possible configurations:

$$z(\theta_0) = \sum_{\mathbf{S}} \exp\left\{ h \sum_{i \in \mathcal{V}} I_1(S_i) + \tau_0 \sum_{<i,j> \in \mathcal{E}} (\omega_i + \omega_j) I_{-1}(S_i) I_{-1}(S_j) \right.$$
$$\left. + \tau_1 \sum_{<i,j> \in \mathcal{E}} (\omega_i + \omega_j) I_1(S_i) I_1(S_j) \right\}. \quad (2)$$

Note that it is computationally prohibitive to evaluate $z(\theta_0)$ when n is large. For instance, there are over 10 billion possible configurations when a graph has 30 nodes. Here, τ_0 and τ_1 assign weights to the 2-cliques in which both nodes are negative and positive genes, respectively; ω_i is a function of d_i and E_i, reflecting a weight we assign to node i. The details of the function ω_i will be described later in Sect. 2.2 when we define methods of combining biological pathways.

The probability measure in (1) directly considers the topological structure of a pathway. The first term is the sum over all the 1-cliques; the second sum and the third sum are taken over all the 2-cliques that contain both of two nodes labeled as -1 and labeled as $+1$, respectively. Positive τ_0 and τ_1 will put more weights on the 2-cliques in which all of the included nodes have the same labels, which is desirable in our context. The parameter h determines the marginal probability of S_i when $\tau_0 = \tau_1 = 0$, i.e., if all nodes are isolated, which indicates that they are independent:

$$\mathbb{P}(S_i = 1|h, \tau_0 = \tau_1 = 0) = \frac{\exp(h)}{\exp(h) + 1}.$$

There is an attractive feature of the Gibbs measure, that is, a sample from Gibbs measure has the local Markov property. This property defines an MRF on S, which by definition is $Pr(S_i|S_{\nu-i}) = Pr(S_i|S_{N_i})$, where $\mathcal{V} - i$ denotes all the nodes but i, and N_i is the set of all immediate neighbors of node i. This property can be asserted by the Hammersley–Clifford theorem [5]. We use an MRF to model the interactions between genes that are directly linked.

Theorem 1 (Hammersley–Clifford Theorem) *The spatial random vector,* $\mathbf{S}$, *under the Gibbs measure, is a Markov random field and thus satisfies*

$$\mathbb{P}(S_i|S_{\nu-i}, \theta_0) = \mathbb{P}(S_i|S_{N_i}, \theta_0).$$

Also, the conditional distribution of an MRF has a logistic regression form as shown below [10]:

$$\begin{aligned}\text{logit}(\mathbb{P}(S_i|S_{N_i}, \theta_0)) = h - \tau_0 &\sum_{<i,j>\in\mathcal{E}} (\omega_i + \omega_j) I_{-1}(S_i) I_{-1}(S_j) \\ &+\tau_1 \sum_{<i,j>\in\mathcal{E}} (\omega_i + \omega_j) I_1(S_i) I_1(S_j), \quad i = 1, \ldots, n. \quad (3)\end{aligned}$$

Equivalently, (3) can be written as a system of linear equations:

$$\begin{aligned}\text{logit}(\mathbb{P}(S_i|S_{N_i}, \theta_0)) &= \beta_{i0} + \beta_{i1} S_1 + \cdots + \beta_{in} S_n, \\ i &= 1, \ldots, n, \quad (4)\end{aligned}$$

where

$$\beta_{i0} = h$$

$$\beta_{ij} = \begin{cases} 0 & \text{if } i = j \text{ or } <i,j> \notin \mathcal{E} \\ (\omega_i + \omega_j)\{\tau_1 I_1(S_j) + \tau_0 I_{-1}(S_j)\} & \text{if } <i,j> \in \mathcal{E}. \end{cases}$$

The Markov property implies that the conditional distribution of S_i, given all the other node labels in the network, is equivalent to the conditional distribution of

S_i given all its immediate neighbors. If S_i and S_j are not neighbors, then they are conditionally independent. Now, we give an interpretation of ω_i in (1). From (4), it is obvious that the conditional probability of S_i depends on the weighted sum of its neighbors. Moreover, S_i has different weights depending on the sizes of cliques used to describe the structure of the graph in the probability measure.

2.2 Combine Multiple Pathways

In Eq. (1), the weight of S_i is

$$(\omega_i + \omega_j)\tau_1 \quad \text{if } S_i = S_j = +1,$$
$$(\omega_i + \omega_j)\tau_0 \quad \text{if } S_i = S_j = -1.$$

Here, $(\omega_i + \omega_j)$ is the sum of weights over all the nodes in the same 2-cliques. Recall that in the combined graph shown in Fig. 5, a pair of nodes can be linked by more than one edge, which may indicate the strength of relation between the neighboring nodes. The weights of nodes and edges are related to the number of neighbors and edges that nodes have in the combined graph. Next, we will present four different probability measures in which ω_i and the weights of edges are set in different ways.

Method 1 In this method, if two or more edges are between two neighboring genes, we only count them once. We set ω_i to be the logarithm of d_i, the number of neighbors of S_i. As a result, a gene that interacts with many other genes in the pathway has a large weight because it may play a central role in a biological process, and thus it is likely to have a large influence. However, a gene with one neighbor is assigned with 0. Thus, its effect has been reduced. The probability measure and the logistic form of the first method are identical to the equations shown in (1) and (3), respectively.

In a combined graph, if multiple edges are present between a pair of nodes, one could assign a weight to this link, in addition to the weights $(\omega_i + \omega_j)$ that are based on the nodes. In Methods 2 through 4 below, we define the weight of the link between nodes i and j as $(E_{ij})^2 \cdot (AE/TE)$, where E_{ij} is the number of edges linking nodes i and j,

$$AE = \frac{\sum_{<i,'j'>\in\mathcal{E}_1} E_{i'j'}^2 + \cdots + \sum_{<i,'j'>\in\mathcal{E}_g} E_{i'j'}^2}{g},$$

$$TE = \sum_{<i,'j'>\in\mathcal{E}_{CP}} E_{i'j'}^2, \ \mathcal{E}_{CP} \text{ denotes the edge set of the combined pathway.}$$

Note that E_{ij}, the number of edges between two nodes in the combined pathway, never decreases as more pathways are added. To regularize the growth of the edge weights, we multiply $(E_{ij})^2$ by a normalizing factor (AE/TE). The probability measure of $\mathbf{S}$ thus becomes

$$\mathbb{P}(\mathbf{S}|\theta_0) = \frac{1}{z(\theta_0)} \exp\left\{ h \sum_{i\in\mathcal{V}_{CP}} I_1(S_i) + \tau_0 \sum_{<i,j>\in\mathcal{E}_{CP}} (\omega_i+\omega_j) I_{-1}(S_i) I_{-1}(S_j) E_{ij}^2 (\frac{AE}{TE}) \right.$$
$$\left. + \tau_1 \sum_{<i,j>\in\mathcal{E}_{CP}} (\omega_i+\omega_j) I_1(S_i) I_1(S_j) E_{ij}^2 \left(\frac{AE}{TE}\right) \right\}. \quad (5)$$

The above probability measure also defines an MRF. The corresponding logistic form is

$$\text{logit}(\mathbb{P}(S_i|S_{N_i}, \theta_0)) = h - \tau_0 \sum_{<i,j>\in\mathcal{E}_{CP}} (\omega_i + \omega_j) I_{-1}(S_i) I_{-1}(S_j) E_{ij}^2 \left(\frac{AE}{TE}\right)$$
$$+ \tau_1 \sum_{<i,j>\in\mathcal{E}_{CP}} (\omega_i + \omega_j) I_1(S_i) I_1(S_j) E_{ij}^2 \left(\frac{AE}{TE}\right),$$
$$i = 1, \ldots, n. \quad (6)$$

The system of linear equations of (6) is

$$\text{logit}(\mathbb{P}(S_i|S_{N_i}, \theta_0)) = \beta_{i0} + \beta_{i1} S_1 + \cdots + \beta_{in} S_n,$$
$$i = 1, \ldots, n, \quad (7)$$

where

$$\beta_{i0} = h$$

$$\beta_{ij} = \begin{cases} 0 & \text{if } i = j \text{ or } < i, j > \notin \mathcal{E}_{CP} \\ (\omega_i + \omega_j)\{\tau_1 I_1(S_j) + \tau_0 I_{-1}(S_j)\} E_{ij}^2 (\frac{AE}{TE}) & \text{if } < i, j > \in \mathcal{E}_{CP}. \end{cases}$$

Methods 2 through 4 differ in the definition of ω_i, the weight assigned to node i. The motivation is to give more credit to the nodes that have more neighbors or more total number of edges in the combined graph.

Method 2 $\omega_i = \log(\frac{E_i}{g})$, where E_i is the total number of edges of node i.

Method 3 $\omega_i = \log(d_i)$, where d_i is the size of neighborhood of node i.

Method 4 $\omega_i = \log(E_i)$.

The probability measures in (1) and (5) both define an MRF that can be applied to describe the pathway topology. The MRF will be treated as a prior distribution under a Bayesian model to help us integrate the topological structure of biological pathways and prior biology knowledge in the Bayesian framework later (the details of Bayesian framework will be shown in Sect. 2.4).

2.3 Likelihood Function

We follow the method proposed by Chen et al. [10] to form a likelihood function. The evidence about disease association status or DE status, which is gathered from biological experiments, can be summarized by p-values at gene level. For gene i, its p-value can be converted to a response variable y_i through

$$y_i = \Phi^{-1}(1 - p_i),$$

where p_i is the p-value and $\Phi(\cdot)$ is the cumulative distribution function of $\mathcal{N}(0, 1)$. Note that a small value of p_i corresponds to a large value of y_i. Assume y_i are conditionally independent given S, the status of all genes. The null hypothesis is that the gene is unrelated to the disease. Under the null case where $S_i = -1$, the distribution of y_i is standard normal distribution. Therefore, the density of y_i is $f_0(y_i) \sim \mathcal{N}(0, 1)$. When the alternative hypothesis is true, that is, $S = +1$, the distribution of y_i is assumed to follow a normal distribution with the mean μ_i and the variance σ_i^2, where μ_i and σ_i are unknown. To account for the variations of μ_i and σ_i, prior distributions need to be assigned to μ_i and σ_i. We employ conjugate priors $\mu_i|\sigma_i^2 \sim \mathcal{N}(\bar{\mu}, \frac{\sigma_i^2}{a})$ and $\sigma_i^2 \sim$ Inverse Gamma$(\frac{\nu}{2}, \frac{\nu d}{2})$ for efficient computations. Define $\theta_1 = (\bar{\mu}, a, \nu, d)$ and $\mathbf{y} = (y_1, \ldots, y_n)$. Under this prior setting, the marginal density of y_i is

$$\begin{aligned}
f_1(y_i|S_i = 1, \theta_1) &= \int\int \frac{1}{\sqrt{2\pi\sigma_i^2}} \exp[\frac{-(y_i - \mu_i)^2}{2\sigma_i^2}] \frac{\sqrt{a}}{\sqrt{2\pi\sigma_i^2}} \exp\left[\frac{-a(y_i - \bar{\mu})^2}{2\sigma_i^2}\right] \\
&\quad \times \frac{(\nu d/2)^{\nu/2}}{\Gamma(\nu/2)} (\sigma_i^{-2})^{\nu/2-1} \exp\left[-(\sigma_i^{-2})\frac{\nu d}{2}\right] d\mu_i d(\sigma_i^{-2}) \\
&= \int \frac{1}{\sqrt{2\pi\frac{a+1}{a}\sigma_i^2}} \exp[\frac{-a(y_i - \bar{\mu})^2}{2(a+1)\sigma_i^2}] \frac{(\nu d/2)^{\frac{\nu}{2}}}{\Gamma(\nu/2)} (\sigma_i^{-2})^{\nu/2-1} \exp\left[\frac{-\nu d\sigma_i^{-2}}{2}\right] d(\sigma_i^{-2}) \\
&= \frac{1}{\sqrt{2\pi}} \frac{\sqrt{a}}{\sqrt{a+1}} \frac{(\nu d/2)^{\frac{\nu}{2}}}{\Gamma(\nu/2)} \int (\sigma_i^{-2})^{\frac{\nu+1}{2}} \exp\left[-\sigma_i^2\{\frac{\nu d}{2} + \frac{a(y_i - \bar{\mu})^2}{2(a+1)}\}\right] d(\sigma_i^{-2}) \\
&= \frac{1}{\sqrt{2\pi}} \frac{\sqrt{a}}{\sqrt{a+1}} \frac{(\nu d/2)^{\nu/2}}{\Gamma(\nu/2)} \Gamma(\frac{\nu+1}{2}) \cdot \{\frac{\nu d}{2} + \frac{1}{2}\frac{a}{a+1}(y - \bar{\mu})^2\}^{-\frac{(1+\nu)}{2}} \\
&= \pi^{-1/2}(\nu d)^{\nu/2} \frac{\sqrt{a}}{\sqrt{a+1}} \frac{\Gamma((\nu+1)/2)}{\Gamma(\nu/2)} \left(\frac{a}{a+1}(y_i - \bar{\mu}^2 + \nu d)\right)^{-(1+\nu)/2}.
\end{aligned} \tag{8}$$

Therefore, the likelihood function of $\boldsymbol{y}$ is

$$f(\boldsymbol{y}|\mathbf{S}, \theta_1) = \prod_{j:S_j=-1} f_0(y_j) \times \prod_{j:S_j=+1} f_1(y_j|S_j = 1, \theta_1). \tag{9}$$

2.4 Posterior Probability Under Bayesian Framework

Under a Bayesian framework, the MRF is the prior probability describing the topological structures of the biological pathways, and the likelihood function in Eq. (9) presents the evidence from biological experiments. Thus, the posterior probability of $\mathbf{S}$, given the observed data $\boldsymbol{y}$, is

$$\begin{aligned} \mathbb{P}(\mathbf{S}|\boldsymbol{y}, \theta_0, \theta_1) &= \frac{f(\boldsymbol{y}|\mathbf{S}, \theta_1)\mathbb{P}(\mathbf{S}|\theta_0)}{\sum_{\mathbf{S}} f(\boldsymbol{y}|\mathbf{S}, \theta_1)\mathbb{P}(\mathbf{S}|\theta_0)} \\ &\propto f(\boldsymbol{y}|\mathbf{S}, \theta_1)\mathbb{P}(\mathbf{S}|\theta_0). \end{aligned} \tag{10}$$

Recall that the prior probability introduced in Sect. 2.1 defines an MRF and has a nice conditional probability. Similar to the prior probability, the posterior probability defines an MRF as well. For node i,

$$\begin{aligned} \mathbb{P}(S_i = +1|\boldsymbol{y}, S_{\nu-i}, \theta_0, \theta_1) &\propto f_1(y_i|\theta_1)\mathbb{P}(S_i = +1|S_{\nu-i}, \theta_0) \\ &= f_1(y_i|\theta_1)\mathbb{P}(S_i = +1|S_{N_i}, \theta_0). \end{aligned} \tag{11}$$

The conditional posterior distribution of S_i, given all other nodes, only depends on its neighbors, which means that the posterior distribution leads to an MRF [10]. We use method 1 as an example to show the logistic form of the conditional distribution of S_i:

$$\begin{aligned} \text{logit}(\mathbb{P}(S_i|\boldsymbol{y}, S_{N_i}, \theta_0, \theta_1) = h + \log LR(y_i; \theta_1) - \tau_0 \sum_{<i,j>\in\mathcal{E}_{CP}} (\omega_i + \omega_j) I_{-1}(S_i) I_{-1}(S_j) \\ + \tau_1 \sum_{<i,j>\in\mathcal{E}_{CP}} (\omega_i + \omega_j) I_1(S_i) I_1(S_j), \end{aligned} \tag{12}$$

where

$$LR(y_i; \theta_1) = \frac{f_1(y_i|\theta_1)}{f_0(y_i)},$$

the marginal likelihood ratio. Therefore, (12) integrates the evidence from biological experiments that is reflected by the marginal likelihood ratio and the effect from interactions among neighboring genes in biological pathway reflected by the conditional prior odds. It is easy to see that the posterior conditional logit form in (12) is the same as the prior conditional logit in (3) except its intercept is $h + \log(LR(y_i); \theta_1)$. The observed log-likelihood ratio provides an additive effect to the logit of prior.

We can also rewrite (12) in the form of a system of linear regressions:

$$\text{logit}(\mathbb{P}(S_i | \mathbf{y}, S_{N_i}, \theta_0, \theta_1)) = \beta_{i0} + \beta_{i1} S_1 + \cdots + \beta_{in} S_n, \quad i = 1, \ldots, n, \tag{13}$$

where

$$\beta_{i0} = h + \log LR(y_i; \theta_1),$$

$$\beta_{ij} = \begin{cases} 0 & \text{if } i = j \text{ or } < i, j > \notin \mathcal{E}_{CP}, \\ (\omega_i + \omega_j)\{\tau_1 I_1(S_j) + \tau_0 I_{-1}(S_j)\} & \text{if } < i, j > \in \mathcal{E}_{CP}. \end{cases}$$

The posterior probabilities of other three priors proposed in Sect. 2.1 have similar logistic regression forms. As mentioned before, the differences among Method 2, Method 3, and Method 4 are the definitions of ω_i.

2.5 Monte Carlo Markov Chain (MCMC) Simulation

As the number of genes becomes very large, it is prohibitive to calculate the posterior probability directly. But the posterior distribution has a nice closed-form conditional distribution, due to the Markov property. It is easier to sample from the conditional distribution using the Gibbs sampling [9]. The Gibbs sampler is one of the MCMC algorithms, and it can generate a sequence of samples from the conditional distributions.

In our context, the specific steps are described as the following: we start by setting the initial values of $\mathbf{S}$, $\mathbf{s}^{(0)} = (s_1, \ldots, s_n)$. Here, the upper case $\mathbf{S}$ is to denote a random vector and use the lower case $\mathbf{s}^{(k)}$ to denote a realization of the random vector in the kth iteration. The elements of the vector $\mathbf{s}^{(k)}$ are $+1$s and -1s. At iteration k, we update the labels sequentially for $i = 1, \ldots, n$ based on

$$\begin{aligned} &\text{logit}(\mathbb{P}(s_i^{(k)} | \mathbf{y}, s_1^{(k)}, \cdots, s_{i-1}^{(k)}, s_i^{(k-1)}, \cdots, s_n^{(k-1)}, \theta_1, \theta_0) \\ &= \beta_{i0} + \beta_{i1} s_1^{(k)} + \cdots + \beta_{i,i-1} s_{i-1}^{(k)} + \beta_{i,i+1} s_{i+1}^{(k-1)} + \cdots + \beta_{in} s_n^{(k-1)}. \end{aligned}$$

When performing the Gibbs sampling, we recommend to restart the simulation multiple times with different initial values to reduce the influence of initial values and ignore a number of simples from beginning (the so-called burn-in period).

2.6 Making Inference Based on the Marginal Posterior Probability

In GWAS and mRNA expression studies, a set of genes is identified as candidates that are very likely to be associated with diseases or differentially expressed. Therefore, we want to include as many truly positive genes among the candidates as possible. Following [10], we describe a method that can be used to rank order genes. The inference of gene status is based on $m_i = \mathbb{P}(S_i = 1|\boldsymbol{y}, \theta_0, \theta_1)$, the mean of the marginal posterior probability of S_i. A decision rule in the form $\delta(m_i) = I(m_i \geq m^*)$ is considered, where $I(\cdot)$ is an indicator function and m^* is a decision threshold. Here, m^* can facilitate deciding the status of a gene as below:

$$\delta(m_i) = \begin{cases} 1 & m_i \geq m^* \\ 0 & m_i < m^*. \end{cases}$$

If $\delta(m_i)$ is 1, the decision is positive, indicating that gene i is considered to be associated with the disease or differentially expressed; otherwise, gene i is identified as a negative gene. To find the decision threshold m^*, a 0–1 loss function, which is widely used in classification problem, is employed. In our context, a 0–1 loss function is defined by $L(\boldsymbol{S}, \delta) = \sum_{i=1}^{n} |I_1(S_i) - \delta(m_i)|$. This loss function penalizes equally the false positive and false negative errors. Note that $L(\boldsymbol{S}, \delta)$ is a random variable because it is a function of the random vector $\boldsymbol{S}$ and a decision function $\delta(\cdot)$, which depends on $E[\boldsymbol{S}|y]$ and m^*. We consider the expected loss with respect to the posterior distribution of $\boldsymbol{S}$:

$$E\{L(\boldsymbol{S}, \delta)|\boldsymbol{y}, \theta_0, \theta_1\} = \sum_{i=1}^{n} |I_1(S_i) - \delta(m_i)| \cdot \mathbb{P}(S_i|\boldsymbol{y}, \theta_0, \theta_1). \tag{14}$$

Then, m^* is sought to minimize the expected loss:

$$\begin{aligned} m^* &= \underset{m}{\text{argmin}}\, E\{L(\boldsymbol{S}, \delta)|\boldsymbol{y}, \theta_0, \theta_1\} \\ &= \underset{m}{\text{argmin}} \sum_{i=1}^{n} |I_1(S_i) - \delta(m_i)| \cdot \mathbb{P}(S_i|\boldsymbol{y}, \theta_0, \theta_1). \end{aligned} \tag{15}$$

To find the solution, look at the loss incurred by gene i: $[1 - \delta(m_i)] \cdot m_i + \delta(m_i) \cdot (1 - m_i)$. To minimize it, $\delta(m_i)$ should be 1 if $m_i \geq 0.5$ and 0 otherwise. Therefore, the expected loss in Eq. (14) can be minimized when $m^* = 0.5$. For other possible decision rules, please see [10].

3 Simulation Studies

Two simulation studies are carried out to examine how the values of (h, τ_1, τ_0) affect the network and evaluate the performances of the proposed methods. A small combined network that only contains 10 nodes is used to explore the effect of prior settings. A relatively large combined network having 27 nodes is used to evaluate the performance of combined network based on the control of false positive rates and false discovery rates.

4 10-Node Network

A 10-node network is used to study the effects of hyper-parameters h, τ_1, and τ_0. In the network shown in Fig. 6, Graph A has 6 nodes, and Graph B has 10 nodes. Combined together, there is a total of 10 nodes in the network. Nodes $(1, 2, 4, 10)$ are labeled as $+1$ (in red color) and nodes $(5, 6, 7, 8, 9)$ are labeled as -1 (in blue color). Graph A and Graph B share 4 positive nodes $(1, 2, 3, 4)$. In addition, Graph B has one more positive node (Node 10) than Graph A. After combining the two graphs based on the common nodes, we can obtain a combined graph in which multiple edges exist. Compared to the single graph A or B, some neighbors are connected by two edges. Consequently, neighboring nodes with identical labels have reinforced relationship if connected by multiple edges. The more edges the neighboring genes share, the stronger the relationship they have. As a result, it is more likely for the neighboring genes to have the same status. To conduct a fair comparison between using only Graph A or B and using combined 10-node

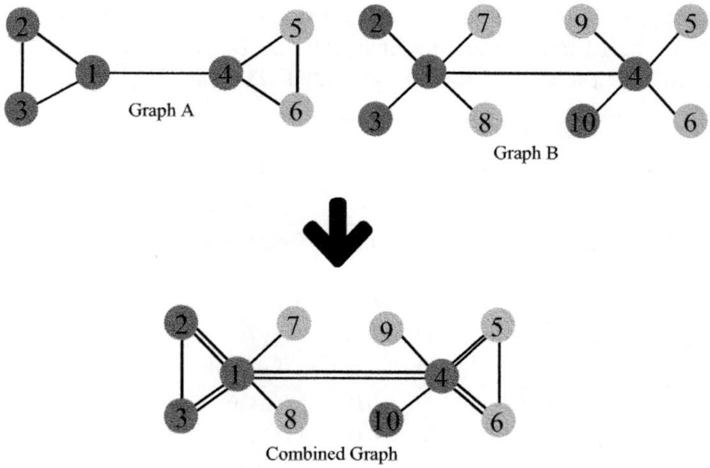

Fig. 6 Simulated 10-node networks and combined network

network, the same set of nodes has to appear in both Graphs A and B, as do in the combined graph. Therefore, the nodes in Graph B but not in Graph A are added as singletons to Graph A.

When $S = +1$, to simulate different levels of the power of the statistical tests, p-values are calculated from two-sided z-scores drawn from $\mathcal{N}(0.5, 1)$, $\mathcal{N}(1, 1)$, and $\mathcal{N}(1.5, 1)$, corresponding to the power of 0.08 (weak), 0.16 (median), and 0.32 (strong), respectively, for the tests. When $S = -1$, p-values are sampled from Uniform$(0, 1)$.

To study the effects of hyper-parameters (h, τ_1, τ_0), Table 1 lists four main groups of prior settings. They are chosen to control the prior mean $\mathbb{P}(S_i = +1)$ to be around 0.05, 0.15, 0.25, and 0.4, respectively, for the four groups. The average values of $\mathbb{P}(S_i = +1)$ are listed in the column $\mathbb{E}[\Pr(S_i = 1)]$. Under each main group, there are two subgroups. The difference of the two subgroups is in the average probability of $\mathbb{P}(S_i = S_j = +1)$, shown in the column $\mathbb{E}[\Pr(S_i = S_j = 1)]$. The values of $(\bar{\mu}, a, v, d)$ in likelihood function are set to be (3,1,10,1).

One thousand datasets are simulated for every prior setting. For the 10-node network, the posterior probability can be calculated directly from the global measure without using the Gibbs sampling. This is because there are only 1024 configurations in total, and it is not computation-intensive to evaluate the normalizing term in the global measure in Eq. (10). To rank the genes based on p-values or marginal posterior $P(S_i = +1|y)$ from the proposed methods, we can calculate true positive rate and false positive rate:

$$\text{true positive rate} = \frac{\text{number of true positives}}{\text{number of true positives } + \text{ number of false positives}},$$

$$\text{false positive rate} = \frac{\text{number of false positives}}{\text{number of true positives} + \text{ number of false positives}}.$$

By varying the cutoff values, we can plot true positive rate versus false positive rate to draw the receiver operating characteristic (ROC) curve. Finally, the area under the ROC curve (AUC) can be calculated. The value of AUC is 0.5 without

Table 1 Prior settings for the 10 nodes combined network

		Parameters			Prior mean	
Group	Subgroup	h	τ_1	τ_0	$\mathbb{E}[\Pr(S_i = 1)]$	$\mathbb{E}[\Pr(S_i = S_j = 1)]$
1	a	-3.000	0.100	0.001	0.0483	0.0029
	b	-2.750	0.150	0.005	0.0616	0.0051
2	a	-2.000	0.200	0.001	0.1351	0.0275
	b	-2.000	0.250	0.005	0.1397	0.0322
3	a	-1.250	0.100	0.001	0.2430	0.0717
	b	-1.500	0.250	0.005	0.2329	0.0861
4	a	-0.500	0.050	0.005	0.3956	0.1703
	b	-1.000	0.250	0.010	0.3660	0.1965

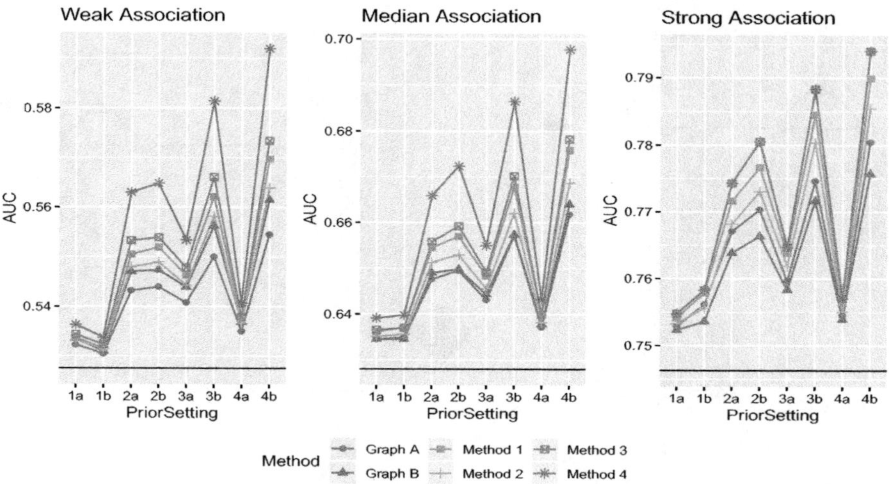

Fig. 7 AUC of the 10-node pathway. Graph A and Graph B are referring to methods based on single pathways A and B, respectively. Methods 1–4 are the proposed ones to combine both pathways. The black horizontal lines indicate AUC based on p-values only

any models, and a value of the AUC higher than 0.5 means that the performance of the model is better. The AUCs calculated using only the p-values are 0.5276, 0.6281, and 0.7463, corresponding to weak, median, and strong associations. Fig. 7 shows the performance of proposed methods.

First of all, in Fig. 7, the values of AUC from Bayesian models (Graph A, Graph B, and Methods 1–4) are larger than the values obtained using p-values alone (the black horizontal lines), no matter using a single pathway (Graph A and Graph B) or the combined one (Methods 1–4). Using the combined graph outperforms the single graph, especially in prior setting 2, prior setting 3, and prior setting 4. In general, the values of AUC that are corresponding to subgroup (b) are higher than those to subgroup (a). The reason is that (h, τ_1, τ_0) in subgroup (b) are larger than the ones in subgroup (a). So, priors in subgroup (b) encourage nodes labeled as $+1$. In general, the value of τ_1, which is the weight of linked truly associated or equally expressed genes, should be larger than τ_0.

5 27-Node Network

The proposed methods are also applied to two large networks and the combined network in Fig. 8. There are 21 nodes in Graph A and 24 nodes in Graph B. Nodes 1, 2, 3, 4, 5, 6, 19, 22, and 23 are considered as true positive genes (in red color), and the others are negative genes (in blue color). One positive node (#19) and two negative nodes (#20 and #21) in Graph A are not presented in Graph B. On the other

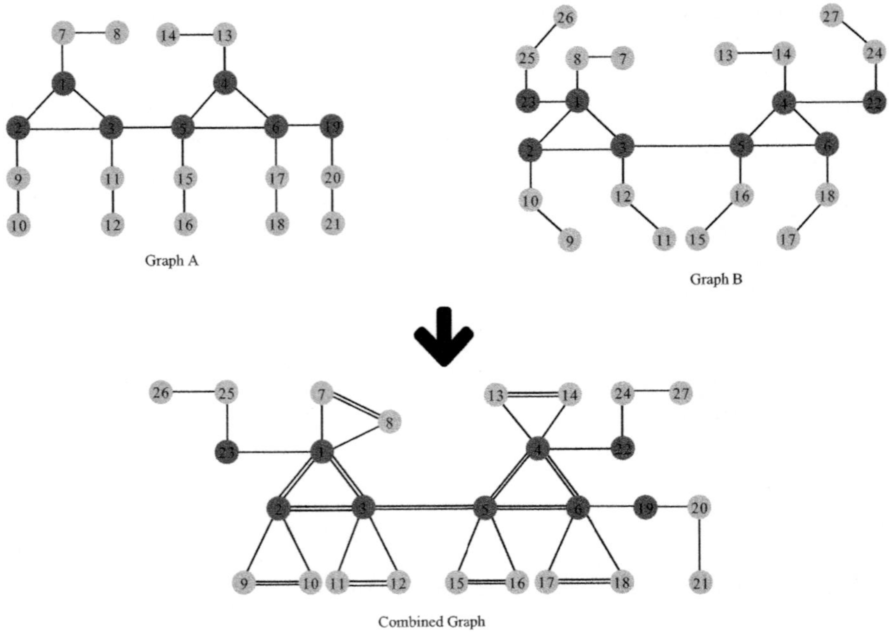

Fig. 8 Simulated 27-node networks and the combined network

Table 2 Prior settings for the combined 27-node pathway

Group	Subgroup	Parameters			Prior mean	
		h	τ_1	τ_0	$\mathbb{E}[\Pr(S_i = 1)]$	$\mathbb{E}[\Pr(S_i = S_j = 1)]$
1	a	-3.000	0.100	0.001	0.0470	0.0031
	b	-2.750	0.150	0.005	0.0626	0.0061
2	a	-2.000	0.200	0.001	0.1414	0.0308
	b	-2.000	0.250	0.005	0.1533	0.0434
3	a	-1.250	0.100	0.001	0.2491	0.0767
	b	-1.500	0.250	0.005	0.2602	0.1139
4	a	-0.500	0.050	0.005	0.3991	0.1740
	b	-1.000	0.250	0.010	0.4184	0.2686

hand, two other positive nodes (#22 and #23) and four negative ones (#24, #25, #26, and #27) in Graph B are not in Graph A. When they are combined together, we obtain a 27-node network. The prior settings are the same as that chosen for 10-node networks. Table 2 shows the average prior probabilities $\mathbb{P}(S_i = 1)$ and the average prior probabilities $\mathbb{P}(S_i = S_j = 1)$.

The same method is applied to simulate p-values, that is, they are computed from two-sided z-scores drawn at random from $\mathcal{N}(1, 1)$, $\mathcal{N}(1.5, 1)$, and $\mathcal{N}(2, 1)$

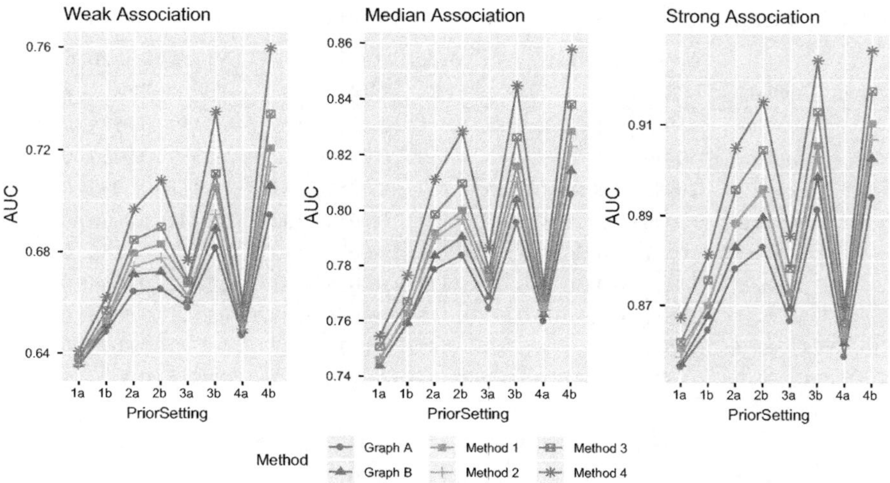

Fig. 9 AUC of the 27-node pathway. Graph A and Graph B refer to methods based on single pathways A and B, respectively. Methods 1–4 are the proposed ones to combine both pathways. The black horizontal lines indicate AUC based on p-values only

when $S = +1$, and p-values are sampled from Uniform(0,1) when $S = -1$. The AUC is computed for each group of prior settings to evaluate the performances of the proposed methods. We simulate 100 datasets and run a Gibbs sampler with 10 restarts where each restart contains 1000 iterations (the first 100 are burn-ins). For each simulated dataset, we calculate the value of AUC. Fig. 9 shows the average values of AUC of the 100 simulations for all scenarios. The values of AUC computed from p-values alone are 0.6367, 0.7489, and 0.8483, corresponding to weak, median, and strong tests, respectively. Form the figure, similar observations can be drawn as from the 10-node network.

In addition to comparisons based on the AUC, next we evaluate the performances of the proposed methods in terms of false positive rate (FPR), true positive rate (TPR), and false discovery rate (FDR). We apply the decision rule $\delta(m_i)$ to the marginal posterior probability with a cutoff $m^* = 0.5$. Table 3 lists the average FPR, TPR, and FDR of 100 datasets with 8 different prior settings. We also compare the proposed methods with the p-value method with a cutoff value of 0.05.

In Table 3, for each prior setting, the proposed methods that make use of multiple networks have higher TPR and lower or equal FDR than using a single network. For prior setting groups 1, 2, and 3, the FPR of the proposed methods is much lower than 0.05, making the TPR worse than the method of p-value only. However, the prior setting 4b controls FPR at $\sim$0.05, and it has a higher TPR and a lower FDR than using p-value alone.

Table 3 Average false positive rate (FPR), true positive rate (TPR), and false discovery rate (FDR)

Group	Method	Weak association			Median association			Strong association		
		TPR	FPR	FDR	TPR	FPR	FDR	TPR	FPR	FDR
	p-Value	0.1578	0.0528	0.4238	0.3111	0.0528	0.2567	0.5189	0.0528	0.1549
1a	Graph A	0.0489	0.0056	0.6183	0.1100	0.0056	0.3278	0.2389	0.0056	0.0979
	Graph B	0.0489	0.0056	0.6183	0.1078	0.0056	0.3278	0.2411	0.0056	0.0979
	Method 1	0.0500	0.0056	0.6167	0.1122	0.0056	0.3278	0.2444	0.0056	0.0979
	Method 2	0.0511	0.0056	0.6067	0.1111	0.0056	0.3278	0.2411	0.0056	0.0979
	Method 3	0.0511	0.0056	0.6067	0.1133	0.0056	0.3178	0.2422	0.0056	0.0979
	Method 4	0.0511	0.0056	0.6067	0.1167	0.0056	0.3178	0.2511	0.0056	0.0879
1b	Graph A	0.0567	0.0072	0.5783	0.1311	0.0072	0.2775	0.2722	0.0072	0.0748
	Graph B	0.0578	0.0072	0.5683	0.1333	0.0078	0.2792	0.2811	0.0078	0.0757
	Method 1	0.0567	0.0072	0.5783	0.1367	0.0078	0.2787	0.2956	0.0078	0.0752
	Method 2	0.0567	0.0072	0.5783	0.1344	0.0072	0.2770	0.2867	0.0072	0.0740
	Method 3	0.0578	0.0072	0.5773	0.1389	0.0072	0.2750	0.3033	0.0072	0.0740
	Method 4	0.0600	0.0072	0.5673	0.1456	0.0072	0.2750	0.3200	0.0078	0.0643
2a	Graph A	0.0900	0.0183	0.4625	0.2111	0.0183	0.2235	0.4167	0.0183	0.0869
	Graph B	0.0911	0.0178	0.4575	0.2144	0.0183	0.2018	0.4244	0.0194	0.0904
	Method 1	0.0956	0.0183	0.4508	0.2278	0.0189	0.1910	0.4622	0.0228	0.0976
	Method 2	0.0933	0.0183	0.4608	0.2144	0.0178	0.2143	0.4400	0.0183	0.0836
	Method 3	0.1022	0.0178	0.4454	0.2233	0.0178	0.1900	0.4667	0.0194	0.0754
	Method 4	0.1078	0.0183	0.4425	0.2511	0.0183	0.1756	0.4900	0.0194	0.0615
2b	Graph A	0.0922	0.0183	0.4525	0.2133	0.0189	0.2185	0.4400	0.0206	0.0889
	Graph B	0.0944	0.0178	0.4508	0.2167	0.0178	0.1943	0.4522	0.0194	0.0870
	Method 1	0.1033	0.0189	0.4435	0.2344	0.0200	0.1782	0.4822	0.0261	0.1041
	Method 2	0.1033	0.0178	0.4404	0.2167	0.0178	0.2177	0.4633	0.0183	0.0832
	Method 3	0.1100	0.0189	0.4392	0.2511	0.0183	0.1781	0.4889	0.0200	0.0649
	Method 4	0.1200	0.0189	0.4292	0.2933	0.0194	0.1687	0.5378	0.0222	0.0661
3a	Graph A	0.1356	0.0350	0.4195	0.2811	0.0361	0.2200	0.5022	0.0361	0.1202
	Graph B	0.1344	0.0356	0.4249	0.2856	0.0361	0.2177	0.5067	0.0383	0.1245
	Method 1	0.1400	0.0361	0.4205	0.2978	0.0378	0.2209	0.5222	0.0394	0.1225
	Method 2	0.1389	0.0356	0.4230	0.2867	0.0356	0.2155	0.5089	0.0361	0.1188
	Method 3	0.1422	0.0361	0.4224	0.2967	0.0356	0.2094	0.5189	0.0367	0.1184
	Method 4	0.1489	0.0356	0.4143	0.3156	0.0356	0.2010	0.5322	0.0367	0.1160
3b	Graph A	0.1322	0.0317	0.4226	0.2911	0.0322	0.1930	0.5211	0.0322	0.1045
	Graph B	0.1344	0.0317	0.4253	0.3000	0.0322	0.2042	0.5278	0.0339	0.1073
	Method 1	0.1522	0.0333	0.4028	0.3311	0.0361	0.2048	0.5656	0.0394	0.1131
	Method 2	0.1400	0.0311	0.4208	0.3100	0.0317	0.1964	0.5322	0.0317	0.1004
	Method 3	0.1489	0.0311	0.4108	0.3456	0.0317	0.1739	0.5778	0.0317	0.0944
	Method 4	0.1622	0.0322	0.4003	0.3933	0.0333	0.1675	0.6267	0.0339	0.0906

(continued)

Table 3 (continued)

Group	Method	Weak association			Median association			Strong association		
		TPR	FPR	FDR	TPR	FPR	FDR	TPR	FPR	FDR
4a	Graph A	0.2089	0.0689	0.4314	0.3867	0.0700	0.2772	0.5989	0.0706	0.1828
	Graph B	0.2100	0.0678	0.4244	0.3867	0.0672	0.2681	0.5967	0.0667	0.1744
	Method 1	0.2133	0.0694	0.4206	0.3911	0.0694	0.2719	0.6011	0.0700	0.1802
	Method 2	0.2089	0.0672	0.4288	0.3867	0.0672	0.2706	0.6011	0.0678	0.1770
	Method 3	0.2133	0.0672	0.4238	0.3967	0.0678	0.2565	0.6044	0.0672	0.1748
	Method 4	0.2144	0.0683	0.4248	0.4056	0.0683	0.2549	0.6056	0.0678	0.1753
4b	Graph A	0.1789	0.0456	0.3974	0.3844	0.0467	0.2107	0.5989	0.0478	0.1287
	Graph B	0.1822	0.0489	0.4124	0.3889	0.0506	0.2161	0.6167	0.0528	0.1332
	Method 1	0.2022	0.0528	0.3817	0.4389	0.0544	0.1998	0.6644	0.0594	0.1413
	Method 2	0.1800	0.0467	0.4134	0.4056	0.0478	0.1956	0.6256	0.0489	0.1243
	Method 3	0.2011	0.0494	0.3961	0.4444	0.0506	0.1937	0.6589	0.0528	0.1251
	Method 4	0.2522	0.0506	0.3425	0.4989	0.0533	0.1758	0.7133	0.0544	0.1219

Table 4 Details of lung cancer datasets

Dataset name	Number of controls	Number of cases
CL	17	65
Moff	27	52
NCIU133A	18	86
NCILungU133A	44	131

6 Lung Cancer Data

We used four mRNA microarray datasets of lung adenocarcinoma [43] to evaluate the performances of the proposed methods. Data were pre-processed and patients were grouped to two categories, labeled as cases and controls, according to their survival times. For details of the data processing, please see [11]. Each of the datasets has 12,992 genes. Table 4 contains information of the data example. Two-sample t-tests were used to obtain p-values for all genes in all four datasets.

We used 59 lung cancer genes [11] as true positive genes in our analysis. However, this set has a much smaller size than the number of genes in the study. To find additional "positive" genes, CL, Moff, and NCIU133A were used as discovery datasets. For every gene, we used Fisher's Method to combine the three p-values from the three discovery sets to obtain an overall p-value. Then, we defined new positive genes by controlling the FDR under 0.15 using the Benjamini–Hochberg procedure [4]. As a result, among the 12,992 genes, a total of 1044 (or 8.0%) are positive genes in the end.

We extracted 528 biological pathways from KEGG (http://www.kegg.jp), GennMapp (http://genmapp.org), and BioCarta (http://www.biocarta.com) that contained 3735 unique genes, among which 301 ones (or 8.1%) are in the positive set. We found that 379 pathways had at least one lung cancer-associated gene. Finally, we

Table 5 Information of 3 biological pathways

Pathway name (short name)	Number of genes	Number of true positive genes under an FDR cutoff of 0.15
GM human integrin-mediated cell adhesion (adhesion)	118	10
GM human regulation of actin cytoskeleton (regulation)	206	12
GM human signaling of hepatocyte growth factor receptor (HGFR)	120	11

Table 6 AUC of single- and combined-pathway analyses for 14 positive genes under FDR cutoff of 0.15

	Group							
Method	1a	1b	2a	2b	3a	3b	4a	4b
Adhesion	0.5851	0.6425	0.6437	0.6586	0.6400	0.6550	0.6465	0.6693
Regulation	0.5743	0.6516	0.6738	0.7042	0.6448	0.6432	0.5945	0.5438
PGFR	0.5762	0.6650	0.6460	0.6773	0.6752	0.6821	0.6590	0.6894
Method 1	0.5768	0.6511	0.6555	0.6899	0.6641	0.6714	0.5745	0.5768
Method 2	0.5869	0.6722	0.7041	0.7175	0.7050	0.7057	0.7162	0.6920
Method 3	0.5859	0.6749	0.7033	0.7058	0.7068	0.7031	0.6952	0.6586
Method 4	0.5879	0.6835	0.7047	0.6971	0.6929	0.6913	0.6701	0.6362

chose three GennMapp (GM) pathways that were enriched with true positive genes. Table 5 shows details about these three pathways.

The combined pathway had 256 distinct genes, 14 of which were associated with lung cancer (Table 5). We used p-values of dataset NCILungU133A as our test data. However, this test set was missing 18 of the 256 genes in the combined gene pathway. After these 18 genes were removed, the combined pathway has 238 genes including 14 positive genes. To conduct a fair comparison between using a single pathway versus using multiple ones, the same genes had to appear in both the single pathway and the combined one. Therefore, the genes that were in the combined pathway but not in the single pathway were added as singletons to each single pathway.

The same 8 sets of prior parameters (Table 1) were used in our analysis. Use Gibbs sampling to draw random samples from the posterior distribution. Restart the Gibbs sampler 50 times and iterate 1000 times (the first 300 were burn-ins) for each restart. Calculate AUC for all methods. The AUC based on the p-values is 0.5663. Table 6 and Fig. 10 show the values of the AUC for 3 single pathways and 4 proposed methods on the combined pathway.

The black horizontal line in Fig. 10 represents the value of AUC obtained from p-values alone. In general, incorporating pathways, using either a single pathway or the combined one, outperformed the one using p-value only. Comparing the performance of using the combined pathway to one single pathway, the AUCs of Methods 2, 3, and 4 are higher than using a single pathway in all settings. However,

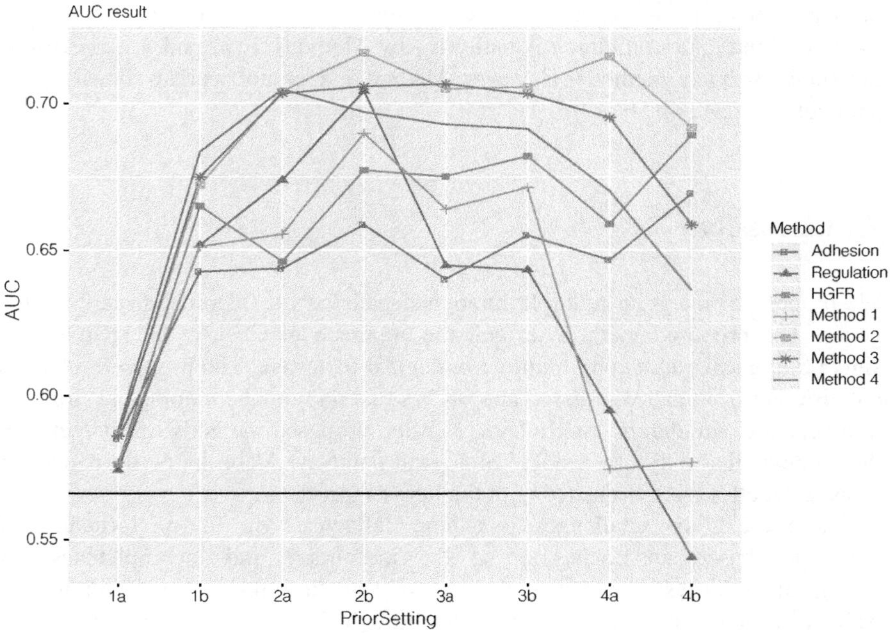

Fig. 10 AUC of single- and combined-pathway analyses with 3 GennMapp pathways to identify 14 positive genes (under an FDR cutoff of 0.15). Adhesion, Regulation, and HGFR refer to the 3 single-pathway analyses. Methods 1–4 are the proposed methods to combine the 3 pathways

Table 7 AUC of single- and combined-pathway analyses for 8 positive genes under FDR cutoff of 0.10

	Group							
Method	1a	1b	2a	2b	3a	3b	4a	4b
Adhesion	0.6285	0.6970	0.7128	0.6967	0.7122	0.7174	0.7011	0.7476
Regulation	0.6114	0.6739	0.6728	0.6938	0.6516	0.6527	0.6177	0.5747
PGFR	0.6084	0.6788	0.6549	0.6755	0.7057	0.6989	0.6736	0.7698
Method 1	0.6120	0.6663	0.6413	0.6905	0.7076	0.6935	0.6133	0.6087
Method 2	0.6302	0.7326	0.7302	0.7258	0.7505	0.7269	0.7644	0.7399
Method 3	0.6274	0.7457	0.7337	0.7122	0.7571	0.7370	0.7454	0.7166
Method 4	0.6293	0.7579	0.7446	0.7253	0.7435	0.7217	0.7255	0.6859

Method 1 does not work well. One possible reason is that there are more shared edges between two nodes in the combined network, but Method 1 only gives weight to the neighbor nodes and does not consider the edges between the nodes.

To examine the impact of selecting positive genes, we further chose a smaller set of positive genes by controlling the FDR at 0.10 instead of 0.15, and it produced 660 positive genes. In the 3 pathways considered above, 8 genes are in the positive set, and the AUC based on the p-values is 0.6571. We reconducted the analysis, and Table 7 reports values of the AUC for the pathway analysis. With the exception of prior parameter 1a, in general, the pathway-based analyses are better than using p-value alone, and combining 3 pathways by Methods 2, 3, and 4 outperforms the single-pathway methods. However, Method 1 does not work well with prior parameters 4a and 4b.

7 Discussion

We propose to integrate multiple biological pathways to identify disease-related genes. The proposed methods extend the approach of Chen et al. [10] from a single biological pathway to multiple biological pathways. The proposed methods are different from pathway-based approaches that do not take topological structure into account. Simulation studies show that the proposed methods can outperform the methods that only use a single biological pathway. Also, the performances of proposed methods are evaluated with the lung cancer data.

There are some challenges that have influences on the performance of topological-based approaches. First, the inaccuracy and incompleteness of biological pathways can lead to the loss of statistical power. In the biological pathways, some genes interact with others through chemical compounds. However, biological pathways extracted from online databases will lose such gene–compound interactions if we focus on genes. For example, gene NOD2 has been identified significantly associated with Crohn' s disease [16]. However, NOD2 indirectly interacts with other genes in the Inflammatory Bowel Disease pathway, and it becomes an isolated gene in the pathway extracted from KEGG. When we apply the proposed approaches, NOD2 has been removed because of the loss of compound mediated interactions. A number of isolated genes can lead to the loss of information about gene–gene interactions. Moreover, it can reduce the statistical power of topological-based approaches. Second, the inconsistency of biological pathways from different data bases [14, 31] can lead to inconsistent conclusions. For instance, gene ontology (GO) [1] defines different pathways for apoptosis in different cell types. Alternatively, KEGG only defines a single pathway for apoptosis. The different definitions of biological pathways in different data bases can affect the results of the approaches. Third, the choices of biological pathways have an influence on the results. When we choose biological pathways that are used to generate combined pathway, we choose the ones that are related to the disease. In general, opinions from experts and external resources are required. Fourth, as the size of biological pathway increases, the computational task will become more intensive.

There is a limitation that may affect the performance of the proposed approaches. The prior setting varies with the sizes and structures of biological pathways. For estimating the hyper-parameters, in the Supplementary Text S2 of [10], the authors described a conditional empirical Bayes approach, which can be readily applied to this chapter. For the future work, distributions may be considered to the hyper-parameters to account for the variability of these parameters.

Acknowledgments This work was partially supported by the National Institutes of Health [grant R15GM131390 to X.W.].

References

1. Ashburner, M., Ball, C.A., Blake, J.A., Botstein, D., Butler, H., Cherry, J.M., Davis, A.P., Dolinski, K., Dwight, S.S., Eppig, J.T., et al.: Gene ontology: tool for the unification of biology. Nat. Genet. **25**(1), 25–29 (2000)
2. Bair, E., Hastie, T., Paul, D., Tibshirani, R.: Prediction by supervised principal components. J. Am. Stat. Assoc. **101**(473), 119–137 (2006). http://www.jstor.org/stable/30047444
3. Barabási, A.L., Gulbahce, N., Loscalzo, J.: Network medicine: a network-based approach to human disease. Nat. Rev. Genet. **12**(1), 56–68 (2011)
4. Benjamini, Y., Hochberg, Y.: Controlling the false discovery rate: a practical and powerful approach to multiple testing. J. R. Stat. Soc. Ser. B Methodol. **57**(1), 289–300 (1995). http://www.jstor.org/stable/2346101
5. Besag, J.: Spatial interaction and the statistical analysis of lattice systems. J. R. Stat. Soc. Ser. B Methodol. **36**(2), 192–236 (1974)
6. Bokanizad, B., Tagett, R., Ansari, S., Helmi, B.H., Draghici, S.: SPATIAL: A System-level PAThway Impact AnaLysis approach. Nucl. Acids Res. **44**(11), 5034–5044 (2016)
7. Buniello, A., MacArthur, J.A.L., Cerezo, M., Harris, L.W., Hayhurst, J., Malangone, C., McMahon, A., Morales, J., Mountjoy, E., Sollis, E., et al.: The NHGRI-EBI GWAS catalog of published genome-wide association studies, targeted arrays and summary statistics 2019. Nucl. Acids Res. **47**(D1), D1005–D1012 (2019)
8. Bush, W.S., Moore, J.H.: Genome-wide association studies. PLoS Comput. Biol. **8**(12), e1002822 (2012)
9. Casella, G., George, E.I.: Explaining the Gibbs sampler. Am. Stat. **46**(3), 167–174 (1992)
10. Chen, M., Cho, J., Zhao, H.: Incorporating biological pathways via a Markov random field model in genome-wide association studies. PLoS Genet. **7**(4), 1–13 (2011). https://doi.org/10.1371/journal.pgen.1001353
11. Chen, M., Zang, M., Wang, X., Xiao, G.: A powerful Bayesian meta-analysis method to integrate multiple gene set enrichment studies. Bioinformatics (Oxford, England) **29**, 862–869 (2013). https://doi.org/10.1093/bioinformatics/btt068
12. Chen, X., Wang, L., Hu, B., Guo, M., Barnard, J., Zhu, X.: Pathway-based analysis for genome-wide association studies using supervised principal components. Genet. Epidemiol. **34**(7), 716–724 (2010)
13. Cookson, W., Liang, L., Abecasis, G., Moffatt, M., Lathrop, M.: Mapping complex disease traits with global gene expression. Nat. Rev. Genet. **10**(3), 184–194 (2009)
14. Creixell, P., Reimand, J., Haider, S., Wu, G., Shibata, T., Vazquez, M., Mustonen, V., Gonzalez-Perez, A., Pearson, J., Sander, C., et al.: Pathway and network analysis of cancer genomes. Nat. Methods **12**(7), 615 (2015)
15. Dutta, B., Wallqvist, A., Reifman, J.: Pathnet: a tool for pathway analysis using topological information. Source Code Biol. Med. **7**(1), 1 (2012)
16. Franke, A., McGovern, D.P., Barrett, J.C., Wang, K., Radford-Smith, G.L., Ahmad, T., Lees, C.W., Balschun, T., Lee, J., Roberts, R., et al.: Genome-wide meta-analysis increases to 71 the number of confirmed Crohn's disease susceptibility loci. Nat. Genet. **42**(12), 1118–1125 (2010)
17. Freytag, S., Manitz, J., Schlather, M., Kneib, T., Amos, C.I., Risch, A., Chang-Claude, J., Heinrich, J., Bickeböller, H.: A network-based kernel machine test for the identification of risk pathways in genome-wide association studies. Hum. Hered. **76**(2), 64–75 (2014)

18. Hindorff, L.A., Sethupathy, P., Junkins, H.A., Ramos, E.M., Mehta, J.P., Collins, F.S., Manolio, T.A.: Potential etiologic and functional implications of genome-wide association loci for human diseases and traits. Proc. Natl. Acad. Sci. **106**(23), 9362–9367 (2009)
19. Hou, J., Acharya, L., Zhu, D., Cheng, J.: An overview of bioinformatics methods for modeling biological pathways in yeast. Brief. Funct. Genomics **15**(2), 95–108 (2016)
20. Hou, L., Chen, M., Zhang, C.K., Cho, J., Zhao, H.: Guilt by rewiring: gene prioritization through network rewiring in genome wide association studies. Hum. Mol. Genet. **23**(10), 2780–2790 (2014)
21. Jassal, B., Matthews, L., Viteri, G., Gong, C., Lorente, P., Fabregat, A., Sidiropoulos, K., Cook, J., Gillespie, M., Haw, R., Loney, F., May, B., Milacic, M., Rothfels, K., Sevilla, C., Shamovsky, V., Shorser, S., Varusai, T., Weiser, J., Wu, G., Stein, L., Hermjakob, H., D'Eustachio, P.: The reactome pathway knowledgebase. Nucl. Acids Res. **48**, D498–D503 (2020). https://doi.org/10.1093/nar/gkz1031
22. Jin, L., Zuo, X.Y., Su, W.Y., Zhao, X.L., Yuan, M.Q., Han, L.Z., Zhao, X., Chen, Y.D., Rao, S.Q.: Pathway-based analysis tools for complex diseases: a review. Genomics Proteomics Bioinformatics **12**(5), 210–220 (2014)
23. Kanehisa, M., Goto, S., Sato, Y., Kawashima, M., Furumichi, M., Tanabe, M.: Data, information, knowledge and principle: back to metabolism in KEGG. Nucl. Acids Res. **42**(D1), D199–D205 (2014)
24. Kanehisa, M., Sato, Y., Kawashima, M., Furumichi, M., Tanabe, M.: KEGG as a reference resource for gene and protein annotation. Nucl. Acids Res. **44**(D1), D457–D462 (2016)
25. Krauss, G.: Biochemistry of Signal Transduction and Regulation. Wiley, London (2006)
26. Lin, Z., Li, M., Sestan, N., Zhao, H.: A markov random field-based approach for joint estimation of differentially expressed genes in mouse transcriptome data. Stat. Appl. Genet. Mol. Biol. **15**(2), 139–150 (2016)
27. Liu, J., Peissig, P., Zhang, C., Burnside, E., McCarty, C., Page, D.: Graphical-model based multiple testing under dependence, with applications to genome-wide association studies. In: Proceedings of the Conference on Uncertainty in Artificial Intelligence, vol. 2012, p. 511. NIH Public Access (2012)
28. Liu, L., Lei, J., Roeder, K., et al.: Network assisted analysis to reveal the genetic basis of autism. Ann. Appl. Stat. **9**(3), 1571–1600 (2015)
29. Loscalzo, J., Kohane, I., Barabasi, A.L.: Human disease classification in the postgenomic era: a complex systems approach to human pathobiology. Mol. Syst. Biol. **3**(1), 124 (2007)
30. Luo, L., Peng, G., Zhu, Y., Dong, H., Amos, C.I., Xiong, M.: Genome-wide gene and pathway analysis. Eur. J. Hum. Genet. **18**(9), 1045–1053 (2010)
31. Mitrea, C., Taghavi, Z., Bokanizad, B., Hanoudi, S., Tagett, R., Donato, M., Voichita, C., Draghici, S.: Methods and approaches in the topology-based analysis of biological pathways. Front. Physiol. **4**(278), 1–22 (2013)
32. Mokry, M., Middendorp, S., Wiegerinck, C.L., Witte, M., Teunissen, H., Meddens, C.A., Cuppen, E., Clevers, H., Nieuwenhuis, E.E.: Many inflammatory bowel disease risk loci include regions that regulate gene expression in immune cells and the intestinal epithelium. Gastroenterology **146**(4), 1040–1047 (2014)
33. Mourad, R., Sinoquet, C., Leray, P.: Probabilistic graphical models for genetic association studies. Brief. Bioinform. **13**(1), 20–33 (2012)
34. Nica, A.C., Dermitzakis, E.T.: Using gene expression to investigate the genetic basis of complex disorders. Hum. Mol. Genet. **17**(R2), R129–R134 (2008)
35. Pan, W.: Relationship between genomic distance-based regression and kernel machine regression for multi-marker association testing. Genet. Epidemiol. **35**(4), 211–216 (2011). https://doi.org/10.1002/gepi.20567
36. Pan, W., Kim, J., Zhang, Y., Shen, X., Wei, P.: A powerful and adaptive association test for rare variants. Genetics **197**(4), 1081–95 (2014). https://doi.org/10.1534/genetics.114.165035
37. Pan, W., Kwak, I.Y., Wei, P.: A powerful pathway-based adaptive test for genetic association with common or rare variants. Am. J. Hum. Genet. **97**(1), 86–98 (2015). https://doi.org/10.1016/j.ajhg.2015.05.018

38. Pavlopoulos, G.A., Secrier, M., Moschopoulos, C.N., Soldatos, T.G., Kossida, S., Aerts, J., Schneider, R., Bagos, P.G.: Using graph theory to analyze biological networks. BioData Mining **4**(1), 1 (2011)
39. Rapin, N., Bagger, F.O., Jendholm, J., Mora-Jensen, H., Krogh, A., Kohlmann, A., Thiede, C., Borregaard, N., Bullinger, L., Winther, O., et al.: Comparing cancer vs normal gene expression profiles identifies new disease entities and common transcriptional programs in AML patients. Blood **123**(6), 894–904 (2014)
40. Ripke, S., O'Dushlaine, C., Chambert, K., Moran, J.L., Kähler, A.K., Akterin, S., Bergen, S., Collins, A.L., Crowley, J.J., Fromer, M., et al.: Genome-wide association analysis identifies 14 new risk loci for schizophrenia. Nat Genet. **45**(10), 1150–1159 (2013)
41. Rodchenkov, I., Babur, O., Luna, A., Aksoy, B.A., Wong, J.V., Fong, D., Franz, M., Siper, M.C., Cheung, M., Wrana, M., Mistry, H., Mosier, L., Dlin, J., Wen, Q., O'Callaghan, C., Li, W., Elder, G., Smith, P.T., Dallago, C., Cerami, E., Gross, B., Dogrusoz, U., Demir, E., Bader, G.D., Sander, C.: Pathway commons 2019 update: integration, analysis and exploration of pathway data. Nucl. Acids Res. **48**, D489–D497 (2020). https://doi.org/10.1093/nar/gkz946
42. Shannon, P., Markiel, A., Ozier, O., Baliga, N.S., Wang, J.T., Ramage, D., Amin, N., Schwikowski, B., Ideker, T.: Cytoscape: a software environment for integrated models of biomolecular interaction networks. Genome Res. **13**(11), 2498–2504 (2003)
43. Shedden, K., Taylor, J.M.G., Enkemann, S.A., Tsao, M.S., Yeatman, T.J., Gerald, W.L., Eschrich, S., Jurisica, I., Giordano, T.J., Misek, D.E., Chang, A.C., Zhu, C.Q., Strumpf, D., Hanash, S., Shepherd, F.A., Ding, K., Seymour, L., Naoki, K., Pennell, N., Weir, B., Verhaak, R., Ladd-Acosta, C., Golub, T., Gruidl, M., Sharma, A., Szoke, J., Zakowski, M., Rusch, V., Kris, M., Viale, A., Motoi, N., Travis, W., Conley, B., Seshan, V.E., Meyerson, M., Kuick, R., Dobbin, K.K., Lively, T., Jacobson, J.W., Beer, D.G.: Gene expression-based survival prediction in lung adenocarcinoma: a multi-site, blinded validation study. Nat. Med. **14**, 822–827 (2008). https://doi.org/10.1038/nm.1790
44. Slenter, D.N., Kutmon, M., Hanspers, K., Riutta, A., Windsor, J., Nunes, N., Mélius, J., Cirillo, E., Coort, S.L., Digles, D., et al.: Wikipathways: a multifaceted pathway database bridging metabolomics to other omics research. Nucl. Acids Res. **46**(D1), D661–D667 (2018)
45. Song, G.G., Lee, Y.H.: Pathway analysis of genome-wide association study on asthma. Hum. Immunol. **74**(2), 256–260 (2013)
46. Tarca, A.L., Draghici, S., Khatri, P., Hassan, S.S., Mittal, P., Kim, J.S., Kim, C.J., Kusanovic, J.P., Romero, R.: A novel signaling pathway impact analysis. Bioinformatics **25**(1), 75–82 (2009)
47. Wei, P., Pan, W.: Bayesian joint modeling of multiple gene networks and diverse genomic data to identify target genes of a transcription factor. Ann. Appl. Stat. **6**(1), 334 (2012)
48. Wu, M.C., Kraft, P., Epstein, M.P., Taylor, D.M., Chanock, S.J., Hunter, D.J., Lin, X.: Powerful SNP-set analysis for case-control genome-wide association studies. Am. J. Hum. Genet. **86**(6), 929–942 (2010)
49. Wu, M.C., Lee, S., Cai, T., Li, Y., Boehnke, M., Lin, X.: Rare-variant association testing for sequencing data with the sequence kernel association test. Am. J. Hum. Genet. **89**(1), 82–93 (2011). https://doi.org/10.1016/j.ajhg.2011.05.029
50. Zalkin, H., DAGLEY, S., Nicholson, D.E.: An Introduction to Metabolic Pathways. Wiley, London (1971)
51. Zhi, W., Minturn, J., Rappaport, E., Brodeur, G., Li, H.: Network-based analysis of multivariate gene expression data. In: Statistical Methods for Microarray Data Analysis: Methods and Protocols, pp. 121–139 (2013)

A Nested Clustering Method to Detect and Cluster Transgenerational DNA Methylation Sites via Beta Regressions

Jiajing Wang, Hongmei Zhang, and Shengtong Han

1 Introduction

For many diseases, e.g., asthma, genetic variances could only explain a small fraction of disease heritability [1, 2]. Various explanations for the missing heritability phenomenon have been suggested, including much larger numbers of variants of small effect yet to be found; low power to detect gene–gene interactions; and inadequate accounting for shared environment among relatives [3]. The transgenerational transmission of epigenetic markers such as DNA methylation is one possible mechanism explaining the missing heritability. DNA methylation (DNAm), which occurs predominantly at Cytosines within CG dinucleotide (CpG sites), has been found to be inherited through generations [4] and to be associated with health outcomes, including allergic and autoimmune diseases [5], such as asthma and eczema during childhood [6] and adolescence. We may expect that asymmetric transmission patterns of DNA methylation from parents to offspring in the general population is beneficial to disease prediction and prevention [7]. Learning the patterns of DNA methylation transmission at different CpG sites is thus greatly needed. However, to our knowledge, currently available approaches detect patterns based on candidate CpG sites selected by size of correlations between offspring and

J. Wang
Department of Mathematical Sciences, University of Memphis, Memphis, TN, USA
e-mail: jwang13@memphis.edu

H. Zhang (✉)
Division of Epidemiology, Biostatistics, and Environmental Health, School of Public Health, University of Memphis, Memphis, TN, USA
e-mail: hzhang6@memphis.edu

S. Han
School of Public Health, University of Wisconsin-Milwaukee, Milwaukee, WI, USA

Y. Zhao, (Din) D.-G. Chen (eds.), *Modern Statistical Methods for Health Research*, Emerging Topics in Statistics and Biostatistics,
https://doi.org/10.1007/978-3-030-72437-5_20

each parent [8] without formally assessing heritability. Doing so may potentially mis-classify non-transmitted CpG sites as being transmitted and vice versa. There is a desire to sort out CpG sites that are transmitted from one generation to the next at the population level and among the transmitted CpGs to study the transmission patterns. For both tasks, detecting transmission status and transmission patterns, the concept of probabilistic clustering analyses can be applied.

Classic clustering methods are separated by unsupervised approaches and the model-based approaches. Unsupervised approaches, such as K-means algorithms, or various hierarchical clustering methods, are not able to evaluate the strength of inheritance while clustering. Research findings showed that model-based clustering techniques are often superior to non-parametric approaches [9]. The existing model-based clustering methods, such as the Bernoulli–lognormal mixture model [9] and recursively partitioned beta mixture model [10], focus on associations among individual subjects and are not able to identify the transmission patterns at the population level. To the best of our knowledge, very limited contribution has been made to this field except for the work in [8], which focuses on transmission patterns detection only and does not assess the status of transmission.

In this chapter, we propose a nested Bayesian clustering method to infer transmission status, and among the transmitted CpG sites, we examine DNAm heterogeneity via clustering CpG sites showing different transmission patterns. The two-step clustering is fulfilled using beta regression [11] and taking into account the association between offspring's mean DNA methylation and parents' mean DNA methylation, i.e., associations in DNAm at the population level. To identify the transmitted CpG sites, an indicator variable is used to infer transmission status. Among the transmitted CpG sites identified in the first step, we group the transmitted CpG sites and assign those CpG sites into a cluster showing unique transmission patterns in DNA methylation from parents to their offspring.

The remainder of this chapter is organized as follows. Section 2 introduces the nested Bayesian clustering method based on beta regressions. The model assumptions, setting of priors, conditional posterior distributions, and detailed procedure are described in this section. We demonstrate and evaluate the applicability of the method through simulations in Sect. 3. Section 4 discusses a real data application. We summarize our method and findings in Sect. 5.

2 Model

2.1 Model Assumption

Suppose there are I triads (each triad consists of one child and the child's two parents) and J CpG sites that are common to all triads. We assume that all CpG sites are independent of each other. Let $Z1_{ij}$ and $Z2_{ij}$ denote DNA methylations at CpG site j for the ith child's mother and father, respectively, and y_{ij} be the DNA methylation level at site j of the child. The range of DNA methylation is between 0 and 1, and the distribution of DNA methylation at a CpG site can be reasonably fit by a Beta distribution [10],

$$Z1_{ij} \sim Beta\left(\alpha_j^M, \beta_j^M\right), \; Z2_{ij} \sim Beta\left(\alpha_j^F, \beta_j^F\right),$$

where $0 < Z1_{ij}, Z2_{ij} < 1$, and α_j^M, β_j^M, α_j^F, and β_j^F are the unknown scale parameters, $i = 1, \cdots, I$, $j = 1, \cdots, J$. Similarly,

$$y_{ij} \sim Beta\left(\alpha_j^0, \beta_j^0\right), \quad (1)$$

where $0 < y_{ij} < 1$, and α_j^0 and β_j^0 are the two unknown scale parameters in the Beta distribution.

2.2 *Identify the Transmission Status*

DNA methylation of offspring at certain CpG sites can be potentially inherited from parents. We examine this at the population level. That is, if at CpG site j, DNA methylation of a child is expected to be transmitted from their parents, then we have the following beta regression applied to mean DNA methylation,

$$O_j = \gamma_{0j} + \gamma_{1j} M_j + \gamma_{2j} F_j, \quad (2)$$

where $O_j = logit(\frac{\alpha_j^0}{\alpha_j^0+\beta_j^0}) = log(\alpha_j^0) - log(\beta_j^0)$, $M_j = log(\alpha_j^M) - log(\beta_j^M)$, and $F_j = log(\alpha_j^F) - log(\beta_j^F)$ denote the logit transformed mean DNA methylations at CpG site j for child, father, and mother, respectively. Under this context, the distribution of a child's DNA methylation depends on their parents' DNA methylation, and (1) should be rewritten as

$$y_{ij} | Z1_{ij}, Z2_{ij} \sim Beta\left(\alpha_j^0, \beta_j^0\right).$$

However, not all CpG sites transmit DNA methylation from parents to offspring. To incorporate this concept into the regression model (2), we introduce an indicator variable into the model to denote transmission status,

$$O_j = (\delta_j \gamma_{0j} + (1 - \delta_j)\gamma_j) + \gamma_{1j} \delta_j M_j + \gamma_{2j} \delta_j F_j, \quad (3)$$

where $\boldsymbol{\delta} = (\delta_1, \delta_2, \cdots, \delta_J)^T$ is a $J \times 1$ vector denoting transmission status of each CpG site $j = 1, \cdots, J$. If $\delta_j = 0$, CpG site j is not transmitted from parents to their offspring and the average DNA methylation of a child is determined by γ_j.

Otherwise, DNA methylation at CpG site j is transmitted from the parents, and transmission patterns are determined by $\boldsymbol{\gamma}_j^{tr} = (\gamma_{0j}, \gamma_{1j}, \gamma_{2j})$, where γ_{1j} represents the strength of maternal transmission and γ_{2j} the strength of paternal transmission. Note that the patterns focus on transmission strengths (slopes) rather than non-transmission-related portions in DNA methylation (intercepts).

A Bayesian approach is applied to infer transmission status δ_j of each CpG site and, for transmitted sites, the patterns of transmission. Frequentist approaches, e.g., via the expectation–maximization algorithm as in [8], can also be used to infer the parameters. The advantage of Bayesian approach exists in its ability to easily introduce prior knowledge into the estimation process. We start the Bayesian inference from specifying prior distributions of the parameters, δ_j and γ_j. For δ_j, we assume a Bernoulli distribution, $\delta_j | p_j \sim Bernoulli(1, p_j)$, with $\boldsymbol{p} = (p_1, \cdots, p_j, \cdots, p_J)$ denoting a vector of transmission probabilities for each of the J CpG sites. For γ_j, a non-informative prior is selected, $N(0, a)$, a normal distribution with mean 0 and variance a. The variance is assumed to be known and large, e.g., $a = 100$. For regression coefficients of transmitted CpGs, $\boldsymbol{\gamma}_j^{tr}$, we discuss in the next section its setting in the context of clustering and related specification of prior distributions.

2.3 Clustering the Transmitted CpG Sites

Among the transmitted CpGs, we further group the CpG sites showing similar transmission patterns. Under the context of clustering, Eq. (3) is revised to the following

$$O_j = \gamma_{0k} + \gamma_{1k} M_j + \gamma_{2k} F_j,$$

where the strength of transmission in cluster k is determined by $\boldsymbol{\gamma}_k^{tr} = (\gamma_{0k}, \gamma_{1k}, \gamma_{2k})$, representing the clustering of $\boldsymbol{\gamma}_j^{tr}$ across J CpG sites. All CpG sites in cluster k share the same transmission pattern from the parents to their offspring. The parameters γ_{1k} and γ_{2k} represent the strength of maternal transmission and paternal transmission for CpGs in cluster k, respectively. For these regression coefficients, the same non-informative prior distribution as that for γ_j is selected, i.e., $N(0, a)$ with a large and known.

The cluster assignment of CpG j is determined by $\boldsymbol{\mu}_j = (\mu_{j1}, \mu_{j2}, \cdots, \mu_{jK})^T = (0, 0, \cdots, 1, 0, \cdots, 0)^T$, a $K \times 1$ vector, and $\mu_{jk} = 1$ indicates CpG site j belonging to cluster k. Denote by π_k the probability of a site falling into cluster k. We assume the prior distribution of μ_{jk} as $Mult(1, \pi)$ (Multinomial distribution), where $\boldsymbol{\pi} = (\pi_1, \pi_2, \cdots, \pi_K)$ with $0 \le \pi_k \le 1$, $k = 1, 2, \cdots, K$, $\sum_{k=1}^K \pi_k = 1$. For the distribution of its hyper-prior, π, we assume $\pi \sim Dir(\mathbf{1})$ with $\mathbf{1}$ being a vector of 1 with length K, a Dirichlet distribution with parameter 1, which is equivalent to a Multivariate uniform distribution.

2.4 The Likelihood Function and the Posterior Distribution

Let $\theta = (\boldsymbol{\alpha}, \boldsymbol{\beta}, \boldsymbol{\delta}, \boldsymbol{\mu}, \gamma_j, \boldsymbol{\gamma}^{tr}, j = 1, \cdots, J)$ denote a collection of all parameters, where $\boldsymbol{\alpha} = (\boldsymbol{\alpha}^{\mathbf{0}}, \boldsymbol{\alpha}^{M}, \boldsymbol{\alpha}^{F})$ with $\boldsymbol{\alpha}^{\mathbf{0}} = (\alpha_1^0, \alpha_2^0, \cdots, \alpha_J^0)$, $\boldsymbol{\alpha}^{M} = (\alpha_1^M, \alpha_2^M, \cdots, \alpha_J^M)$, $\boldsymbol{\alpha}^{F} = (\alpha_1^F, \alpha_2^F, \cdots, \alpha_J^F)$. Analogous to $\boldsymbol{\alpha}$, parameter $\boldsymbol{\beta}$ has the same structure, $\boldsymbol{\beta} = (\boldsymbol{\beta}^{\mathbf{0}}, \boldsymbol{\beta}^{M}, \boldsymbol{\beta}^{F})$ with $\boldsymbol{\beta}^{\mathbf{0}} = (\beta_1^0, \beta_2^0, \cdots, \beta_J^0)$, $\boldsymbol{\beta}^{M} = (\beta_1^M, \beta_2^M, \cdots, \beta_J^M,)$ and $\boldsymbol{\beta}^{F} = (\beta_1^F, \beta_2^F, \cdots, \beta_J^F)$. For the transmission status, $\boldsymbol{\delta} = (\delta_1, \delta_2, \cdots, \delta_J)^T$ is a $J \times 1$ vector, and $\boldsymbol{\mu} = (\boldsymbol{\mu_1}, \boldsymbol{\mu_2}, \cdots, \boldsymbol{\mu_J})^T$ with $\boldsymbol{\mu_j} = (\mu_{j1}, \mu_{j2}, \cdots, \mu_{jK})^T = (0, 0, \cdots, 1, 0, \cdots, 0)^T$ is a $K \times 1$ vector denoting cluster assignment. Finally, for non-transmitted CpG site j, parameter γ_j is the average DNA methylation of a child. Among the transmitted CpG sites, parameter $\boldsymbol{\gamma}^{tr}$ is a collection of regression coefficients, $\boldsymbol{\gamma}^{tr} = (\boldsymbol{\gamma}_1^{tr}, \boldsymbol{\gamma}_2^{tr}, \cdots, \boldsymbol{\gamma}_K^{tr})$ with $\boldsymbol{\gamma}_k^{tr} = (\gamma_{0k}, \gamma_{1k}, \gamma_{2k})$, $k = 1, 2, \cdots, K$. Denote by $Y = (y_{ij}, Z1_{ij}, Z2_{ij})$, $i = 1, 2, \cdots, I$, $j = 1, 2, \cdots, J$. The likelihood of θ is

$$L(\theta|Y) \propto \prod_{i=1}^{I}\prod_{j=1}^{J}(\prod_{k=1}^{K} I(\delta_j = 1)p(y_{ij}|Z1_{ij}, Z2_{ij}, \theta)^{\mu_{jk}}$$
$$p(Z1_{ij}|\theta)p(Z2_{ij}|\theta) + (1 - I(\delta_j = 1))p(y_{ij}|\theta)).$$

The joint posterior distribution of $\boldsymbol{\theta}$ is then given as

$$p(\theta|Y) \propto p(\boldsymbol{\theta})\prod_{i=1}^{I}\prod_{j=1}^{J}(\prod_{k=1}^{K} I(\delta_j = 1)p(y_{ij}|Z1_{ij}, Z2_{ij}, \theta)^{\mu_{jk}}$$
$$p(Z1_{ij}|\theta)p(Z2_{ij}|\theta) + (1 - I(\delta_j = 1))p(y_{ij}|\theta)),$$

with the prior of $\boldsymbol{\theta}$ as defined in earlier sections.

Markov Chain Monte Carlo (MCMC) simulations from the joint posterior distribution are implemented to draw posterior inferences. Specifically, we utilize the Gibbs sampler with Metropolis–Hastings steps to sample from the full conditional posterior distributions of each parameter, which are then used to infer the parameters of interest. In the following, we list the conditional posterior distributions with $(\cdot)$ denoting data and other parameters to be conditional on.

For parameter δ_j, representing transmission status of CpG sites, we have the following conditional posterior distribution:

$$\delta_j|(\cdot) \sim Bernoulli(p_{post}). \tag{4}$$

Since

$$p(\delta_j = 1|(\cdot)) \propto p(\boldsymbol{\theta})\prod_{i=1}^{I}\prod_{k=1}^{K} p(y_{ij}|Z1_{ij}, Z2_{ij}, \theta)^{\mu_{jk}} p(Z1_{ij}|\theta)p(Z2_{ij}|\theta) = a,$$

and

$$p(\delta_j = 0|(\cdot)) \propto p(\boldsymbol{\theta})\prod_{\boldsymbol{i=1}}^{\boldsymbol{I}} p(y_{ij}|\theta) = b,$$

parameter p_{post} in (4) is defined as

$$p_{post} = \frac{a}{a+b}.$$

Among the transmitted CpG sites, the conditional posterior of μ_j is a Multinomial distribution with π_k in $\boldsymbol{\pi} = (\pi_1, \pi_2, \cdots, \pi_K)$ determined by

$$\begin{aligned}\pi_k|(\cdot) = p(\mu_{jk}|(\cdot)) \propto \prod_{i=1}^{I} & p\left(y_{ij}|Z1_{ij}, Z2_{ij}, \boldsymbol{\alpha_j}, \boldsymbol{\beta_j}, \boldsymbol{\gamma_k^{tr}}, \delta_j, \mu_{jk}\right) \\ & p\left(Z1_{ij}|\alpha_j^M, \beta_j^M\right) p\left(Z2_{ij}|\alpha_j^F, \beta_j^F\right) p\left(\boldsymbol{\gamma_k^{tr}}|\delta_j\right) \\ & p(\mu_{jk}|\boldsymbol{\pi})p(\pi_k).\end{aligned}$$

The conditional posterior distribution of $\boldsymbol{\gamma_j}$ for the non-transmitted CpG sites is

$$P(\gamma_j|(\cdot)) \propto \prod_{i=1}^{I} p\left(y_{ij}|\alpha_j^0, \beta_j^0, \gamma_j\right) p(\gamma_j|\delta_j),$$

and the conditional posterior distribution of the transmission patterns $\boldsymbol{\gamma_k^{tr}} = (\gamma_{mk}, m = 0, 1, 2)$ for the transmitted CpG sites is defined as

$$\begin{aligned}P(\gamma_{mk}|(\cdot)) \propto \prod_{i=1}^{I}\prod_{j=1}^{J} & p\left(y_{ij}|Z1_{ij}, Z2_{ij}, \boldsymbol{\alpha_j}, \boldsymbol{\beta_j}, \boldsymbol{\gamma_k^{tr}}, \delta_j, \mu_{jk}\right) \\ & p(Z1_{ij}|\alpha_j^M, \beta_j^M)p\left(Z2_{ij}|\alpha_j^F, \beta_j^F\right) p(\gamma_{mk}).\end{aligned}$$

The conditional posterior distributions of γ_j and γ_k^{tr} are not in the standard form, and to sample γ_j and γ_k^{tr}, we apply the Metropolis–Hastings algorithm and take the normal distribution as the proposal distribution. With all the conditional posterior distributions defined, for a given K, we apply the Gibbs sampler to sequentially sample from each distribution to determine each CpG site's transmission status as well as cluster assignment among the transmitted CpGs. Since clustering of CpG sites happens after we determine the transmission status of each CpG site, we denote this as a nested clustering method.

To determine the number of clusters K, we implement the Bayesian information criterion (BIC) introduced in [8] constructed via the likelihood calculated using posterior estimates of the parameters. A scree plot of BICs for different values of K and a sharp decrease in BIC followed by a flatten pattern indicate an optimal selection of K.

3 Simulation Study

This section, via simulation, demonstrates and evaluates the proposed method by using 100 Monte Carlo (MC) replicates and assesses its sensitivity and specificity to cluster detections.

3.1 Simulation Scenarios

We generate 100 Monte Carlo (MC) replicates. Each MC replicate represents DNA methylation of 650 CpG sites from 100 triads. DNA methylation data is simulated using beta distributions. The scale parameters in the beta distribution are generated from truncated normal distributions for each CpG site, which potentially results in unique patterns of data at each CpG site. Out of 650 CpG sites, about 500 transmitted CpG sites are equally assigned into 2 clusters with coefficients $\boldsymbol{\gamma}_1^{tr} = (-4.2, 1.2, 2.5)$, $\boldsymbol{\gamma}_2^{tr} = (-2.7, 3, 2.5)$, representing CpG sites paternal- and maternal-dominated transmission, respectively. To assess the sensitivity and specificity of the method with respect to different transmission patterns, for another set of 100 MC replicates, we assign the 500 transmitted CpG sites into 3 clusters. In this scenario, the first two clusters have the same setting as before. For the third cluster, the coefficients are chosen as $\boldsymbol{\gamma}_3^{tr} = (-8, 1, 1)$, that is, parental transmission is evenly distributed between mother and father. These two scenarios are constructed based on different transmission patterns.

To summarize our results, for each MC replicate, we calculate the rate of accuracy of detected transmission status, record the number of clusters identified, and calculate the sensitivity ($Se = TP/(TP + FN)$) and specificity ($Sp = TN/(TN + FP)$) of clustering, where "TP" denotes true positives (correct cluster identification), "FN" denotes false negatives, "TN" denotes true negatives, and "FP" denotes false positives. Medians of these statistics along with IQR (25th percentile–75th percentile) across the 100 MC replicates are summarized and used to assess the robustness of the method as well as the uncertainty of the inferred statistics. As noted earlier, the number of clusters is determined by use of the scree plot of BICs with each BIC corresponding to a specific number of clusters. As an illustration, Fig. 1 shows the pattern of BIC from one MC replicate, from which we infer 2 clusters.

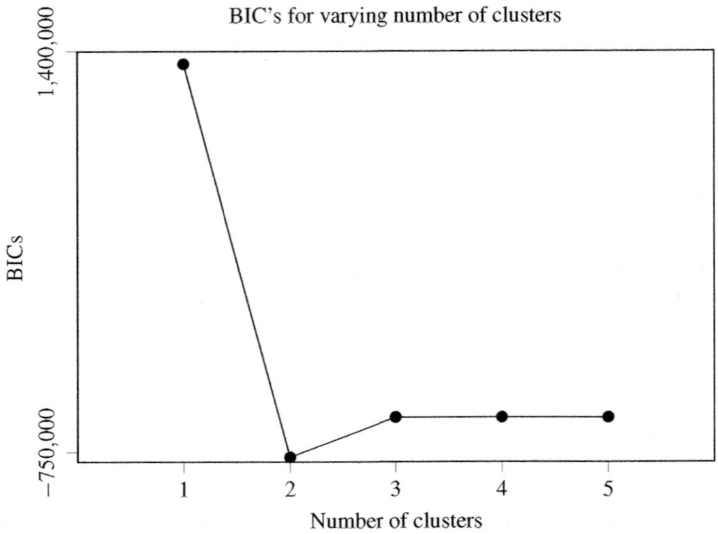

Fig. 1 BIC values for a varying number of clusters in the simulated data with 650 CpG sites in one MC replicate. The best number of clusters is achieved at $K = 2$

Table 1 The occurrence frequency of each cluster number over 100 MC replicates

		Underlying truth:	2 clusters	
Number of candidate clusters (K)	2	3	4	5
Frequency	59	9	19	12
		Underlying truth:	3 clusters	
Number of candidate clusters (K)	2	3	4	5
Frequency	17	56	15	12

3.2 Results

We discuss findings from the fully Bayesian sampling scheme discussed in Sect. 2. In total, we run one chain with 20,000 MCMC iterations and use the last 1000 iterations to draw inferences on the parameters. In the process of inferring transmission patterns, i.e., estimating $\boldsymbol{\gamma}_k^{tr}$ for cluster k, rather than drawing posterior samples for each component in $\boldsymbol{\gamma}_k^{tr}$, we utilize linear regressions based on CpGs assigned to cluster k to improve sampling efficiency.

Summarizing the result across the 100 MC replicates, the uncertainty on the number of clusters is shown in Table 1 as the frequency for each cluster number over the 100 MC replicates in the two- and three-cluster situations. In both situations, the numbers of clusters inferred are correct; the median of number of clusters is 2 with a 95% empirical interval of $(2, 5)$ when the underlying true number of clusters is 2, and for the three-cluster situation, these two statistics are 3 and $(2, 5)$. The rate of accuracy of transmission status, and sensitivity and specificity of clustering are

Table 2 Summary of rate of accuracy of transmission status and sensitivity and specificity of clustering across 100 MC replicates for both two- and three-cluster situations

			Two clusters	Three clusters
Transmission status	Accuracy	Median	0.9985	1.000
		IQR	(0.9954,1)	(0.9938,1)
Cluster 1	Sensitivity	Median	0.9960	1.000
		IQR	(0.9921,1)	(0.9939,1)
	Specificity	Median	0.9796	0.9881
		IQR	(0.9684,0.9842)	(0.9762,0.9939)
Cluster 2	Sensitivity	Median	0.9796	0.9750
		IQR	(0.9684,0.9842)	(0.9426,0.9850)
	Specificity	Median	0.9960	1.000
		IQR	(0.9921,1)	(0.9970,1)
Cluster 3	Sensitivity	Median	–	1.000
		IQR	–	(1,1)
	Specificity	Median	–	1.000
		IQR	–	(1,1)

IQR stands for 25th percentile–75th percentile. Each MC replicate presents DNA methylation of 650 CpG sites from 100 triads generated. Out of 650 CpG sites, about 500 CpG sites are equally assigned into two or three clusters, respectively

summarized in Table 2. Overall, regardless of the underlying truth on the number of clusters, high accuracy, sensitivity, and specificity are observed, indicating the effectiveness of the proposed method and its potential to handle a combination of different transmission status.

3.3 *Further Assessment of the Method*

In the above analysis, we focus on the assessment of the method on its ability to deal with different transmission patterns. In this section, to further assess the proposed method, we compare with the approach by Han et al. [8], from which the proposed approach is extended. Furthermore, to demonstrate properties reflected by finite samples, we examine how the results of clustering and detection of transmission are affected by different sample sizes and different numbers of CpG sites. The two-cluster situation is considered in this section. To compare with the method in [8], we use data simulated following the scenario in Sect. 3.1 for two clusters, but we assume DNA methylation at all CpG sites was transmitted and set the number of clusters as three (denote this situation as S0). To evaluate the performance of our method with different sample sizes and numbers of CpG sites compared to the settings in Sect. 3.1, we considered the following three situations, and for each situation, 100 MC replicates are simulated:

S1. Decreasing the sample size from 100 to 85.

S2. Increasing the sample size from 100 to 200. S1 and S2, along with the setting used in Sect. 3.1, are used to assess the impact of sample sizes on the inference of clustering and transmission status.

S3. Increasing the number of CpG sites to 1500 and equally assigning the 1000 transmitted CpGs to two clusters (500 CpG sites in each cluster). This is to assess the influence of larger number of CpG sites.

The results of S0–S3 are summarized in Table 3. Under S0 assuming DNA methylation at all CpG sites is transmitted, the approach in Han et al. groups the CpG sites into two clusters in most of the MC replicates. In particular, all the non-transmitted CpG sites are assigned into one cluster, leading to low sensitivity or specificity. Although this might be due to large variations in the data, the results emphasize the need to take into account DNA methylation transmission status. Turning to the impact of sample sizes and numbers of CpG sites, as the sample size increases (from 85 [S1] to 100 [S0], and then to 200 [S2]), the overall sensitivity and specificity increase. Similar patterns are observed when increasing the number of CpG sites, which is understandable, since a larger number of CpG sites are equivalent to having a larger sample size in terms of parameter estimation. All these findings support the large sample properties on parameter inferences.

4 Real Data Analysis

We applied the proposed nested clustering method to DNA methylation data measured in two generations for a random subset of participants in a birth cohort located on the Isle of Wight, United Kingdom [12]. The methylation level for each queried CpG is presented as beta values. The beta values represent the ratio of the methylated (M) probe intensities to the sum of methylated (M) and unmethylated (U) probe intensities (beta=M/(U+M+C) with constant C=100 introduced for the situation of too small M+U). In total, DNA methylation at more than $450K$ CpG sites is available.

In this chapter, DNA methylation at 4063 CpGs on autosomes in 41 triads is included and selected based on potential inheritance measured by correlations in DNA methylation between a parent and his/her offspring. A CpG site will be excluded for further consideration if the mother–child or father–child correlation in DNA methylation is <0.5. Although DNA methylation at these 4063 candidate CpG sites shows a potential of inheritance, uncertainty of inheritance and effects of both maternal and paternal CpGs on their offspring DNA methylation (instead of individual effects) are not considered by simple correlations. We use these 4063 CpGs as candidate sites to infer status of transmission as well as clustering transmittted CpG sites.

The nested clustering method discussed in Sect. 2 is applied to identify transmitted CpG sites at the population level and assign the transmitted CpG sites to different

Table 3 Results (accuracy, sensitivity, and specificity) from Han et al.'s approach (S0) and from settings with sample size and number of CpG sites different from those in Sect. 3.1 (S1 to S3), summarized across 100 MC replicates

			S0	S1	S2	S3
Transmission	Accuracy	Median		0.9985	1.000	0.9987
		IQR		(0.9969, 1)	(0.9996,1)	(0.9950,1)
Cluster 1	Sensitivity	Median	1	0.9960	1.000	0.9961
		IQR	(1, 1)	(0.9920,1)	(0.9960,1)	(0.9942,0.9980)
	Specificity	Median	0.3758	0.9688	0.9959	0.9781
		IQR	(0.3621, 0.3951)	(0.9540,0.9763)	(0.9919,0.9961)	(0.9724,0.9838)
Cluster 2	Sensitivity	Median	0	0.9688	0.9959	0.9781
		IQR	(0, 0)	(0.9540,0.9763)	(0.9919,0.9961)	(0.9724,0.9838)
	Specificity	Median	0.9999	0.9960	1.000	0.9961
		IQR	(1, 1)	(0.9920,1)	(0.9960,1)	(0.9942,0.9980)

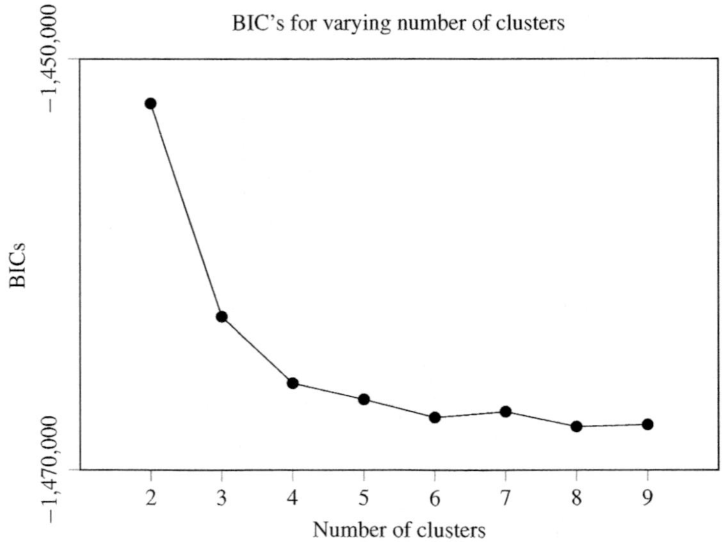

Fig. 2 BIC values for a varying number of clusters for the IOW real data with 4063 CpG sites and 41 triads after screening by a cut-off at 0.5 in correlation. The BIC curve decreases sharply and then reaches stable at K=5

Table 4 Coefficient estimation of 3837 CpGs identified as transmitted sites

Cluster index(k)	$\hat{\gamma_{0k}}$(CI)	$\hat{\gamma_{1k}}$(CI) maternal transmission	$\hat{\gamma_{2k}}$(CI) paternal transmission	No. of CpG sites
1	0.24	0.52	0.52	422
	(0.23, 0.25)	(0.47, 0.56)	(0.47, 0.57)	
2	0.08	0.60	0.43	643
	(0.07, 0.08)	(0.55, 0.63)	(0.39, 0.47)	
3	0.55	0.53	0.49	177
	(0.53, 0.57)	(0.42, 0.65)	(0.37, 0.61)	
4	−0.06	0.64	0.39	1054
	(−0.07, −0.06)	(0.60, 0.69)	(0.34, 0.43)	
5	−0.32	0.57	0.50	1541
	(−0.33, −0.31)	(0.55, 0.60)	(0.48, 0.53)	

CI denotes the 95% credible interval

clusters. The scree plot of BIC, which is used to estimate the number of clusters, is displayed in Fig. 2. The plot indicates that the best number of clusters is achieved at $K = 5$. The estimated coefficients with their 95% credible intervals, which are used to explain the transmission strength, and the number of transmitted CpG sites included in each cluster are summarized in Table 4.

Of the 4063 candidate CpGs, 3837 CpG sites are identified as transmitted sites. Recall that the parameter γ_{1k} represents the strength of maternal transmission and the γ_{2k} is for the strength of paternal transmission. Among the 5 identified clusters, the first cluster containing 422 CpG sites shows an even transmission strength between mothers and fathers, indicating parents have the same contribution to offspring's DNA methylation. Cluster 3 also shows a similar transmission strength between the parents, indicated by the overlapping credible intervals. The remaining clusters are mainly maternal-transmission-dominated, as indicated by larger estimates of γ_{1k} as well as non-overlapping credible intervals.

With 3837 of the 4063 CpGs identified as potentially transmitted CpGs, DNA methylation at some CpGs is likely not transmitted based on our approach although the correlation is 0.5 or larger. This is likely due to large uncertainties in the data as well as the consideration of effects from both parents in our transmission assessment.

5 Summary and Discussion

As epigenetic markers such as DNA methylation allow us to better explain the phenomenon of disease heritability, we propose a nested clustering method in a Bayesian framework to identify the transmitted CpG sites and study the asymmetric transmission pattern of DNA methylation from parents to offspring in a general population. In the simulation study, our proposed approach can effectively identify the transmitted CpG sites and clusters with high accuracy, sensitivity, and specificity. As a demonstration, we apply the method to a triad DNA methylation data set.

In the real data application, among the 3837 CpGs identified as transmitted sites, most of the CpGs are clustered into maternal-transmission-dominated clusters, which is consistent with the findings in [8] for the transmitted CpGs. The maternal importance in epigenetic transmission between generations has been recognized [13, 14], supporting the findings in this chapter. It is suggested that during the prenatal period, the biological inheritance of phenotype from one generation to the next can be a result of the transplacental passage of nutrients, metabolic signals, and toxins in utero [13, 15]. We did not identify any paternal-transmitted CpG sites, which was different from Han et al.'s study [8]. Since Han et al. pre-assumed transmissions, that is, DNA methylation at all the 4063 candidate CpG sites was transmitted, their identified paternal-transmission-dominated CpGs could have been mis-classified. It is worthy noting that in our approach DNA methylation transmission from parents to offspring is defined based on means of Beta distribution.Thus the transmission is at the population level rather than DNA methylation transmission within each individual family. For transmission at the individual level, a different modeling based on regression of individual DNA methylation measures is required. It will be interesting to extend the approach to further incorporate transmission assessment at the individual level.

The strength of the proposed approach exists in its ability to detect inheritability. The idea of nested clustering can be applied to other situations, e.g., in multi-level designs. The method has the potential to be generalized to incorporate non-linear transmissions, although computation can be more challenging.

Funding
This study is supported by the National Institutes of Health research funds R01AI121226 (MPI: H. Zhang and J. W. Holloway) and R01 AI091905 (PI: W. Karmaus).

Program and Data Availability
Programs for data simulations and nested clustering, along with a read me document, are available online. For readers with interest in the real data, please contact the corresponding author.

References

1. Ober, C., Hoffjan, S.: Asthma genetics 2006: the long and winding road to gene discovery. Genes Immun. **7**(2), 95 (2006)
2. Weiss, S.T., Raby, B.A., Rogers, A.: Asthma genetics and genomics 2009. Curr. Opin. Genet. Dev. **19**(3), 279–282 (2009)
3. Manolio, T.A., Collins, F.S., Cox, N.J., Goldstein, D.B., Hindorff, L.A., Hunter, D.J., McCarthy, M.I., Ramos, E.M., Cardon, L.R., Chakravarti, A., et al.: Finding the missing heritability of complex diseases. Nature **461**(7265), 747 (2009)
4. Bégin, P., Nadeau, K.C.: Epigenetic regulation of asthma and allergic disease. Allergy Asthma Clin. Immunol. **10**(1), 27 (2014)
5. Martino, D., Kesper, D.A., Amarasekera, M., Harb, H., Renz, H., Prescott, S.: Epigenetics in immune development and in allergic and autoimmune diseases. J. Reprod. Immunol. **104**, 43–48 (2014)
6. Zhang, X., Biagini Myers, J.M., Burleson, J.D., Ulm, A., Bryan, K.S., Chen, X., Weirauch, M.T., Baker, T.A., Butsch Kovacic, M.S., Ji, H.: Nasal DNA methylation is associated with childhood asthma. Epigenomics **10**(5), 629–641 (2018)
7. Lockett, G.A., Holloway, J.W.: Genome-wide association studies in asthma; perhaps, the end of the beginning. Curr. Opin. Allergy Clin. Immunol. **13**(5), 463–469 (2013)
8. Han, S., Zhang, H., Lockett, G.A., Mukherjee, N., Holloway, J.W., Karmaus, W., et al. Identifying heterogeneous transgenerational DNA methylation sites via clustering in beta regression. Ann. Appl. Stat. **9**(4), 2052–2072 (2015)
9. Siegmund, K.D., Laird, P.W., Laird-Offringa, I.A.: A comparison of cluster analysis methods using DNA methylation data. Bioinformatics **20**(12), 1896–1904 (2004)
10. Houseman, E.A., Christensen, B.C., Yeh, R.-F., Marsit, C.J., Karagas, M.R., Wrensch, M., H.H. Nelson, Wiemels, J., Zheng, S., Wiencke, J.K., et al.: Model-based clustering of DNA methylation array data: a recursive-partitioning algorithm for high-dimensional data arising as a mixture of beta distributions. BMC Bioinf. **9**(1), 365 (2008)
11. Ferrari, S., Cribari-Neto, F.: Beta regression for modelling rates and proportions. J. Appl. Stat. **31**(7), 799–815 (2004)
12. Arshad, S.H., Hide, D.W.: Effect of environmental factors on the development of allergic disorders in infancy. J. Allergy Clin. Immunol. **90**(2), 235–241 (1992)
13. Ho, D.H.: Transgenerational Epigenetics: The Role of Maternal Effects in Cardiovascular Development (2014)
14. Curley, J.P., Mashoodh, R., Champagne, F.A.: Epigenetics and the origins of paternal effects. Horm. Behav. **59**(3), 306–314 (2011)
15. Pembrey, M., Saffery, R., Bygren, L.O., et al. Human transgenerational responses to early-life experience: potential impact on development, health and biomedical research. J. Med. Genet. **51**(9), 563–572 (2014)

Detecting Changepoint in Gene Expressions over Time: An Application to Childhood Obesity

Sunil Mathur and Jing Sun

1 Introduction

There has been a rapid rise in obesity in the USA, and recent studies have suggested that 31.7% of children 2–19 years of age are overweight, of whom 18.4% are obese [1–3]. Obesity in children has been linked to many physical, psychological, and social problems such as cardiovascular disease, diabetes, sleep apnea and respiratory problems, and osteoarthritis [4–9], which have resulted in premature deaths in children [10, 11]. Obesity is a complex disorder that is affected by many interacting genetic and non-genetic factors [12].

In genome-wide association, studies scans are performed on several hundred thousands of genetic markers across several thousands of individuals' complete sets of DNA to find gene variations that may be related to obesity. These studies have found that common genetic variants in the FTO gene are associated with significant changes in BMI [13–16]. The FTO variant [NM_001080432] [17] which came as a consequence of T2D GWA studies [18, 19] operates through insulin resistance. In addition to several variants of FTO such as rs8050136 and rs3751812 [14, 17] and MC4R (melanocortin-4 receptor) [20] that have been identified as associated with childhood obesity, there are more than 30 candidate genes on 12 chromosomes that are associated with body mass index [14, 21–24].

Many biological systems are dynamic systems; temporal profiles of gene expression levels during a given biological process can provide information on how gene

S. Mathur (✉)
Department of Mathematics and Statistics, Texas A&M University, Corpus Christi, TX, USA
e-mail: Sunil.Mathur@tamucc.edu

J. Sun
Department of Biostatistics and Epidemiology, Augusta University, Augusta, GA, USA
e-mail: Jing.Sun@Augusta.edu

Y. Zhao, (Din) D.-G. Chen (eds.), *Modern Statistical Methods for Health Research*,
Emerging Topics in Statistics and Biostatistics,
https://doi.org/10.1007/978-3-030-72437-5_21

expression levels evolve. Also, it is of interest to know how gene expressions change at a given time point in a given biological process. We find that most of the genes evolve and may not express the same way as they did after a certain point of time. These changes to gene expression may be due to certain events such as adverse environmental conditions. Mathur proposed a procedure to compare several genes at a time instead of pair-wise comparisons [25].

Regression modeling of gene expression trajectories has been proposed as an important alternative to clustering methods for analyzing the expression patterns of cell cycle-related genes. The analysis of gene expression data obtained from experiments can be useful to identify the regulatory relationship between genes. Genes with a common functional role have similar expression patterns across different biological experiments. These similar expression patterns are perhaps due to the co-regulation of genes in the same functional group. Most of the existing methods available for the identification of the regulatory relationships are either made for comparing two genes at a time or methods that are not computationally efficient in the identification of the regulatory relationships. However, due to the nature of the genes, the expression levels may change after some time, and the model fitted initially may not be able to explain the behavior after that time point. Thus, it is not always true that the same linear model will hold good for the entire data set. A good model should be flexible in nature to explain the entire data set. Changepoint detection is estimating the point at which the statistical properties of a sequence of observations change [26]. The change could be in the intercept, slope, or both. Most of the time, it is observed that changepoint is suspected but is not caught by usual statistical models. A time series of scatterplot or a linear regression line may show such changepoint and highlight a possible break in an expected linear trend over time or a covariate X. With this kind of observed discontinuity in the trend at a given point, say c, necessitates further investigation. Therefore, there is a clear need and motivation to develop a method that can confirm quantitatively such a departure from the linear trend at that specific point c. A two-line model was introduced, with an F-test to detect a change in the regression coefficient [27]. A test was proposed based on maximum F statistics to detect the changepoint in the two-phase linear regression model [28]. Reeves and colleagues [29] compared eight undocumented changepoint detection methods. The differences in assumptions among these eight methods and guidelines for which methods work best in different situations have been discussed. The method integrates a Box-Cox power transformation procedure into a common trend two-phase regression model-based test. Murakami [30] used the combination of the Wilcoxon and Mood statistics to the changepoint setting and introduced a nonparametric location-scale statistic for detecting a changepoint. Nosek and Szkutnik [31] proposed a new changepoint detection test based on the likelihood ratio in a two-phase linear regression model with inequality constraints.

Most of the methods available in the literature assume the normality of errors in the model. In practice, this assumption may not be always true, and methods based on this assumption, if not true, will eventually produce misleading results. In this article, we propose to use a rank-based estimator of regression coefficients to develop a nonparametric test to detect unknown changepoint. The article is organized as follows. In Sect. 2, we provide background, and in Sect. 3, we propose a new test and investigate its properties. In Sect. 4, we report the simulation study's results. We used a data set to illustrate the testing procedure in Sect. 5. The discussion about the proposed test is presented in Sect. 6.

2 Background

The simple linear regression model is given by

$$Y_i = \beta_0 + \beta_1 X_i + \varepsilon_i, i = 1, \ldots, n. \tag{1}$$

We make the following assumptions [29]:

1. Under the null hypothesis of a homogeneous series (no changepoints), the series of interest Y_t can be adequately described by a regression equation with error terms that are independent and identically distributed (IID) normal random variables.
2. Over the period examined, Y_t has at most one changepoint.
3. Except where noted, the procedures examined are being applied directly to Y_t.

The two-phase linear regression model with a single regressor and single changepoint is given by

$$Y_i = \begin{cases} \alpha_1 + \beta_1 X_i + \varepsilon_i \text{ , if } i < c \\ \alpha_2 + \beta_2 X_i + \varepsilon_i \text{ , ifi} > c \end{cases}, \tag{2}$$

where ε_i is the zero-mean independent random error with a constant variance σ^2. Let there be a single unknown changepoint c, and then the null hypothesis which we wish to test is given by.

$$H_0 : \alpha_1 = \alpha_2 = \alpha \text{ and } \beta_1 = \beta_2 = \beta \text{ Vs.} H_a : \alpha_1 \neq \alpha_2 \text{ and } \beta_1 \neq \beta_2.$$

Under H_0, the model in Eq. (1) reduces to

$$Y_i = \alpha + \beta X_i + \varepsilon_i, i = 1, \ldots, n, \tag{3}$$

where Y is the response variable, X is the independent variable,α and β are the unknown regression coefficients, and ε_i is the error term. To test the null hypothesis H_0, assuming normality for the error terms, Lund and Reeves [28] proposed an F-test based on least squares estimators of the parameters involved and is given by

$$F(c) = \frac{(\text{SSE}_{\text{reduced}} - \text{SSE}_{\text{full}})/2}{\text{SSE}_{\text{full}}/(n-4)}, \tag{4}$$

where SSE_{full} is the error sum of squares for the full model

$$SSE_{full} = \sum_{X_i<c} \left(Y_i - \hat{a}_1 - \hat{\beta}_1 X_i\right)^2 + \sum_{X_i>c} \left(Y_i - \hat{a}_2 - \hat{\beta}_2 X_i\right)^2 \quad (5)$$

and $SSE_{reduced}$ is the error sum of squares for this reduced model. Mathematically,

$$SSE_{reduced} = \sum_{i=1}^{n} \left(Y_i - \hat{\alpha} - \hat{\beta}\, x_i\right)^2 \quad (6)$$

Note that, under the null hypothesis of no changepoint and assuming normal errors ε, F, given by (4), follows the F distribution of 2 numerator degrees of freedom and (n–4) denominator degrees of freedom.

A general linear test statistic F should be small when there is no changepoint. So the goal is to figure out when F achieves its maximum value for all possible values of c.

Hence, the changepoint can be identified at

$$\hat{c} = \arg\max F(c), \quad (7)$$

provided the *maxF*(c) is large enough to guarantee that it is not due to chance. Practically, max$F$(c) is compared to a critical value obtained from its sampling distribution. Lund and Reeves [28] reported quantiles from the distribution of max$F$(c) for different sample sizes but assumed normality of errors. In practice, errors are seldom normal. Non-normality of errors seriously affects the least squares estimates of the parameters, and hence tests based on it may not provide valid results. Rank-based estimation is robust to the non-normality of errors and performs better than least squares in such situations [32].

3 Proposed Method

We propose a new procedure for the identification of changepoint in a two-phase linear regression model with a single regressor using rank-based estimation.

Let us denote the ith residual expressed as $y_i - (\alpha + \beta x_i)$. The rank-based estimate of regression coefficients is obtained by minimizing [32]

$$\sum_{i=1}^{n} \left[\text{rank}\left(_i \lceil \hat{e}_i \rceil\right)\right] \lceil \hat{e}_i \rceil \quad (8)$$

where $\hat{e}_i = y_i - \left(\hat{a} + \hat{\beta} x_i\right)$.

It is equivalent to minimize

$$\sum_{i=1}^{n}\left[\text{rank}\left(y_i - x_i\hat{\beta}\right) - \frac{n+1}{2}\right]\left(y_i - \hat{\beta}x_i\right), \tag{9}$$

as α doesn't affect the minimizer.

The rank-based estimation assumes that the errors have asymmetric distribution. α is estimated as the median of the differences $d_i = y_i - \beta x_i$.

Let

$$A_{ij} = \frac{(\hat{e}_i + \hat{e}_j)}{2} \text{ for } 1 \leq \text{i} \leq j \leq n$$

and

$$k_1 = \text{the closest integer to } \frac{1}{2} + a\text{–}(1.645)b,$$

$$k_2 = \text{the closest integer to } \frac{1}{2} + a + (1.645)b,$$

where

$$a = \frac{n\,(n+1)}{4} \text{and } b = \sqrt{\frac{n\,(n+1)\,(2n+1)}{24}}.$$

$$\text{Define } f = \sqrt{\frac{n}{n-5}} \text{and } \hat{\tau} = f\frac{\sqrt{n}\left[A_{(k_2)} - A_{(k_1)}\right]}{2(2.1645)}, \tag{10}$$

where and $A_{(1)} \leq A_{(2)} \leq \ldots \leq A_{(N)}$ are the following $N = \frac{n(n+1)}{2}$ numbers in increasing order.

To test H_0, McKean and Hettmansperger [33] proposed a nonparametric test statistic (based on rank estimators $\hat{e}_i$ of the parameters involved in the regression model) given by

$$T(c) = \frac{(\text{SRWR}_{\text{reduced}} - \text{SRWR}_{\text{full}})}{\hat{\tau}} \tag{11}$$

where the notation SMWR is defined by

$$\text{SRWR} = \frac{\sqrt{12}}{n+1}\sum_{i=1}^{n}\left(\text{rank}\left(\hat{e}_i\right) - \frac{1}{2}(n+1)\right)\hat{e}_i;\text{ with } \hat{e}_i = y_i - \left(\hat{a} + \hat{\beta}x_i\right).$$

We use the short form SRWR for the sum of rank-weighted residuals. $SRWR_{reduced}$ and $SRWR_{full}$ are calculated by applying the nonparametric regression method to the reduced model and full model, respectively. SRWR measures the goodness of fit of the model to the data.

We define

$$T^2(c) = \left[\frac{(SRWR_{reduced} - SRWR_{full})}{\hat{\tau}}\right]^2 \tag{12}$$

The smaller values of the test statistic T^2 indicate that the reduced model is the true model and there is no changepoint in the data. On the other hand, if the difference between $SRWR_{full}$ and $SRWR_{reduced}$ is large, it indicates that the two-phase linear model is an appropriate fit to the data and there is a change at c. Under H_0, the asymptotic distribution of T is chi-square distribution with 2 degrees of freedom [33]. Using this fact, we propose a rank-based test to detect the undocumented changepoint which is analogous to Lund and Reeves [28] least squares-based test.

We propose the changepoint as

$$\tilde{c} = \arg\max T^2(c), \tag{13}$$

provided that arg max T is large enough to guarantee that it is not just due to chance.

We need to calculate T^2 for all possible values of c and then figure out when T^2 achieves its maximum value. We could calculate the P-value and confidence interval of c by a permutation test based on the specific sample.

If τ is unknown, it is estimated from the data based on the full model. Here, the full model involves two phases. We assume that τ remains the same in each phase and we estimate it using the formula

$$\hat{\tau} = \left[\frac{(n_1 - 2)\,\hat{\tau}_1^2 + (n_2 - 2)\,\hat{\tau}_2^2}{n_1 + n_2 - 4}\right]^{\frac{1}{2}} \tag{14}$$

$\hat{\tau}_1$ and $\hat{\tau}_2$ are obtained by Eq. (10) for the first and second phases separately.

The algorithm for detecting undocumented changepoint is shown below:

1. Choose c as $2, 3, \ldots, n-1$.
2. Compute the test statistics $T(c)$.
3. The changepoint is $\tilde{c} = \arg\max T(c)$.

4 Power Comparisons

The critical values of T statistic are estimated under the finite sample size by Monte Carlo simulation studies. The simulations are based on 10,000 repetitions. Throughout the simulations, the significance level set as 0.05. L-R present Lund and Reeves method and PM present our proposed method. X was fixed from 0 to 1 with an interval of $1/n$. The simulation results are listed in Table 1.

Table 1 can be used to get the critical values of the L-R and PM tests based on different sample sizes with different error distributions when X was fixed from 0 to 1 with an interval of $1/n$. It is interesting to note that, in general, the critical value for Lund and Reeves method decreases with the increase of sample size, while the critical value of the proposed method increases with the increase in the sample size.

When the independent variable X was generated randomly from $N(0,1)$, the critical values for different error distributions are shown in Table 2.

Table 1 Critical value under the null hypothesis when X is fixed

Test	Error	$n = 20$	$n = 60$	$n = 100$
L-R	Normal (0,1)	7.933	6.975	6.860
PM		7.021	7.512	7.81
L-R	Laplace (0,1)	10.129	8.935	8.662
PM		8.07	8.910	9.123
L-R	Student t (2)	18.145	19.059	20.545
PM		11.01	12.74	13.783
L-R	Student t (4)	10.259	9.465	9.756
PM		7.987	8.723	8.987
L-R	Mixture ($P = 0.9$)	17.867	15.761	15.021
PM		10.314	11.765	12.312
L-R	Mixture ($P = 0.75$)	15.284	11.560	10.967
PM		11.109	12.678	12.678

Table 2 Critical value under the null hypothesis when X was generated randomly from the normal distribution

Test	Error	$N = 20$	$N = 60$	$N = 100$
L-R	Normal (0,1)	7.689	6.677	6.631
PM		7.012	7.412	7.987
L-R	Laplace (0,1)	9.681	8.307	8.180
PM		8.012	8.793	8.912
L-R	Student t (2)	17.788	15.515	16.373
PM		11.213	12.567	13.891
L-R	Student t (4)	10.125	8.789	8.908
PM		7.987	8.546	8.768
L-R	Mixture ($P = 0.9$)	17.188	13.894	13.565
PM		10.567	11.897	12.098
L-R	Mixture ($P = 0.75$)	15.113	11.072	10.049
PM		11.654	12.678	13.456

Table 3 Power comparison between Lund and Reeves method and the proposed method

Error	Δ_1	Δ_2	Power		CRB (%)	
			L-R	PM	L-R	PM
Normal	0	0	0.0467	0.0512	0.0044	0.0061
	2	−1.33	0.831	0.8312	0.2630	0.2513
	5	−3.33	1	0.9997	0.6772	0.6243
Laplace (0,1)	0	0	0.0499	0.0491	0.0013	0.0021
	2	−1.33	0.3999	0.5561	0.0895	0.1454
	5	−3.33	0.991	0.9979	0.5231	0.5561
Students t (2)	0	0	0.0478	0.0512	0.0001	0.0008
	2	−1.33	0.0599	0.1811	0.0035	0.0312
	5	−3.33	0.4616	0.9341	0.1874	0.4123
Students t (4)	0	0	0.0483	0.0431	0.0007	0.0019
	2	−1.33	0.3725	0.5134	0.0905	0.1354
	5	−3.33	0.9891	0.9989	0.5240	0.5812
Mixture ($P = 0.9$)	0	0	0.0497	0.0491	0.0000	0.0004
	2	−1.33	0.0751	0.2531	0.0050	0.0512
	5	−3.33	0.5825	0.9871	0.0411	0.2134
Mixture ($P = 0.75$)	0	0	0.0796	0.051	0.0005	0.0004
	2	−1.33	0.1314	0.1981	0.0119	0.0351
	5	−3.33	0.6116	0.9231	0.2041	0.4154

Table 2 can be used to get the critical values of the L-R and PM tests based on different sample sizes with different error distributions when the independent variable X was generated randomly from $N(0,1)$. It is interesting to note that, in general, the critical value for Lund and Reeves method decreases with the increase of sample size, while the critical value of the proposed method increases with the increase in the sample size. We compared the power and the accuracy of the T statistic with the F statistics. Table 3 presents the comparison of results for the different error distributions as n equals 60 and X follows the normal distribution. We used different error distributions as normal distribution with mean 0 and standard deviation 1, Laplace distribution with location 0 and scale 1, Student t distribution with 2 and 4 degrees of freedom, and Gaussian mixture distribution with $P = 0.9$ and 0.75 in which the first component is a normal distribution with mean 0 and standard deviation 1 and the second component is a normal distribution with mean 0 and standard deviation $\sqrt{5}$. Here Δ_1 indicates the change of slope and Δ_2 represents the change of intercept. For our study we kept $\Delta_1 = 0, 2, 5$, respectively, and Δ_2 was chosen by $0, -1.33, -3.33$, respectively. We set the changepoint in the middle of the data. Also set β_1 as 1, so $\beta_2 = 1, 3, 6$ *as* $\Delta_1 = 0, 2, 5$. We set $\alpha_1$as 0,so $\alpha_2 = 0, -1.33, -3.33$ *as* $\Delta_2 = 0, -1.33, -3.33$.

Also, we investigate the accuracy of detecting a changepoint by confidence region bound (CRB).

Table 4 Power comparison between Lund and Reeves method and proposed method when X was fixed

Error	Δ_1	Δ_2	Power		CRB (%)	
			L-R	PM	L-R	PM
Normal	0	0	0.0518	0.0491	0.0044	0.0051
	2	−1.33	0.1535	0.1621	0.0189	0.0217
	5	−3.33	0.7656	0.7891	0.1386	0.1203
Laplace (0,1)	0	0	0.0468	0.0498	0.0013	0.0022
	2	−1.33	0.0671	0.512	0.0043	0.0071
	5	−3.33	0.2802	0.4931	0.0375	0.0812
Students t (2)	0	0	0.0486	0.0489	0.0000	0.0001
	2	−1.33	0.0483	0.0497	0.0000	0.0004
	5	−3.33	0.0476	0.0929	0.0000	0.0101
Students t (4)	0	0	0.0508	0.0512	0.0003	0.0013
	2	−1.33	0.0609	0.1102	0.0014	0.0062
	5	−3.33	0.2266	0.5128	0.0316	0.0677
Mixture ($P = 0.9$)	0	0	0.0534	0.0489	0.0000	0.001
	2	−1.33	0.0562	0.0492	0.0002	0.0017
	5	−3.33	0.0626	0.2456	0.0023	0.0371
Mixture ($P = 0.75$)	0	0	0.0502	0.0559	0.0001	0.0001
	2	−1.33	0.0521	0.0789	0.0002	0.0011
	5	−3.33	0.0633	0.1134	0.0020	0.0106

$$\text{CRB} = \text{Number of times that identified change point in } [c - 5\%N, \text{c} + 5\%N] \tag{15}$$

CRB is one of the power measures, which equals the number of times that identify the changepoint and locate the changepoint within ±5% sample size of the true location.

The results are given in Table 3 which indicate that the powers of both statistics increase as the change of slope becomes larger. When the error was non-normal distribution, the T statistic was more powerful and more accurate for detecting a changepoint than the F statistic. Furthermore, the F test proposed by Lund and Reeves did not reach the desired power of one as quickly as the proposed test. Also, the T statistic performs similar to the F test when the error distribution is the normal distribution. Thus, the proposed T statistic could detect the changepoint precisely for various error distributions, and hence the T statistic was more suitable than the F statistics when the error distribution is unknown.

When X was fixed from 0 to 1 with an interval of $1/n$, the results were very similar to the results obtained using $n = 60$. Table 4 simulation results are based on 10,000 repetitions, and sample size n equals 100. Other settings are the same as the above simulations.

The proposed method is more powerful than the Lund-Reeves method under various error distributions, and the proposed method will be able to detect the changepoint much better than the Lund-Reeves method.

5 Application to the Obesity Problem

Leptin-specific patterns of gene expression in white adipose tissue were studied by Soukas and colleagues [34]. Leptin, a hormone that regulates body weight by decreasing food intake and increasing energy expenditure, was administered to Ob/ob mice that carry leptin mutations and are obese and hyperphagic. When leptin was administered to lean and ob/ob mice, it activated a novel metabolic program that depletes adipose tissue. When animals are treated with leptin, it voluntarily decreases their food intake, whereas a novel metabolic program selectively depletes body adipose stores [35]. The changes in the gene expression levels of white adipose tissue due to the exposure of exogenous leptin were measured in groups of ob/ob and wild-type mice. A phosphate-buffered saline (PBS) group served as a control. The level of expression for all genes at each time point was measured as a fold change value relative to the wild-type sample. Data were filtered based on fold change and abundance (average difference change) values. Northern blotting was used as a criterion for inclusion, establishing a boundary above which detected fold changes were quantitatively reliable. A total of 410 genes satisfied these criteria in the experiments with ob/ob mice. In a cluster of genes, leptin specifically repressed genes upregulated in the ob/ob animal, whereas pair feeding had no effect. We would like to detect the point at switching between expression levels when leptin specifically repressed expression of genes. The proposed T statistic is applied to the data pertaining to leptin-specific patterns of gene expression in white adipose tissue and analyzed the patterns of gene expression in white adipose tissue in the presence or absence of leptin to detect the changepoint at which gene expression levels started switching due to the presence of leptin.

The changepoint has been marked as red in the Graph 1. The P-value is calculated based on 10,000 permutations and no changepoint model as Eq. (15). The residuals have been calculated based on the no changepoint model, and then all possible values of the test statistics have been calculated under all possible rearrangements of the residuals for the no changepoint model. When we applied the Lund and Reeves method to the same data, the changepoint detected was 5.10 and the $F_{\text{Max}} = 3.700$. The bootstrap P-value is 0.001. The value of the proposed test statistic $T^2(c) = 1.48$. The bootstrap P-value is 0.001. Based on the simulation results, the changepoint we detected should be more accurate.

In order to detect the change-point, we fit the reduced model for gene expression (Y_i) and days (X_i) as

$$\hat{Y}_i = -0.171 + 0.066X_\text{i} \tag{16}$$

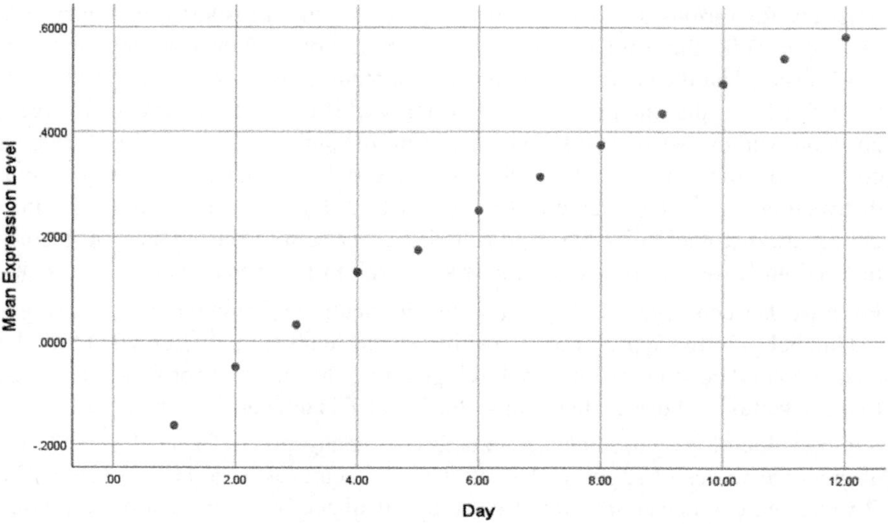

Graph 1 The patterns of gene expression in white adipose tissue in the presence of leptin

Using the proposed method, we find the changepoint as 4.05 with the P-value <0.001 and the 95% confidence interval as (4.0304, 4.0694) (based on 10,000 permutations).

Thus, the best fitting full model for the T statistic is

$$Y_i = \begin{cases} -0.2552 + 0.097X_i, & \text{if } X_i < 4 \\ -0.1021 + 0.0580X_i, & \text{if } X_i > 4 \end{cases} \tag{17}$$

Thus, there is significant evidence to show the linear relationship between the gene expression levels and the number of days of leptin treatment. These results indicate that leptin treatment of wild-type and ob/ob mice changes the gene expression levels starting from day 4.05. Also, leptin treatment of wild-type and ob/ob mice reduces food intake, body weight, and adipose tissue mass [35].

6 Discussion

In this paper, we proposed a nonparametric procedure for detecting the undocumented changepoint problem. By Monte Carlo simulation studies, the critical values of the T statistic were estimated under finite sample sizes. In addition, the power and the accuracy of detecting the changepoint were investigated by using the T and F statistics. The proposed procedure outperforms its competitor, while the changepoint detection procedure based on the F test is found to be suboptimal when the error distribution is non-normal. Thus, the T statistic could detect the changepoint precisely for various distributions. It is shown [38] that in general, as n increases (e.g., $n = 500$), the estimates of the changepoint approach to the true parameter much faster than the coefficient parameter estimates. Also, empirical coverages of the estimates of the true parameters show that the estimates have very high percent coverage within two standard deviations from the simulated sample means which confirms the n-consistency of the changepoint estimator. Under H_0, the asymptotic distribution of T is chi-square distribution with 2 degrees of freedom [33]. Since chi-square distribution has an exponential tail, for some fixed number of degrees of freedom k, we can show that $\lim_{n\to\infty} \frac{T_{\max}}{\ln n} = c$, almost surely (c being a constant). For a weaker convergence, we see that the distribution of centered $T_{\max}$ converges to Gumbel [39]. In the presence of positive autocorrelation, it is natural that [36] the changepoint detection procedures developed for independent error series may lead to the detection of false changepoints [29, 37]. If T is not concave, then one can use minimization of $\tilde{c} = \text{argmin} T^2(c)$ to detect the changepoint. Then calculate T^2 for all possible values of c, and figure out when T^2 achieves its minimum value. The P-value and confidence interval of c can be calculated by a permutation test based on the specific sample. The proposed method can be applied to solve biology and public health problems such as childhood obesity.

In this paper, the proposed method is to detect the slope and intercept changes, but it also can extend to detect the variance changes in the data sets. In the future, we need to consider the limiting distribution of the T statistic under the null hypothesis and develop a GLM-based nonparametric changepoint detection procedure. Furthermore, when more than one undocumented changepoint is present in the data, the proposed method needs to be modified.

Acknowledgments The authors would like to thank Dr. Yichuan Zhao for inviting us to present the work at the workshop. The authors would like to thank the reviewers for providing their constructive feedback which led to a significant improvement in the paper.

References

1. Ogden, C.L., Carroll, M.D., Curtin, L.R., Lamb, M.M., Flegal, K.M.: Prevalence of high body mass index in US children and adolescents, 2007–2008. JAMA. **303**(3), 242–249 (2010)
2. Ogden, C.L., Carroll, M.D., Flegal, K.M.: High body mass index for age among US children and adolescents, 2003–2006. JAMA. **299**(20), 2401–2405 (2008)
3. Ogden, C.L., Flegal, K.M., Carroll, M.D., Johnson, C.L.: Prevalence and trends in overweight among US children and adolescents, 1999–2000. JAMA. **288**(14), 1728–1732 (2002)
4. Daniels, S.R.: The consequences of childhood overweight and obesity. Futur. Child. **16**(1), 47–67 (2006)
5. Dietz, W.H.: Health consequences of obesity in youth: childhood predictors of adult disease. Pediatrics. **101**(Supplement 2), 518–525 (1998)
6. Freedman, D.S., Khan, L.K., Dietz, W.H., Srinivasan, S.R., Berenson, G.S.: Relationship of childhood obesity to coronary heart disease risk factors in adulthood: the Bogalusa Heart Study. Pediatrics. **108**(3), 712–718 (2001)

7. Kiess, W., Galler, A., Reich, A., Müller, G., Kapellen, T., Deutscher, J., Raile, K., Kratzsch, J.: Clinical aspects of obesity in childhood and adolescence. Obes. Rev. **2**(1), 29–36 (2001)
8. Must, A., Strauss, R.S.: Risks and consequences of childhood and adolescent obesity. Int. J. Obes. Relat. Metabol. Dis. **23**, S2–S11 (1999)
9. Tauman, R., Gozal, D.: Obesity and obstructive sleep apnea in children. Paediatr. Respir. Rev. **7**(4), 247–259 (2006)
10. Flegal, K.M., Graubard, B.I., Williamson, D.F., Gail, M.H.: Excess deaths associated with underweight, overweight, and obesity. JAMA. **293**(15), 1861–1867 (2005)
11. Fontaine, K.R., Redden, D.T., Wang, C., Westfall, A.O., Allison, D.B.: Years of life lost due to obesity. JAMA. **289**(2), 187–193 (2003)
12. Han, J.C., Lawlor, D.A., Kimm, S.: Childhood obesity. Lancet. **375**(9727), 1737–1748 (2010)
13. Cecil, J.E., Tavendale, R., Watt, P., Hetherington, M.M., Palmer, C.N.A.: An obesity-associated FTO gene variant and increased energy intake in children. N. Engl. J. Med. **359**(24), 2558–2566 (2008)
14. Grant, S.F.A., Li, M., Bradfield, J.P., Kim, C.E., Annaiah, K., Santa, E., Glessner, J.T., Casalunovo, T., Frackelton, E.C., George Otieno, F.: Association analysis of the FTO gene with obesity in children of Caucasian and African ancestry reveals a common tagging SNP. PLoS One. **3**(3), e1746 (2008)
15. Hotta, K., Nakata, Y., Matsuo, T., Kamohara, S., Kotani, K., Komatsu, R., Itoh, N., Mineo, I., Wada, J., Masuzaki, H.: Variations in the FTO gene are associated with severe obesity in the Japanese. J. Hum. Genet. **53**(6), 546–553 (2008)
16. Scuteri, A., Sanna, S., Chen, W.-M., Uda, M., Albai, G., Strait, J., Najjar, S., Nagaraja, R., Orrú, M., Usala, G.: Genome-wide association scan shows genetic variants in the FTO gene are associated with obesity-related traits. PLoS Genet. **3**(7), e115 (2007)
17. Frayling, T.M., Timpson, N.J., Weedon, M.N., Zeggini, E., Freathy, R.M., Lindgren, C.M., Perry, J.R.B., Elliott, K.S., Lango, H., Rayner, N.W.: A common variant in the FTO gene is associated with body mass index and predisposes to childhood and adult obesity. Science. **316**(5826), 889–894 (2007)
18. Burton, P.R., Clayton, D.G., Cardon, L.R., Craddock, N., Deloukas, P., Duncanson, A., Kwiatkowski, D.P., McCarthy, M.I., Ouwehand, W.H., Samani, N.J.: Genome-wide association study of 14,000 cases of seven common diseases and 3,000 shared controls. Nature. **447**(7145), 661–678 (2007)
19. Zeggini, E., Weedon, M.N., Lindgren, C.M., Frayling, T.M., Elliott, K.S., Lango, H., Timpson, N.J., Perry, J.R.B., Rayner, N.W., Freathy, R.M.: Replication of genome-wide association signals in UK samples reveals risk loci for type 2 diabetes. Science. **316**(5829), 1336–1341 (2007)
20. Loos, R.J.F., Lindgren, C.M., Li, S., Wheeler, E., Zhao, J.H., Prokopenko, I., Inouye, M., Freathy, R.M., Attwood, A.P., Beckmann, J.S.: Common variants near MC4R are associated with fat mass, weight and risk of obesity. Nat. Genet. **40**(6), 768–775 (2008)
21. Bochukova, E.G., Huang, N.I., Keogh, J., Henning, E., Purmann, C., Blaszczyk, K., Saeed, S., Hamilton-Shield, J., Clayton-Smith, J., O'Rahilly, S.: Large, rare chromosomal deletions associated with severe early-onset obesity. Nature. **463**(7281), 666–670 (2009)
22. Hardy, R., Wills, A.K., Wong, A., Elks, C.E., Wareham, N.J., Loos, R.J.F., Kuh, D., Ong, K.K.: Life course variations in the associations between FTO and MC4R gene variants and body size. Hum. Mol. Genet. **19**(3), 545–552 (2010)
23. Walley, A.J., Asher, J.E., Froguel, P.: The genetic contribution to non-syndromic human obesity. Nat. Rev. Genet. **10**(7), 431–442 (2009)
24. Walters, R.G., Jacquemont, S., Valsesia, A., De Smith, A.J., Martinet, D., Andersson, J., Falchi, M., Chen, F., Andrieux, J., Lobbens, S.: A new highly penetrant form of obesity due to deletions on chromosome 16p11. 2. Nature. **463**(7281), 671–675 (2010)
25. Mathur, S.K.: A run-based procedure to identify time-lagged gene clusters in microarray experiments. Stat. Med. **28**(2), 326–337 (2009)

26. Killick, R., Eckley, I.A., Jonathan, P., Chester, U.K.: Efficient detection of multiple change-points within an oceano-graphic time series. Proceedings of the 58th world science congress of ISI (2011)
27. Julious, S.A.: Inference and estimation in a changepoint regression problem. J. Roy. Statis. Soc.: Ser. D. **50**(1), 51–61 (2001)
28. Lund, R., Reeves, J.: Detection of undocumented changepoints: a revision of the two-phase regression model. J. Clim. **15**(17), 2547–2554 (2002)
29. Reeves, J., Chen, J., Wang, X.L., Lund, R., Qi Qi, L.: A review and comparison of changepoint detection techniques for climate data. J. Appl. Meteorol. Climatol. **46**(6), 900–915 (2007)
30. Murakami, H.: A nonparametric location–scale statistic for detecting a change point. Int. J. Adv. Manuf. Technol. **61**(5–8), 449–455 (2012)
31. Nosek, K., Szkutnik, Z.: Change-point detection in a shape-restricted regression model. Statistics. **48**(3), 641–656 (2014)
32. Birkes, D., Dodge, Y.: Alternative methods of regression, vol. 190. John Wiley & Sons, New York (2011)
33. McKean, J.W., Hettmansperger, T.P.: Tests of hypotheses based on ranks in the general linear model. Commun. Statis. Theory Methods. **5**(8), 693–709 (1976)
34. Soukas, A., Cohen, P., Socci, N.D., Friedman, J.M.: Leptin-specific patterns of gene expression in white adipose tissue. Genes Dev. **14**(8), 963–980 (2000)
35. Halaas, J.L., Boozer, C., Blair-West, J., Fidahusein, N., Denton, D.A., Friedman, J.M.: Physiological response to long-term peripheral and central leptin infusion in lean and obese mice. Proc. Natl. Acad. Sci. **94**(16), 8878–8883 (1997)
36. Entringer, S., Buss, C., Wadhwa, P.D.: Prenatal stress and developmental programming of human health and disease risk: concepts and integration of empirical findings. Curr. Opin. Endocrinol. Diab. Obes. **17**(6), 507 (2010)
37. Lund, R., Wang, X.L., Qi Qi, L., Reeves, J., Gallagher, C., Feng, Y.: Changepoint detection in periodic and autocorrelated time series. J. Clim. **20**(20), 5178–5190 (2007)
38. Koul, H.L., Qian, L.: Asymptotics of maximum likelihood estimator in a two-phase linear regression model. Journal of Statistical Planning and Inference. **108**(1–2), 99–119 (2002)
39. Embrechts, P., Klüppelberg, C., Mikosch, T.: Modelling extremal events: for insurance and finance. Vol. 33. Springer Science & Business Media. (2013)

Index

Y. Zhao, (Din) D.-G. Chen (eds.), *Modern Statistical Methods for Health Research*, Emerging Topics in Statistics and Biostatistics,
https://doi.org/10.1007/978-3-030-72437-5

Q

R

S

Printed by Printforce, the Netherlands